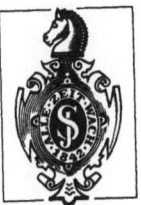

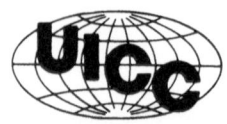
International Union Against Cancer

Treatment and Rehabilitation Programme

Chairman: Ismail Elsebai

Project on Prospects of Treatment

Ian Magrath (Chairman)
K. Cowan, M. Israel, T. Kinsella, L. Liotta, M. Lippmann,
D. Longo, C. Meyers, V. Narayanan

New Directions in Cancer Treatment

Edited by Ian Magrath

With 71 Figures, 12 in Color

Springer-Verlag
Berlin Heidelberg New York
London Paris Tokyo

UICC, Rue du Conseil-Général 3, CH-1205 Geneva

Editor:

IAN MAGRATH
National Institutes of Health
National Cancer Institute
Lymphoma Biology Section
Pediatric Branch
Bethesda, MD 20892, USA

ISBN-13:978-3-540-19063-9   e-ISBN-13:978-3-642-83405-9
DOI: 10.1007/978-3-642-83405-9

Library of Congress Cataloging-in-Publication Data
New directions in cancer treatment/edited by Ian Magrath.
        p.   cm.
    "UICC (International Union against Cancer) treatment and
Rehabilitation Programme"—P. facing t.p.
    Includes bibliographies and index.
    ISBN-13:978-3-540-19063-9 (U.S.)
    1. Cancer—Treatment. I. Magrath, Ian. II. UICC Treatment and
Rehabilitation Programme.
    [DNLM: 1. Neoplasms—therapy.   QZ 266 N5317]
RC270.8.N48   1988
616.99'406—dc19
DNLM/DLC
                                        88-24915

Typesetting: Asco Trade Typesetting Ltd., Hong Kong

2121/NY30-543210

Foreword

During the last few decades, there has been a tremendous improvement in the treatment of cancer. There is evidence that this trend is continuing, based on the achievements resulting from the combined efforts of clinicians and basic research workers. This book is an example of such interaction and collaboration. It was prepared by authors representing both areas of work.

Most of the work reported in this book is not merely theoretical, but has been experimentally successfully tested and sometimes applied clinically. This work has, however, not yet been generalized and practiced on a wide scale.

Some of the results reported here relate to new aspects and open new horizons for future progress.

This book will be of great value for both clinicians and basic research workers.

UICC
Treatment and Rehabilitation Programme
ISMAIL ELSEBAI
Chairman

Preface

The three main approaches to the treatment of cancer are surgery, radiotherapy, and chemotherapy. Today, all malignant neoplasms are managed by one or more of these modalities, with varying success rates depending on the type of tumor, its degree of spread, and the knowledge and skill with which the treatment plan has been designed and executed. In the United States of America and in Europe, approximately half of all cancer is presently curable, but this has been the case for approximately 20 years. Although major progress has been made in the treatment of specific cancers, the 5-year survival rate for all cancers in US Whites, for example, has increased by only approximately 10% since 1960. One interpretation of the apparent lack of progress overall in recent years is that available approaches to cancer treatment are being employed at a close to optimal level. It is true, of course, that results of treatment in the larger cancer centers may be better for some diseases than those achieved in smaller units or nonspecialist hospitals with more limited resources and expertise. It is also true that major progress in the management of some diseases, such as the hemopoietic neoplasms and testicular cancer, has occurred in recent years. It would seem, however, that even if every cancer patient were to profit to the full from modern approaches to treatment, the overall results, measured in terms of the percentage of patients cured of their disease, would not differ significantly from those currently being obtained, since so little progress in the management of the common cancers, such as lung, breast, and colon, has occurred.

When viewed from the standpoint of the world as a whole, it is clear that only a fraction of patients world-wide are receiving the benefits of modern cancer therapy, and a major goal, which would result in the saving of millions of lives every year, must be to provide improved cancer treatment to the developing countries. This would not necessarily mean the simple transplantation of Western expertise to those areas of the world that lack it, but rather a planned campaign whereby the problems relevant to the developing world are addressed. Yet at the same time, notwithstanding the major advances that have been made, the deficiencies of the current approaches to cancer treatment must be recognized and rectified if overall results are to be improved.

One of the major handicaps to rapid improvements in cancer therapy is that all modern approaches have been initially empirical. Whereas, with luck, empirical approaches may prove to be highly successful, when they fail, the course of action is not at all clear, and improvements are dependent upon the whims of chance. But some treatment approaches have proved to be highly effective in specific, often uncommon diseases, and attempts have been made to expand these glimmers of light into therapeutic principles. Further, enormous progress has been made in the understanding of the biology of cancer, and the possibility exists of developing rational approaches to treatment based on the new knowledge of the nature of the cellular and biochemical changes that result in neoplastic growth. These same advances in understanding may be even better utilized by applying them to the prevention of cancer, but that is not the subject of this book.

The objective of this volume is to examine current trends in research relevant to or applied directly to cancer treatment. As such, it covers a broad area, and in philosophy includes attempts to improve current modalities as well as totally novel approaches which would have been inconceivable even 10 years ago. It also contains rather more speculative material than is usual for a book on cancer treatment, but this is entirely justifiable since new ideas are sorely needed. It is hoped that this volume will be read both by physicians engaged in the treatment of patients with cancer, particularly those responsible for clinical research in this area, and by scientists working in fields impinging upon the understanding of cancer and its treatment. One increasing disadvantage faced by cancer research is that there is a widening gap between clinicians and basic scientists. The language of the latter increasingly deals in terms of molecular structure and molecular interactions, whereas the physician still deals mainly in terms of histology, clinical staging, and pharmacology. There is a need to bring these two worlds into closer apposition, and it is to be hoped that this volume, if only in a small way, will help to bring this about.

IAN MAGRATH

Contents

Biological Approaches to Therapy

X

Potential Approaches

Therapeutic Trends in Specific Neoplasms

Contributors

K.H. Antman, Dana-Farber Cancer Institute, Division of Medicine, Boston, MA 02115, USA

F.R. Appelbaum, University of Washington, The Fred Hutchinson Cancer Research Center, Division of Oncology, Seattle, WA 98104, USA

S.D. Averbuch, Department of Neoplastic Diseases, The Mount Sinai School of Medicine, New York, NY 10029, USA

S. Aznavoorian, National Institutes of Health, National Cancer Institute, Laboratory of Pathology, Betheda, MD 20892, USA

K.D. Bagshawe, Charing Cross Hospital, Department of Medical Oncology, London W6 8RF, UK

R.W. Baldwin, University of Nottingham, Cancer Research Campaign Laboratories, Nottingham NG7 2RD, UK

D.E. Bergsagel, Ontario Cancer Research Institute, Toronto, Ontario M4X 1K9, Canada

G.J. Bosl, Memorial Sloan-Kettering Cancer Center, Department of Medicine, Genitourinary Section, Solid Tumor Service, New York, NY 10021, USA

V.S. Byers, University of Nottingham, Cancer Research Campaign Laboratories, Nottingham NG7 2RD, UK

G.P. Canellos, Dana-Farber Cancer Center, Division of Clinical Oncology, Boston, MA 02115, USA

J.W. Clark, Frederick Cancer Research Facility, Clinical Research Branch, Biological Response Modifiers Program, Frederick, MD 21701-1013, USA

R.L. Comis, Fox Chase Cancer Center, Philadelphia, PA 19111, USA

K.H. Cowan, National Institutes of Health, Pharmacology Branch, Bethesda, MD 20892, USA

E.T. Creagan, Mayo Clinic, Department of Medical Oncology, Rochester, MI 55905, USA

G.J. D'Angio, Children's Hospital of Philadelphia, Children's Cancer Research Center, Philadelphia, PA 19104, USA

T.F. DeLaney, National Cancer Institute, Radiotherapy Branch, Bethesda, MD 20892, USA

R.F. Diaz, Methodist Hospital, Minneapolis Radiation Oncology, Department of Radiation Therapy, St. Louis Park, MN 55426, USA

M.C. Favrot, Centre Léon Bérard, F-69373 Lyon-Cédex 08, France

A. Fojo, National Cancer Institute, Medicine Branch, Bethesda, MD 20892, USA

B.A. Fraass, Department of Radiation Oncology, University of Michigan, Ann Arbor, MI 48109, USA

B.L. Gallie, University of Toronto, Hospital for Sick Children Research Institute and Departments of Ophthalmology and Pediatrics, Toronto, Ontario M5G 1X8, Canada

R.I. Glazer, National Institutes of Health, Laboratory of Biological Chemistry, Bethesda, MD 20892, USA

L.G. Gomella, National Cancer Institute, Surgery Branch, Bethesda, MD 20892, USA

R.G. Gray, Vincent T. Lombardi Cancer Research Center, Division of Medical Oncology, Washington, DC 20007, USA

N.H. Greig, National Institutes of Health, Laboratory of Neurosciences, Bethesda, MD 20892, USA

R.B. Herberman, Pittsburgh Cancer Center, Pittsburgh, PA 15215, USA

S.J. Horning, Stanford University Medical School, Stanford University Medical Center, Division of Oncology, Stanford, CA 94305, USA

S.P. Ivy, National Cancer Institute, Clinical Pharmacology Branch, Bethesda, MD 20892, USA

C. Jacobs, Stanford University Medical School, Stanford University Medical Center, Division of Oncology, Stanford, CA 94305, USA

A.M. Keenan, Hospital of the University of Pennsylvania, Nuclear Medicine/Radiology, Philadelphia, PA 19104, USA

T.J. Kinsella, University of Wisconsin School of Medicine, Department of Human Oncology, Madison, WI 53792, USA

E. Kohn, National Institutes of Health, National Cancer Institute, Laboratory of Pathology, Bethesda, MD 20892, USA

S.M. Larson, National Institutes of Health, Department of Nuclear Medicine, Clinical Center, Bethesda, MD 20892, USA

B. Leyland-Jones, National Institutes of Health, Cancer Therapy Evaluation Program, Bethesda, MD 20892, USA

A.S. Lichter, University of Michigan, Department of Radiation Oncology, Ann Arbor, MI 48109, USA

W.M. Linehan, National Cancer Institute, Surgery Branch, Bethesda, MD 20892, USA

M.P. Link, Stanford University School of Medicine, Stanford University Medical Center, Department of Pediatrics, Stanford, CA 94305, USA

L.A. Liotta, National Cancer Institute, Laboratory of Pathology, Bethesda, MD 20892, USA

M.E. Lippman, National Cancer Institute, Medicine Branch, Bethesda, MD 20892, USA

D.L. Longo, Frederick Cancer Research Facility, Clinical Research Branch, Biological Response Modifiers Program, Frederick, MD 21701-1013, USA

J.S. Macdonald, University of Kentucky, Lucille Parker Mackay Cancer Center, Lexington, KY 40502, USA

I.T. Magrath, National Cancer Institute, Lymphoma Biology Section, Pediatric Branch, Bethesda, MD 20892, USA

D.L. McShan, University of Michigan, Department of Radiation Oncology, Ann Arbor, MI 48109, USA

J.S. Miser, Mayo Clinic, Pediatrics, Hematology, Oncology, Rochester, MI 55905, USA

C.E. Myers, National Cancer Institute, Medicine Branch, Bethesda, MD 20892, USA

V. Narayanan, National Cancer Institute, Drug Synthesis and Chemistry Branch, Bethesda, MD 20892, USA

R.F. Ozols, National Cancer Institute, Medicine Branch, Bethesda, MD 20892, USA

G.L. Peck, National Cancer Institute, Dermatology Branch, Bethesda, MD 20892, USA

C. Perez-Tamayo, University of Michegan, Department of Radiation Oncology, Ann Arbor, MI 48109, USA

T. Philip, Centre Léon Bérard, F-69373 Lyon-Cédex 08, France

R. Pinkerton, The Hospital for Sick Children, Department of Haematology and Oncology, London WC1N 3JH, UK

D.G. Poplack, National Cancer Institute, Leukemia Biology Section, Pediatric Branch, Bethesda, MD 20892, USA

I.C. Quirt, The Princess Margaret Hospital, Ontario Cancer Research Institute, Toronto, Ontario M4X 1K9, Canada

C.N. Robertson, National Cancer Institute, Section of Urology, Surgery Branch, Bethesda, MD 20892, USA

H.I. Robins, Wisconsin Clinical Cancer Center, Divisions of Clinical Oncology and Radiation Oncology, Madison, WI 53792, USA

N.E. Rothschild, Vincent T. Lombardi Cancer Research Center, Division of Oncology, Washington, DC 20007, USA

L. Rubinstein, National Cancer Institute, Cancer Therapy Evaluation Program, Bethesda, MD 20892, USA

D.S. Sarnoff, National Cancer Institute, Dermatology Branch, Bethesda, MD 20892, USA

G. Sarosy, National Cancer Institute, Cancer Therapy Evaluation Program, Bethesda, MD 20892, USA

W.F. Sindelar, National Cancer Institute, Surgery Branch, Bethesda, MD 20892, USA

M.L. Stracke, National Cancer Institute, Laboratory of Pathology, Bethesda, MD 20892, USA

A. Surbone, National Cancer Institute, Clinical Pharmacology Branch, Bethesda, MD 20892, USA

R.K. TenHaken, University of Michigan, Department of Radiation Oncology, Ann Arbor, MI 48109, USA

W.J. Urba, National Cancer Institute, Biological Response Modifiers Program, Frederick Cancer Research Facility, Frederick, MD 21701-1013, USA

K. Weeks, University of Michigan, Department of Radiation Oncology, Ann Arbor, MI 48109, USA

U.M. Wewer, National Cancer Institute, Laboratory of Pathology, Bethesda, MD 20892, USA

G. Wilding, Wisconsin Clinical Cancer Center, Department of Human Oncology, Madison, WI 53792, USA

P.V. Woolley, Georgetown University Hospital, Division of Oncology, Washington, DC 20007, USA

D.C. Wright, National Institutes of Health, Clinical Neurosurgery Section, Surgical Neurology Branch, Bethesda, MD 20892, USA

1. New Directions in Cancer Treatment: An Overview

I.T. Magrath

Introduction

In the first half of this century, effective cancer therapy was only available for patients with localized tumors amenable to surgery or to the evolving modality of irradiation. There were no available methods to eradicate disseminated disease, which is present at the time of diagnosis in some 30% of patients with invasive cancer. Many of the remaining percentage of patients will subsequently relapse with metastatic disease after loco-regional therapy. Since the 1950s there has been a dramatic broadening of the range of proven or potential methods of cancer therapy, which currently includes such disparate approaches as tumor bombardment with subatomic particles on the one hand, and attempts to manipulate biochemical pathways related to cell proliferation or differentiation on the other. Particulary gratifying is the demonstration that at least some patients with widely disseminated tumors are curable with modern approaches to therapy. In fact a high proportion of patients with certain cancers such as choriocarcinoma, testicular cancer, many lymphomas and leukemias, and a number of childhood neoplasms—at one time uniformly fatal—can now expect to be cured, although many other cancers remain refractory to treatment except when disease is localized. These promising results have their foundations in the numerous conceptual and technological advances of recent years. Some of these have had a direct impact on therapeutic strategies, such as the development of the linear accelerator and new cytotoxic drugs, but others have had a more indirect influence, including improvements in methods of conducting and evaluating clinical trials, vastly improved imaging techniques and advances in supportive care, particularly that of the febrile neutropenic patient. The development of the microchip has had a major impact upon all aspects of cancer treatment and research, because of the resulting enormous increase in our capacity to store and analyze large quantities of information by computer, a trend equally important to data management in clinical trials, therapeutic planning in radiotherapy, tomographic and magnetic resonance imaging, and molecular biology. Progress in immunology and cell biology, closely linked with the development of the new field of molecular genetics, has led not only to increased accuracy and objectivity with regard to the diagnosis of at least some neoplastic diseases, a critically important prerequisite for the refinement of treatment strategies, but also to new approaches to cancer imaging and therapy.

1

Moreover, the discovery that drugs can cure some types of disseminated cancer (a major step forward that has been taken in the last 25 years or so) has provided a foundation upon which much more systematic approaches to the identification or synthesis of either totally new drugs or analogues with a higher therapeutic index are being constructed.

In spite of the major advances which have been made in the understanding and treatment of cancer, carrying with them the implicit promise that almost all cancers will ultimately be curable or preventable, there remains at present a considerable way to go before this goal is accomplished. This has led to an unreasonable degree of pessimism in those with a perspective limited to the clinical arena or with unrealistic expectations of the speed at which new knowledge and technology can be translated into improvements in the results of treatment of all cancer [1]. At present approximately 49% of all cancer is curable in the United States and Europe. This has been achieved by progress in the application of each of the three major treatment modalities—surgery, radiation, and chemotherapy—and also by judicious combinations of two or more of these modalities. It would appear that the major principles of cancer treatment using the three primary modalities have already been established and further progress in the results achieved with these treatment methods will, to a large extent, be made by refinement of treatment strategies, such as the development of more effective, less toxic chemotherapeutic agents and the improvement of radiation therapy techniques (both are subjects discussed in later chapters of this book). However, a number of totally novel forms of therapy are under investigation or at early stages of preclinical development. Many of these have only been made possible by progress in understanding the biology of neoplastic and nonneoplastic growth. At the present time, we are only at the very beginning of this era of understanding the cause and nature of cancer. Thus, it is not possible to predict with any degree of accuracy which areas of research are likely to be most fruitful, and it seems likely that at present we cannot even perceive the nature of some of the approaches to cancer treatment that will be used in the future. Insights into the pathogenesis of neoplasia have, however, provided substantial grounds for optimism even though a great deal of work both in the laboratory and in the clinic remains to be done.

This chapter will outline briefly some of the more promising recent trends in the treatment of cancer by radiation or chemotherapy, i.e., by traditional methods, as well as some potentially revolutionary approaches, based on our increased understanding of the nature of neoplastic cells and host–tumor interactions. This will provide a framework for the more detailed discussions which follow. A basic theme which runs throughout all approaches to cancer treatment will recur again and again: namely, the goal of achieving the highest therapeutic index possible, i.e., maximal tumor-cell elimination with minimal toxicity to normal tissues. Although a number of advances have been made in surgical oncology, such as, for example, the advent of limb-sparing procedures for extremity sarcomas and the use of the CO_2 laser, surgery will not be discussed as a separate modality. Another area which is not within the scope of this book, that

2

of supportive care, has nonetheless been crucial to the development of modern intensive chemotherapy regimens. In recent years, a large number of powerful new antibiotics, including antiviral compounds, have become available, and the principles of broad-spectrum antibiotic coverage of the febrile neutropenic patient along with empiric antifungal treatment in persistently febrile patients have been firmly established. This, coupled with improved blood product transfusion capabilities, particularly the administration of platelets to profoundly thrombocytopenic patients, has led to the ability to administer intensive chemotherapy with a much wider safety margin. There is no question that the ancillary components of the management of cancer—diagnosis, the determination of the extent of disease, and supportive care—have a crucially important role to play in the achievement of improved therapeutic results. This should not be forgotten when the primary treatment modalities themselves are considered.

Radiation Therapy

Conceptually, the irradiation of tumors resembles surgery with regard to its objectives, i.e., the eradication of local disease. The potential advantages of extenal beam irradiation over surgery include: the treatment of bodily regions which cannot be surgically removed or the removal of which would result in major disability; the possibility of encompassing a wider area around the tumor than with surgery; and the capacity to treat multiple areas, including metastatic disease, simultaneously. An extension of the concept of irradiation as local therapy has been the development of treatment plans which include anatomical regions likely to be involved by tumor spread, such as regional lymph nodes, or areas highly likely to be the site of cryptic metastatic tumor, including the nervous system or lungs. This form of treatment is usually known as "prophylactic," since, although it is based on the assumption that micrometastases exist, disease is not detectable at these sites at the time of therapy. The concept of irradiating areas at high risk for disease extension has been maximally developed in Hodgkin's disease, where there has been sufficient success with extended field or total nodal irradiation for there to be controversy over whether radiation or chemotherapy provides optimal treatment for some subgroups of patients with widespread tumor.

Radiation, like chemotherapy, cannot be delivered without exacting a price in terms of normal-tissue toxicity. Thus, for the optimal delivery of radiation, close attention must be paid to the dose delivered to irradiated normal structures. Normal-tissue toxicity is the limiting factor in all treatment protocols involving radiation, and this problem is often exacerbated where radiation is combined with chemotherapy. A number of drugs may give rise to worsening of radiation-induced toxicity of normal tissues when administered with radiation, or even the recall of local toxicity when a drug is administered after the completion of radiation therapy (for example actinomycin D, adriamycin (doxorubicin), methotrexate).

Further developments in radiation therapy can be achieved only by altering the delivery schedule (dose rate and size of dose fractions), by improving treatment planning so that more normal tissue is spared, by altering the nature of the radiation used (an area currently under exploration in a number of centers using particle beam radiation such as protons, neutrons, and pi-mesons), or by combining radiation with other modalities in an attempt to increase specificity for neoplastic tissue.

Attempts to Improve the Therapeutic Index of Conventional Radiation Therapy

Relatively little investigation has been carried out on dose rate and fractioning. This is partly due to the practical difficulties of increasing the dose rate beyond one fraction per day, although there may be some advantage, in selected tumors, of hyperfractionation (several smaller fractions per day) or accelerated fractionation [1]. Much more effort has been put into the problem of limiting the irradiation of normal tissue surrounding the tumor. Clearly, if only tumor and no normal tissue were included in the radiation field—an unattainable theoretical ideal—radiation therapy would be extremely simple, since whatever dose of radiation necessary to cause 100% tumor-cell kill could be delivered with impunity. While it is possible that further technological advances resulting in improved beam characteristics will lessen scatter outside the intended radiation volume, it is unlikely that major improvements in the therapeutic index will come simply from the development of better radiation sources and beam collimation.

Intraoperative Irradiation. A more imaginative attempt to approach the theoretical ideal situation as closely as possible is the technique of intraoperative irradiation. Unfortunately, while high doses of radiation can be delivered to well-defined tumorous areas at the time of surgery, and particularly vulnerable normal structures such as bowel, ovaries, etc., can be removed from the radiation field, only tumors in certain anatomical situations are amenable to intraoperative therapy. This method also has the disadvantages that usually, because of the need for a major surgical procedure, only single high doses of radiation can be delivered, and that normal tissues can only be partially removed from the path of the radiation beam.

Field Planning from Three-Dimensional Imaging. A different approach to the problem of maximizing the dose to the tumor and minimizing the dose to normal tissue, and one which holds considerable promise, is the utilization of three-dimensional planning to better define the precise volume to be irradiated. This is accomplished by making extensive use of both new imaging techniques, such as computerized tomographic scanning, magnetic resonance imaging, and imaging with monoclonal antibodies, coupled to the enormous ability of the computer to

4

transform multiple two-dimensional slices (even when obtained from different imaging devices) into three-dimensional images. This, combined with computerized calculation of optimal beam angles and intensities, and the ability to control precisely, again by computer, the rotation of the beam and/or the patient in several planes during therapy, (generating, thereby, truly curved fields), considerably lessens the irradiation of uninvolved tissue. This new technology, when fully developed, will presumably give the highest possible therapeutic indexes using conventional external beam irradiation. Although complex, the extensive computerization may eventually permit more accurate treatment to be delivered at all radiation oncology centers, even in smaller units where the radiotherapists may be less experienced. Carefully designed computer programs could even indicate where brachytherapy (implantation of radioactive wires, needles, etc.) would be preferable to external beam therapy and what kind of external beam (electrons, gamma rays, etc.) would be optimal, at least in terms of the physical constraints imposed by the tumor shape and volume.

Radiation Sensitizers and Protectors. A variety of drugs able to sensitize tumor tissue to radiation (such as halogenated pyrimidines, nitroimidazoles, sulfhydryl compounds and inhibitors of DNA repair) or protect normal tissues from radiation (WR-2721 and cysteamline-related thiophosphates) have been examined, with some promising results. Perhaps new agents of this kind will be developed which will prove more effective than those currently undergoing clincial testing.

Multimodality Therapy. The possibility that combinations of physical modalities, e.g., hyperthermia, radiation (possibly using novel approaches such as intra-operative irradiation or particle beam irradiation), with drugs (other than cytotoxic drugs) may provide an increased therapeutic index has been explored to a limited extent. The true promise of these techniques cannot, as yet, be estimated. Moreover, since optimal timing and fractionation of radiation may differ when administered in combination with other modalities, numerous empiric trials will be necessary to fully evaluate such combinations.

Targeted Radiation Therapy

With the same goal of sparing normal tissue in mind, but utilizing a completely different approach, attempts have been made to "target" radiation by coupling radionuclides to monoclonal antibodies directed against tumor-associated antigens. Under ideal circumstances, this could result in the delivery of radiation only to tumor tissue, with almost total sparing of normal tissue. In practice, of course, this ideal is unlikely to be attained since no absolutely tumor-specific antigen exists, and, even if it did, it is unlikely that non-specific tissue uptake could ever be reduced to zero. At the present time, the ratio of specific to non-specific binding with most monoclonal antibodies used in vivo is between 2 and 10. A number of problems relating to both the antibody and radionuclide components of the therapeutic medium need to be overcome; these include technical difficulties in the construction of suitable antibody/radioisotope conjugates, tissue distribution of the conjugate, nonspecific binding via the F_c region of the antibody molecules to the reticuloendothelial system, the development of a host immune response against the antibody (since it is normally a foreign protein), and limitations in the radiation dose which can be administered by this route (related to the half-life of the radioisotope used and the type of emitted radiation). However, this is a new field and one in which we may see considerable developments in the future.

A similar approach to targeting therapy with monoclonal antibodies is to use radioactive compounds which are selectively taken up by tumor tissue. The most obvious example is the use of radioactive isotopes of iodine for the treatment of thyroid carcinoma. Recently, responses have been seen in pheochromocytoma, medullary thyroid carcinoma, and neuroblastoma to therapeutic doses of iodo-131-meta-iodobenzylguanidine (MIBG), a drug taken up by tissues which synthesize catecholamines [2]. Such radionuclides can be of value in diagnosis, treatment, and follow-up, and although their effect is at present mainly palliative, further exploration of this approach would appear worthwhile.

Alternatives to Photon Therapy

Particle beam irradiation, with the exception of electron therapy, is an area of radiation therapy still being researched. Progress is hindered by the fact that there are relatively few centers able to generate fast neutrons, negative pi-mesons (pions), or ion beams with appropriate energies, that also have the facilities for treating patients. The potential advantage of these particle beam irradiation therapies is largely derived from their minimal dependence (unlike photons) on the presence of oxygen, and—since they all are densely ionizing in tissue—improved depth dose distribution, so that higher doses can be delivered to the target tissue with less irradiation to surrounding tissue. In anatomical locations where the radiation field must conform precisely to the tumor volume, such as in the eye, where preservation of vision is an objective (e.g., uveal melanomas), or with para-CNS sarcomas abutting critical normal structures, helium ion or proton irradiation may be the treatment of choice [3,4]. In less critical regions a combination of particle therapy with improved definition of the tumor volume provided by three-dimensional treatment planning might be of particular benefit, although only very few specialized centers have this dual capability at present [5]. Fast neutrons appear to provide an advantage over photon and electron techniques in some well-defined series of patients with locally extensive salivary gland tumors or slow growing, well-differentiated soft tissue sarcomas and in some melanoma patients [6].

Much work remains to be done to determine the role of these newer types of irradiation. Optimal fractionation schedules may differ for different types of radiation, and combinations of different types of beam, e.g., photons and neutrons, could have advantages. Two questions that must be asked are whether the potential benefits justify the cost and practical difficulties involved, and how such benefits will compare with those of other approaches to cancer treatment. These questions can only be answered if at least some centers continue to explore alternatives to photons in the practice of radiotherapy.

Systemic Irradiation

The use of systemic irradiation, i.e., irradiation delivered to the entire body and therefore encompassing all tumor cells, however widely metastatic, has had a new lease of life in recent years with the advent of autologous or allogeneic marrow infusion able to "rescue" the patient from therapy which is presumptively totally marrow ablative. Since total body irradiation maximizes the amount of normal tissue included in the radiation field, it has a particularly low therapeutic index. However, its use in combination with chemotherapy has been explored in a number of different tumors. Although encouraging results have been obtained, improvements in the results of treatment protocols utilizing marrow transplantation seem more likely to come from improvements in the preparative chemotherapy regimens used than from advances in the delivery of total body irradiation. Low-dose total body irradiation has been of some value in a small number of tumors, e.g., low grade lymphomas, but has not become standard therapy in any tumor and seems unlikely to do so.

Other Physical Methods

Hyperthermia

It now seems unlikely that hyperthermia will be used as a single treatment modality. Current trends in this field are focusing on combinations of hyperthermia with either radiation or drugs. Although serious acute toxicities have been observed with hyperthermia alone or hyperthermia in combination with, for example, adriamycin, new methods of elevating body temperature appear to be less toxic. It is of interest that a number of drugs have proved to be cytotoxic at an elevated temperature, but not under normothermic conditions. The use of hyperthermia is still experimental, but this modality does represent a unique approach to cancer treatment and may find a role in concert with other therapies.

Photoactivation

The use of light-sensitive compounds such as psoralens [7] or hematoporphyrins—some of which may be preferentially taken up by tumor tissue— to induce tumor toxicity when exposed to light (in the form of laser beams in the case of hematoporphyrin sensitization) is an interesting area for research which may provide a valuable form of therapy for specific kinds of cancer. Examples include some cutaneous neoplasms, cancers of internal body surfaces which can be illuminated with appropriate instruments, and possibly, in the case of laser activation, cancers in anatomical locations where the preservation of function requires that local therapy be applied to the tumor only, with tumor margins measured in millimeters at most (e.g., the eye). The role of photoactivation in the overall schema of cancer treatment, however, has yet to be defined.

Chemotherapy

The treatment of cancer by drugs represents a quite different philosophical approach to that espoused by surgical oncology and, at least for the most part, radiation therapy. Cancer chemotherapy has been primarily directed against tumors which are widespread from the outset, or have a known high propensity to metastasize. However, the regional use of chemotherapy, e.g., in the treatment of tumor in body compartments such as the CNS or peritoneal cavity, or in organs amenable to regional perfusions such as the liver or an extremity, has been under investigation for a long time. The therapeutic index of cancer chemotherapy varies markedly from tumor to tumor and from drug to drug. While a small number of tumors may be curable by chemotherapy alone, even when massive or widely disseminated, in other cancers chemotherapy is largely considered as an adjuvant to surgery or radiation which are used to eradicate known sites of disease. Chemotherapy is also sometimes used as the sole treatment modality in localized tumors when the tumor is highly sensitive to chemotherapy and has a high propensity to spread (e.g., some lymphomas).

Because chemotherapy is a systemic modality the effect of the drugs on normal tissue is of critical importance. Based, to some extent, on principles learned from antimicrobial therapy, there has been a major trend in the past decade towards the use of drug combinations as opposed to single agents. With the exception of some incurable neoplasms which can be controlled for a period of time with single agents and the initial clinical trials of new drugs, single agents are rarely used today except in an experimental setting. The use of drug combinations is based on the principles that (a) multiple drugs are likely to be more effective against cancer cells because of simultaneous damage to several biochemical pathways. (b) resistance is less likely to arise to a drug combination than to an individual drug, and (c) the overall toxicity of the combination regimen will, at worst, be increased within a tolerable range above the level anticipated for a single agent when drugs with different side effects are combined. In a number of malignancies, particularly hemopoietic malignancies, there is no doubt that drug combinations are superior to single-agent therapy and a large amount of clinical chemotherapeutic research is devoted to the development of better drug combinations (i.e., combinations with a higher therapeutic index). Whereas new drug combinations can often be rationalized on the basis of current knowledge, well-designed clinical trials are still necessary to dem-

8

onstrate the superiority of one combination over another, and a large helping of empiricism in such studies is unavoidable. Multiagent regimens fail, all too often, because of the major obstacle to cure by chemotherapy—the development of drug resistance, or, perhaps more accurately, the gradual predominance in a tumor of drug-resistant clones which may have been minimally represented at the start of therapy.

Because of the all too frequent development of drug resistance and the poor responsiveness of some tumors from the outset, for a long time there has been a move toward the development of new agents which might prove to be more effective than existing agents, or at least to be non-cross-resistant alternatives. Three major approaches to dealing with the problem of primary or secondary chemotherapy resistance are being pursued, although the last two are still in their infancy: (a) the development of new drugs, (b) attempts to reverse resistance, and (c) attempts to use the altered biochemistry of drug-resistant cells as a therapeutic target. In addition, maximal exploitation of available drugs is being attempted through the more rational design of drug combinations, the use of pharmacokinetic information, and the exploration of very high-dose therapy.

Drug Screening

The National Cancer Institute of the United States of America has for many years undertaken empirical drug screening programs whereby very large numbers of compounds are examined for cytotoxic activity in selected panels of animal tumors. Recently there has been a trend towards the introduction of drug screening against human tumors in vitro, using the clonogenic assay system or cell lines derived from human tumors (predominantly lung, breast, colon, and CNS tumors, leukemia, and melanoma). Once promising agents are identified, detailed toxicity studies are carried out in animals, and the drugs are finally examined in clinical trials for toxicity (phase I) and activity (phase II). The place of active drugs in cancer treatment is finally examined in phase III trials (usually randomized) in which drug combinations containing the new agent are compared with the best available drug therapy. Whatever the screening method used, this approach to the discovery of potential new agents requires extensive resources and is relatively inefficient. Increased efficiency of preclinical screening has been made possible by improved knowledge of pharmacology and of the biochemical pathways with which drugs interact, as well as the development of computer data bases incorporating structure/activity information so that new compounds can be selected for screening on the basis of the similarity of their structure to drugs of known activity or the uniqueness of their structure.

Drug Design

Now that a sizable chemotherapeutic armamentarium has been built up, increasing efforts are being expended in the design and development of new agents by structural modification of existing drugs (i.e., the development of less toxic or more effective analogues). A number of potentially useful agents which appear to have less of the dose-limiting toxicities of their parent compounds have been developed, good examples being cisplatinum and anthracycline analogues with less renal and cardiac toxicity respectively. As more is learnt of structure-activity relationships, there is likely to be major progress in the ability to synthesize drug analogues with a number of desirable features, such as rapid penetration into the cerebrospinal fluid, or even into specific tumors, based on the biochemistry of the particular tissue, and resistance to enzymatic degradation. It may even be feasible to design drugs which have activity against specific tumors, which have less toxicity, or which interfere with more than one biochemical pathway. A prototype of the latter kind is the drug ara-azacytidine, which combines the biochemical characteristics of two drugs, cytosine arabinoside (ara-C) and 5-azacytidine. This agent has proved to be more active than either ara-C or 5-azacytidine alone in initial animal studies, but whether increased activity will be observed in clinical studies, and whether it will have advantages over the simultaneous or sequenced administration of the individual parent compounds remains to be seen [8].

A more recent approach to the development of chemotherapeutic agents, which is also dependent upon computer-based information, is the attempt to design drugs with particular activities, e.g., the ability to bind to an enzyme (and therefore inhibit the binding of the normal substrate) known to be important in a biochemical pathway involved in cellular proliferation. This has been made possible by the ability to generate, by means of sophisticated computer graphics, representations of the three-dimensional structure of enzymes, and to predict the structure of compounds which will bind to the catalytic regions. This permits the search for, or even the active synthesis of, agents which possess regions with the appropriate structure for the requisite function. Such an approach has already been used in the development of new folate inhibitors, and is likely to be used increasingly as more information becomes available regarding the deranged biochemical pathways of cancer cells. For example, the design of drugs which inhibit oncogene products, possibly even oncogene products which are specific for certain types of tumor, is a potentially very exciting area for future research.

Drug Resistance

In essence, chemotherapy failure is due either to failure of the drug to reach all tumor tissue (or to do so in sufficient concentration) or to the development of drug resistance. In the latter case, tumor will continue to progress in the face of drug concentrations which are normally cytotoxic. This is due either to intrinsic resistance of a proportion of the tumor cells, which may eventually come to predominate in the population, or to the development of resistance after exposure to chemotherapeutic agents. Thus, a worthy parallel endeavor to the development of improved or alternative drugs is the exploration of the mechanisms of drug resistance, in the hope that this knowledge will lead to effective methods of preventing or reversing resistance. Mechanisms of resistance can be simply divided into those which reduce the effective level of a drug in tumor cells (i.e., impair entry, increase elimination, lessen activation, increase inactivation) or those which interfere with the biochemical effect of the drug (e.g., reduce binding of the drug to an enzyme, compensate biochemically for the function that has been impaired by the drug, or directly inhibit the drug effect). Resistance can be associated with increased transcription of a gene involved in one of these processes (in more extreme cases involving amplification of the gene itself), such as the dihydrofolate reductase (DHFR) gene whose product is inhibited by methotrexate, or the multidrug resistance gene which codes for a protein (P170) believed to be involved in the elimination of certain chemicals, including several chemotherapeutic agents, from the cell via a membrane pump. Increased levels of DHFR or P170 means that increased concentrations of cytotoxic drugs will be required to overcome their effect. Increased levels of glutathione, which destroys free radicals (which mediate the cytotoxicity of some drugs), have been associated with resistance to anthracyclines. Sometimes resistance is caused by the structural modification of an important cellular enzyme which is inhibited by a chemotherapeutic agent e.g., (once again) DHFR.

Knowledge of the mechanisms of resistance will hopefully permit the development of methods of avoiding, or lessening the probability of, the development of resistance, or even of increasing the sensitivity of tumor cells to chemotherapeutic drugs, either before or after the acquisition of clinical resistance. When 5-fluorouracil (5-FU) is given before methotrexate, for example, it can induce amplification of the DHFR gene, such that cells become more resistant to subsequently administered methotrexate [9]. Cells which are resistant to methotrexate because of defective polyglutamate formation (methotrexate polyglutamates remain in the cell for longer and increase inhibition of thymidylate synthetase, another important enzyme in the pyrimidline synthesis pathway, as well as prolonging inhibition of DHFR) retain sensitivity to trimetrexate, a lipid-soluble antifolate which does not form polyglutamates. There is some evidence that sequential administration of methotrexate and trimetrexate may decrease the rate of emergence of methotrexate resistance [10].

Resistance may be reversed by agents which inhibit the action of the primary macromolecules involved in the expression of drug resistence (e.g., blocking the function of P170 with verapamil or quinidine, or reducing levels of glutathione with buthionine sulfoximine). It may even prove possible to develop drugs which bind specifically to structurally modified enzymes associated with drug resistance (such as modified DHFR [11]). Finally, the recent cloning of the gene coding for P170 (mdr-1) should permit rapid progress in the understanding of its normal functions and its role in pleiotropic drug resistance.

Rational Drug Combination

Until recently, combination chemotherapy regimens have been designed empirically, paying attention only to the known spectrum of activity and the toxicities of the drugs under consideration. As information regarding biochemical pathways improves, the possibility exists of rationally designing drug combinations to have the maximal effect on a specific intracellular pathway. This approach has, to date, mainly been explored in the case of drugs affecting purine and pyrimidine metabolism, the pathways of which are known in quite substantial detail. One example is the use of 5-FU/leukovorin combinations. It has been shown that complete thymidylate synthetase inhibition by the active metabolite of 5-FU (fluorodeoxyuridine monophosphate) can only be achieved in the presence of a folate cofactor, N^{5-10} methylene tetrahydrofolate [12]. Sensitivity to 5-FU correlates directly with the intracellular folate level of cultured cells, and reduced folates enhance the cytotoxicity of 5-FU in both sensitive and resistant lines [13, 14]. Combinations of drugs acting on the same pathway may prove to be synergistic. This is the case when methotrexate is administered before 5-FU, although administration in the reverse order has the opposite effect (see above). Hopefully, as more information is obtained regarding the mode of action of cytotoxic agents, the design of drug combinations can be based more and more upon the biochemical effects anticipated rather than simply the known spectrum of activity and toxicity of a drug and empirical studies of drug combinations in animal tumors. The latter frequently fail to predict the result in human tumors, the biochemistry of which may differ markedly.

Role of Pharmacokinetics in Cancer Chemotherapy

In recent years, because of the development of improved methods of measuring drug levels, particularly through the use of high-pressure liquid chromatography, pharmacokinetics has played an increasingly important role in the design of chemotherapy protocols. Because of age-related and individual differences in metaoblism and in the absorption (after oral administration) of drugs, standard dosing does not necessarily produce similar serum levels in different individuals. In the future, dosage could be determined on the basis of serum levels attained—a concept which is undergoing preliminary clinical trials. Knowledge of the distribution and true half-life of a drug; its absorption from the gastrointestinal tract, muscle, or subcutaneous tissue; and its protein binding capacity, lipophilicity, and passage across the blood-brain barrier all enable treatment protocols to be designed more rationally, at least with regard to optimal dose, route, and scheduling of administration. Erratic absorption of oral 6-mercaptopurine may be a factor which contributes to the relapse of patients suffering from acute lymphoblastic leukemia while they are on maintenance therapy (probably because of a resultant reduction in the dose intensity delivered to the tumor cells—see below) [15]. Valuable information pertinent to the dose and frequency of administration of ara-C has been gained with knowledge of its rapid deamination in serum and tumor cells [16]. Measurement of serum and CSF methotrexate levels has been instrumental in permitting the safe administration of high-dose methotrexate regimens, including those designed to provide CNS prophylaxis.

Pharmacokinetics provide particularly valuable information with regard to

12

the choice of drug and design of regional chemotherapy regimens (e.g., hepatic artery infusions, intraperitoneal therapy). Clearly, such therapy has very specific indications, such as the presence of hepatic metastases of colorectal cancer, or intraperitoneal spread of ovarian cancer or cancer of the colon (see below).

Concept of Dose Intensity

Because the development of chemotherapy regimens has for the large art been empirical and has also been influenced by practical issues such as the need for hospitalization, a number of basic aspects of the design of chemotherapy regimens have not been given the attention they deserve. One such issue is the question of dose intensity—the amount of drug delivered per unit time. Is it more likely that cure will result from high doses given at relatively long intervals or from lower doses given frequently, or are these two approaches equivalent so long as the same dose per unit time is given? There is no absolute answer to this question, since efficacy is often influenced by the pharmacology of the cytotoxic drug in question. In the case of ara-C, for example, the effect on the tumor is clearly schedule-dependent. There is good evidence, however, that for several drugs, e.g., mitoxantrone in breast cancer and VP16 in lung cancer, there is a linear relationship between the response rate and the dose intensity (at least over a part of the dose-intensity range), suggesting that the most important factor which determines the outcome of therapy (at least the initial response rate) is often dose intensity rather than schedule [17].

This concept has important implications for the design of phase I and II studies. In the case of drugs with a steep slope of the linear dose-intensity–response relationship, small increments in dose intensity may have a significant effect on response. For mitoxantrone given every 3 weeks, for example, the response rate in patients with advanced breast cancer increased by almost 20% for an approximate increment in *received* dose intensity from 4 to 4.5 mg/m^2 per week. Knowledge of the slope of the line representing the dose-intensity–response relationship permits better assessment of the therapeutic gains which might be achieved by further increase of dose intensity, and, coupled with knowledge of the schedule-dependency of toxicity, may permit schedules to be designed which maximize dose intensity, and therefore response, and keep toxicity within acceptable limits. Low-dose continuous infusions, as sometimes employed for 5-FU in colorectal cancer, for example, may allow more drug to be administered per unit time, yet result in less toxicity. Preliminary information appears to confirm that low-dose continuous infusions result in a higher response rate in patients with colon cancer (see Woolley, this volume).

Another concept resulting from dose-intensity analysis is that larger tumors require a higher dose intensity. Whereas for low-burden tumors, an increment in dose intensity may not result in any improvement, for high-burden tumors significant benefit could result. This is consistent with the finding that relatively low-dose adjuvant therapy is of considerable value in some diseases, while higher dose intensities may be curative in an adjuvant setting, even where the tumor is relatively resistant or incurable by chemotherapy alone (e.g., osteogenic sarcoma).

Although calculation of dose intensity for combination chemotherapy regimens is more difficult, this can be done by relating the dose intensities of each drug in any given regimen to that of the dose intensity of the drug in a standard regimen in which the component drugs are of approximately equal activity, and averaging the resultant dose intensities. Such calculations yield dose-intensity–response relationships as seen for single agents. Moreover, when the range of dose intensities of the individual agents is sufficiently different in a series of regimens of similar average dose intensity, the relatively activity of one of the agents can be determined by plotting dose intensity of the agent in question against response rate [17]. These kinds of calculations could be useful in the design of drug combinations which should clearly contain the optimal dose intensities of each drug.

In addition to dose intensity, the duration of treatment is important, the product of these two factors being total dose. Theoretically, and assuming that drug resistance does not arise, there should be an optimal duration of therapy for each tumor, based upon the total tumor burden. To analyze the relative importance of dose intensity and total dose, randomized trials will need to be conducted in which either dose intensity or total dose is fixed, with the other factor as a variable [18].

Massive Dose Therapy

Some investigators have attempted to improve tumor cell kill by using very high drug doses. In some cases the resultant very high drug levels may result in a more effective drug action; for example, the ability of methotrexate to prevent DHFR from producing reduced folates is dependent upon a large excess of free drug in the cell. Similarly, very high levels of circulating ara-C will swamp the available deaminases present in normal serum and tumor cells which rapidly break down this drug. Moreover, high intracellular levels compete effectively with intracellular deoxycytidine triphosphate pools for incorporation into DNA. Very high drug levels may also increase penetration into tumor cells and may have other effects which increase tumor cytoxicity. High levels of methotrexate, for example, can increase the formation of methotrexate polyglutamates, which appear to be of significance to the cytotoxic effect of methotrexate, and provide a basis for selectivity of drug action, since bone marrow cells and intestinal epithelial cells do not accumulate polyglutamates. In the case of S-phase agents, duration of exposure to the drug is critically important with regard to toxicity to the normal cells, and extraordinarily high doses of these drugs, with the attendant theoretical advantages, can be administered to patients for short periods, measured in some cases in days (e.g., ara-C), without causing lethal toxicity. High-dose therapy is sometimes carried out in conjunction with "marrow rescue," whereby autologous marrow, stored (cryopreserved) prior to the administration of the high-dose drug therapy, or allogeneic bone marrow is

14

reinfused into the patient to permit marrow recovery after what is believed to be a lethal dose of drug (with or without total body irradiation) has been administered. Marrow rescue is logical where myelosuppression is the major form of toxicity of the drug in question. In protocols incorporating very high drug doses, however, alternative toxicities may sometimes prove to be dose-limiting, e.g., liver toxicity with the nitrosoureas, cerebellar toxicity with high-dose ara-C, and the potential for cardiac toxicity with very high-dose cyclophosphamide. These extramedullary toxicities essentially limit the drugs which can be used in very high dosage to alkylating agents, methotrexate, ara-C, and VP16. Moreover, if the concept of dose intensity is correct, very high-dose chemotherapy may offer advantages over more conventional dosage schemes only when sufficient total drug can be administered in a single chemotherapy cycle for destruction of the total tumor burden (a single cycle of treatment may also lessen the probability that drug resistance will arise), or when there are particular pharmacologic or biological advantages. The latter may exist in certain chronic malignancies such as chronic myeloid leukemia (CML) or follicular lymphomas, particularly small cleaved-cell follicular lymphomas. These tumors may differ from others in that there is a population of tumor stem cells which, while retaining sensitivity to chemotherapy over long periods, appear, like bone marrow stem cells, to be impossible to eliminate with conventional drug regimens. These tumor stem cells continually replenish the tumor cell pool. Cure may only be accomplished by total ablation of these tumor stems cells, a process which appears to be possible, at least in the case of CML (see chapter 45), by massive therapy, usually involving total body irradiation followed by hemopoietic reconstitution.

Regional Chemotherapy

While chemotherapy is rightly considered as systemic therapy, like radiation, exposure of normal cells limits its efficacy. Two potential means of achieving high tumor drug levels while keeping systemic drug exposure to a minimum are being studied. The first is regional chemotherapy, in which intra-arterial infusion (in the case of the liver, portal vein infusion is also used) or intracavitary instillation can, when appropriate drugs and anatomical situations are chosen, increase the differential concentration of drugs between the regional tumor and the serum [19]. With arterial infusion, the differential concentration is inversely proportional to the ratio of the arterial blood flow to the cardiac output, since the venous return from the tumor will provide the systemic concentration. Where systemic clearance is high, or there is a significant "first pass" effect, i.e., elimination of drug from the bloodstream before the systemic circulation is reached, as occurs in hepatic artery infusion of 5-FU, a significant concentration gradient can be established. Although arterial perfusion has been under exploration for many years, however, it has not become a standard therapeutic approach, with the possible exception of the control of hepatic metastases of colorectal cancer using 5-FU. It would appear that in general, pharmacologic advantages are minor or insignificant.

The use of intraperitoneal infusions for tumors confined to the abdomen has met with some success when the tumor nodules are small and drugs with slow egress from the peritoneal compartment but rapid systemic clearance are chosen. This approach could prove to be of value when large molecules, e.g., protein-drug conjugates, are used, for these penetrate more deeply into the tumor since they do not readily enter tumor capillaries.

Targeted Chemotherapy

The second method of diminishing systemic toxicity is to use targeted therapy, in which the tumor uptake of the drug is much greater than uptake into other body cells, or in which the drug has a relatively specific effect because of the functional activity and resultant biochemical pathways of the normal and tumor tissue. Ortho para'DDD, for example, causes necrosis of the normal adrenal cortex and is active against adrenal carcinoma, while streptozotocin causes specific toxicity of pancreatic islet tissue and functional islet cell tumors. In the absence of selective uptake on a biochemical basis, improved specificity can be achieved by coupling the drug to a molecule that will selectively bind or be taken up by the tumor cell. One potential benefit of efficient targeting would be that highly toxic drugs or toxins could be used in place of chemotherapeutic agents without risking systemic toxicity. The most widely explored method to date, although still in its early stages of development, has been the coupling of drugs to monoclonal antibodies which bind specifically to tumor cells (see below).

Chemotherapy of Pharmacologic Sanctuaries

An area which has become of increasing importance as improvements in systemic therapy are made is the therapy of tumors in body sites less accessible to chemotherapeutic agents, e.g., the central nervous system. In several diseases, spread into the CNS has become an increasingly frequent reason for failure, so that the development of more effective therapy for brain and meningeal involvement will have an impact upon a wide range of neoplasms. Special characteristics, primarily lipid solubility, are required of drugs which cross the blood-brain barrier—which is composed of two lipid bilayers—and toxicity considerations differ for this body compartment so that direct intrathecal injection is possible only with a very limited number of drugs. New compounds able to cross the blood-brain barrier are being developed and evaluated (e.g., phenylhydantoin mustard), while oxazaphosphorines not requiring activation in the liver (hydroperoxycyclophosphamide) have recently been administered directly into the CSF without major toxicity [20].

Recently intraocular recurrences in acute lymphoblastic leukemia have focused attention on the eye as a sanctuary site, [21] while the testis has for long been recognized as a potential sanctuary, depending upon the drugs being used for treatment. There has, however, been less clinical research directed toward the testis as a pharmacologic sanctuary because of its amenability to local therapy.

Reduction or Abrogation of Toxic Side Effects

If the toxic side effects of a drug can be reduced, higher doses can be given, so increasing its antitumor efficacy. While some drug analogues appear to have less toxicity in general than the parent compound at an equally tumor-toxic dose, and others may be less toxic with regard to a specific side effect, an alternative to the development of new agents is the employment of a method, or additional agent, to lessen a particular toxicity. For example, hyperchloremic hydration considerably lessens the nephrotoxic effect of cisplatin, allowing more drug to be administered [22]. Similarly, sodium thiosulfate or diethyldithiocarbamate can abrogate both the nephrotoxicity, and, in higher dosage, the cytotoxicity of cis-platin. Sodium thiosulfate can also be used to prevent systemic toxicity when cisplatin is used for regional therapy (e.g., intraperitoneal instillation) [23]. Recently a protective effect of ICRF-187 against adriamycin-induced cardiac toxicity was reported [24].

Another example of an increased therapeutic index as a consequence of reduction in regional toxicity is provided by dimercaptoethanesulfonate (mesna) [25]. This sulfhydryl compound is able to protect the renal tract (particularly the bladder) against the chemical irritation induced by the oxazaphosphorines. Mesna, which is almost exclusively excreted by the kidney, is inactive in serum, but binds to urinary acrolein and the 4-hydroxy oxazaphosphorine metabolites which yield acrolein, the agent believed to be primarily responsible for the production of cystitis. Clearly, mesna fulfills many of the requirements for an ideal regional protective agent, since it exerts an effect only in urine and does not influence systemic cytotoxicity. Its use has permitted reintroduction of ifosfa-mide, an oxazaphosphorine which may be more effective than cyclophospha-mide, at least in some tumors, but whose dose-limiting side effect in the absence of mesna is hemorrhagic cystitis. High-dose cyclophosphamide, as given in marrow transplantation preparative regimens, is also more safely administered with mesna uroprotection.

Biological Approaches to Therapy

Progress in the fields of developmental biology, immunology, and molecular genetics has led to the realization that the pathogenesis of individual cancers can and will be comprehended in the near future. In some cases, e.g., Burkitt's lymphoma, CML, and to a lesser extent other hemopoietic neoplasms, Wilms' tumor, and retinoblastoma, there is already quite detailed knowledge of the somatic genetic changes which have induced neoplastic behavior. At the same time, information regarding the regulation of cell differentiation and prolifera-tion, the derangement of which is a quintessential aspect of neoplasia, is rapidly accumulating. These exciting developments in the biological sciences have pro-vided impetus, and some of the tools, to begin to consider therapeutic interven-tions based on a view of cancer as a genetically induced derangement of cellular behavior, which might in some circumstances be correctable and in others provide a target for truly tumor-specific therapy. The same techniques which have permitted an increased understanding of cancer have led to the development of new and more objective methods of diagnosis and made possible new treatment approaches using, for example, molecularly cloned cytokines or cell clones. The present blossoming of clinical trials to examine the efficacy of biological response modifiers has largely been made possible by the ability to produce large quantities of cytokines by recombinant DNA techniques. These same molecules, particularly interleukins and hemopoietic growth factors, have made it possible to expand clones of cells in vitro which can be used in adoptive immunotherapy, and raise the possibility of ultimately replacing entire normal hemopoietic lineages destroyed by intensive chemotherapy.

Immunotherapy

For a long time, the realization that the immune system provides defenses against a broad range of microorganisms and even cells derived from other individuals has stimulated efforts to divert this natural defense system toward the treatment of cancer. Empirical attempts at nonspecific immunotherapy have met with little success in the past, but the recent ability to raise and purify monoclonal antibodies coupled with significant advances in the understanding of the numerous regulatory factors elaborated by lymphoid cells and macrophages has led to a resurgences of interest in this area.

Monoclonal Antibodies. Antibodies produced by a single clone of mouse (rarely other species) lymphocytes fused to a plasmacytoma cell line to permit continued survival and production of the antibody have led to the recognition of a series of lineage-specific and differentiation-specific antigens, as well as many others, which, while associated with specific cell lineages (e.g., T lymphocytes) are not exclusively expressed on such cells. These antigens provide valuable diagnostic aids as well as potential targets for therapeutic approaches. It should be noted that, with the exception of the antigen receptors of B- and T-cell lymphoid neoplasms (which are clone-specific), no truly tumor-specific antigens have been recognized in man. This is of significance to therapy in which antibodies directed against these antigens are used, since the consequences of effects on normal cells must always be considered.

The simple binding of a monoclonal antibody to a surface receptor of a tumor cell will, by itself, rarely lead to cell death, although some antibodies are cytotoxic in vitro in the presence of complement. It is theoretically possible, however, that monoclonal antibody binding alone could have therapeutic value if the target antigen (more specifically, epitope) were carefully selected. This is based upon the assumption that some surface antigens may be obligately expressed (e.g., an essential growth factor receptor), so that dividing tumor cells must always possess them, and deprivation of the binding of the appropriate ligand would have a detrimental effect on the tumor. Appropriate antibodies could prevent the binding of the ligand to the receptor, by binding to the ligand itself

18

or to the cell-surface receptor. This approach has been shown to be theoretically possible by the demonstration that antibodies against the peptide bombesin (which acts as a growth factor for small cell lung cancer) can inhibit the growth of small-cell lung cancer cell lines and xenografts [26]. Many cell surface antigens, however, as has been shown in a number of clinical trials, may be down-regulated (modulated) with no apparent harm to the tumor cell, so that they can be useful as targets only when the monoclonal antibody is conjugated to a toxin, drug, radioisotope, or possibly cytokine capable of causing cell death. Such approaches to cancer therapy are in their infancy. Numerous problems still remain to be surmounted, such as the destruction of heterologous antibody molecules by the patient's immune system, penetration of the antibody molecules to all tumor-bearing sites, modulation of the target antigen (if initial binding does not result in cell death), the blocking of monoclonal antibodies by circulating antigens, and possible side effects due to nonspecific uptake of antibodies by other organs (especially liver). Whether some of these problems can be overcome, for example, by the use of human or hybrid (mouse variable region, human F_c region) monoclonal antibodies, which would not excite a significant host immune response against them, by antibody "cocktails" containing several antibodies which react with different antigens on the neoplasm, or by the simultaneous use of agents which enhance antigen expression to avoid the problem of modulation remains to be seen.

Adoptive Immunotherapy. For many years the theoretical possibility of boosting the host immune response against tumor cells has been discussed, and numerous approaches have been attempted in preclinical and clinical trials. The essential failure of nonspecific immune stimulants, such as BCG (bacille Calmette-Guérin), led for a time to disillusionment with the whole concept of immunotherapy, but the recent definition of a number of molecules which are involved in the regulation of the immune response has rejuvenated this field. Highly purified lymphokines—molecules which regulate the proliferation and function of lymphocytes—are now available in large quantities through recombinant DNA technology which has permitted the cloning and expression of their genes in bacterial systems (or, more rarely, in mammalian cells). This in turn has raised the possibility of manipulating the immune system in a very precise way, either in vivo, by administering the purified molecules directly to the patient, or by expanding selected cell populations in vitro with the aid of lymphokines prior to reinfusing them into the patient. In practice, there is much to be learnt about the actions of the many lymphokines, and ongoing clinical trials still have a large element of empiricism. Among the more promising approaches is the use of interleukin-2 (IL-2). Numerous studies are currently exploring the use of this agent alone and in combination with LAK cells (lymphokine activated killer cells) or with TIL cells (tumor infiltrating lymphocytes), which are expanded in vitro by the use of IL-2 and then administered to the patient along with additional IL-2 to maintain the proliferation of the responsive cells in vivo. Although the LAK cell/IL-2 regimen, as originally reported (bolus doses of IL-2 3 times daily), is toxic, resulting in marked fluid retention, hypotension, and liver and renal impairment, responses, including complete responses, have been observed

19

in tumors for which there is no other effective therapy, such as metastatic renal cell cancer and melanoma (with response rates of 33% and 23% respectively) [27]. A much less toxic regimen involving the constant infustion (5-day cycles) of a lower dose of IL-2 with LAK cell reinfusion was recently reported [28]. A similar response rate was observed although no complete responses were seen. In this study there was a good correlation between the initial and rebound (in response to IL-2) lymphocyte counts and the chance of responding. Patients more likely to respond to this approach would appear to be those with relatively small tumor burdens, a good performance status, and good preservation of peripheral lymphocyte counts. In such patients, the value of reinfused, in vitro-stimulated lymphoid cells is not clear, and, indeed, responses have been observed with IL-2 alone (e.g., 31% in patients with melanoma [26]). These results clearly demonstrate that lymphokine therapy, with or without LAK cells, can be of therapeutic value and provide incentive for the further exploration of this approach. It is possible that adoptive immunotherapy may prove to be of value when combined with monoclonal antibodies directed at cell-surface receptors (some cells are capable of killing antibody-coated cells), or even in combination with cytotoxic drugs such as cyclophosphamide. Synergism between adoptive immunotherapy and cyclophosphamide has been demonstrated in animal experiments.

Cytokines: Cellular Regulatory Factors

Lymphokines belong to the broader class of cytokines, molecules involved in cellular differentiation and proliferation in all tissues. In order to exert their effects, the cytokines must bind specifically to high-affinity cell-surface receptors, which are present on most malignants cells as well as on a variety of normal tissue. Molecular cloning has made available large quantities of such molecules, and thus detailed in vitro studies and clinical trials can be carried out.

Interferons and Tumor Necrosis Factor. Prominent among the cytokines are the interferons. Some tumors have shown good responses to these cytokines, such as follicular lymphomas and hairy-cell leukemia. α-Interferon is currently one of the most effective therapies for the latter disease. Whether the effect is mediated via a direct action on the tumor cells themselves, or via other cells such as lymphocytes and macrophages, is not know. Few trials have been performed to date with other interferons, including τ-interferon, which is showing considerable promise in preclinical studies.

Another cytokine which has shown considerable promise in preliminary animal studies is tumor necrosis factor (TNF), a pleiotropic molecule normally produced by macrophages. TNF has a variety of actions on different cell types, among them the induction of hemorrhagic necrosis in some animal tumors, cytostasis, and differentiation induction. TNF-α has been shown to directly inhibit the transcription of the c-*myc* oncogene in the HL60 cell line derived from human promyelocytic leukemia cells [29]. Clinical trials with TNF are currently under way.

20

It is possible that cytokines will have synergistic effects on tumors when used in combination with each other (TNF and τ-interferon, for example, are synergistic in some systems), or possibly in combination with chemotherapy [30] or monoclonal antibodies. At present such combination studies remain largely empirical, but IL-2, for example, can enhance antibody dependent cellular cytotoxicity in vitro [31].

Hemopoietic Colony Stimulating Factors. Of particular interest has been the recent availability of purified hemopoietic growth factors, again due to recombinant DNA technology. Factors such as granulocyte macrophage-colony stimulating factor (GM-CSF) are able to stimulate phagocytic cell production in vitro and in vivo. One of the most important potential uses of these factors is the shortening of the period of granulocytopenia after chemotherapy. Since this is a dose-limiting side effect with so many chemotherapeutic agents, the hemopoietic growth factors may considerably increase the total dose of chemotherapeutic agents which can be administered in a given period. This is critically important in rapidly growing tumors, where tumor regrowth can occur prior to marrow recovery. Increased dose rate could also be of major benefit in high-dose chemotherapy protocols where the marrow recovery time may be unacceptably long, thus exposing the patient to a serious risk of infections. Thus as well as permitting an increased dose intensity, hemopoietic growth factors may reduce the infectious complication rate in neutropenic patients by shortening the period of neutropenia.

One possible problem with such factors is that they may increase growth rates of hemopoietic tumors. Careful preclinical testing will be needed to ensure that administration of such hemopoietic factors will not stimulate tumor growth.

Hemopoietic factors could also be used in the growth of bone marrow in vitro prior to its use to reconstitute hemopoiesis after ablative therapy. If such techniques could be perfected, they might also have application in reducing myelosuppression in response to chemotherapy. For example, autologous marrow could be grown ex vivo in the presence of gradually increasing concentrations of chemotherapeutic drugs to which it would become resistant. This marrow could then be reinfused into the patient who could be treated at higher dose intensity with the same chemotherapeutic agents. A possible problem with this approach is the observation that bone marrow never seems to lose its sensitivity to chemotherapeutic drugs, so that the ability to induce chemotherapy resistance simply by drug exposure in vitro would be questionable.

The demonstration that cloned colony stimulating factors such as GM-CSF can activate neutrophils and macrophages and enhance antibody-dependent cell mediated cytotoxicity in vitro provides a rational basis for the combination of these factors with appropriate monoclonal antibodies for the treatment of specific tumors. Further, the enhancement of LAK or TIL cell dependent tumor cell killing represents yet another novel use of these molecules which is currently undergoing preliminary exploration.

Growth Factors and Growth Inhibitory Factors. A number of factors produced by normal cells have been shown to exert an effect on cell proliferation [32].

21

Growth factors and their receptors may sometimes be relevant to the pathogenesis of cancer, and some oncogenes appear to be altered growth factors or growth factors receptors [e.g., epidermal growth factor receptor (*erb*-B), and platelet-derived growth factor (*sis*)]. Cancer cells may become independent of some exogenous growth factors because of activation of a growth factor receptor or post-receptor pathway, or autologous production of the factor itself. Some factors which are stimulatory for some cell types are inhibitory for others (e.g., the transforming growth factor TGF-β inhibits the proliferation of breast cancer cells). The possible role of these molecules in various cancers is being investigated; this being made feasible by the availability of purified recombinant molecules. Soluble receptor molecules or analogues of growth factors could be used to inhibit growth factor binding, while growth inhibitory factors could have a direct role in cancer therapy. As yet, clinical studies using such molecules have not been reported, but their pleiotropic actions cause problems similar to those arising from the use of interferons.

Hormone Therapy

Hormone therapy is not a new approach to cancer treatment, but the understanding of the mode of action of hormones in a variety of hormone-responsive tumors, notably breast and prostate, is being rapidly elucidated. While the hormone dependency of these tumors can be exploited therapeutically by the deprivation of the relevant hormone (e.g., by gonadotropin secretion blockers to prevent androgen production in patients with prostatic cancer), new information on the mode of action of hormones on such tumors could lead to the development of alternative approaches. Hormones induce the expression of a number of genes, including, in some cases, growth factors or, possibly, their receptors. For example, estrogens induce TGF-α production in hormone-responsive breast cancer cell lines. Hormone receptors, or hormone-induced surface proteins, growth factors, or growth-factor receptors could provide targets for therapeutic attempts, e.g., with monoclonal antibodies or modified growth factors, possibly coupled to toxins or radionuclides. A combination of anti-hormone and anti-growth factor therapy could have additive or synergistic value. Once again, the potential effects on normal tissue must be carefully explored and taken into consideration in contemplating such treatment approaches.

Inhibition of Angiogenesis

Tumors, like normal tissues, require a blood supply in order to proliferate. The marked variations in tumor vascularity are believed to be due to differences in the ability of neoplastic tissue to induce capillary growth by production of angiogenesis factors. A novel approach to cancer treatment is to inhibit angiogenesis, and thereby impair tumor growth. The demonstration that heparin, normally released by mast cells on the edges of vascularizing tumors, can potentiate angiogenesis, whereas heparin in conjunction with corticosteroids is antiangiogenetic, led to the discovery that heparin fragments without anticoagulant activity could also inhibit angiogenesis in the presence of corticosteroids. The treatment of tumor-bearing mice with oral heparin (which results in the release of heparin fragments into the bloodstream) and corticosteroids can eliminate some tumors [33]. It has also been shown that metastasis occurs only after vascularization of implanted tumors in experimental animals. Antiangiogenesis could also be accomplished by antibodies or new drugs directed against angiogenesis factors or the receptors for such factors on endothelial cells. Such agents could provide a new approach to cancer treatment, but no clinical studies have been reported so far.

Prevention of Metastases

New understanding of the mechanisms whereby cancer cells metastasize from the primary site (or even from a secondary site) may lead to novel means of preventing spread. While such therapy could be of major benefit as ancillary treatment of localized tumors, it is not clear that it could replace adjuvant chemotherapy, since the latter is based on the assumption that subclinical metastasis has already occurred. However, a small number of metastases which subsequently became clinically apparent in a favorable site could be dealt with by local therapy (e.g., wedge resection of pulmonary metastases and antimetastatic therapy could have a role in preventing further metastasis). Whether antimetastatic therapy will ever be of value in human tumors remains to be seen. The process of metastasis is complex, requiring the penetration of cells through the extracellular matrix (epithelial basement membrane and stroma) and into a capillary. Intravasation and extravasation of tumor cells requires penetration of the endothelial basement membrane, and the establishment of a metastatic colony also requires penetration of perivascular interstitial stroma. The process of metastasis therefore requires that the tumor cells have the ability to attach to and degrade connective tissue-matrix components, including various collagens, laminin, fibronectin, proteoglycans, and glycoproteins [34]. Effective antimetastatic therapy would require attack on one or more of the three main steps of metastasis, e.g., the prevention of attachment to laminin and fibronectin by means of drugs or monoclonal antibodies directed toward the relevant receptors; the targeting of protease inhibitors to tumor cells to prevent local hydrolysis of the matrix; or interference with the process of migration of the tumor cell, possibly by interfering with its recognition of chemotactic signals. Considerably more work with in vitro and animal models will be required before clinical trials can be contemplated.

Approaches Based on an Understanding of Molecular Pathogenesis

In recent years there has been dramatic progress in the understanding of the pathogenesis of cancer at a biochemical level. Cancer is emerging as a somatic, genetic disorder caused by highly specific alterations in the structure and func-

23

tion of relevant genes, frequently as a result of chromosomal translocation. An understanding of these molecular aberrations is likely to lead to new approaches to cancer therapy. Ultimately, cancer is a disorder of cellular differentiation, proliferation, and migration. Thus, future approaches to cancer treatment may be directed toward rectifying these disorders, either by means of relatively empirical treatment, or by utilizing approaches directed toward tumor-specific biochemical lesions produced by specific somatic genetic disorders. The latter provide hope of ultimately developing truly tumor-specific therapy. Although we are at the beginning of a new era in the comprehension of the molecular pathology of cancer, it is appropriate to begin considering how this new information may be utilized in the development of novel approaches to cancer treatment.

Induction of Differentiation in Tumor Cells. The possibility of inducing differentiation in tumor cells and therefore rendering them nonneoplastic has been a theoretical goal since the immaturity of most tumor cells was recognized. Because of major progress in understanding the biology of differentiation, this approach may become a practical proposition in the future. Such attempts may involve the use of drugs, including cytotoxic agents and differentiation-inducing agents (the latter include such compounds as the vitamin A analogues, i.e., retinoids), but the possibility that cellular regulatory factors which act on normal cells by influencing physiological pathways will be synthesized and used as drugs in cancer treatment is a real one. Moreover, the particular approach employed could be tailored to specific tumors once the mechanism of impairment of differentiation has been elucidated.

Development of Tumor Specific Therapy. Once the deranged biochemical mechanisms associated with specific cancers have been unraveled, the possibility of directing highly specific therapy toward the particular cancer exists. This is because the molecular lesion is unique to each type of cancer cell. Potential approaches include the development of peptides or drugs with highly specific properties, e.g., the ability to inhibit an abnormal oncogene product but not the normal equivalent; the use of antisense oligonucleotides, possibly inserted into tumor cells by means of retrovirus vectors, which specifically inhibit translation of an abnormal oncogene messenger RNA; or the development of a means to bypass the biochemical abnormality of the tumor cell (e.g., by provision of a missing molecule). These approaches are in their infancy, and, moreover, can only be explored in the handful of neoplasms for which detailed information is available.

Molecular Approaches to the Amelioration of Toxicity

One of the major toxicities encountered in the chemotherapeutic treatment of cancer is myelosuppression. Possible methods of lessening this have been discussed above. An alternative approach, which could abrogate marrow toxicity altogether, is to render bone marrow totally resistant to chemotherapy. The removal of normal bone marrow cells from a patient, insertion of drug-resistance genes (e.g., multiple copies of a DHFR gene, particularly one which binds methotrexate poorly), and reinfusion of the marrow cells should result in an increased tolerance of the appropriate drug once the resistant cells have become predominant in the marrow. To date, only preclinical studies of the feasibility of this form of "gene therapy" have been carried out. Whether similar methods could be applied to the amelioration of other forms of toxicity remains to be seen.

This brief overview of selected new approaches to cancer treatment has hopefully indicated that the empirical approach to cancer treatment is likely to be gradually complemented by approaches based on new understanding of the mechanisms of oncogenesis, the interactions between cancer cells and the tumor-bearing host, and the mechanisms whereby currently available therapies kill tumor cells, or conversely, tumors cells become resistant to their effects. The possibilities for developing new approaches to therapy are numerous, and it is extremely likely that many of those discussed will not prove feasible, while other approaches not yet conceived of may ultimately become routine. It seems likely that no single approach will provide an all-encompassing solution to treating cancer, and that therapeutic approaches will become increasingly specific for indivdual cancers and for smaller and smaller subcategories of currently accepted disease entities. Even the newest of approaches, if successful, are likely to be used initially in addition to more conventional methods. It is, however, the very diversity of current therapies which promotes optimism. Ultimately, it would seem that an understanding of the nature of cancer, that is, of the precise chain of events leading to the conversion of a normal cell into a neoplastic cell, will prove to be the most fruitful step in developing not only effective, but minimally toxic methods of treatment (and prevention) which are aimed at the root cause of the neoplastic process rather than at its manifestations. A few years ago such a statement would have appeared fatuous. In the second half of the 1980s, however, we have entered an era in which understanding the detailed biochemistry of cancer is becoming a reality. It is inconceivable that this knowledge will not have a major impact on the prevention and treatment of cancer in the future.

References

1. Peters LJ, Ang KK (1986) Unconventional fractionation schemes in radiotherapy. In: DeVita VT Jr, Hellman S, Rosenberg SA (eds) Important advances in oncology 1986. Lippincott, Philadelphia: 269–86
2. Hoefnagel CA, Voute PA, Marcuse HR (1988) Radionuclide diagnosis and therapy of neural crest tumors using iodine-131 metaiodobenzylguanidine. J Nucl Med 28: 308–14
3. Saunders WM, Char DH, Quivey JM et al. (1985) Precision, high dose radiotherapy: helium ion treatment of uveal melanoma. Int J Radiat Oncol Biol Phys 11: 227–233
4. Verney LJ, Munzenrider JE (1982) Proton beam therapy. Annu Rev Biophys Bioeng 11: 331–357
5. Chu JC, Richter MP, Sontag MR et al. (1987) Practice of 3-dimensional treatment planning at the Fox Chase Cancer Center, University of Pennsylvania. Radiother Oncol 8: 137–43

6. Wambersie A, Battermann JJ (1985) Review and evolution of clinical results in the EORTC Heavy-Particle Therapy Group. Strahlentherapie 161: 746–55

7. Gasparro FP, Chan G, Edelson RL (1985) Phototherapy and photopharmacology. Yale J Biol Med 58: 519–534

8. Driscoll JS, Johns DG, Plowman J (1985) Comparison of the activity of arabinosyl-5-azacytosine, arabinosyl cytosine, and 5-azacytidine against intracerebrally implanted L1210 leukemia. Invest New Drugs 3: 331–334

9. Schuetz JD, Westin EH (1986) Fluorodeoxyuridine (FdUrd) induced amplification of dihydrofolate reductase (DHFR) with methotrexate (MTX) resistance: a potential factor in the interaction between methotrexate and fluoropyrimidines (abstract). Proc Am Assoc Cancer Res 27: 9 (abstract No 34)

10. Sobrero AF, Bertino JR (1986) Alternating trimetrexate (TMQ) with methotrexate delays the onset of resistance to antifolates in vitro and in vivo (abstract). Proc Am Assoc Cancer Res 27: 269 (abstract No 1067)

11. Bertino JR, Mini E, Sobrero A et al. (1985) Methotrexate resistant cells as targets for selective chemotherapy. Adv Enzyme Regul 24: 3–11

12. Santi DV, McHenry CS, Sommer H (1974) Mechanism of interaction of thymidylate synthetase with S-fluorodeoxyuridylate. Biochemistry 13: 471–481

13. Evans RM, Laskin JD, Hakala MT (1981) Effect of excess folates and deoxyinosine on the activity and site of action of 5-fluorouracil. Cancer Res 41: 3288–3295

14. Waxman S, Bruckner H (1982) The enhancement of 5-fluorouracil antimetabolic activity by leucovorin, menadione and alpha-tocopherol. Eur J Cancer Clin Oncol 18: 685–692

15. Zimm S, Collins JM, Riccardi R et al. (1983) Variable bioavailability of oral mercaptopurine. Is maintenance chemotherapy in acute lymphoblastic leukemia being optimally delivered? N Engl J Med 308: 1005–1009

16. Chao DL, Kimball AP (1972) Deamination of arabinosyladenine by adenosine deaminase and inhibition by arabinosyl-6-mercaptopurine. Cancer Res 32(8): 1721–1724

17. Hryniuk WM (1987) Average relative dose intensity and the impact on design of clinical trials. Semin Oncol 14: 65–74

18. Hryniuk W (1986) Is more better? J Clin Oncol 4: 621–622

19. Howell SB (1984) Intraarterial and intracavitary cancer chemotherapy. Martinus Nijhoff, Boston

20. Arndt C, Colvin M, Balis F et al. (1987) Intrathecal administration of 4-hydroperoxy-cyclophosphamide (hpc) Proc Annu Meet Am Assoc Cancer Res 28: 439 (abstract)

21. Bunin N, Rivera G, Goode F, Hustu H O (1987) Ocular relapse in the anterior chamber of the eye in childhood acute lymphoblastic leukemia. J Clin Oncol 5: 299–303

22. Ozols RF, Corden BJ, Jacob J, Wesley MN, Ostchega Y, Young RC (1984) High dose cisplatin in hypertonic saline. Ann Intern Med 100: 19

23. Markman M, Cleary S, Howell SB (1985) Nephrotoxicity of high-dose intracavitary cisplatin with intravenous thiosulfate protection. Eur J Cancer Clin Oncol 21: 1015–1018

24. Green MD (1987) Rationale and strategy for prevention of anthracycline cardiotoxicity with the bisdioxopiperazine ICRF-187. Pathol Biol (Paris) 35: 49–53

25. Brock N, Pohl J, Stekar J, Sheef W (1982) Studies on the urotoxicity of oxazaphosphorine cytostatics and its prevention. III. Profile of action of sodium 2-mercaptoethane sulphonate (mesna). Eur J Cancer Clin. Oncol 18: 1377

26. Carney DN, Cuttitta F (1986) Interruption of small cell lung cancer (SCLC) growth by a monoclonal antibody to bombesin. 5th NCI-EORTC symposium on new drugs in cancer therapy. October 22–24, 5th Amsterdam (abstract)

27. Rosenberg SA, Lotze MT, Muul L et al. (1987) A progress report on the treatment of 157 patients with advanced cancer using lymphokine-activated killer cells and interleukin-2 or high-dose interleukin-2 alone. Engl J Med 316: 889–897

28. West WW, Tauer KW, Yanell JR et al. (1987) Constant infusion recombinant interleukin-2 in adoptive immunotherapy of advanced cancer. N Engl J Med 316: 898–905

29. Krönke M, Schlüter C, Pfizenmaier K (1987) Tumor necrosis factor inhibits MYC expression in HL-60 cells at the level of mRNA transcription. Proc Natl Acad Sci USA 84: 469–473

30. Wanatabe N, Niitsu Y (1986) Anti-tumor effect and the mechanism of action of human recombinant TNF. Gan To Kagaku Ryoho 13: 1322–1328
31. Shilone E, Eisenthal A, Sachs D, Rosenberg SA (1987) Antibody dependent cellular cytotoxicity mediated by murine lumphocytes activated in recombinant interleukin-2. J Immunol 138: 1992–1998
32. Goustin AS, Leof EB, Shipley GD, Moses H (1986) Growth factors and cancer. Cancer Res 46: 1015–1029
33. Folkman J (1985) Angiogenesis and its inhibitors. In: deVita VT Jr, Hellman S, Rosenberg SA (eds) Important advances in oncology 1985: 42–62 Lippincott Philadelphia
34. Liotta LA (1985) Mechanisms of cancer invasion and metastasis. In: deVita VT Jr, Hellman S, Rosenberg SA (eds) Important advances in oncology 1985: 28–41, Lippincott Philadelphia

Physical Approaches to Therapy

2. New Approaches in Radiation Therapy

T.J. Kinsella

Introduction

According to recent statistics from the American Cancer Society, over 850 000 cases of invasive cancers are diagnosed yearly in the United States. Approximately 70% of these patients will present with locoregional disease potentially amenable to curative treatment using surgery, radiation therapy, or combined modality therapy. However, in spite of current treatment strategies, up to 30% of these patients will develop recurrent local disease which, in the majority, will lead ultimately to death. In addition, acute and late radiation damage to normal tissues can occur following high-dose external beam therapy used in definitive radiation therapy or as adjunctive therapy in combination with surgery and/or chemotherapy. We now realize that the radiation tolerance of some normal tissues can be modified in combined modality therapy due to additive or synergistic effects of surgery and, particularly, chemotherapy with radiation therapy.

While radiation therapy is a major treatment modality for many cancers, present-day clinical practice has been determined largely by empiricism from experience accumulated over the last 50–60 years. Such clinical experience has resulted in an arbitrary classification of tumors as being radioresponsive (e.g., lymphoma and seminoma), moderately radioresponsive (e.g., squamous cell carcinoma and adenocarcinoma), and poorly radioresponsive (e.g., melanoma and glioblastoma). Obviously, within each tumor type, many other factors can influence radiocurability, including tumor size, histological grade, and anatomical location.

Although radiotherapy has been shown to be effective in sterilizing many cancers, the biological mechanism(s) of this process are not completely understood. Over the last two decades, a considerable amount of work has been done on defining the inherent radiosensitivity of both normal and tumor cells [1–10]. Other biological factors felt to be important include repair of radiation damage, reoxygenation of hypoxic cells, redistribution of cycling cells, and recruitment of noncycling cells into the cell cycle. Collectively, these have been referred to as the four R's of fractionated radiotherapy [11]. Pathophysiological considerations such as tumor blood flow and the immunocompetence of the host may also be important in determining the radiation response, although these have not been studied as thoroughly in the radiobiology laboratory.

Today, clinical radiation therapy involves the use of high-energy linear

Table 1. Normal tissue reactions to radiation

	Acute	Intermediate	Late
Structure at risk	Actively proliferating cell renewal systems	Slowly proliferating cell renewal systems	Endothelium and connective tissue
Regions at risk	Gut, skin, marrow	Lung, heart, liver, kidney	All
Dependent variables	Dose rate, fractionation	Fractionation, total effective dose	Total effective dose

accelerators, which generate megavoltage photons. Radiation treatment planning using simulators, computerized tomographic (CT) scanning, and computers allows the radiation oncologist to define more precisely the tumor volume and then to determine how to deliver a homogeneous dose to this volume with relative sparing of adjacent normal tissues. The major parameters of a treatment course of external beam irradiation are the total dose, the number of treatment fractions (usually 1 fraction/day × 5 days/week), and the dose rate (usually 1.8–2.0 Gy/fraction). For most common carcinomas, the total dose is often 45–50 Gy for microscopic residual disease and 60–75 Gy for gross residual disease of intact tumors. The use of brachytherapy techniques employing interstitial or intracavitary applicators for such sites as the cervix can permit delivery of higher total doses (> 80 Gy) to a precisely defined "boost" volume.

The choice of optimal radiation therapy is often limited by consideration of acute and, more importantly, late effects of treatment on normal tissues (Table 1). Often, the tolerance of multiple normal tissues must be weighed in designing radiation treatment. Acute effects occur in rapidly proliferating tissues (e.g., bone marrow, skin, intestine, bladder, and the epithelium of the aerodigestive tract) and are believed to result from a disruption of homeostasis in these cell-renewal systems. Recruitment of noncycling cells into active proliferation and reduction of the mean cell cycle time are characteristic responses of these cell-renewal systems to fractionated irradiation. Typically, acute damage is self-limited and completely reversible within a short period (a few days to a week), although a reduction in the dose rate is often necessary. While normal and tumor cells of the same tissue probably sustain similar radiation damage, normal tissues appear more effective at cell recruitment and at acceleration of the division of cells already in cycle.

Late radiation injury is infrequent, but often progressive in nature, leading to considerable morbidity and even mortality. The mechanism(s) of late injury are not completely understood. Most likely, it results from injury to the supporting tissue stroma with secondary parenchymal damage. A progressive, obliterative arteritis of small arteries and arterioles associated with fibrosis of connective tissue is found histologically. The total radiation and the volume of normal tissue irradiated are the major variables determining late radiation injury.

Theoretical curves depicting the probability of tumor control and the risk of a major complication are plotted as a function of the total radiation dose in Fig. 1.

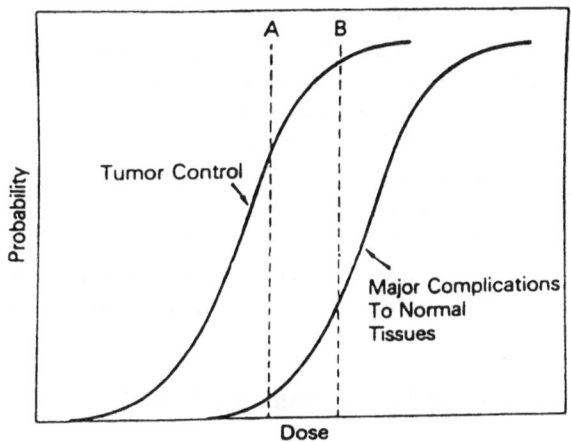

Fig. 1. Theoretical curves depicting the probability of tumor control and the risk of a major complication to normal tissues related to the radiation dose. The distance separating the curves represents the therapeutic gain

Although both curves have a sigmoid distribution, their relationship will vary according to the normal tissue and tumor type. The distance separating the curves represents the therapeutic gain. Therapeutic gain can be realized by increasing the probability of tumor control, reducing the risk of major complications, or, ideally, both. However, if the curves are shifted equally in the same direction, there is no therapeutic gain, merely a modification of radiation response. The difference between treatment programs A and B in Fig. 1 is an improvement in tumor control with program B, but at a higher risk of complications. In addition to considering the probability of incurring a major complication, the probability of treating it effectively is an integral part of the initial treatment decision. Thus, if a radiation complication is manageable, the higher dose (program B) should be used to maximize tumor control and the higher complication rate be accepted.

While it is felt that the tolerance of normal tissues and "resistant" tumor cell populations have limited the radiocurability of certain tumors, especially at higher clinical stages, research in radiobiology and radiation physics is providing ways of increasing cure while limiting morbidity. It is the intent of this chapter to review the state-of-the-art information on several innovative approaches in radiation oncology and to speculate on areas of future research. Topics included in this review are radiobiology and tumor biology, radiation sensitizers and protectors, combined modality therapy, systemic use of radiation, and particle beam radiation therapy.

Radiobiology and Tumor Biology

It is important to define carefully terms used to describe the clinical response of tumors to radiation therapy. Traditionally, there has been some confusion with the terms "radiosensitive" and "radioresponsive." The term "radioresponsive" is used to describe a tumor in which obvious shrinkage of a tumor mass occurs after some modest dose of radiation therapy has been applied. Thus, when a tumor mass shrinks during the course of treatment, it is considered "radio-responsive." Shrinkage of a tumor is a gross and complex manifestation of many factors, including cell death, change in cell-cycle distribution, and possibly a change in tumor vascularity, which are difficult to assess as independent variables. If the rate of cell division is very slow, then the expression of cell death may evolve over many weeks or even months, which is the clinical observation of traditionally poorly "radioresponsive" tumors, such as sarcomas.

Sublethal Radiation Damage Repair

The term "radiosensitive" refers specifically to cell survival data obtained from in vitro and in vivo experiments using mammalian cells and tissues including both normal tissues and tumors. Likewise, "radioresistant" refers to data similarly derived from cell-survival analysis. A typical radiation survival curve for a "sensitive" and a "resistant" cell population is shown in Fig. 2. The cell-survival data are plotted as a logarithm of survival versus radiation dose on a linear scale. Radiation dose is expressed in terms of Gray (Gy), which has recently been adopted in preference to the rad (1 Gy = 100 rad). The radiation survival curve is characterized normally by two parameters.

Following low radiation doses, the survival curves of most mammalian cells, including cultured human tumor lines, have a "shoulder" which is interpreted to show that cells can repair some amount of radiation damage (sublethal damage)

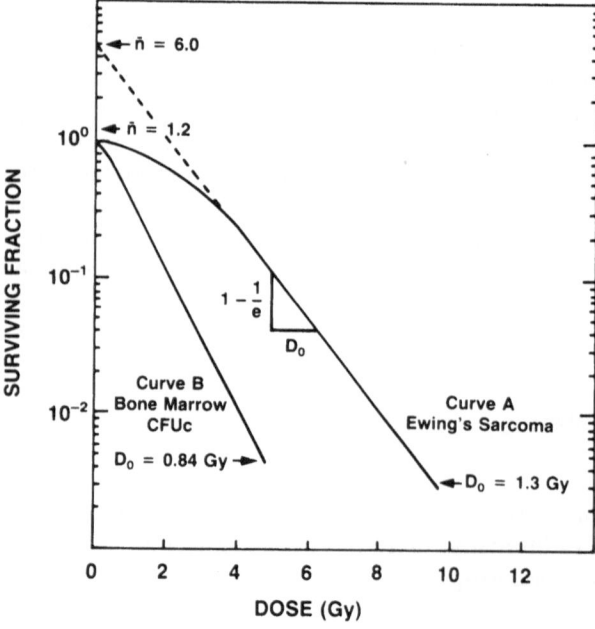

Fig. 2. X-ray survival curves of human Ewing's sarcoma cells and human hematopoietic bone marrow precursor cells (CFU-C) (adapted from [9]). Radiation survival curve parameters $\bar{n}$ and D_0 are indicated on the graph. Note the increased sensitivity of the bone marrow CFU-C compared with the tumor line. In general, hematopoietic cells are sensitive to X-rays; however, other normal tissues exhibit X-ray sensitivity closer to that for tumor cell lines

before additional radiation results in cell death. The width of the shoulder is a relative measure of the extent of the given cell population to repair sublethal damage and is described by the term $\bar{n}$ which is obtained when the exponential straight line portion of the curve is extrapolated to zero dose. As illustrated in Fig. 2, the Ewing's sarcoma line appears to be more capable of sublethal damage repair than the human bone marrow CFU-C (colony-forming unit-culture) ($\bar{n}$ = 6.0 for Ewing's sarcoma line cells, compared with 1.2 for CFU-C). For most mammalian cells, the $\bar{n}$ value ranges between 2 and 10.

The second parameter of radiation survival is a measure of the slope of the exponential portion of the survival curve and is expressed as the D_o. By definition, the D_o is actually the reciprocal of the slope and is the dose which will reduce survival to 37% along any straight portion of the curve. Again, most mammalian cells, including both normal and tumor cells, reveal a rather narrow range of D_os of 1–2 Gy. In general, it is felt that the $\bar{n}$ value may be a more relevant determinant for correlating clinical radioresponsiveness or curability, since the usual radiation doses used in the clinic are within the range of those found on the shoulder of the survival curve.

There are a number of general characteristics of sublethal damage repair, including completion of repair within 2–4 h from irradiation, sustained repair capability with multiple or fractionated irradiation (as long as the interval between fractions is >4 h), and repair during protracted low dose-rate (0.2–1 Gy/h) irradiation. Some laboratory studies have demonstrated a greater capacity of certain normal cells to repair sublethal damage compared with tumor cells of similar tissue origin [12].

Potentially Lethal Radiation Damage Repair

A second type of radiation repair that has been described is called potentially lethal damage repair (PLDR) [13, 14]. This repair is observed in vitro when cells are irradiated in dense plateau conditions and held in this "nutrient-depleted" environment for several hours after irradiation before subculturing and cloning at low cell densities. Also, PLDR has been observed in murine tumor systems in vivo. It is assumed that in many human carcinomas and sarcomas, a variable proportion of the cell population may be in a "nutrient-depleted" state (acidic pH; noncycling) and may repair potentially lethal damage. Indeed, some investigators argue that the extent of PLDR may correlate, at least in part, with the radiocurability of certain human tumors [15, 16]. An important question which remains is the influence or extent of PLDR following conventionally (2 Gy) fractionated irradiation in the clinic.

Mechanisms of Radiation Damage

While these processes of sublethal and potentially lethal damage repair have been demonstrated in normal and malignant human cells, the molecular mechanisms responsible for repair are not completely understood. A large amount of experimental evidence supports the hypothesis that radiation produces many of its effects by damaging DNA [17, 18]. Radiation may damage the DNA in the genome directly or indirectly. Direct radiation damage occurs when radiation is absorbed by DNA and results in strand breaks. It has been estimated that a dose of 1 Gy delivered to a mammalian cell should lead to 3×10^5 bond-breaking absorption events [17]. Yet, this dose of radiation would result in only 20%–30% cell kill in a typical mammalian cell population in vitro. Elution studies show that about 40 double-strand breaks and 1000 single-strand breaks in the DNA will be registered with this dose, but most breaks will be rejoined (repaired) within a few minutes to a few hours of radiation. Clearly, this suggests that only a minority of direct DNA breaks can result in lethality. However, there are some cell lines that lack virtually any ability to repair sublethal and potentially lethal radiation damage. Cultured skin fibroblasts and lymphocytes from patients with the autosomal recessive disease, ataxia telangiectasia (AT), are exquisitely sensitive to X-rays ($D_0 = 0.4$–0.5 Gy $\bar{n} = 1.0$) and show no radiation repair in vitro [19, 20]. These types of repair of cellular damage, while operationally defined, appear nonetheless real and should serve as a framework for future work on the molecular biology of DNA radiation damage and repair (e.g., identifying repair genes, amplifying them, and finally characterizing them via an appropriate cloning vector).

Indirect damage to DNA following radiation results when reactive chemicals (free radicals) are produced intracellularly by the interaction of secondary electrons and the cellular solvent, water. These products of water excitation and ionization, principally hydroxyl radicals and peroxides, are estimated to result in 70%–80% of radiation damage, with direct DNA effects accounting for the other 20%–30% [18]. These highly reactive products of hydrolysis can migrate and cluster, making repair more difficult. However, the reactive species can be scavenged or inactivated by repair enzymes, such as glutathione peroxidase and polymerases, and other smaller molecules which may contribute hydrogen atoms for the termination of free radical reactions. Investigations are under way comparing indirect radiation damage and repair in normal and malignant cells.

Heterogeneity of Radiation Response

Heterogeneity in the intrinsic radiation response of subpopulations derived from human tumor cells has been reported, as well as differences in the radiosensitivity of primary tumor cells versus metastatic tumor cells in experimental animal systems [7, 8, 10]. There is good reason to believe that the generation of heterogeneity among tumor cells may be a factor determining clinical radiation response [21]. The development of substantial resistance to chemotherapeutic drugs within stem-cell populations of tumors is well recognized [22]. The study of tumor-cell heterogeneity to radiation is an expanding area of research with many unanswered questions. Further studies are needed to examine whether the heterogeneity of radiation sensitivity within a tumor-cell population is related entirely to intrinsic differences in radiosensitivity. Most likely, cell-kinetic and microenvironmental factors (PO_2, pH, etc.) are important variables of the clinical radiation response. The interaction of these factors in determining radiation response is an active area of experimental research.

It is well established that cell-cycle kinetics influence the radiation response [23, 24]. In general, cells are most radiosensitive in G_2/M phase and most radioresistant in late S phase. The radiosensitivity of Go (noncycling) cells is more difficult to assess, since the most reliable assay of clonogenic survival requires that cells attempt proliferation (cell division) before reproductive death can be ascertained. Some in vivo studies indicate greater radiosensitivity of proliferating cells than of nonproliferating (Go) cells [25]. On the other hand, radiation clearly affects cell kinetics of several well-regulated normal tissues (bone marrow, bowel) and some experimental tumors [25, 26], although these data are less clear. With substantial radiation-induced cell kill, increased cell proliferation can result which may be mediated through changes in cell-cycle duration, recruitment of Go cells into the cell cycle, or a change in cell loss.

One major difficulty in unraveling the interaction of cell kinetics and radiation in human tumors involves differentiating the cell kinetics of truly clonogenic or stem cells from the kinetics of the total cell population. Difficulties also exist in repeatedly monitoring cell kinetics during a course of fractionated radiation therapy. However, a number of invasive and noninvasive techniques are being developed which may be applied to investigating the interaction of cell kinetics and radiation, including positron emission tomography with [11C] thymidine and cell-sorting techniques using a thymidine analogue (bromodeoxyuridine, BUdR) and fluorescent-tagged anti-BUdR monoclonal antibody to distinguish cycling and noncycling cells [27, 28].

At present, clinical studies are under way using some of these in vitro and in vivo techniques to better understand the contribution of radiation damage repair and cell-cycle effects on the response of some tumors, including small-cell lung carcinoma, Ewing's sarcoma, adult soft-tissue sarcomas, and high-grade brain tumors [8, 9, 21, 27, 28]. Such studies may result in an alteration of radiation dose fractionation and total dose for specific tumor types over the next few years.

Radiation Sensitizers and Protectors

In the design of a clinical strategy to modify radiation response, the effect on both tumor and normal cells (or tissues) must be considered. If a clear advance in clinical radiation therapy is to result, then there must be a substantial differential effect resulting in sensitization of the tumor, protection of normal tissues, or, ideally, both. At present, there are two classes of chemical radiosensitizers and one class of chemical radioprotector which have been developed in the radiobiology laboratory and are being studied in clinical trials.

Hypoxic Cell Sensitizers

The concept of a chemical radiosensitizer of hypoxic cells dates from the initial observations by Gray, Thomlinson, and coworkers that oxygen has a major effect on cellular radiation response [29]. As the oxygen concentration is reduced, there is a corresponding decrease in radiosensitivity such that at very low concentrations (<0.1% oxygen), mammalian cells are approximately 3 times more resistant to X-rays than in fully oxygenated conditions (20% oxygen). It is now recognized that the population of hypoxic cells within rodent tumors and possibly in some human tumors can vary from 1% to 20% [30].

Initial attempts at increasing the oxygen concentration in tumors employed hyperbaric oxygen. Some clinical trials showed an improvement in local control and survival in traditionally moderately responsive tumors such as advanced cervix and head and neck cancers [31]. However, technical difficulties in administering hyperbaric oxygen and the observed adverse physiological changes in tumor blood flow in some tumor sites led to a major effort to develop drugs which could mimic oxygen and thus act as chemical radiosensitizers of hypoxic tumor cells.

Over the last decade, the 5-nitro- and 2-nitroimidazole drugs have been found to have potential as clinical radiosensitizers. The first prospective randomized clinical trial using metronidazole, a 5-nitroimidazole, and an unconventional radiation fractionation scheme (9 fractions over 3 weeks to a total dose of 30 Gy) compared with the unconventional radiation therapy alone in patients with glioblastoma showed that the addition of the sensitizer [32] increased survival. However, it must be realized that the combination of metronidazole and unconventional radiation was not better in terms of survival compared with historical controls using conventional radiation alone. A subsequent randomized, prospective trial in glioblastoma patients using conventional radiation as the control showed there was no advantage in using the combination of metronidazole and unconventional fractionation [33]. Moderate to severe gastrointestinal and peripheral nerve toxicity limited the frequency and duration of administration of metronidazole.

Further in vitro and in vivo work established that the 2-nitroimidazoles were superior to the 5-nitro compounds as hypoxic cell sensitizers based on a higher electron affinity and lipophilicity [34, 35]. Misonidazole (Ro-07-0582) was selected for clinical use and has undergone extensive phase I to III testing by the Radiation Therapy Oncology Group (RTOG) and others [36]. Attempts to reduce neurotoxicity using the concomitant administration of dexamethasone or pyridoxine have shown some promise in early testing [37, 38].

Although these clinical results with misonidazole are not very encouraging, it is not certain whether the role of hypoxic cell sensitizers in clinical radiotherapy has been assessed adequately. A recent review of the experimental data on misonidazole indicates that, with the dose schedules used clinically, the expected therapeutic gain was more in the range of 1.1–1.2 rather than >1.5 as initially projected [39]. Whether a 10%–20% effect on a subpopulation of tumor cells (i.e., the hypoxic cells) could be detected clinically is questionable. More recently, potentially superior hypoxic-cell sensitizers have been started in phase I clinical trials [40]. A less neurotoxic drug than misonidazole is SR 2508, permitting over 3 times more drug to be administered. A second compound, Ro-03-8799, produces a sensitizer-enhancement ratio almost 4 times greater than misonidazole for the same administered dose. In addition, this new sensitizer produces some acute neurotoxicity, but no cumulative neurotoxicity is evident in the available phase I testing [41].

Halogenated Pyrimidines as Sensitizers

A second class of radiosensitizers is the halogenated pyrimidine analogues, principally BUdR and iododeoxyuridine (IUdR). These compounds are analogues of the nucleoside thymidine and have been recognized as in vitro radiosensitizers for over 20 years [42, 43]. Although the exact mechanism of radiosensitization is not clearly understood, it most likely results from direct incorporation of these analogues into DNA, replacing thymidine. Exponentially growing cells in culture exposed to BUdR or IUdR prior to X-irradiation may show a change in both the shoulder width ($\bar{n}$) and slope (D_o) of the radiation survival curve. An approximate linear relationship is found for thymidine replacement by these drugs, with 40% thymidine replacement resulting in an enhancement ratio of 3–4 [42].

Based on these experimental studies, two clinical trials using selective intra-arterial infusions of BUdR and conventional fractionated X-irradiation were performed in the 1960s. Japanese investigators reported an improvement in survival in a one-arm study of approximately 200 patients with primary brain tumors, half of whom had high-grade gliomas [44]. Catheter-related problems resulting in sepsis, brain abscesses, and arterial emboli were found in about 15% of patients, but no enhancement of radiation injury to normal brain tissue was reported. However, in a small randomized prospective trial at Stanford University, of patients with advanced head and neck cancers, comparing the combined modality experimental approach to radiation therapy alone, no improvement in local control was found but there was enhancement of damage to normal tissue in the ipsilateral oropharyngeal cavity with combined radiation-sensitizer treatment [45]. In retrospect, the latter trial was not an optimal test of this combined approach, since the oropharyngeal mucosa is mitotically active and would be expected to incorporate BUdR to an extent as great as, or probably greater than the adjacent squamous cell carcinoma. Because of these conflicting studies, clinical interest in the halogenated pyrimidine analogues as radiosensitizers diminished in the 1970s.

Over the last 4 years, investigators at the National Cancer Institute have initiated phase I/II studies of both BUdR and IUdR given as constant intravenous infusions for up to 2 weeks [46]. The clinical strategy is to attempt to maximize tumor incorporation using two separate 2-week infusions prior to and during X-irradiation. Patients with glioblastoma multiforme and unresectable high-grade bone and soft tissue sarcomas have been selected for study, since both tumor types are considered to be poorly radioresponsive and the normal tissues surrounding these tumors (normal brain, muscle, bone) do not contain a large proliferating cell component.

Pharmacological studies reveal steady arterial levels of $1-5 \times 10^{-6}$ molar at the maximum tolerable doses of both BUdR and IUdR given by continuous intravenous infusion [47, 48]. Incorporation of BUdR into human dividing cells in vivo was measured by comparing the survival curves of patients' bone marrow (CFU-Cs) prior to and following the 14-day infusion [49]. Radiation enhancement ratios of 1.5–2.2 were found at the higher infusion levels of BUdR, suggesting that enhancement of dividing tumor cells was clearly possible. Subsequently, direct tumor cell incorporation into a variety of human tumors, including glioblastoma multiforme, chondrosarcoma, melanoma, and poorly differentiated adenocarcinoma has been demonstrated by tissue biopsy following administration of the sensitizer and histological staining using a specific monoclonal antibody against BUdR and IUdR [50, 51]. In these tumor specimens, up to 50%–70% of cells are counterstained with the monoclonal antibody.

Tumor response to this combined sensitizer-radiation approach has been dramatic in several patients, with some glioblastoma patients surviving for more than 2 years and some high-grade sarcoma patients having a complete response for up to 2 years. Systemic toxicity, primarily to the bone marrow, has been the dose-limiting factor, but marrow recovery is prompt and most patients receive two 2-week infusions [50, 52]. In general, the toxicity to local normal tissue in this combined modality approach has been acceptable.

These phase I and II results of the halogenated pyrimidine analogues are encouraging and further clinical trials are planned. More quantitative information on thymidine replacement in tumor cells is needed using such methods as cesium chloride gradients and high-performance liquid chromatography assays. With this information, attempts to enhance incorporation of these sensitizers by blocking endogenous thymidine synthesis using coadministration of fluorodeoxyuridine (FUdR) seems reasonable. Additionally, a direct, continuous intraarterial infusion might allow for up to 1 log greater tumor concentrations of the drug compared with the presently used continuous intravenous infusion [47].

New Potential Radiosensitizers

In the future, two additional classes of potential radiosensitizers may undergo clinical testing. There is currently a great deal of interest in the role that cellular sulfhydryl compounds, particularly glutathione (GSH), may play in the radiation response of mammalian cells, including human tumor cell lines, in vitro and in vivo [53]. By depleting cellular GSH levels using such drugs as diamide, which binds GSH, or buthionine-sulfoximide (BSO), which blocks GSH synthesis, the in vitro radiation survival curve is shifted to the left, suggesting sensitization, particularly for hypoxic cells [54, 55]. Interestingly, this same approach of GSH depletion can increase the in vitro sensitivity of tumor cells made resistant to such drugs as melphalan and cis-platinum compounds [56, 57]. Cross-sensitization of drug-resistant cancer cells to radiation by BSO administration opens up interesting avenues for future clinical research into combined chemotherapy and radiation therapy [57].

The second class of future radiosensitizers are the metabolic inhibitors of PLDR as previously described [13, 16]. Agents such as dactinomycin, β-arabinofuranosyladenine (β-ARA-A), and other purine nucleoside analogues have been shown to inhibit PLDR in vitro and in vivo [58, 59]. If further experimental studies of these PLDR inhibitors show positive results, these drugs may enter clinical trials.

Radioprotective Drugs

Over the last 5 years, considerable progress has been made in the experimental and clinical testing of radioprotective drugs in radiation therapy. The prototype drug is WR-2721 [S-2-(3-aminopropylamino)-ethylphosphorothioic acid], which has undergone clinical testing in the USA and Japan [60, 61]. Three factors have been recognized which may explain the ability of a drug like WR-2721 to preferentially protect normal tissues: decreased blood flow and/or vascularity, which limits drug access to the tumor; differences in tumor-cell-membrane permeability to these drugs; and the decreased protection afforded hypoxic cells (primarily in tumors) by these compounds.

However, the relative importance of these factors in man is not known. Experimentally, a number of thiophosphate drugs have been identified which have comparable radioprotection of normal tissues without protection of solid tumors. One problem in further clinical investigation of these compounds is a lack of a sensitive assay for plasma or tissue levels of WR-2721 and its metabolites. Moreover, there are differences in phase I studies of WR-2721, regarding the maximum tolerated single dose, that need to be resolved before multiple dose and phase II testing can proceed [60, 61]. Of major importance if clinical application is to be successful will be to establish the optimal timing of radioprotective drug administration in relation to the delivery of radiation.

Combined Modality Treatment with Chemotherapy and Surgery

Combination of Radiation and Chemotherapy

Over the last 15 years, there has been increasing use of a combination of modalities in the clinical treatment of cancer. It is instructive to approach the idea of combined modality treatment with cytotoxic drugs and radiation using the concepts proposed by Steel and Peckham [62]. An improvement in the therapeutic gain can be realized in a variety of ways: enhancement of tumor response (similar to the use of the radiosensitizers described previously); minimization of normal tissue damage (similar to the use of thiophosphate derivatives like WR-2721); spatial cooperation, which requires radiation to eradicate local disease and cytotoxic drugs to treat gross and/or microscopic metastatic foci; and toxicity independence, which requires the use of cytotoxic drugs and drug scheduling that do not enhance radiation injury to normal tissues.

The majority of experimental studies of combined chemotherapy and radiation have been directed toward enhancement of tumor response using tumor cells grown in monolayers, as multicellular spheroids, or more commonly in vivo in mice [63–65]. However, it is obvious that there is a need for better and more diverse tumor models. Recently, there has been a shift to the use of human tumor cells grown and treated in vivo as xenografts using nude mice, or in vitro using semisolid medium cultures or human tumor-cell spheroids. Cell-kinetic-directed therapy should also be developed in a fashion similar to that described by Barranco et al. [66]. In order to develop more effective drug-radiation protocols for human cancer treatment, it is also important to develop noninvasive techniques to monitor physiological and biochemical states of the tumor as well as of normal tissues. The technology of nuclear magnetic resonance spectroscopy is evolving to monitor parameters such as the inorganic phosphate to adenosine triphosphate ratios in various in vivo tumors which can then be correlated with more traditional techniques (such as tumor regression measurements) to elucidate more effective drug-radiation sequences [67].

In the clinic, numerous protocols have been devised both for single drug and combination chemotherapy regimens combined with radiation therapy. Combined modality therapy made up of combination chemotherapy and radiation has been particularly successful for such tumors as Wilms' tumor and childhood sarcomas [68, 69]. For adult solid tumors, combined modality therapy has made recent progress in squamous cell carcinomas arising in the head and neck area as well as in the anus [70, 71]. Improvements in locoregional control and disease-free survival in these childhood and adult cancers is most likely due to spatial cooperation. However, clear improvements in cures using combined modality therapy may be fraught with unexpected late effects, such as second neoplasms. The difficulty of investigating clinically the multiplicity of drug combinations and drug-radiation sequencing to improve tumor response, yet limit both acute and late damage, necessitates increased experimental studies using appropriate human tumor and normal tissue assays.

Combination of Radiation and Surgery

Historically, radiation therapy has sometimes been used as a modality for sparing normal tissues, for example in the larynx for treatment of early stage laryngeal carcinomas that would otherwise be ablated by surgical resection. More recently, the combination of radiation therapy and less aggressive (function-sparing and cosmetic) surgery has achieved locoregional control as satisfactory as more radical surgery alone for some tumors. The treatment of early-stage breast cancer and soft tissue sarcomas of the extremities in adults are two examples where combined modality therapy has been found to be equivalent to radical surgery in recent randomized, prospective trials [72, 73].

The basic rationale for combining surgery and radiation therapy is that radiation can sterilize minimal gross or microscopic residual disease with acceptable toxicity. An analysis of patterns of failure for many tumors, including gastric carcinoma, pancreatic carcinoma, rectal carcinoma, and retroperitoneal sarcomas, reveals that locoregional failure can vary from 30% to 70% following "complete" resection. While the use of radiation therapy as a postoperative adjunctive treatment may be effective in reducing local failure at some sites, the total dose of radiation is usually limited to 45–50 Gy, primarily because of bowel tolerance [74].

Recently, there has been increasing interest in the USA in the use of intraoperative radiation therapy (IORT) to treat abdominal, pelvic, and retroperitoneal tumors. The present interest in IORT is based on the work of Abe and co-workers in Japan [75]. The strategy of IORT is quite simple. It involves the use of a large single dose of radiation delivered at the time of surgical exploration to a tumor or a tumor bed and potential areas of locoregional spread. The use of IORT may improve the therapeutic gain of tumor control in relation to normal tissue toxicity for two major reasons. First, the extent of tumor can be more precisely defined at surgery and the tumor can be directly irradiated. Second, all or part of sensitive normal tissues (small bowel, liver, stomach, ureter, etc.) may be excluded from the treatment volume by operative mobilization, customized lead shielding, and the selection of appropriate electron beam energies. The concept of IORT is similar, in some aspects, to the use of interstitial or intracavitary radiation (brachytherapy), where a large dose can be delivered to a specified tumor volume with relative sparing of adjacent normal tissue. Intraoperative radiation therapy may have an advantage over brachytherapy techniques in that it provides a more homogeneous dose distribution, especially to large volumes ($> 5\,cm^3$), although the dose rate used for IORT (2–10 Gy/min) may be less biologically advantageous to irradiated normal tissues.

When used as an adjunct to surgical resection, IORT requires that the tumor volume may include some intact normal tissues such as blood vessels and peripheral nerves as well as extensively manipulated tissues such as anastomosed vessels and gastrointestinal suture lines. Since the radiation tolerance of these tissues to large single doses of IORT was not known, investigators at the National Cancer Institute performed dose-tolerance experiments using large animals to provide guidelines for clinical doses [76]. Both clinical and histological changes caused by IORT in doses up to 50 Gy were studied. The animal data indicate that intact blood vessels tolerate up to 50 Gy without loss of structural integrity. Vascular anastomoses heal after doses of 45 Gy, although fibrotic strictures can develop with time and lead to growth of collateral vessels around the anastomoses. Intestinal suture lines heal after doses of 45 Gy. However, bile duct fibrosis and stenosis develop at doses above 20 Gy, and biliary-enteric anastomoses fail to heal at any dose level. Ureteral irradiation leads to stenosis and sometimes occlusion at doses of 30 Gy or more. Finally, peripheral nerve (e.g., femoral or sciatic nerve) can show evidence of nerve loss with clinical paresis and paresthesia at 25–30 Gy.

The clinical studies of IORT both in Japan and in the USA have concentrated on locally advanced malignancies of the abdomen, pelvis, and retroperitoneum. Over 1000 patients have been treated in Japan and approximately 400 in the USA. Preliminary results indicate that it is technically feasible to combine IORT and a major surgical resection and that the acute morbidity is quite acceptable [75, 76]. Additionally, IORT may be combined with moderate dose (45–50 Gy) external beam irradiation for unresectable tumors such as pancreatic carcinoma and locally advanced rectal carcinoma. Early phase I/II clinical trials indicate some benefit of using IORT in the treatment of gastric, rectal, cervical, and bladder carcinomas [77, 78]. Randomized prospective trials are under way at the National Cancer Institute comparing surgical resection and IORT (with moderate dose external beam irradiation) with resection and high-dose postoperative external beam irradiation in gastric carcinoma and retroperitoneal sarcomas [78].

In the future, experimental and clinical studies of IORT for mediastinal, lung, and brain tumors should be performed. Radiobiologic studies of acute and late IORT-induced normal tissue toxicity are necessary in these sites to guide subsequent clinical studies and to minimize the likelihood of late complications of treatment.

Systemic Radiation Therapy

Radiation therapy may be used as a systemic agent to prepare patients for organ transplantation and sustained immunosuppression. Since total lymphoid irradiation (TLI) causes immunosuppression in patients with Hodgkin's disease [79, 80], there has been considerable recent interest in TLI for the treatment of autoimmune disease and organ transplantation [81–83]. Total body irradiation (TBI) has been used mainly for bone marrow transplantation in acute and chronic leukemias and aplastic anemia [84, 85]. High-dose TBI has also been used as a systemic cytotoxic agent for the treatment of childhood sarcomas and small cell carcinoma of the lung [9, 86].

Total Lymphoid Irradiation

TLI has been used in the treatment of early stage Hodgkin's and non-Hodgkin's lymphomas for over two decades. While such treatment is effective in curing many patients, it was noted to cause a marked depression in the peripheral blood lymphocyte count, which recovered gradually over 1–2 years [79, 80]. A persistent depression of T-cell count and a reversal of the normal T-cell/B-cell ratio were noted with long-term follow-up. Functionally, delayed hypersensitivity responses were absent, although the clinical sequelae of severe bacterial or viral infections were uncommon. Moreover, not a single case of radiation-induced leukemia has been reported in Hodgkin's-disease patients treated with TLI alone [87, 88].

The immunosuppressive effects of TLI have been examined extensively in animal models of organ transplantation and autoimmune diseases [89–91]. Successful engraftment of skin, bone marrow, and hearts was performed using various immunosuppression regimens including TLI. The results of human trials using TLI for preparing prospective renal transplant recipients show that the addition of TLI to conventional immunosuppressive agents (prednisone and azathioprine) resulted in an approximately two fold improvement (78% vs 36%) in 2-year graft survival in patients who had previously rejected a renal transplant [83]. Based on the successful treatment of a systemic lupus glomerulonephritis-like disease in NZB/NZW F_1 mice [90], TLI has been used as therapy for refractory autoimmune diseases in man. Preliminary studies performed in patients with refractory rheumatoid arthritis at Harvard University show objective responses in the majority of cases [82].

Clinical investigations of the value of TLI in autoimmune diseases like rheumatoid arthritis and systemic lupus erythematosus need to be continued. Similarly, the use of TLI for kidney and heart transplantation should be evaluated objectively. Continued studies in small laboratory animals should be helpful in defining the mechanisms of immune alteration induced by TLI. Defining these mechanisms may ultimately permit the development of more effective transplantation programs in man.

Total Body Irradiation

Over the last decade, total body irradiation (TBI) has played a crucial role in bone marrow transplantation for leukemias, lymphomas, congenital hematopoietic disorders, and immunodeficiency syndromes. There are several methods of delivering TBI. The most experience has been with single fraction TBI (7.5–10 Gy) given at a low-dose rate (0.05 Gy/min) and at a moderate-dose rate (0.26 Gy/min) [85]. However, because of a high rate of interstitial pneumonitis and an unacceptably high recurrence rate in certain leukemia patient groups, trials of fractionated TBI were initiated which suggest an improvement in survival with a decreased risk of pneumonitis [92, 93]. When multiple daily fractions of TBI are administered, the interval between fractions should be long enough to allow for complete repair of sublethal damage in the critical normal tissues (e.g., in the lung and gut).

In future, more rigid guidelines for the clinical use of TBI need to be established. TBI studies should explore the types of drugs and timing of their administration necessary for preparation of the patient before radiation and marrow transplantation. Obviously, certain drugs which enhance pulmonary or gastrointestinal complications should be avoided. Finally, with more successful transplantation regimens, an assessment of other late effects including endocrine dysfunction, sterility, and carcinogenesis will be necessary.

Therapy with Radionuclides

The last area to be discussed in this section is the evolving field of radionuclides targeted to antibodies for systemic therapy. In the past, both beta-emitting isotopes such as phosphorus-32 and gamma-emitting isotopes such as iodine-131 have been used therapeutically for specific clinical situations, such as the treatment of polycythemia vera and thyroid cancer [94]. In other situations, such as the treatment of ovarian cancer, isotopes have been bound to colloids for intraperitoneal injection, although the range of the beta particles in tissue is only 3–5 mm, which may allow treatment of microscopic peritoneal deposits but certainly not of gross disease [96]. Further, the use of an intraperitoneal radioisotope such as colloidal chromic phosphate is limited to situations in which the regional draining lymphatics (peritoneal, diaphragmatic) are obstructed and there is free circulation within the peritoneal cavity [95]. Finally, attempts at localization of liver tumors by direct intra-arterial infusion of yttrium-90 microspheres have had limited success [96].

So far, a diverse array of systemically infused monoclonal and polyclonal radiolabeled antibodies have been demonstrated to localize primary and metastatic sites [97, 98]. While much of the effort has been directed at diagnostic scanning, the potential for tumor therapy, especially with alpha particles, is quite attractive [99, 100]. The determination of dose distribution, toxicity, and tumor response following administration of these isotopes needs to be refined further. Efforts should be concentrated on the dose administered and its relationship to the tumor-saturation dose rather than simply on dose escalation.

Particle Beam Radiation Therapy

Interest in the clinical investigation of particle beam radiation therapy is based on two theoretical advantages over conventional photon (or X-ray) irradiation. The first is the improved physical dose distribution provided by certain particles (protons, pions, helium ions), which allows an increase in the radiation dose to a well-defined tumor volume while sparing adjacent normal tissues (e.g., bowel, spinal cord) which typically limit the dose of external photon irradiation. The second theoretical advantage involves several in vitro and in vivo radiobiological observations of particle beam irradiation, which include less dependence on the presence of molecular oxygen for cell kill, less variability in cell kill based on the cell-cycle position, and less repair of sublethal and potentially lethal radiation damage.

The clinically attractive physical properties of particle beams relate to the pattern of energy deposition on a microscopic scale (termed linear energy transfer or LET). Neutrons, which are uncharged particles, are attenuated exponentially in matter in a similar fashion to 4–6 MV X-rays, but have significantly greater biological effects for the same physical dose. In comparison with the exponential attenuation of neutron and X-ray or photon beams, charged particles such as protons, helium ions, pions, and a number of heavy ions, have a discrete range of penetration determined by their initial momentum and modified slightly by different tissues (muscle, fat, bone) in the body. When a charged particle reaches the end of its path, an intense burst of ionization called the Bragg peak occurs. The ionization in this Bragg peak is considerably more dense than anywhere along the path of a charged particle and enhances the radiobiological effects in this defined peak. By selecting charged particle beams with the correct initial incident energy or by interposing absorbing material between the beam source and the patient, it is theoretically possible to make the tumor volume in the patient conform to the range of the Bragg peak.

Probably the most important biological property of these types of high LET radiation compared to conventional X-rays is their greater effectiveness in killing cells in an oxygen-poor environment. As previously mentioned, mammalian cells are approximately 3 times more resistant to killing by X-rays when the oxygen concentration is lowered to < 0.1% than in fully oxygenated conditions (20% oxygen). Since the proportion of hypoxic cells in rodent tumors and possibly in some human tumors may be as high as 30%, the observed poor response of some tumors to X-rays may be explained by the presence of these "resistant" hypoxic cells. With some high LET irradiation, there does not appear to be any difference in cell kill under hypoxic compared with under normal oxygen conditions.

In order to take advantage of the physical and biological potential of particle beam irradiation, very sophisticated and costly treatment planning is required. An important consideration in particle beam irradiation, particularly for charged particles, is the correction of dose calculations for tissue density inhomogeneities. Modern CT scanners provide a good first approximation of tissue densities for both normal and tumor tissues. In the case of neutron beams, a determination of tissues with high lipid concentrations (brain, spinal cord, adipose tissue) is necessary since there is preferential absorption of energy from neutrons in hydrogenated materials.

The clinical application of particle beam irradiation is hampered by several problems. A major logistical problem results from the considerable distance of most particle beam therapy facilities from clinical centers. In the USA, three cyclotrons for neutron irradiation have been recently installed in or adjacent to major medical centers to facilitate clinical research. In Europe, several institutions have participated in neutron trials for many years, although most equipment had poor neutron beam characteristics. For charged particle treatment, clinical research is severely hampered by the physical limitations of the equipment and the fact that sophisticated treatment planning has only recently been developed. As a result, only a small number of patients can be treated annually with each charged particle beam. Clinically, the Harvard cyclotron is used for proton beam irradiation and the Lawrence Berkley cyclotron for helium ion therapy. Pion radiotherapy clinical studies are being carried out at Los Alamos in the USA, in British Columbia, and at the Swiss Institute of Nuclear Physics (SIN).

The preliminary clinical data on particle radiation therapy have been recently reviewed, and the reader is referred to two excellent reviews for more detail [101, 102]. Briefly, there is unequivocal evidence that the unique dose distribution of these particles can provide clear-cut advantages in certain clinical situations such as ocular melanoma and paraspinal soft tissue sarcomas. However, these documented advantages of particle radiation therapy over conventional photon irradiation are limited to date. While the preliminary results of neutron therapy are not as encouraging as might have been expected from preclinical studies, it is important to point out that neutron therapy systems designed specifically for patients did not become operational in the USA until late 1983. Thus, the clinical research program to evaluate the role of neutrons in cancer therapy with adequate treatment systems will need to run for several more years before firm conclusions can be drawn.

References

1. Barranco SC, Romsdahl MM, Humphrey RM (1971) The radiation response of human malignant melanoma cells grown in vitro. Cancer Res 31: 830–833
2. Weichselbaum RR, Epstein J, Little JB, Kornblith PL (1976) In vitro cellular radiosensitivity of human malignant tumors. Eur J Cancer 12: 47–51
3. Smith IE, Courtenay VC, Mills J, Peckham MJ (1978) In vitro radiation response of cells from four human tumors propagated in immune suppressed mice. Cancer Res 38: 390–392
4. Arlett CF, Harcourt SA (1980) Survey of radiosensitivity in a variety of human cell strains. Cancer Res 40: 926–932
5. Fertil B, Malaise EP (1981) Inherent cellular radiosensitivity as a basic concept for human tumor radiotherapy. Int J Radiat Oncol Biol Phys 1: 621–629
6. Weichselbaum RR, Malcolm AW, Little JB (1982) Fraction size and the repair of potentially lethal radiation damage in a human melanoma cell line. Radiology 1425: 225–227
7. Leith JT, Dexter DL, de Wyngaert JK, Zeman EM, Chu MY, Calabresi P, Glicksman AS (1982) Differential responses to X-irradiation of subpopulations of two heterogeneous human carcinomas in vitro. Cancer Res 42: 2556–2561
8. Carney DN, Mitchell JB, Kinsella TJ (1983) In vitro radiation and chemotherapy sensitivity of established cell lines of human small-cell lung cancer and its large-cell morphological variants. Cancer Res 43: 2806–2811.
9. Kinsella TJ, Mitchell JB, McPherson S, Miser J, Triche T, Glatstein E (1984) In vitro radiation studies on Ewing's sarcoma cell lines and human bone marrow: application to the clinical use of total body irradiation (TBI). Int J Radiat Oncol Biol Phys 10: 1005–1011
10. Mitchell JB, Morstyn G, Russo A, Carney DN (1985) The in vitro radiobiology of human lung cancer. Cancer Treat Symp 2: 3–11
11. Withers HR (1975) The four R's of radiotherapy. Adv Radiat Biol 5: 241–271
12. Hall EJ (1978) Radiobiology for the radiologist. Harper and Row, Hagerstown, MD, pp 136–139
13. Little JB (1969) Repair of sublethal and potential lethal radiation damage in plateau phase cultures of human cells. Nature 224: 804–806
14. Little JB, Hahn GM, Frindel E, Tubiana M (1973) Repair of potentially lethal radiation damage in vitro and in vivo. Radiology 106: 689–694

15. Weichselbaum RR, Little JB (1983) X-ray sensitivity and repair in human tumor cells. In Steel GG, Adams GE, Peckham MJ (eds) The biological basis of radiotherapy. Elsevier, Amsterdam, pp 113–121
16. Weischselbaum RR, Little JB (1982) The differential response of human tumours to fractionated radiation may be due to a postirradiation repair process. Br J Cancer 46: 532–537
17. Elkind MM (1979) DNA repair and cell repair: are they related? Int J Radiat Oncol Biol Phys 5: 1089–1094
18. Elkind MM (1980) Cells, targets and molecules in radiation biology: the Ernst W. Bertmer memorial award lecture. In: Meym R, Withers HR (eds) Radiation biology in cancer research. Raven, New York, pp. 71–93
19. Taylor AMR, Harnden DG, Arlett CF, Harcourt SA, Lehmann AR, Stevens S, Bridges BA (1975) Ataxia telangiectasia: a human mutation with abnormal radiation sensitivity. Nature 258: 427–429
20. Cox R (1982) A cellular description of the repair defect in ataxia telangiectasia. In: Lehman A (ed) Ataxia telangiectasia. Wiley, Bristol, pp 141–153
21. Wilson RE, Antman KH, Brodsky G, Greenberger JS (1984) Tumor-cell heterogeneity in soft tissue sarcomas as defined by chemoradiotherapy. Cancer 53: 1420–1425
22. Goldie JH, Coldman AJ, Gudauskas GA (1982) Rationale for the use of alternating non-cross-resistant chemotherapy. Cancer Treat Rep 66: 439–449
23. Terasima R, Tolmach LJ (1963) X-ray sensitivity and DNA synthesis in synchronous populations of HeLa cells. Science 140: 490–492
24. Mitchell JB, Bedford JS, Bailey SM (1979) Dose-rate effects in mammaliam cells in culture. III. Comparison of cell killing and cell proliferation during continuous irradiation for six different cell lines. Radiat Res 79: 537–551
25. Kallman RF, Combs CA, Franko AJ (1980) Evidence for the recruitment of non-cycling clonogenic tumor cells. In: Meyn R, Withers HR (eds) Radiation biology in cancer research. Raven, New York, pp 394–414
26. Denekamp J, Fowler JF (1977) Cell proliferation kinetics and radiation therapy. In Becker FF (ed) Cancer: a comprehensive treatise, vol 6. Plenum, New York, pp 101–137
27. Brownell GI, Budinger TF, Lauterbur PC (1982) Positron tomography and nuclear magnetic resonance imaging. Science 215: 619–626
28. Morstyn G, Hsu SM, Kinsella T, Gratzner H, Russo A, Mitchell JG (1983) Bromodeoxyuridine in tumors and chromosomes detected with a monoclonal antibody. J Clin Invest 72: 1844–1850
29. Thomlinson RH, Gray LH (1955) The histological structure of some human lung cancers and the possible implications for radiotherapy. Br J Cancer 9: 539–549
30. Brown JM (1979) Evidence for acutely hypoxic cells in mouse tumors and a possible mechanism of reoxygenation. Br J Radiol 52: 650–656
31. Dische S (1979) Hyperbaric oxygen: the Medical Research Council trials and their clinical significance. Br J Radiol 51: 888–894
32. Urtasun RC, Band P, Chapman JD, Feldstein KL, Mielke B, Fryer C (1976) Radiation and high dose metronidazole (Flagyl) in supratentorial glioblastomas. N Engl J Med 293: 1364–1369
33. Urtasun R, Feldstein ML, Partington JL, Tanasichuk H, Miller JDR, Russell DB, Agboola A, Mielka B (1984) Radiation and nitroimidazoles and supratentorial high-grade gliomas: a second clinical trial. Br J Cancer 46: 101–108
34. Adams GE, Flockhart IR, Smithen CE, Stratford IJ, Wardman P, Watts ME (1976) Electron-affinic sensitization. VIII: a correlation between structures, one-electron reduction potentials, and efficiencies of nitroimidazoles as hypoxic cell radiosensitizers. Radiat Res 67: 9–20
35. Fowler JF, Denekamp J (1979) A review of hypoxic cell radiosensitization in experimental tumors. Pharmacol Ther 7: 413–444
36. Phillips TL, Wasserman TD (1984) Promise of radiosensitizers and radioprotectors in the treatment of human cancer. Cancer Treat Rep 68: 291–201
37. Urtasun RC, Tanasichuk H, Fulton D (1982) High dose misonidazole with dexamethasone rescue: a possible approach to circumvent neurotoxicity. Int J Radiat Oncol Biol Phys 8: 365–369

38. Eifel PJ, Brown DM, Lee WW, Brown JM (1983) Misonidazole neurotoxicity in mice decreased by administration with pyridoxine. Int J Radiat Oncol Biol Phys 9: 1513–1519
39. Brown JM (1984) Clinical trials of radiosensitizers: what should we expect? Int J Radiat Oncol Biol Phys 10: 425–429
40. Coleman CN (1985) Hypoxic cell radiosensitizers: expectations and progress in drug development. Int J Radiat Oncol Biol Phys 11: 323–329
41. Roberts JT, Bleehen NM, Workman P, Walton MI (1984) A phase I study of the hypoxic cell radiosensitizer RO-03-9877 in man. Int J Radiat Oncol Biol Phys 10: 1755–1758
42. Djordjevic B, Szybalski W (1960) Genetics of human cell lines. III. Incorporation of 5-bromo and 5-iododeoxyuridine into the deoxyribonucleic acid of human cells and its effect on radiation sensitivity. J Exp Med 112: 509–351
43. Kaplan HS, Smith KC, Tomlin PA (1962) Effect of halogenated pyrimidines on radiosensitivity of E. Coli. Radiat Res 16: 98–113
44. Hoshino T, Sano K (1969) Radiosensitization of malignant brain tumors with bromouridine (thymidine analog). Acta Radiol Ther Phys Biol 8: 15–26
45. Bagshaw MA, Doggett RLS, Smith KC, Kaplan HS, Nelsen TS (1967) Intra-arterial 5-bromodeoxyuridine and X-ray therapy. Radiology 99: 886–894
46. Kinsella TJ, Mitchell JB, Russo A, Morstyn G, Glatstein E (1984) The use of halogenated thymidine analogs as clinical radiosensitizers: rationale, current status and future prospects. Int J Radiat Oncol Biol Phys 10: 1399–1406
47. Russo A, Gianni L, Kinsella TJ, Klecker RW, Jenkins J, Rowland J, Glatstein E, Mitchell JB, Collins J, Myers CE (1984) A pharmacologic evaluation of intravenous delivery of BUdR to patients with brain tumors. Cancer Res 44: 1702–1705
48. Klecker RW, Jenkins J, Kinsella TJ, Fine R, Strong JM, Collins JM (1985) Clinical pharmacology of 5-iodo-2'deoxyuridine and 5-iodouracil and endogenous pyrimidine modulation. Clin Pharmacol Ther
49. Mitchell JB, Kinsella TJ, Russo A, McPherson S, Rowland J, Kornblith P, Glatstein E (1983) Radiosensitization of hematopoietic precursor cells (CFUc) in glioblastoma patients receiving intermittent intravenous infusions of bromodeoxyuridine (BUdR). Int J Radiat Oncol Biol Phys 9: 457–463
50. Kinsella TJ, Mitchell JB, Russo A, Morstyn G, Hsu SM, Rowland J, Glatstein E (1984) Continuous intravenous infusion of bromodeoxyuridine (BUdR) as a clinical radiosensitizer. J Clin Oncol 2: 1144–1150
51. Kinsella TJ, Russo A, Mitchell JB, Rowland J, Jenkins J, Schwade J, Myers CE, Collins J, Speyer P, Kornblith P, Smith B, Kufta C, Glatstein E (1984) A phase I study of intermittent intravenous BUdR with conventional irradiation. Int J Radiat Oncol Biol Phys 10: 69–76
52. Kinsella TJ, Russo A, Mitchell JB, Collins J, Klecker R, Rowland J, Jenkins J, Glatstein E (1985) Phase I study of intravenous infusions of iododeoxyuridine (IUdR) as a clinical radiosensitizer. Int J Radiat Oncol Biol Phys 11: 1579–1585
53. Bump EA, Yu NY, Brown JM (1982) Radiosensitization of hypoxic tumor cells by depletion of intracellular glutathione. Science 217: 544–545
54. Harris JW (1983) Cellular thiols in radiation and drug response. In: Nygaard OF, Simic M (eds) Radioprotectors and anticarcinogens. Academic, New York, pp. 255–274
55. Mitchell JB, Russo A, Biaglow JE (1983) Cellular glutathione depletion by diethyl maleate or buthionine sulfoximine: no effect on the oxygen enhancement ratio. Radiat Res 96: 422–428
56. Green JA, Vistica DC, Young RC, Hamilton TC, Rogan AM, Ozols RF (1984) Melphalan resistance in human ovarian cancer: characterization of drug resistant cell lines and potentiation of melphalan cytotoxicity by glutathione depletion. Cancer Res 44: 5427–5431
57. Louie KG, Behrens BC, Kinsella TJ, Hamilton TC, Grotzinger KR, McKoy WM, Winker MA, Young RC, Ozols RF (1985) Radiation survival parameters of antineoplastic drug-sensitive and resistant human ovarian cancer cell lines and their modification by buthionine sulfoximine. Cancer Res 45: 211–2115
58. Nakatsugawa S, Sugahara T, Kumar A (1982) Purine nucleoside analogues inhibit the repair of radiation-induced potentially lethal damage in mammalian cells in culture. Int J Radiat Biol 41: 343–346

50

59. Nakatsugawa S, Kumar A, Ono K (1982) Increased tumor curability by radiotherapy combined with PLDR inhibiters in murine cancer. In: Prospective methods of radiation therapy in developing countries, IAEA-TECDOR 2666 International Atomic Energy Agency, Vienna, pp 77–86

60. Tanaka Y, Sugahara T (1979) Clinical experience of chemical radiation research protection in tumor radiotherapy in Japan. In: Brady L (ed) Radiation sensitizers. Masson, New York, pp 421–425

61. Blumberg A, Nelson D, Gramrowski M (1982) Clinical trials of WR-2721 with radiation therapy. Int J. Radiat Oncol Biol Phys 8: 561–564

62. Steel GG, Peckham MJ (1979) Exploitable mechanisms in combined radiotherapy-chemotherapy: the concept of additivity. Int J. Radiat Oncol Biol Phys 5: 85–91

63. Steel GG, Hill RP, Peckham MJ (1978) Combined radiotherapy-chemotherapy of Lewis lung carcinoma. Int J. Radiat Oncol Biol Phys 4: 49–52

64. Looney WB, Ritenhour ER, Hopkins HA (1981) Solid tumor models for the assessment of different treatment modalities. XVI. Sequential combined modality therapy. Cancer 47: 860–869

65. Berry RJ (1982) Interaction of drugs and radiation—promise or pitfall? Clin Radiol 33: 121–129

66. Barranco SC, May JT, Boerwinkle W (1982) Enhanced cell killing through the use of cell kinetics directed treatment schedules for two-drug combinations in vitro. Cancer Res 42: 2894–2898

67. Evanochko WT, No TC, Lilly MB, Lawson AJ, Corbett TH, Durant JR, Glickson JD (1983) In vivo ^{31}P, NMR study of the metabolism of murine mammary 16/C adenocarcinoma and its response to chemotherapy, X-radiation and hyperthermia. Proc Natl Acad Sci USA 80: 334–338

68. D'Angio GJ, Evans A, Breslow N (1981) The treatment of Wilms' tumor: results of the second national Wilms' tumor study. Cancer 47: 2302–2311

69. Kinsella TJ, Glaubiger D, Deisseroth A, Makuch R, Waller B, Pizzo P, Glatstein E (1983) Intensive combined modality therapy including low dose TBI in high-risk Ewings's sarcoma patients. Int J Radiat Oncol Biol Phys 9: 1955–1960

70. Al-Sarraf M, Jacobs J, Kinzie J, Marchial V, Velez-Garcia E, Glick J, Fu K (1983) Combined modality therapy utilizing single high intermittent dose of cis-platinum and radiation in patients with advanced head and neck cancer. Proc Am Soc Clin Oncol 2: 159

71. Cummings BJ, Rider WD, Harwood AR, Keane TJ, Thomas GM, Erlichman C, Fine S (1982) Combined radical radiation therapy and chemotherapy for primary squamous cell carcinoma of the anal canal. Cancer Treat Rep 66: 48–492

72. Fisher B, Bauer M, Margolese R, Poisson R, Pilch Y, Redmon C, Fisher E (1985) Five-year results of a randomized clinical trial comparing total mastectomy and segmental mastectomy with or without radiation in the treatment of breast cancer. N Engl Med 312: 665–673

73. Rosenberg SA, Tepper J, Glatstein E (1982) The treatment of soft-tissue sarcomas of the extremities: prospective randomized trial of (1) limb-sparing surgery plus radiation therapy compared to amputation and (2) the role of adjuvant chemotherapy. Ann Surg 196: 305–315

74. Kinsella TJ, Bloomer WD (1980) Bowel tolerance to radiation therapy. Surg Gynecol Obstet 151: 273–284

75. Abe M, Takahashi M (1981) Intraoperative radiotherapy: the Japanese experience. Int J Radiat Oncol Biol Phys 7: 863–868

76. Sindelar WF, Kinsella TJ, Tepper J, Travis EL, Rosenberg SA, Glatstein E (1983) Experimental and clinical studies with intraoperative radiotherapy. Surg Gynecol Obstet 157: 205–219

77. Gunderson LL, Tepper JE, Biggs PJ, Goldson A, Martin JK, McCullough EC, Rich TA, Shipley WU, Sindelar WF, Wood WC (1983) Intraoperative ± external beam irradiation. In: Hickey RC (ed) Current problems in cancer. Year Book Medical Publishers, Chicago; pp 42–60

78. Kinsella TJ, Sindelar WF (1985) Intraoperative radiation therapy. In: De Vita VT, Hellman S, Rosenbery SA (eds) Principles and practice of oncology. Lippincott, Philadelphia; pp 2293–2304

79. Fuks Z, Strober S, Bobrove AM, Kaplan HS (1976) Long-term effects of radiation on T and B lymphocytes in peripheral blood of patients with Hodgkin's disease. J Clin Invest 58: 803–814

80. Engleman EG, Benike CJ, Hoppe RT, Kaplan HS (1980) Autologous mixed lymphocyte reaction in patients with Hodgkin's disease: evidence for a T-cell defect. J Clin Invest 66: 149–158

81. Schurman DJ, Hirshman HP, Strober S (1981) Total lymphoid and local joint irradiation in the treatment of adjuvant arthritis. Arthritis Rheum 24: 38–44.

82. Trentham DE Belli JA, Anderson RJ (1981) Clinical and immunological effects of fractionated total lymphoid irradiation in refractory rheumatoid arthritis. N Engl J Med 305: 976–982

83. Najarian JS, Ferguson RM, Sutherland DER (1982) Fractionated total lymphoid irradiation as preparative immunosuppression in high risk renal transplantation: clinical and immunological studies. Ann Surg 196: 442–452

84. Storb R, Thomas ED, Weiden PL (1978) One hundred and ten patients with aplastic anemia treated by marrow transplantation in Seattle. Transplant Proc 10: 135–140

85. Thomas ED, Buckner CD, Clift RA (1979) Marrow transplantation for acute non-lymphoblastic leukemia in first remission. N Engl J Med 301: 597–599

86. Glode LM, Robinson WA, Hartmann DW, Klein JJ, Thomas MR, Morton N (1982) Autologous bone marrow transplantation in the therapy of small cell carcinoma of the lung. Cancer Res 42: 4270–4275

87. Coleman CN, Williams CJ, Flint A (1977) Hematologic neoplasia in patients treated for Hodgkin's disease. N Engl J Med 297: 1249–1252

88. Tester WJ, Kinsella TJ, Waller B, Makuch RW, Kelley PA, Glatstein E, De Vita VT (1984) Second malignant neoplasms complicating Hodgkin's disease: the National Cancer Institute experience J Clin Oncol 2: 762–769

89. Slavin S, Reitz B, Bieber CP (1978) Transplantation tolerance in adult rats using total lymphoid irradiation: permanent survival of skin, heart, and marrow allografts. J Exp Med 147: 700–707

90. Kotzin BL, Strober S (1979) Reversal of MZB/NZW disease with total lymphoid irradiation. J Exp Med 150: 371–378

91. Koretz SH, Gottlieb MS, Strober S (1981) Organ transplantation in mongrel dogs using total lymphoid irradiation. Transplant Proc 13: 443–445

92. Thomas ED, Clift RA, Hersman J (1982) Marrow transplantation for acute non-lymphoblastic leukemia in first remission using fractionated or single dose irradiation. Int J Radiat Oncol Biol Phys 8: 817–821

93. Shank B, Simpson L (1982) The role of total body irradiation in bone marrow transplantation for leukemia. Bull NY Acad Med 58: 763–777

94. Reinhard EH (1975) Polycythemia. In: Beeson PB, McDermott W (eds) Textbook of medicine. Saunders, Philadelphia, pp 40–58

95. Leichner PK, Rosenshein NB, Leibel SA (1980) Distribution and tissue dose of intraperitoneally administered radioactive chromic phosphate in New Zealand white rabbits. Radiology 134: 729–734

96. Ariel IM, Padula G (1978) Treatment of metastatic cancer to the liver from primary colon and rectal cancer by the intra-arterial administration of chemotherapy and radiotherapy isotopes. Prog Clin Cancer 7: 247–263

97. Goldenburg DM, Decand F, Kim E (1978) Use of radiolabelled antibodies to carcinoembryonic antigen for the detection and localization of diverse cancers by external photoscanning. N Engl J Med 298: 1384–1388

98. Ballou B, Levine G, Hakala TR (1979) Tumor location detected with radioactively labelled monoclonal antibody and external scintigraphy. Science 206: 844–847

99. Ettinger DS, Order SE, Wharam MD (1982) Phase I–II study of isotopic immunoglobulin therapy for primary liver cancer. Cancer Treat Rep 66: 289–297

100. Order SE (1982) Monoclonal antibodies' potential role in radiation therapy and oncology. Int J Radiat Oncol Biol Phys 8: 1193–1201

101. Parker RG (1985) Particle radiation therapy. Cancer 55: 2240–2245

102. Pistenma DA (1985) Particle beam radiation therapy In: De Vita VT, Hellman S, Rosenburg SA (eds) Principles and practice of oncology. Lippincott, Philadelphia, pp 2280–2292

3. Radiotherapy Treatment Planning: Past, Present, and Future

A.S. Lichter, B.A. Fraass, D.L. McShan, R.F. Diaz, R.K. TenHaken,
C. Perez-Tamayo, and K. Weeks

Introduction

Radiation therapy treatment planning has made tremendous strides over the last two decades. With the application of modern imaging modalities, faster computers, advanced graphics techniques, and new calculational algorithms, treatment planning is ready to progress to new levels of sophistication. This chapter will summarize the progress made in clinical treatment planning and highlight where the field may be heading over the next decade.

Historical Perspective

When radiation was initially used therapeutically in the first half of this century, machine energy was low, the penetrating power of the beams was modest, and most radiotherapy prescriptions were based on the dose applied to the skin (formerly the "skin erythema dose," later the "applied dose" or "given dose"). Since the skin was the site of maximum dose build-up and was frequently the dose-limiting structure in radiotherapy treatment, the practice of basing prescriptions on skin dose was logical and warranted. While radiation depth dose curves were measured and the dose from combinations of beams could be calculated, for the first 50 years of radiotherapy there was little treatment planning as we know it today.

Several factors combined to change the importance of treatment planning and tissue/tumor dose calculation. In the 1950s Cobalt-60 units became available and for the first time radiotherapists had a reliable machine that could produce high energy photons with a significant amount of skin sparing. Instead of skin, the dose to underlying structures became the dose limiting factor and calculation of dose to major organs became increasingly important. The simulator was popularized as a tool for increasing the accuracy of set-up, leading to increased demand for precision [1]. The rad (r) replaced the Roentgen (R) as the unit of radiation dose. Since the Roentgen was a unit of exposure and the rad a unit of absorbed dose in tissue (radiation absorbed dose), calculating doses to specified targets became more common.

The methods used by physicists and dosimetrists in the 1950s and 1960s to calculate the relative dose at a *point* inside the patient were rather straightforward and have changed little to the present time. Tables of percentage depth dose were created by direct measurement of beam attenuation in water; corrections for field size, blocks, and distance to the body surface were made, and the calculations were done using reference tables and simple multiplication of the appropriate factors [2]. However, when it was necessary to calculate a *dose distribution* over a cross-section of the patient, early efforts at treatment planning became very cumbersome. It was necessary to take a precalculated isodose curve, place it underneath a paper containing the external contour of the patient, and to trace the beam data onto the contour. This was done for all beams, and then the doses were summed at points of beam intersection to create the isodose plan (Fig. 1). If a comparison of several beam configurations was wanted, the dosimetrist might spend hours or days planning a single case.

The advent of the computer dramatically changed radiotherapy treatment planning. After creating a computerized model of the fall-off of radiation intensity with depth in tissue and storing this information in a computer for a variety of field sizes, one could place beams on a contour of the patient using the computer. The computer rapidly summed the doses throughout the irradiated area, adding together the contribution of all beams and then displaying the resultant dose distribution. What used to take hours by hand took minutes by computer, and accuracy was increased since many more data points could be sampled. The first computerized dosimetry systems were developed in the late 1950s [3], and development continued into the early 1960s [4, 5]. These were experimental systems, but once it became clear that computerized dosimetry was reliable and accurate, commercial manufacturers entered the market. By the mid-1970s computerized dosimetry was the standard worldwide.

The 1960s and 1970s produced other significant changes in the field of radiation oncology. Simulators became widely used as radiotherapists were designing more sophisticated treatment plans with custom-shaped shielding blocks. The mantle field for treating Hodgkin's disease is a good example of a then new treatment approach that demanded a simulator for optimal results [6]. Linear accelerators began to replace the Cobalt-60 machine as the main treatment unit in radiotherapy. The added precision of these machines further enhanced the radiotherapist's ability to deliver dose to a precise volume of tissue. Computers became faster and less expensive, allowing for greater flexibility in designing calculational algorithms. Computerized dosimetry systems also became more sophisticated; for example, being able to calculate the influence of inhomogeneous tissue density on the dose distribution [7, 8].

It was into this rapidly expanding field of radiotherapy treatment planning that the computed tomogram (CT) made its entry, and radiotherapists wasted little time before recognizing and taking advantage of its potential [9–12]. CT provided the anatomic information on patient shape, location of tumor and target volume, and location of normal anatomic structures. Furthermore, CT performed these tasks on multiple parallel slices and gave information on tissue

Fig. 1. Treatment planning as formerly done, manually. The isodose curve from the anterior field is traced on to the patient contour (*dotted lines* in *upper figure*). The posterior field is also traced (*dashed lines* in *middle figure*). Finally, the two-field dose distribution is summed where the isodose lines cross, showing the composite dose distribution (*solid line* in *lower panel*)

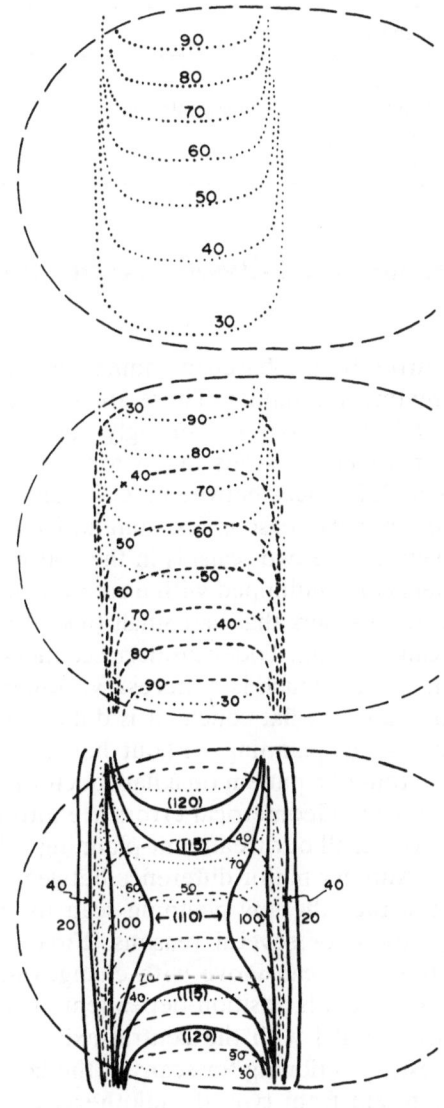

density differences as well. Much as with the first computerized planning systems themselves, the first CT treatment planning systems were developed as one-of-a-kind demonstration systems, usually in academic departments. A series of studies in the literature demonstrated the advantages of these systems [13–16], and illustrated treatment planning superimposed on the CT scan itself for greater accuracy and visual impact. Today most commercial treatment planning companies market systems with the capability to treatment plan directly on top of CT data.

Table 1. Differences between diagnostic and radiotherapy planning CT scans

Diagnostic	Treatment planning
Round couch	Flat couch
Position for best diagnostic information	Must duplicate treatment position
No breathing	Quiet breathing
No external marks	External markers define a coordinate system

Standard CT-Based Treatment Planning

Currently, CT-based planning represents the state of the art for radiotherapy treatment planning. There are a variety of ways in which this art is being practiced today. We feel strongly that the most accurate CT treatment planning is performed on scans taken for the specific purpose of radiotherapy planning. The differences between a CT scan taken for diagnostic reasons and one taken for therapy reasons are summarized in Table 1. The most obvious difference between the two scans is in the couch configuration. Virtually all diagnostic scanners come equipped with a round couch. This type of couch was necessary with early scanners that had small (40cm) apertures so that patients could fit into the scanning ring. Today modern scanners have large apertures of 70cm or more and the round couch is unnecesary; however, it persists. Radiotherapy patients are treated on a flat couch. It is difficult to use a round-couch CT scan for therapy treatment planning without having to make an estimate of how the external contour of a patient on a flat couch will align with the contour in the round-couch CT scan. Geometrical errors are introduced in this estimating process. Thus we perform all our treatment-planning CT scans using a flat-couch insert (Fig. 2).

Another major difference between the two types of scans is patient position. In a radiotherapy planning scan the patient must be aligned in the treatment position for several reasons. First, certain organs, especially intraabdominal structures, can move with changes in position. Second, the external shape of the patient is position-dependent. Third, it is important to obtain CT slices that are parallel with the central axis of the treatment beam. Characteristic diagnostic positioning for scans of the head and brain, for example, are significantly different from typical radiotherapy treatment positions (Fig. 3). While all the anatomic information is present on a diagnostic CT of the head, the relationships between structures can be greatly obscured when the angulation of the head is changed. Fourth, a powerful new tool in radiotherapy treatment planning involves aligning CT cuts with the simulator films to aid design of fields and shielding blocks (see below). This technique cannot be accurately employed if the scan was performed in a position that is different from the treatment position. Finally, the information that pinpoints the location of tumor, target, and normal tissue rarely comes from a single radiographic study, but rather from many different types of studies including CT, magnetic resonance imaging, simulator films, etc. It has become increasingly important to be able to correlate

56

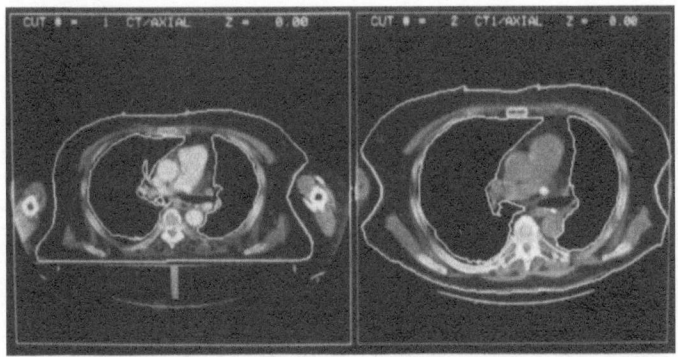

Fig. 2. Differences between a radiotherapy treatment planning scan and a diagnostic CT scan are no more evident than in the couch configuration. Differences in anatomic configuration occur when the patients are scanned on a round couch and treated on a flat one

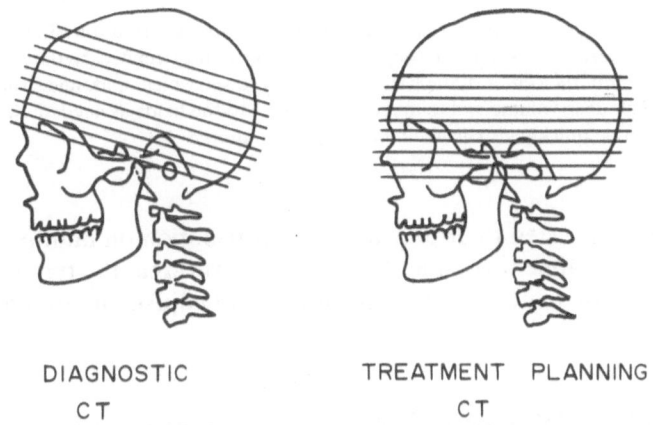

DIAGNOSTIC
C T

TREATMENT PLANNING
C T

Fig. 3. Typical scan positions for a diagnostic versus treatment-planning CT scan of the head. The diagnostic scan is angled so that one can image the entire intracranial content without scanning directly through the orbits. Treatment positions for radiotherapy place the head in a more neutral position. Using the diagnostic information directly for treatment planning purposes becomes difficult since the diagnostic scans do not align with the central axis of the radiotherapy treatment plan

and use many kinds of images. For radiotherapy treatment planning purposes this means that as many imaging studies as possible should be obtained in the treatment position to ensure consistency. This concept is discussed in greater detail later in this chapter.

The standard use of CT images for treatment planning involves the superimposition of a dose distribution directly onto the CT image (Fig. 4). This simple strategy is very sophisticated in its ability to demonstrate proper coverage of the target region and to display doses to normal tissue. Since CT scans are done at multiple levels and radiation treatment covers a volume of tissue, it is a straight-

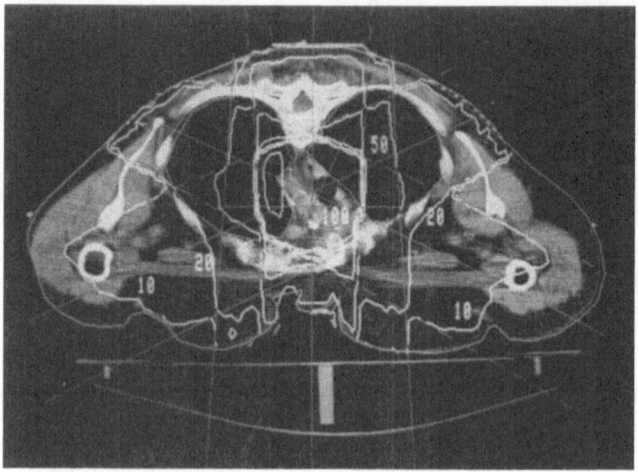

Fig. 4. A CT scan with treatment fields and dose distribution directly superimposed. The numbers are percentages, representing the percentage of dose relative to the point where the treatment beams meet in the center of the patient. It is easy to see which anatomic structures are encompassed by the high-dose volume and to make adjustments to the fields as needed. Similarly, dose to normal tissues can be quickly visualized and adjusted as required

forward step to display the dose distribution on multiple transverse slices within the treatment volume. One then confirms that the tumor and normal tissue doses are adequate at several key levels and adjusts the treatment plan accordingly.

Three-Dimensional CT-Based Treatment Planning

Once multiple CT scans became routinely available to radiotherapists, new horizons opened in the treatment planning field. One of the most obvious new applications involved the integrated display of multiple CT slices stacked in a way that reflected their true geometric relationships (Fig. 5). Simultaneous display of dose distributions on these selected slices creates a better appreciation of the volume being treated. Since CT scans can be reconstructed in the sagittal plane, this sagittal image can then be displayed along with transverse cuts, either in a multiwindow format or directly integrated (Figs. 6, 7). Calculating and displaying dose on the sagittal plane is a complex problem which is addressed separately below. However, this calculational problem can be solved and dose can be displayed on these integrated multiplanar displays as illustrated in Figs. 6 and 7. The saggittal view of the treatment plan is especially useful in following the dose to structures such as the spinal cord that might traverse an entire treatment volume longitudinally at varying depths. Instead of relying on dose displays from

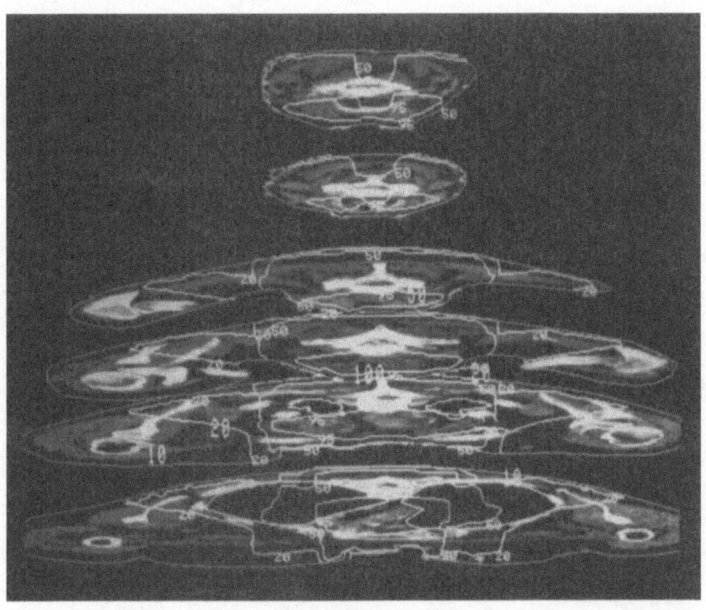

Fig. 5. Multiple CT slices for treatment of carcinoma in the upper esophagus. The dose distribution is displayed on six slices simultaneously. One begins to appreciate the three-dimensionality of radiotherapy treatment planning through such displays. Adjustments to the fields can be monitored on all levels simultaneously

two or three levels in the cord, the dose to this critical structure can be visualized in its entirety using a single display.

Stacking of multiple CT slices has also become the most precise way in which to draw shielding blocks for treatment fields. By drawing the tumor and target volume on multiple consecutive CT slices, one can then display this information with the appropriate divergence, creating a display called the "beam's eye view" (BEV) (Fig. 8) [17, 18]. This is an exciting display which can aid treatment planning in a variety of ways. One can use it to decide upon the overall size of a field. All too frequently the field size that is chosen by studying the simulator film, the diagnostic films, and the diagnostic CT, is too small and would have touched the target volume (i.e., allowed no tumor-free margin) in one or more places. One can also use the display to help choose the best angle to use for the treatment fields. For example, by displaying critical normal tissues as well as the traget, one can immediately recognize the best gantry angle and collimator angle so that the normal tissue is spared (Fig. 9).

Finally, one can use the display to design shielding blocks. The blocks are drawn using the joy stick and cursor, either freehand or, in our system, automatically by selecting a constant margin around the volume—for example, 1 cm (Fig. 10). In our system the block design is fed by computer into an automated block cutting machine (HEK Model MCP-70-SE) and the styrofoam form is

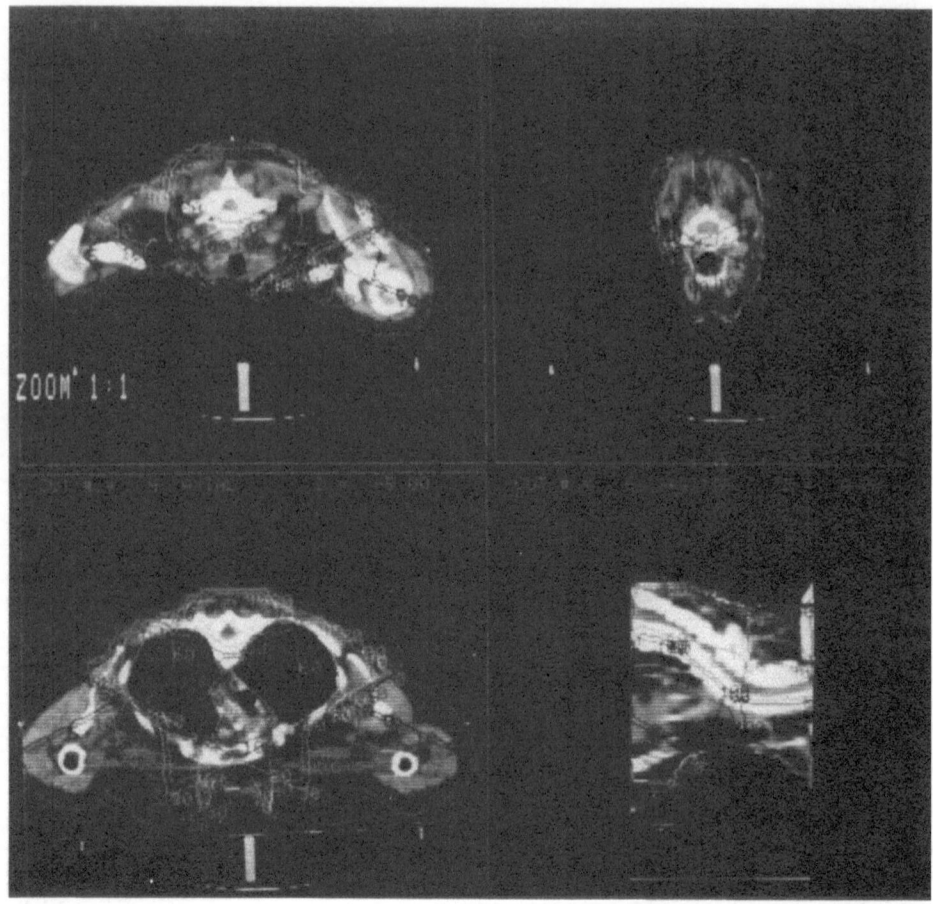

Fig. 6. Multiple CT slices displayed in a multiwindow format. Each color codes for a different dose intensity. The *reddish-brown* coloration indicates full dose; *Green* and *blue* colors are low-dose regions. In the *lower right hand corner* is the saggital dose distribution. The spinal canal and vertebral column can be seen making an S-shaped course through this volume. With special angulation and shielding, the high-dose region is confined in front of the spinal cord. The entire spinal column is in green with a small area of pink, indicating that 60% or less of the dose is going to this structure. To view this figure in color see Color Plates following page 78

fashioned. Alternatively, the block information can be printed on paper and this print-out used as a template for a standard block cutting device. If the field size and location have already been selected, we still use the beam's eye view to verify block design. The simulator film is digitized into the computer system and its size is scaled to correspond to the size of the field on the treatment planning screen. The drawn blocks are then digitized into the system by tracing over the simulator film blocks with the cursor of the digitizer. The blocks appear on the same display with the stacked CT slices and target volumes. Modifications to the block shapes are made, if necessary, and the blocks are then cut from the film in a standard manner.

60

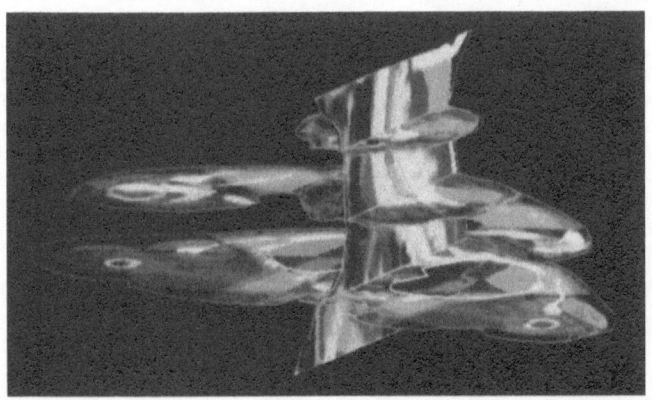

Fig. 7. The same four panels of dose information as in Fig. 6. now integrated into an anatomically correct display. Dose can be seen to spill over from the saggital plane onto the transverse planes and vice versa. This is a further step towards conceptionalizing the three-dimensionality of radiotherapy treatment planning. To view this figure in color see Color Plates following page 78

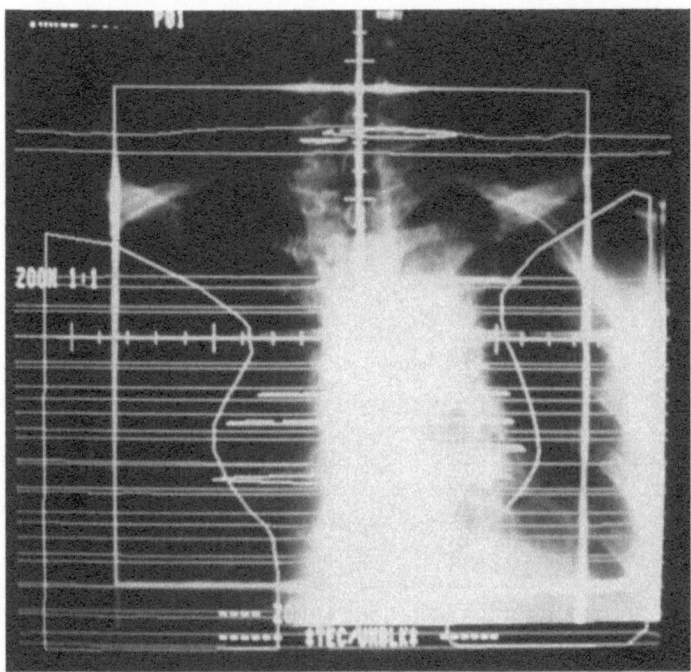

Fig. 8. The "beam's eye view" display. The *blue* lines represent the CT slices. The *pink* outlines represent the target volume on each slice. The *white* lines outline the field size necessary to treat this target volume. Adjustments can be made to the field location and size and block shape to ensure proper coverage of the volume. To view this figure in color see Color Plates following page 78

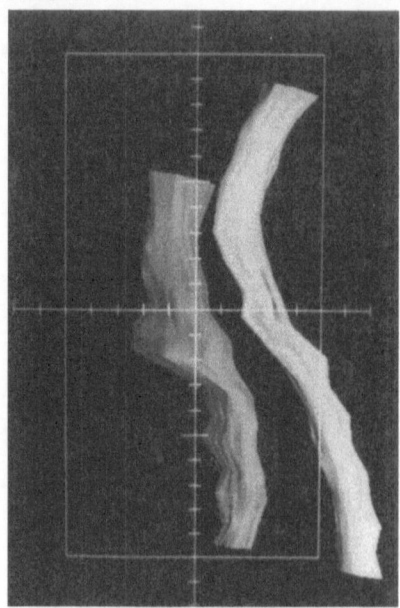

Fig. 9. Beam's eye view display to determine gantry angle. The target (esophagus) is located anterior to the spinal cord. In this illustration, the gantry has been angled so that the target is separated from the spinal cord. A block would then be added to this field to shield the spinal cord while still exposing the target. The rotation of the gantry can be done interactively and the target and spinal cord structures will move relative to one another, allowing the dosimetrist to optimize the gantry angle

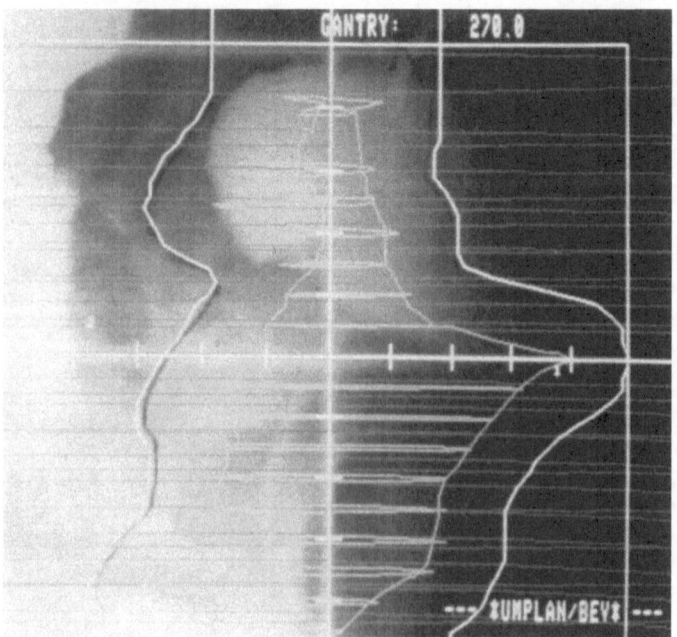

Fig. 10. A block design for the prostate tumor volume. A 1-cm margin has been taken in all directions. This block design superimposed on the CT target volumes is the most accurate way to draw shielding blocks. To view this figure in color see Color Plates following page 78

MRI in Radiotherapy Treatment Planning

Cross-sectional CT scans show the electron density variations across the scanned volume. Often such variations do not differentiate unambiguously between tumor and normal tissue. Imaging modalities which provide further information can have an important place in radiotherapy. Magnetic resonance imaging (MRI) images the presence and/or status of hydrogen in the body. The status is a complex function of local molecular environment, allowing great flexibility in the construction of the images. Clinical experience with MRI has increased rapidly and optimal pulse sequencing techniques are improving our ability to delineate tumor from normal tissue. It is already clear that for certain tumors, MRI data is indispensable. For some tumors, such as primary brain stem gliomas, it is the only imaging modality that can visualize the lesion [18]. MRI can also display sagittal and coronal images that are primary images and not reconstructed images as they are with CT. For visualizing some longitudinal structures, such as the spinal cord or tumors that are oriented logitudinally, the MRI display is superb. However, MRI has several drawbacks as a treatment planning modality. It does not give tissue density information as does CT. Its long image-acquisition time makes the study susceptible to artifacts and inaccuracy due to patient motion. The image can be distorted by nonuniformity of the magnetic field throughout the scanning volume. This is less of a problem with small regions such as the brain, but becomes a big concern for body images.

With these drawbacks and advantages in mind, it appears that the best way to use MRI is to integrate it with CT data whenever the MRI adds information as to tumor location and extent of disease which is missing from CT. This means superimposing the information from the two images, using the CT as the anatomic standard. Correlating these studies is a challenging task. If the images were obtained with external markers on the patient outlining the treatment ports, the job becomes somewhat easier. One then knows which slice on each study corresponds to the central axis of the beam, giving a good start to the process of cross-referencing the studies. One must then superimpose the corresponding scans at each level, quantitating the misregistration and/or distortion between the MRI study and the CT, and then align and "unwarp" the distorted MRI image to match the CT as closely as possible (Fig. 11).

Further checks on the accuracy of the match of the two studies are then performed. For example, a coronal MRI of the thorax is displayed on the screen. We draw the location of the external patient contour and lung from a stacked set of CT scans and superimpose them on the MRI to confirm that the two studies agree on the location of these structures (Fig. 12). This process is repeated for the MRI using the CT as the reference display and the MRI as the overlay. All three major views—sagittal, coronal, transverse—are checked. The planning system has the ability to rotate one data set relative to the other in order to improve the alignment and agreement between the studies. When the best match is achieved, treatment planning can then proceed on the basis of either study interchangeably (Fig. 13). Thus the advantages of both CT and MRI can be integrated and utilized.

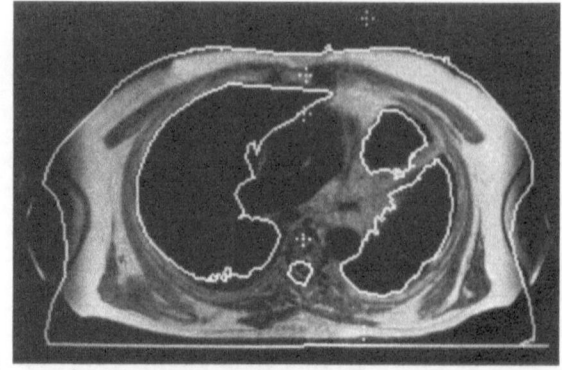

a

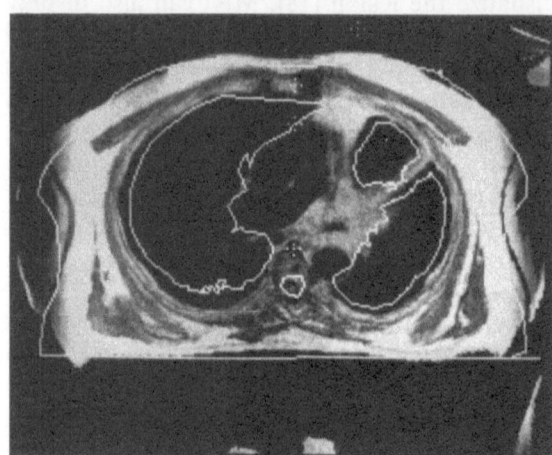

b

Fig. 11a,b. An MRI unwarping sequence. **a** The MR image is overlaid with the CT data from the external contour and lungs. The distortion of MRI is especially severe in the inferior corners of the image. **b** The unwarped image

Three-Dimensional Dose Calculations

Having MRI scans in both sagittal and coronal orientations as well as reconstructed CT images in these and other non-transverse planes was not ideal for radiotherapists because dose could not be calculated or displayed on these images. Most treatment planning systems are set up to calculate dose on transversely-oriented planes only, with the central axis of each beam forced to be coplanar with those transverse planes. In addition, the basic algorithms used to calculate the dose on those planes were predicated on approximations and simplifications which are only appropriate to two-dimensional types of calculations. In order to accurately display dose on planes that are not oriented coplanar with the transverse central axis of the beam, one needs a three-dimensional dose calculation algorithm.

There are several distinct areas in which three-dimensionality must be incorporated into dose calculations. The first is simply the ability to calculate dose

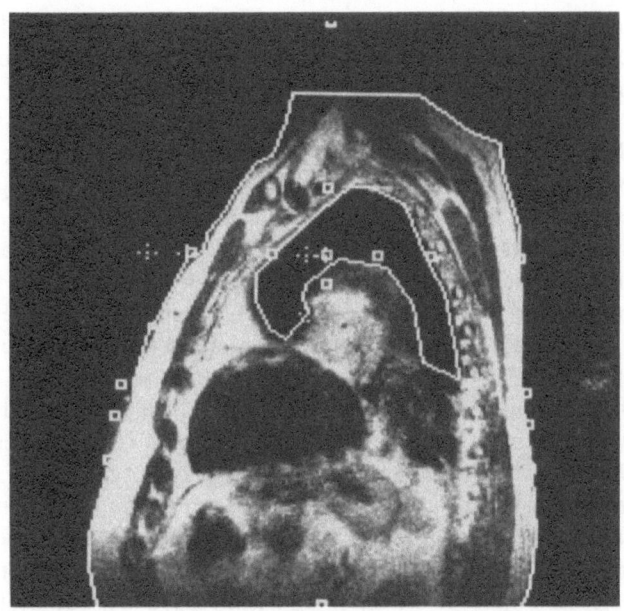

Fig. 12. Data set correlation between CT and MRI. The saggital MRI is displayed. The small boxes indicate location of lung and external contour on multiple CT slices. Notice the excellent agreement between the CT and MRI in this display. All three views (transverse, sagittal, and coronal) are checked in this fashion and adjusted as necessary in order to bring the CT and MRI in perfect alignment

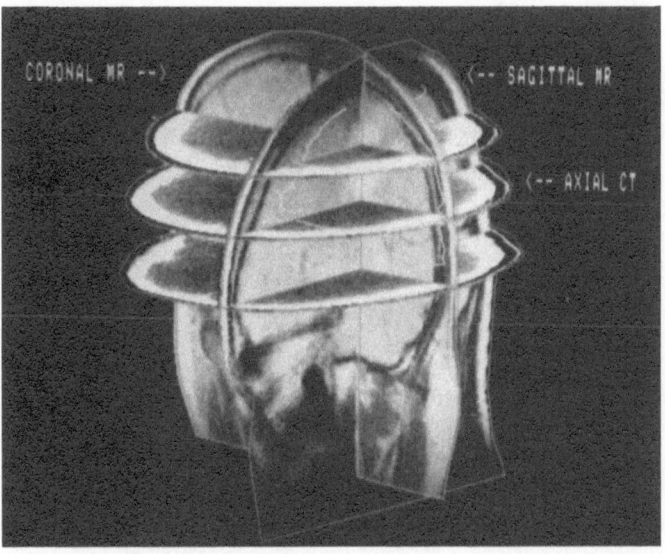

Fig. 13. Once integrated, CT and MR images can be used interchangeably, as on this display where different studies are integrated in a single picture. To view this figure in color see Color Plates following page 78

on a 3D grid of points, even if the way in which the dose is calculated for each point is one-dimensional. Many recent treatment planning systems are capable of volume-type calculations [19].

The second area is that of the beam geometry. Correctly calculating the divergence of the radiation beam and determining the effect of that divergence on transverse or other planes of calculations is a straightforward but very time-consuming part of the dose calculation. Most commercial treatment planning systems do not incorporate this effect, even when calculating dose to off-axis transverse planes. In a 3D planning system, where one is utilizing non-transverse planes and beam's-eye-view type planning, this geometry is critical.

Dose calculations which take into account the shape of the radiation field and shielding blocks which are placed in the field are the third type of three-dimensionality. This added sophistication is required in 3D views of plans in which a coronal image is used to evaluate the dose resulting from a plan, even one as simple as an anterior-posterior opposed pair of fields (Fig. 14). The scatter under blocks and lack of full scatter in the field near blocks must be incorporated once the planning system is used to evaluate those doses. There are several methods by which these effects are taken into account, but most of them are calculationally slow. The algorithm used by our system, on the other hand, accurately incorporates all the effects discussed so far, and requires only 15 seconds per beam per plane to calculate on the VAX 750 (Digital Equipment Corp.)

Incorporation of scatter effects due to missing or low density tissue which is not in the ray line between the radiation source and the point at which dose is being calculated is the final aspect of three-dimensionality which must be

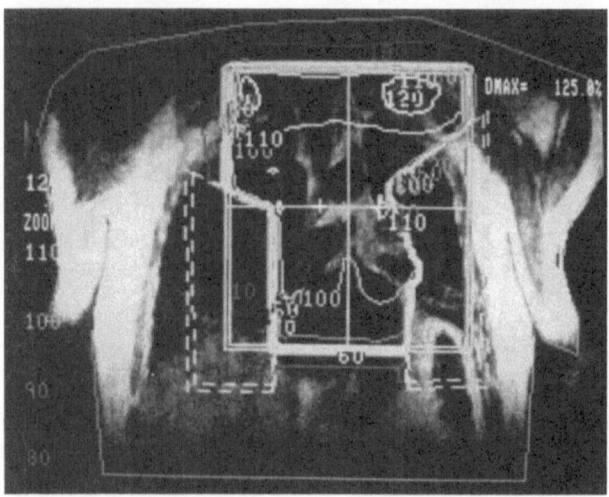

Fig. 14. Dose displayed on a coronal MRI slice in a patient with cancer of the left lung. The full effects of beam diversion, dose near the edges of the blocks, and dose under blocks are completely accounted for in this display. To view this figure in color see Color Plates following page 78

incorporated into the dose calculations. In general, incorporating this effect requires a 3D integration over the whole volume which is irradiated. For electron beams, this is handled fairly well by algorithms such as the 3D version of the pencil beam model which was developed in our department [20]. For photon beams, however, this is a much more difficult project due to the long range of scattered photons and electrons, especially for high energy beams. At the present time, calculational algorithms, such as the Delta Volume method [21], require large amounts of computer time, and are not clinically useful. This is an area of active research in many centers.

The Future of Radiotherapy Treatment Planning

In the near future, three developments will profoundly change the way radiotherapy treatment planning is practiced. These developments are: (1) fully three-dimensional treatment planning, (2) an integrated radiographic display of patient and tumor anatomy, and (3) conformational or dynamic therapy. All three are being practiced on prototype systems today but over the next decade will be refined, "debugged," and made practical and affordable for widespread use.

Fully Three-Dimensional Treatment Planning

Up to now, radiotherapists have been constrained to treat patients with beams that entered the patient at right angles to the central axis of the body. This severely limited the flexibility of the therapist in individualizing treatment to fit a specific anatomic situation. Treatment planning became predictable, and even in the most sophisticated institutions atlases of radiotherapy treatment planning could contain reproductions of treatment plans that would satisfy the vast majority of treatment situations [22]. Why had treatment planning become so rigid in this era of advanced tumor imaging? One can point to several important factors. For one, tumor anatomy could not be displayed in 3D. The inability to visualize the tumor in anything but a transverse display limited the creativity of radiotherapy. Without beam's-eye-view displays it was impossible to visualize how oblique fields entering from a superior direction, for example, would hit the tumor and miss normal structures. In fact, it was difficult to know exactly which structures would be in the beam path. Simulators are relatively bulky pieces of equipment and cannot simulate from many angles that are non-coplanar with the axis of gantry rotation. Thus the beam's-eye-view display becomes even more critical for setting up unusual fields and designing shielding blocks to shape these fields. Finally, dose calculations could not be performed three-dimensionally or displayed superimposed on images obtained in arbitrary planes.

Radiation oncology is now developing solutions to these problems. As

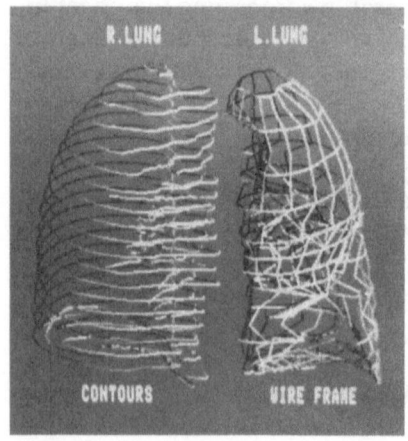
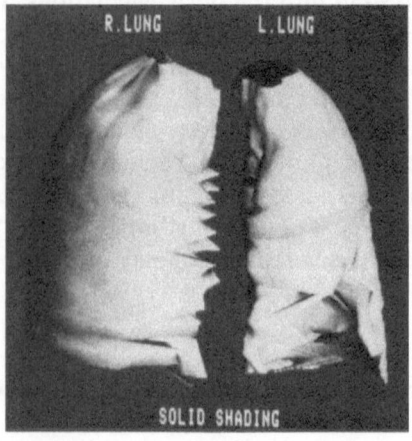

Fig. 15   **Fig. 16**

Fig. 15. The first steps towards solid-surface 3D reconstruction. The right lung has been outlined on consecutive CT slices. The slices have been stacked and shading has been applied to create the 3D effect. The left lung has had a wire frame reconstructed to give further 3D characteristics

Fig. 16. The solid surface has been "tiled" and shaded to create a full 3D effect

pointed out, 3D dose calculation and display are becoming more rapid and more accurate. Calculational speed is increasing due to better software design, faster and more powerful hardware, and in some cases the design of custom chips to calculate dose [21]. The beam's-eye-view display is now available [17, 18]. All that remains is to produce and display the 3D view of patient anatomy and this is now practicable on several prototype treatment planning systems as well as in some commercial graphics display hardware.

The concept of displaying 3D structures is a relatively simple one. If one can stack CT images that have designated structures outlined, then the structures can be given a 3D appearance by connecting outlines from various slices through the use of a "wire frame" (Fig. 15). This gives each structure the appearance of solidity, and one can see through this girder-like frame to visualize other structures. A more realistic 3D form can then be generated from the wire frame display through the use of a graphics technique known as "tiling." Here the individual frames in the wire frame are made solid and these solid tiles are shaded lighter or darker to simulate a light shining on their surface. The tiles that are to be perceived as being closest to the viewer are made lighter, while those that recede into the screen are shaded darker corresponding to their depth into the picture. The result can be very realistic (Fig. 16). By reconstructing solid-surface displays throughout an anatomic region, a full 3D reconstruction can be displayed (Fig. 17).

Having created this 3D picture of the patient's anatomy and the tumor, how can one use it for treatment planning? To begin with, one must be able to display beam positions with respect to the anatomy and target volume. To plan three-

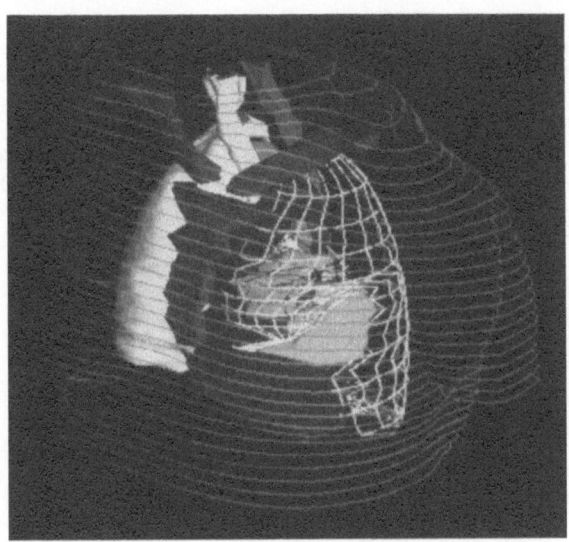

Fig. 17. A complete 3D reconstruction of a lung tumor. The external contour of the patient is seen in *blue* lines. The trachea and lungs are in *white*. The left lung has been made transparent to see the tumor (*pink* structure) and pulmonary arteries (*blue*) through the lung. The heart and aorta are in *red*, the spinal cord in *green*, the esophagus in *yellow*, and the bones of sternum and clavicles in *brown*. The reconstruction can be rotated to view from any angle. Pictured here is the left superior oblique view. To view this figure in color see Color Plates following page 78

dimensionally, the beams must be able to strike and enter the patient from any given angle. Thus the computer planning system must be able to simulate not only different field sizes and gantry angles, the standard functions that are available in 2D treatment planning systems, but must be able to reproduce all motions of the couch (including pedestal angle), and all collimator functions (including collimator angle and asymmetric collimator jaws). Since many of the advanced non-coplanar field arrangements cannot be reproduced on the simulator, all patient setup parameters must be available from the computer plan.

The 3D display should be flexible so that the target region can be easily identifed and visualized. By making some structures "transparent" through the use of wire frames, a centrally located tumor can be visualized. One must also have the ability to cut away any part of the display and view the CT reconstruction on the surface of that cut-away plane so that anatomic relationships are reinforced (Fig. 18). Wedge- or pie-shaped cut outs are frequently made in a trial-and-error fashion until the most useful display is achieved. The display can be rotated in any direction so that the planners can "walk around" the patient while viewing the display. This rotation can be done by precalculating the display in successive increments of 5 or 10 degrees, saving each picture on disk. The replay of these images is then controlled with a joy stick. The ideal way to employ rotation is to do so in real time. Commercial graphics display workstations that can perform this task are becoming available. Industry has been using similar technology for

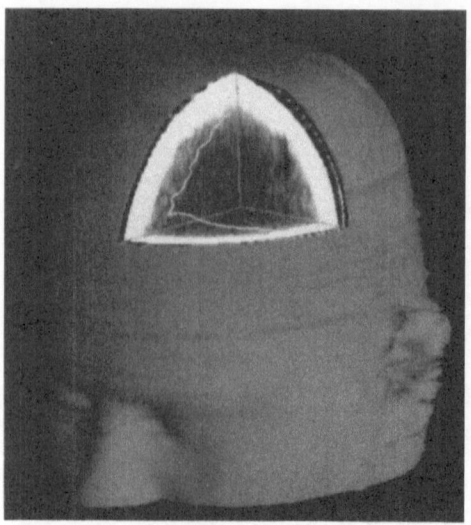

Fig. 18. A 3D reconstruction for a brain tumor case with a wedge-shaped cutout through the target volume. CT data appears on all three surfaces. This cutout can be moved, enlarged, or reoriented until the best reinforcement of internal versus external anatomy is created. To view this figure in color see Color Plates following page 78

several years, but the requirements for treatment planning systems to have this real-time rotational capability are somewhat more complex than is available in CAD/CAM-type systems.

Once the graphics requirements are met, the planning system must then be able to display dose on any of the graphics images created. This requires a fully 3D dose calculational system, the complexities of which have been touched upon above. The dose display also needs to be graphically flexible. For example, it may be advantageous to display a particular isodose level as a solid surface. If one then displays the target volume as a solid of a different color, it is easy to see if the target extends beyond the desired dose region in any direction (Fig. 19). This is the type of detailed error analysis that is almost impossible to perform in a conventional 2D system. The system can also display the dose to a target or normal structure graphically using dose–volume histograms, a function that is essential in a volume-oriented planning system. An example of a dose–volume histogram for a liver is presented in Fig. 20. Since dose–volume histogram analyses of treatment plans for specific sites are not commonly available, there is little information about partial organ radiation tolerances. For example, the whole liver can safely tolerate 30 Gy of conventionally fractionated therapy (10 Gy/ week in five fractions). But how much dose can 70% of the liver take if the other 30% gets no dose, or receives only 10 Gy? The permutations are endless. With a 3D system, it will be possible to assemble clinical experience using dose–volume data for a variety of organs and, in so doing, characterize partial organ toler- ances that have long eluded quantification.

Another developmental area in 3D treatment planning involves the intercom- parison of alternative treatment plans. In a 2D system, one can view two or three rival plans side by side and choose between them with relative ease. How is one going to compare the relative merits of alternative 3D plans? Certainly dose– volume histograms will help, especially for normal tissues. Another display that

Fig. 19. In this four-field boost (anterior, posterior, left and right lateral fields) for prostate cancer, the volume that is encompassed by the 95% isodose line is displayed as a wire frame. To view this figure in color see Color Plates following page 78

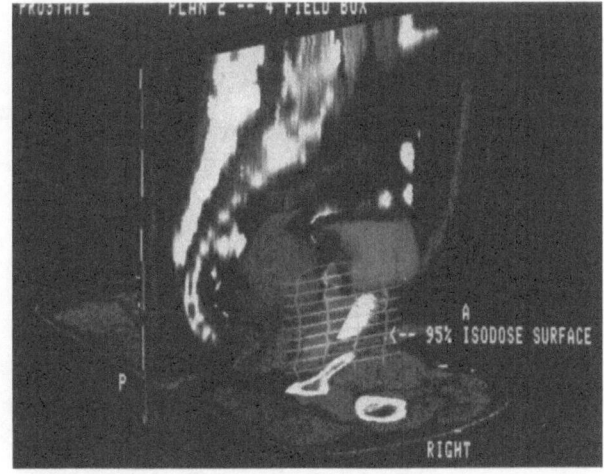

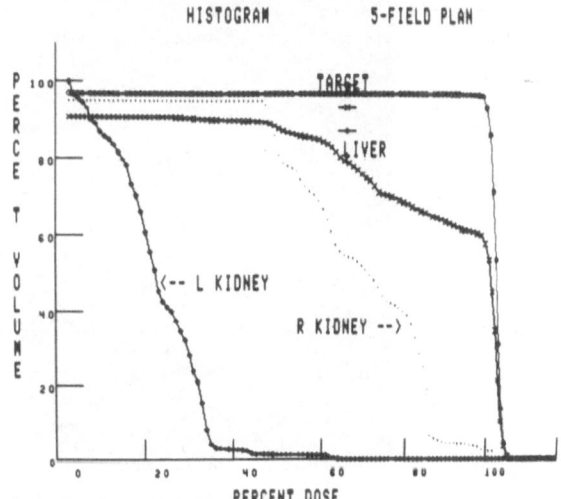

Fig. 20. A dose–volume histogram for a patient with hepatoma. The target volume receives full dose throughout the treatment. The liver receives a partial dose, the left kidney is receiving considerably less than the right kidney as would be expected. By contrasting dose–volume histograms for different treatment configurations, one can choose between rival plans

is worthy of study is the dose-difference display. In this display the dose distribution for one plan is subtracted from another plan and areas of difference, greater or lesser dose, are highlighted in color (Fig. 21). This display can emphasize and quantitiate where plans are different. By combining the dose-difference display with 3D graphics, one has a start on the complex process of 3D plan intercomparison. A great deal of work needs to be done in this area. Simply knowing that two plans differ in dose by a certain amount does not tell you which one is better.

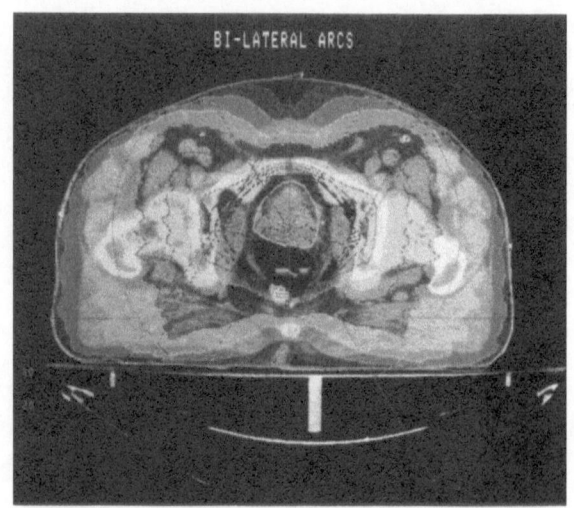

a

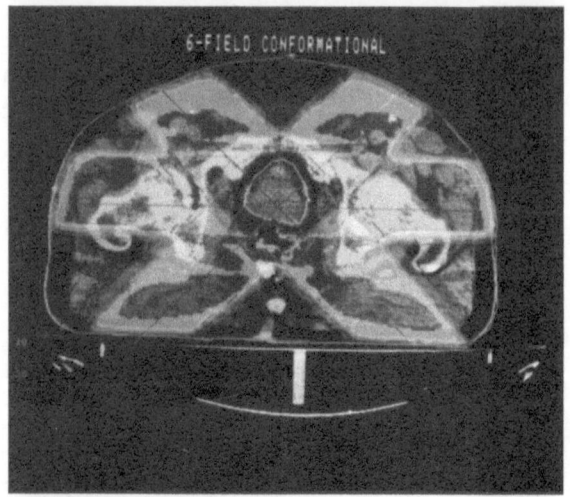

b

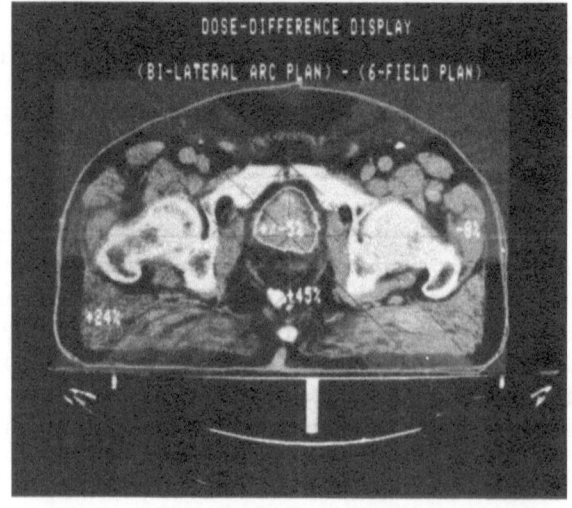

c

Fig. 22. A fully divergent radiograph digitally reconstructed from CT data. This picture has the appearance of the scout view from the CT scan, but with computer techniques, full divergence has been restored to the radiograph. It can thus be compared with simulator films or port films. To view this figure in color see Color Plates following page 78

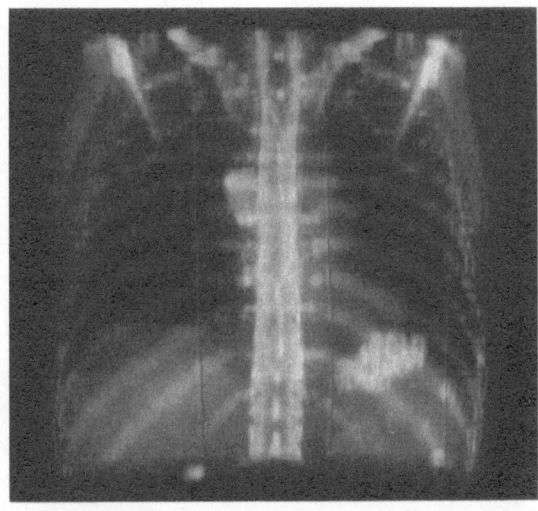

If one plan has an advantage in terms of lung dose while the other is superior in terms of cardiac dose, which one should be chosen?

A final capability needed by the 3D system is the ability to graphically generate a fully divergent radiograph [23]. The scout view of a CT scanner has divergence represented laterally but not in the superior-inferior direction. Reconstructed images that are derived from individual CT slices contain no divergence at all. Radiotherapy simulators and treatment machines have fully divergent beams and thus the planning system must be able to introduce divergence into the CT data. Divergence can be visually taken into account in the stacked CT displays previously illustrated (Fig. 8). One views the central slice edge on, the slices superior to central ray from their underside and slices inferior to central ray from their top side. By projecting the CT information onto a plane located behind the scanned object at a known distance and performing the projection from a set of ray lines originating at a single point, one can produce an image that simulates a divergent radiograph (Fig. 22). The need for these types of films becomes clear when one considers that simulator films of many non-coplanar fields cannot be taken whereas port films on the treatment machine can be obtained. Simulators have image intensifiers that give the device a C-arm configuration, and once the gantry is rotated to an oblique angle the movements of the couch pedestal are severely restricted lest the couch collide with the image intensifier. On linear accelerators without beam stoppers, the freedom of movement is much greater. If one has the ability to create a divergent radiograph from

Fig. 21a–c. Illustration of a dose-difference display. **a** A bilateral arc rotation for the boost treatment in prostate cancer. **b** The same treatment volume approached with a six-field conformational technique. **c** The two plans subtracted from each other and the dose difference displayed. Over the central prostate target volume the dose is within 5% on each plan. However, the bilateral arc plan places 45% more dose in the posterior rectal region compared to the six-field treatment plan at this slice level. The six-field plan is thus clearly superior in terms of dose to normal tissues. To view this figure in color see Color Plates following page 78

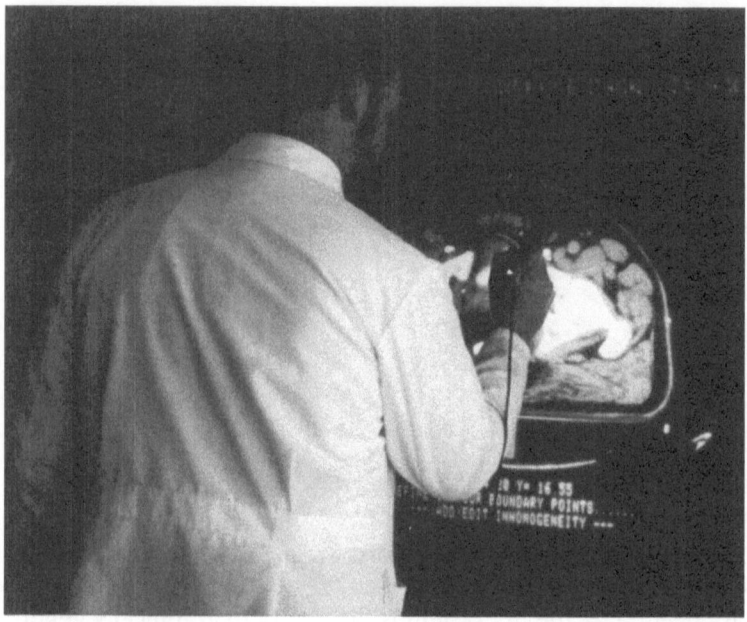

Fig. 23. The back-projection TV system for rapid entry of anatomic structures using CT scans. To view this figure in color see Color Plates following page 78

the CT data, then this image becomes the substitute simulator film to which the port film can be compared for accuracy. In many ways, a 3D treatment planning system requires the therapist to "fly on instruments," to use the aviation analogy, having to perform treatments with fields that cannot be set up and verified in the conventional manner. This will clearly produce a certain level of uneasiness until we become more secure with this new technology and until we can show that the instrument approach is accurate, reliable, and reproducible.

There are many new problems created by 3D treatment planning, aside from the verification issues just discussed, mostly revolving around the issues of speed and cost. Today most prototype fully 3D systems are relatively slow and cumbersome and take a great deal of time to operate, both in terms of data input and calculational speed. For data input, someone must enter the outline of each structure to be displayed into the planning system. For a thorax, where 10–12 structures on a slice can be required for a full anatomic reconstruction, 100 to 200 separate entries are not uncommon, consuming large amounts of time. Such data entry must be made faster. We and others have automated the entry of the external contour and the air-containing structures of lungs and trachea. We have gone further, setting up a back-projection television system which projects the CT image onto a digitizer tablet. Then, with the use of a pen for data entry, one can digitize the outline of structures into the system quickly (Fig. 23). The biggest advance in this area will come from automated structure recognition and data entry for a large number of normal anatomic structures. Such work is under development in both diagnostic and therapeutic radiology departments, and the next few years should witness dramatic progress in this area of research.

The other facet of the time required to perform 3D treatment planning relates to computer calculational speed, both for creating the displays and for calculating the dose. The problems of creating the graphics displays are being rapidly solved by a new generation of graphics display systems specifically designed to deal with 3D structures. These systems are expensive today (ranging from \$60 000 to \$120 000), but their price will surely fall in the next few years. The speed of dose calculation is a different problem. The sheer number of calculations that must be performed is staggering for a fully 3D dose calculation. Of course, much of the complexity of the dose calculation is driven by the level of dose accuracy that one is willing to accept. If one tries to calculate dose to less than a 5% error, especially if inhomogeneity corrections are required, the complexity of the calculation increases dramatically. Our system requires 10 min to calculate each photon beam in a 3D calculation of $(40)^3$ points. At Washington University, a very accurate algorithm called Delta Volume requires about 40 h to calculate the same field using similar computer hardware [21]. This is clearly an area in which different groups will choose a different approach to the tradeoffs involved.

In our opinion, one of the most important characteristics in a treatment planning system is its interactivity. It is very important that the dosimetrist and physician be able to plan in real time for maximum efficiency. It is totally impractical to envision a system wherein a beam configuration is suggested and then hours or days must elapse before dose can be displayed. If a change is then required, several more hours are needed. Such a system will stretch treatment planning for each case over several days and will simply not be used. How can the process be enhanced? The answer lies in several parts. Hardware is becoming faster, so that the brute force necessary to process a complex calculation is at hand. We estimate, for example, that the speed difference between a VAX 750 and a VAX 8800 (Digital Equipment Corp.) will be a factor of about 30. That is, a calculation that takes 30 min on the 750 will take 1 min on the 8800. Right now an 8800 is 10–15 times more expensive, but the cost of this calculational speed will drop dramatically in the future just as it has done in the past. Research is being done to streamline the calculational code so that speed is enhanced [23, 24]. Array processors can further enhance the speed of certain calculations. Finally, we must be creative in setting up systems to create a hierarchy of calculational speed and accuracy. For example, to set up beam configurations and to compare several different set ups, a very coarse calculation grid may be all that is required. Approximations which give limited calculational accuracy could be used to speed the process. Once a plan or two has been chosen, then the full detailed calculation could be performed.

Cost is another serious problem. Three-dimensional treatment planning is very labor-intensive compared to 2D planning, just as CT treatment planning (when done correctly) is more time-consuming and labor-intensive than non-CT planning. The hardware cost for a modern 3D multiuser system can be sizable (Table 2). This all increases patient cost, and the charge for 3D treatment plan-

Table 2. Components and costs of a typical multiuser 3D compatible CT treatment planning system

Item	Description	Approximate cost (in $1 000s)
Computer	32 bit at least 8 megabyte memory > 4 users	30–50
Disk storage	400 megabyte—1 gigabyte	20–50
Tape drive	1600/6250 bits per inch	10–30
Terminals	Several needed	0.8 each
Printer	Gray scale, line drawings	10–30
Digitizer	Digitizer tablet	6
Imaging system	16 bit × 512 × 512 display hardware vector generator joystick/trackball/mouse graphics processor	35–70
TV digitizer	Video digitizer + camera + stand	8
Software	Variable capabilities	30–100
	Total	160–350

ning must be greater than for 2D planning. Is it worth the price? Our patients, hospital administrators, and third party payers will demand an answer. Careful research will be required to answer this question.

An Integrated Radiographic Image of Anatomy and Tumor

Every oncologist depends heavily on radiographic imaging to help delineate the location of primary and metastatic tumors. The number of useful studies has grown in recent years. One now routinely views plain radiographs, CTs, MRIs, isotope scans, contrast studies, ultrasound scans, and even single photon emission computed tomography (SPECT) and positron emission tomograms (PETs). Each of these studies has distinct advantages in displaying tumors and normal structures. Currently we view each of these studies independently, then integrate them in our mind's eye to create the overall image of the patient's disease. Radiation oncologists are particularly dependent on analysis of X-ray and scan data to formulate their treatment.

Others have suggested [25, 26], and our experience with integrating CT and MRI has reinforced the idea, that it might be possible and certainly highly desirable to integrate all imaging into a single display, relating all studies to each other. A patient with a bile duct tumor that is poorly visualized on CT may have his data from cholangiography integrated with and superimposed on the CT image for accurate treatment planning. The data from a PET scan might be overlaid on the MRI and CT images to help differentiate between viable tumor, edema, and necrosis. The distribution of a tagged antibody as seen through the SPECT scanner might be superimposed on the CT or MRI to help calculate the dose to metastatic deposits in liver or lung. It is clear that the technology exists today to produce such integration, and we would predict that this research will result in a powerful diagnostic and therapeutic tool over the next decade.

In principle, a series of closely spaced CT scans spanning an area of interest yields a 3D grid of electron density information which defines the patient's anatomy at a level of resolution sufficient to be useful for radiotherapy planning. However, the CT scans are not always adequate for this purpose by themselves; they are useful if:

1. The patient's position during the CT study is identical to the positioning of the patient during the therapy
2. The patient is adequately marked during the CT study so that patient and beam positioning are not dependent on additional simulation-type procedures or information
3. All the diagnostic information needed to plan the case is directly imaged with the CT data (i.e., no MRI, PET, ultrasound, radiograph, or other imaging information is necessary)
4. The physician and planners have no need to visualize the CT anatomic information in views which are not transverse to the patient (i.e., no use of beam's-eye view or X-ray radiographs)

In practice, qualifications 1, 3, and 4 are never completely satisfied. It is almost always necessary to perform a simulation-type procedure before or after the CT study in order to localize the area of interest for the CT study, mark the patient's skin and verify the immobilization technique, or to verify beam placement and blocks design. In addition, attempting to perform radiation therapy planning with precision forces one to pay careful attention to maintaining a self-consistent set of patient data. One must ensure that the information transmitted to the physician from a simulator film with focused shielding blocks drawn on it agrees with the same information when presented overlaid on a 2D transverse CT slice. Finally, MRIs, ultrasound scans, and radiographs all contribute a great deal of diagnostic information that must be used quantitatively.

Incorporating patient-related data from several different sources is thus essential to the ability to plan treatment accurately in three dimensions. This capability is also the source of a major increase in complexity of the planning system. In order to make quantitative use of the various kinds of data, detailed correlation of the different images and studies into a self-consistent set of anatomically related data is often required. This data set, even in a fully 3D system, will rely heavily on the 2D images from CT, MRI, and radiographs, since a significant learning curve must be overcome before these 2D images will be replaced by 3D ones.

A few details of the method used at the University of Michigan to facilitate the integration of various imaging modalities and the synthesis of 2D gray scale images and 3D graphics are described here to illustrate the complexity of the problem. Patient-related information is stored in several different formats. All gray-scale images used in the planning system, including CT, MRI, PET, digitized radiographs, digitized isodose data, and compound B-mode ultrasound scans, are maintained in a standard image file format. This allows the substitution of one type of image directly for another if the image sets have been aligned (see Fig. 13). A second file maintains the coordinates of the 3D surfaces (see for example Figs. 16, 17) which have been abstracted from serial contours of CT or other data. The final patient-related data file describes the relationships of all the 2D images and contours and the 3D surfaces with each other. Images which come from the same self-consistent set of scans are maintained as a group ("data set"), so that one data set (for example, MRI) can be aligned with another (CT) without worrying about individual slices. Each 2D slice, set of slices, or data set can be translated, rotated, warped, and overlaid with contours and other information from other slices or data sets using a system of reference points and manual or automatic methods of correlation of the various systems.

Each one of the features described above is necessary in order to register and correlate the information in one data set with another, as is illustrated in Fig. 12 for the use of MR and CT images for treatment planning. Overlaying contours abstracted from an axial MRI scan onto the corresponding CT image immediately presents the need for fairly sophisticated methods for comparison and correlation of data from different sources. Patient positioning for different studies (for example, CT, MRI, and simulator localization) can be somewhat variable. Each of the studies may have its own inherent distortions that must be avoided or corrected. Therefore, in order to transfer a target volume from an axial MRI scan to the corresponding CT scan, one is already forced into a system which can overlay information from one type of study on that of another, can unwarp distorted images, and can deal with variable patient positioning and marking. In summary, generation of a self-consistent data set in which geometrically accurate MR and CT images can be interchangeably displayed (as in Fig. 13) requires many sophisticated image correlation tools. Progress in this area has been rapid and over the next decade we predict that this unified radiographic patient image will achieve widespread use not only in radiotherapy but in general diagnostic radiology as well.

Conformational or Dynamic Therapy

The goal of any radiation treatment is to give all the dose to the tumor with no dose going to normal tissue. Since this goal is unattainable, one tries to come as close to the ideal as possible through the use of sophisticated treatment planning. The need for minimizing normal tissue dose can be understood from analysis of the theoretical dose-response curve (Fig. 24). Let us assume for simplicity that the cell density distributions of tumor and normal tissue (P_t and P_n) are homogeneous though not necessarily equal. Similarly the cell killing effects (K_t and K_n) of each treatment fraction (G_t and G_n) are on average relatively time-independent functions during treatment. The result of n identical radiation fractions of equal time increments will result in C_t (C_n) surviving tumor (normal) cells as given by the expressions

$$C_t = P_t G_t^n K_t^n V_t \tag{1}$$

$$C_n = P_n G_n^n K_n^n V \tag{2}$$

Color Plates I–VII

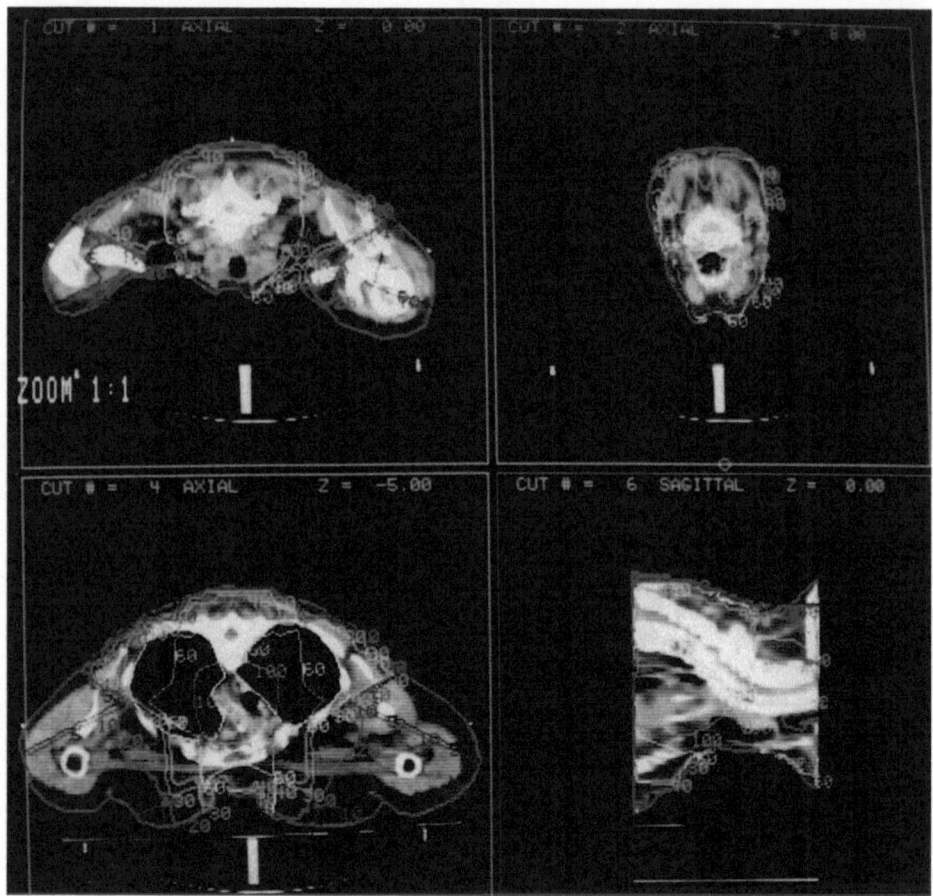

Fig. 6. Multiple CT slices displayed in a multiwindow format. Each color codes for a different dose intensity. The *reddish-brown* coloration indicates full dose; *Green* and *blue* colors are low-dose regions. In the *lower right hand corner* is the saggital dose distribution. The spinal canal and vertebral column can be seen making an S-shaped course through this volume. With special angulation and shielding, the high-dose region is confined in front of the spinal cord. The entire spinal column is in green with a small area of pink, indicating that 60% or less of the dose is going to this structure (see p. 60)

Color Plate I

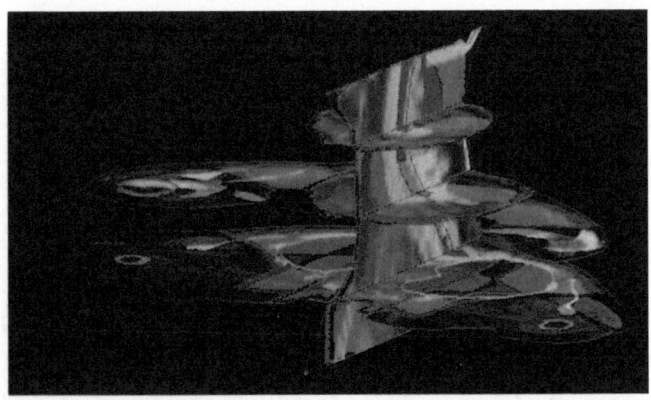

Fig. 7. The same four panels of dose information as in Fig. 6. now integrated into an anatomically correct display. Dose can be seen to spill over from the saggital plane onto the transverse planes and vice versa. This is a further step towards conceptionalizing the three-dimensionality of radiotherapy treatment planning (see p. 61)

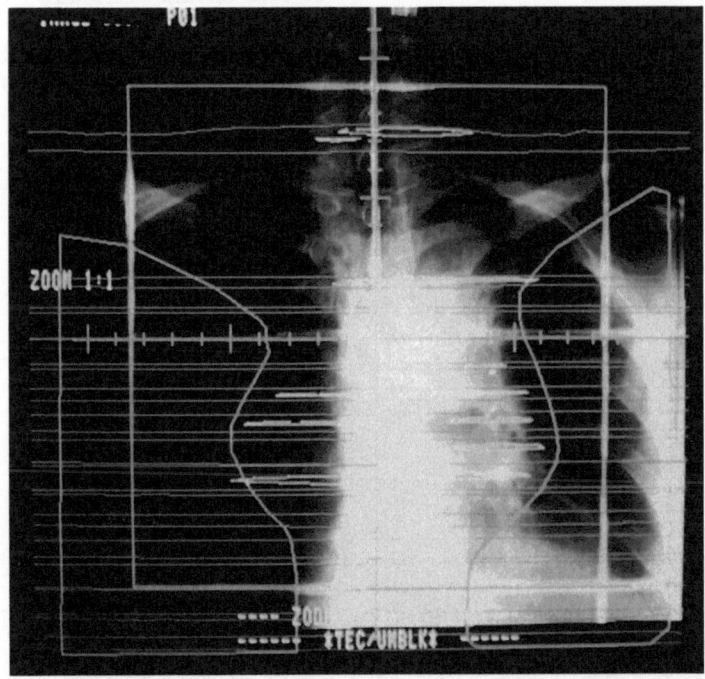

Fig. 8. The "beam's eye view" display. The *blue* lines represent the CT slices. The *pink* outlines represent the target volume on each slice. The *white* lines outline the field size necessary to treat this target volume. Adjustments can be made to the field location and size and block shape to ensure proper coverage of the volume (see p. 61)

Color Plate II

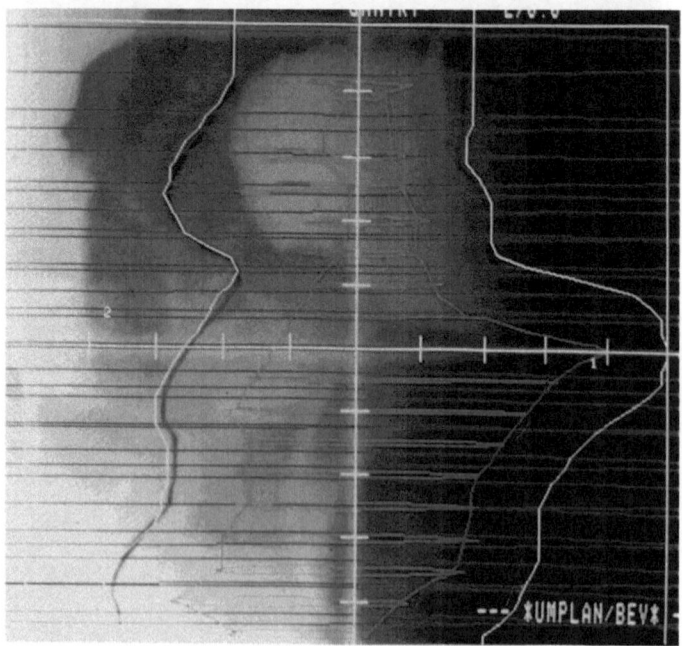

Fig. 10. A block design for the prostate tumor volume. A 1-cm margin has been taken in all directions. This block design superimposed on the CT target volumes is the most accurate way to draw shielding blocks (see p. 62)

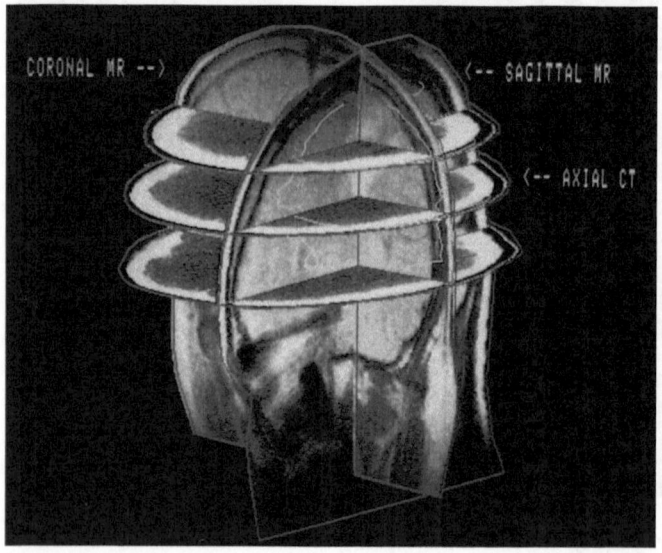

Fig. 13. Once integrated, CT and MR images can be used interchangeably, as on this display where different studies are integrated in a single picture (see p. 65)

Color Plate III

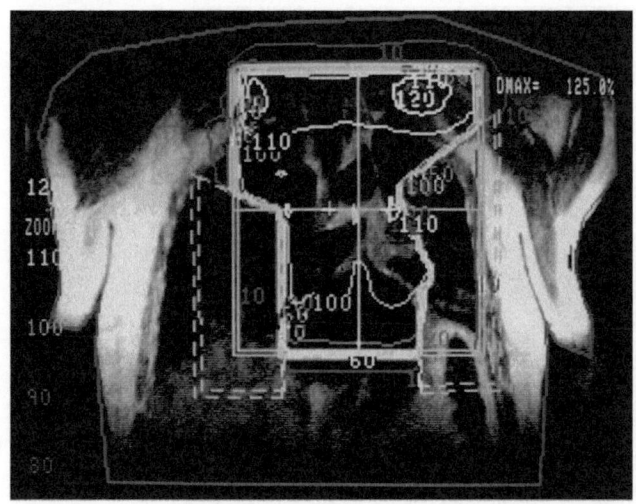

Fig. 14. Dose displayed on a coronal MRI slice in a patient with cancer of the left lung. The full effects of beam diversion, dose near the edges of the blocks, and dose under blocks are completely accounted for in this display (see p. 66)

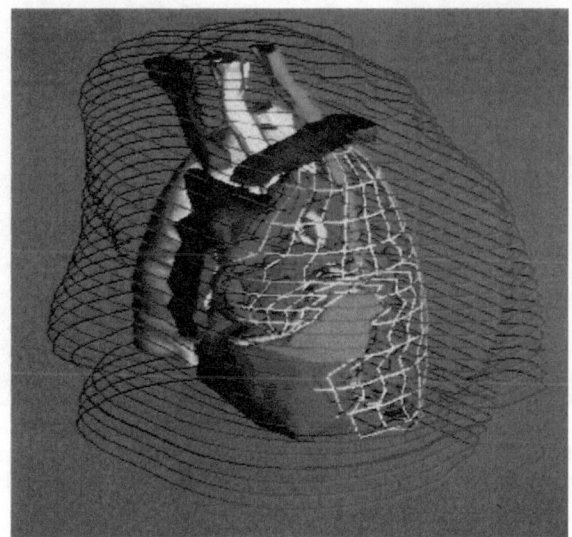

Fig. 17. A complete 3D reconstruction of a lung tumor. The external contour of the patient is seen in *blue* lines. The trachea and lungs are in *white*. The left lung has been made transparent to see the tumor (*pink* structure) and pulmonary arteries (*blue*) through the lung. The heart and aorta are in *red*, the spinal cord in *green*, the esophagus in *yellow*, and the bones of sternum and clavicles in *brown*. The reconstruction can be rotated to view from any angle. Pictured here is the left superior oblique view (see p. 69)

Color Plate IV

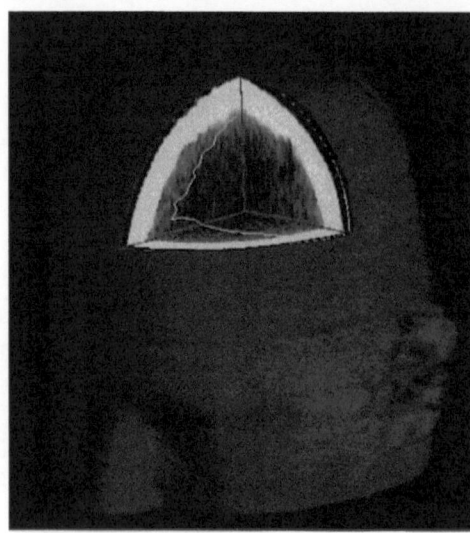

Fig. 18. A 3D reconstruction for a brain tumor case with a wedge-shaped cutout through the target volume. CT data appears on all three surfaces. This cutout can be moved, enlarged, or reoriented until the best reinforcement of internal versus external anatomy is created (see p. 70)

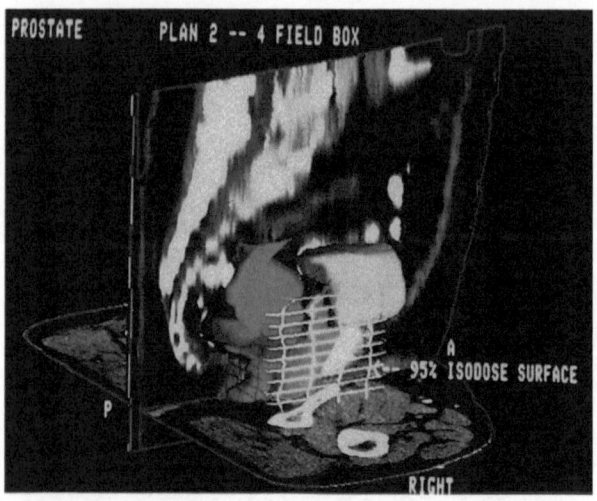

Fig. 19. In this four-field boost (anterior, posterior, left and right lateral fields) for prostate cancer, the volume that is encompassed by the 95% isodose line is displayed as a wire frame (see p. 71)

Fig. 21a–c. Illustration of a dose-difference display. **a** A bilateral arc rotation for the boost treat- ▷ ment in prostate cancer. **b** The same treatment volume approached with a six-field technique. **c** The two plans subtracted from each other and the dose difference displayed. Over the central prostate target volume the dose is within 5% on each plan. However, the bilateral arc plan places 45% more dose in the posterior rectal region compared to the six-field treatment plan at this slice level. The six-field plan is thus clearly superior in terms of dose to normal tissues (see p. 72)

Color Plate V

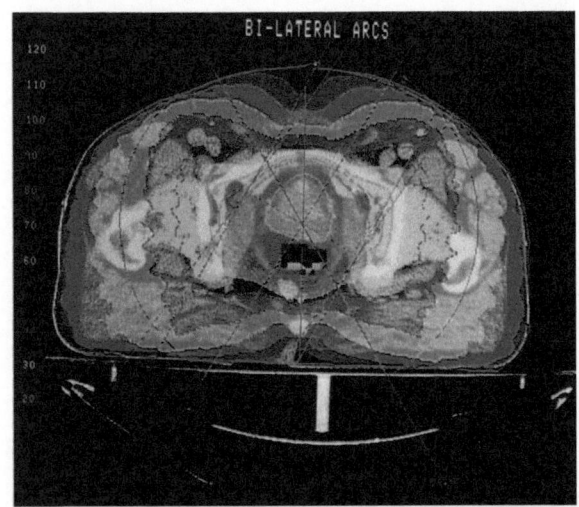

a BI-LATERAL ARCS

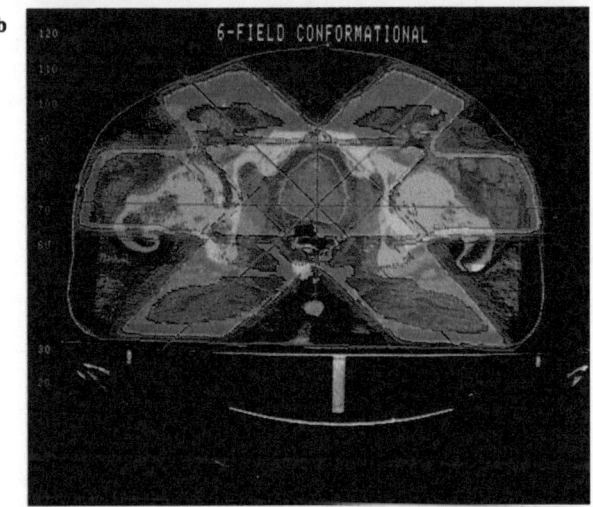

b 6-FIELD CONFORMATIONAL

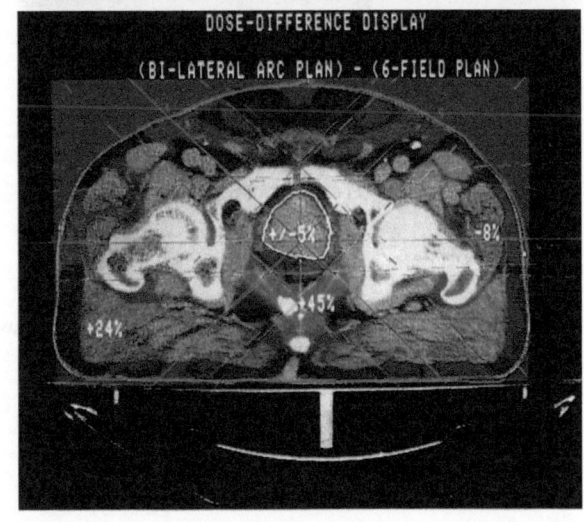

c DOSE-DIFFERENCE DISPLAY
(BI-LATERAL ARC PLAN) - (6-FIELD PLAN)

Color Plate VI

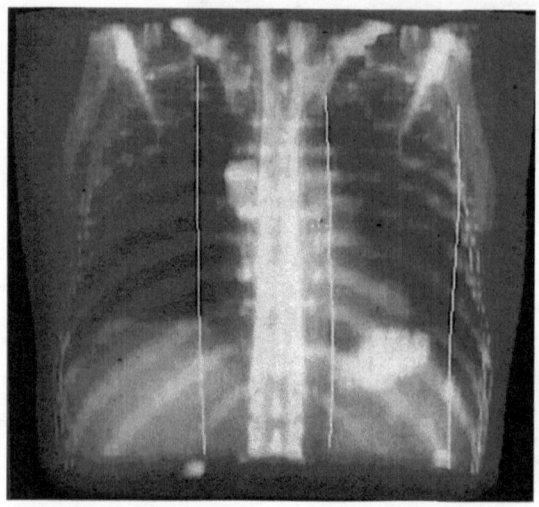

Fig. 22. A fully divergent radiograph digitally reconstructed from CT data. This picture has the appearance of the scout view from the CT scan, but with computer techniques, full divergence has been restored to the radiograph. It can thus be compared with simulator films or port films (see p. 73)

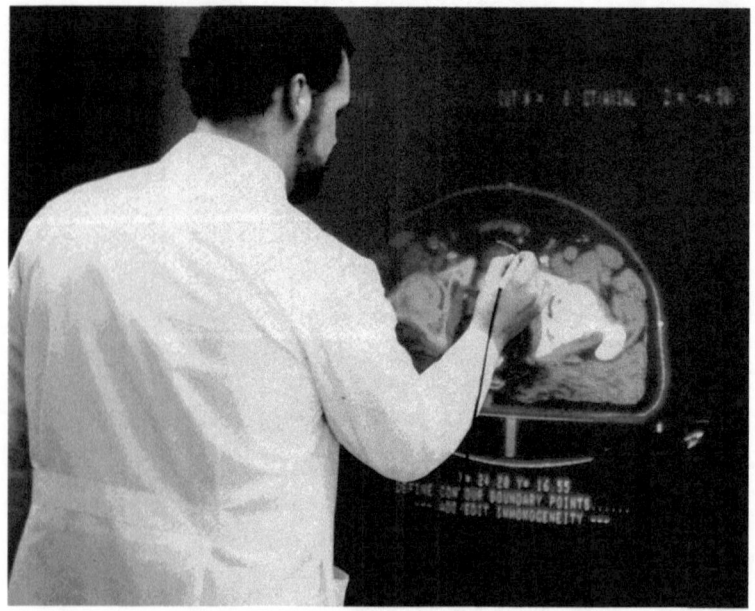

Fig. 23. The back-projection TV system for rapid entry of anatomic structures using CT scans (see p. 74)

Color Plate VII

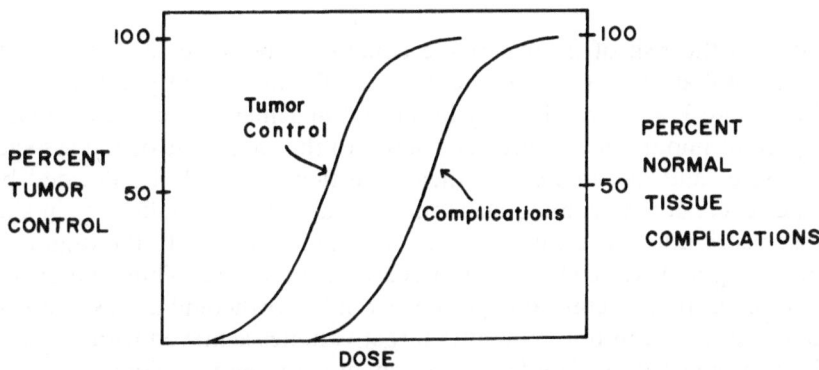

Fig. 24. The theoretical sigmoid curve for tumor control and complications as a function of dose

where V_t and V are the tumor and target volumes respectively, and where we remember that in practice $V_t < V$ due to the need to surround the tumor with a margin of safety. In addition we must pay attention to the 'entrance/exit' volume (V_e) which consists of all irradiated (to a lesser dose) normal tissue outside the target volume. Analogously to the above, we would have for the cells in that volume

$$C_e = P_e \, G_e^n \, K_e^n \, V_e \tag{3}$$

where P_e, G_e, and K_e are suitable averages over the volume V_e. Relative value judgements determine which normal tissue parts of the $V + V_e$ volume are more important; such judgements are usually decided by clinical experience. The practice of radiotherapy has established how far one can go in dose relative to given field sizes in specific anatomic sites before normal tissue tolerance is exceeded with appreciable certainty. This prescribed dose is, in effect, a measure of normal tissue tolerance and, relative to the dose fraction size, establishes the number of fractions permitted. Empirical methods for varying n and the dose/ fraction as well as time spacing between treatments have been developed and are summarized in [27].

C_t has been assumed by many authors [28, 29] to be related to cure via

$$\text{local cure probability} = e^{-C_t}. \tag{4}$$

This is the Poisson expression for the probability of zero survivors when the expected number is C_t. This naturally leads to the sharp dose response curve for cure (local control), as shown in Fig. 24. It is also assumed that a similarly sharp mathematical function holds for normal tissue tolerance. The degree of sharpness of both responses is debatable and will not be addressed here. Regardless, it is clear that in radiotherapy we desire to keep $C_n + C_e$ (surviving normal cell population) as large as possible, simultaneously making C_t (surviving tumor cell population) as small as possible. All things being equal, it is clear from Eq. 1 that the smaller the tumor/target volume, the easier it is to reduce C_t to small final values. Additionally, the smaller V_t and V become, the smaller V_e becomes, thus reducing the risk of normal tissue complications. One sees immediately from Eqs. 1–4 that the need to restrict the target volume tightly to the tumor volume (i.e., make $V = V_t$) can be very important in achieving our stated goal [30]. The degree of importance is directly related to the sharpness of the associated dose responses and the answers to these questions can only be decided by clinical experience. It is becoming clear that our ability and confidence in shaping the dose distributions (i.e., in restricting the target volume to the tumor volume) is increasing and will continue to increase in the future. Thus one expects that a new generation of clinical experience will be forthcoming, based on the higher tumor doses permitted by smaller target volumes achieved with confidence from the new generation of radiation treatment planning techniques.

To date, the best methods devised for restricting and shaping the dose distribution involve the use of multiple fields with beam shaping provided from custom-shaped blocks. If one treats a tumor with anterior-posterior opposed fields, then one creates a block of dose that extends from one side of the body through to the other (Fig. 25a). While some situations demand this approach, in general this treatment technique does not minimize normal tissue exposure. A refinement of this technique is to add lateral or oblique fields to restrict the high dose region to a cube or box shape (Fig. 25b). This is a step in the right direction, but few tumors are cube-shaped and further reduction of the irradiated volume is possible. Another method of restricting dose is to rotate the field, creating a cylinder of dose (Fig. 25c). However, the cylinder must be as large as the largest dimensions of the tumor in any direction, again losing some dose to normal tissue. The ideal field configuration would have the beam aiming at the tumor from multiple directions with the beam shape adjusted at each angle to correspond to the exact shape of the tumor (Fig. 25d). This technique is known as conformational therapy, an idea that has been researched for two decades [31–33].

How many fields are enough? No one has yet studied this question. If one is using a series of fixed fields with shielding blocks, then there is a practical limit to the number of fields possible due to treatment machine time: each time the gantry is moved to a new angle, the technologist must go into the room and change the blocks in the machine head. It is likely that between six and eight fields are all that can be employed in this fashion. We have begun to explore this technique in the treatment of prostate cancer. Our former boost technique involved a bilateral arc rotation, a relatively standard approach. This technique encased the prostate and seminal vesicles in a cylinder of high dose. The cylinder was placed as far anterior as possible in an attempt to protect the rectum (Fig. 21a). Our new technique involves the use of six fixed fields as illustrated (Fig. 21b). The CT scan is used to outline the prostate and seminal vesicle volume on each slice (typically 20–30 slices). The CT data are viewed from the six angles using beam's-eye view. Shielding blocks are drawn using the autoblock function to create a 1.0-cm margin around the target. The patient is set up isocentrically in the exact position used for arc rotation. The six fields are treated independently. A dose difference display (Fig. 21c) comparing the dose from the arc to that from this six-field plan shows the savings in dose to the rectum with the new

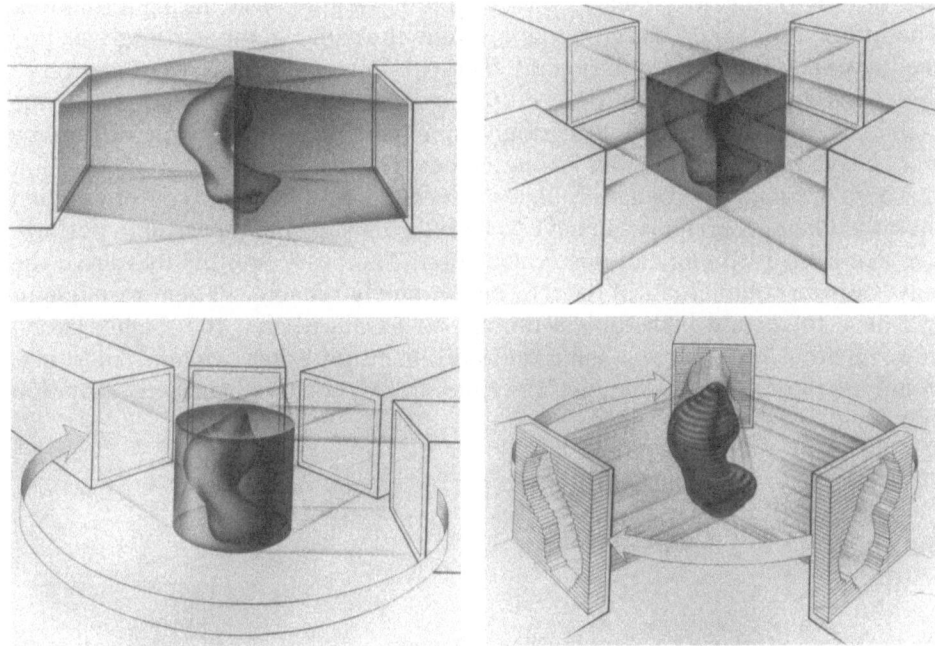

Fig. 25. a A tumor approached with a pair of opposed fields. The tumor volume is adequately covered but large amounts of adjacent tissue are treated. **b** The tumor is now approached with a four-field crossfire technique that creates a box of high dose. The tumor is adequately treated and smaller amounts of normal tissue receive dose compared to the two-field plan illustrated in **a**. **c** A rotation is now used, creating a cylinder of high dose. This further restricts the dose that normal tissue receives but there is still a substantial amount of tissue outside the tumor volume that receives the full tumor dose. **d** A fully conformational treatment. The shape of the field is adjusted through multiple collimator leaves that can move during the rotation. At each angle of treatment, the shape of the individual leaves is adjusted to precisely conform to the tumor shape. In this fashion an extremely tight dose distribution is created and the maximum amount of normal tissue is spared

technique compared to the standard rotational fields. The dose to the target region is preserved, as evidenced by a zero dose difference. Since the rectum is a major source of morbidity in the curative treatment of prostate cancer, it is difficult to discount the importance of a technique which lessens dose to this critical normal structure.

A full rotation can be thought of as a large series of fixed fields strung together. The ultimate conformational therapy would involve a rotation wherein the field shape could be altered while the rotation was in progress, always having the field to conform to the shape of the tumor. Such dynamic conformational therapy is certainly possible [31–33]. The easiest way to visualize accomplishing such therapy is by using a field-shaping collimator that is made up of 30–40 thin leaves, each capable of independent motion. Such multileaf collimators have seen use over the last decade, and at least one commercial manufacturer has made a multileaf system available for sale (Scanditronix AB, Uppsala, Sweden).

By using the beam's-eye-view option in the planning system, one could adjust the location of the 30–40 leaves on a degree-by-degree basis during a rotation. The information could be fed to the machine through a computer interface and the leaves could be driven during the therapy. One could conceive of motion of the couch and non-uniform dose output or gantry speed to further shape the high-dose volume. There is little doubt that some form of this type of therapy will be commercially available within the next decade.

There are many potential problems associated with dynamic conformational therapy. Planning systems will have to be fully 3D and very powerful to perform the treatment planning and dose calculation. The 60–80 motors that drive the leaves of the collimator will have to be extremely reliable. Patient throughput will have to remain high for the therapy to be affordable. It is highly likely, however, that research will solve these problems and that dynamic conformational therapy will become the next major treatment advance in radiation oncology.

Summary

Radiotherapy treatment planning has achieved new levels of sophistication in recent years, and the future for continued improvement is bright. During the next decade, tumor localization will become more precise, using fully 3D displays of integrated radiographic imaging data. Compiling this display will be largely automatic using artificial intelligence concepts and automatic structure recognition computer programs. Radiotherapy treatment will progress to conformational therapy where extremely precise dose distributions will closely follow the contours of the tumor. This will allow increased dose to the tumor without an increase in normal tissue dose. Local control and cure rates will thus be enhanced.

Acknowledgement. We would like to acknowledge the financial support provided by Scanditronix; the figures were produced by their treatment planning system.

References

1. Bornford CK, Craig LM, Hanna FA, et al. (1981) Treatment simulators. Br J Radiol [Suppl] 16: 1–31
2. Johns HE, Cunningham JR (1983) The physics of radiology, 4th edn. Thomas, Springfield, pp 337–339
3. Tsien KC (1955) The application of automatic computing machines to radiation treatment planning. Br J Radiol 28: 432

4. van de Geijn J (1965) The computation of two and three dimensional dose distribution in Co^{60} therapy. Br J Radiol 38: 369–377
5. Sterling TD, Perry H, Katz L (1964) Automation of radiation treatment planning IV. Br J Radiol 37: 544–550
6. Kaplan HS (1980) Hodgkin's disease, 2nd edn. Harvard University Press, Cambridge, Mass., p 376
7. Batho HF (1964) Lung corrections in Cobalt 60 beam therapy. J Can Assoc Radiol 15: 79–83
8. Sontag MR, Cunningham JR (1978) The equivalent tissue-air-ratio method for making absorbed dose calculations in a heterogeneous medium. Radiology 129: 787–794
9. Goitein M (1979) Computed tomography in planning radiation therapy. Int J Radiat Oncol Biol Phys 5: 445–447
10. Lichter AS, Fraass BA, van de Geijn J, Fredrickson HA, Glatstein E (1983) An overview of clinical requirements and clinical utility of computed tomography (CT) based radiotherapy treatment planning. In: Ling CC, Rogers CC, Morton RJ (eds) Computed tomography in radiation therapy. Raven, New York, pp 1–21
11. Van Dyk J, Battista JJ, Cunningham JR, Rider WD, Sontag MR (1980) On the impact of CT scanning on radiation planning. Comput Tomogr 4: 55–65
12. Glatstein E, Lichter AS, Fraass BA, Kelly BA, van de Geijn (1985) The imaging revolution and radiation oncology: use of CT, ultrasound, and NMR for localization, treatment planning and treatment delivery. Int J Radiat Oncol Biol Phys 11: 299–314
13. Ragan DP, Perez CA (1978) Efficacy of CT-assisted two-dimensional treatment planning: analysis of 45 patients. Am J Roentgenol 131: 75–79
14. Goitein M, Wittenberg J, Mendiondo M, Doucette J et al. (1979) The value of CT scanning in radiation therapy treatment planning: a prospective study. Int J Radiat Oncol Biol Phys 5: 1787–1798
15. Lee DJ, Leibel S, Shiels R, Sanders R et al. (1980) The value of ultrasonic imaging and CT scanning in planning the radiotherapy for prostatic carcinoma. Cancer 45: 724–727
16. Lee KR, Mansfield CM, Dwyer SJ, Cox HL, Levine E, Templeton AW (1980) CT for intra-cavitary radiotherapy planning. AJR 135: 809–813
17. McShan DL, Silverman A, Lanza DN, Reinstein LE, Glicksman AS (1979) A computerized three-dimensional treatment planning system utilizing interactive color graphics. Br J Radiol 52: 478–481
18. Goitein M, Abrams M, Rowell D, Pollar H, Wiles J (1983) Multidimensional treatment planning II: beam's-eye-view, back projection and projection through CT sections, Int J Radiat Oncol Biol Phys 9: 789–797
19. Goitein M (1982) Limitations of two-dimensional planning programs. Med Phys 9: 580–586
20. McShan DL, Fraass BA, TenHaken RK, Jost RJ (1985) Three-dimensional electron beam dose calculations and dosimetric evaluations (abstract) Med Phys 12: 507
21. Wong JW, Henkelman RM (1983) A new approach to CT Pixel-based photon dose calculations in heterogeneous media. Med Phys 10: 199–208
22. Order SE, Kopicky J, Leibel SA (1979) Principles of successful treatment planning. Hall, Boston
23. Boyer AL, Mok EC (1984) Photobeam modeling using fourier transform techniques. Proceedings 8th international conference on the use of computers in radiation therapy, Toronto, IEEE Computer Society Press, Silver Spring, MD, pp 14–16
24. Siddon RL (1985) Prism representation: a 3D ray-tracing algorithm for radiotherapy applications. Phys Med Biol 30 (8): 817–824
25. Chen GTY, Kessler M, Pitluck S (1985) Structure transfer in three dimensional medical imaging studies: Proceedings national computer graphics association meeting. IEEE Computer Society Press, Silver Spring MD, pp 171–177
26. Coffey CW, Hines HC, Wang PC, Smith SL (1984) The early applications and potential usefulness of NMR in radiation therapy treatment planning. Proceedings 8th international conference on the use of computers in radiation therapy, Toronto, IEEE Computer Society Press, Silver Spring, MD, pp 173–180
27. Orton CG, Ellis F (1973) A simplification in the use of the NSD concept in practical radiotherapy. Br J Radiol 46:529:537

28. Porter EH (1980) The statistics of dose/cure relationships for irradiated tumors. Br J Radiol 53: 210–227
29. Munro TR, Gilbert CW (1961) The relationship between tumors lethal doses and the radiosensitivity of tumor cells. Br J Radiol 34: 246–251
30. Brahme A (1984) Dosimetric precision requirements in radiation therapy. Acta Radiol 23: 379–391
31. Takahashi S (1962) Conformation radiotherapy rotation techniques as applied to radiography and radiotherapy of cancer. Acta Radiol [Suppl] 242: 57–59
32. Mantel J, Perry H, Weinham JJ (1977) Automatic variation of field size and dose rate in rotation therapy. Int J Radiat Oncol Biol Phys 2: 697–704
33. Levene MB, Kijewski PK, Chin LM, Bjarngard BE, Hellman S (1978) Computer-controlled radiation therapy. Radiology 129: 769–775

4. Hyperthermia as Cancer Therapy: Current Status and Future Prospects

H.I. Robins*

Although hyperthermia is currently an experimental therapeutic modality, anti-cancer effects of elevated (noncauterizing) temperature were first observed in ancient Egyptian times [1]. Hippocrates later incorporated fever therapy into a homeopathic approach to disease. During the nineteenth century, Coley reported an anecdotal series of cancer patients responding to fevers induced by erysipelas and bacterial endotoxins [2], and his observations have stimulated a number of novel approaches to cancer therapy, including immunotherapy and hyperthermia. In 1953, Warren induced "artificial fevers" using diathermy in conjunction with incandescent light bulbs and also described antineoplastic activity [3]. A methodical evaluation of the potential value of hyperthermia has been undertaken only in recent years. The hypothetical basis for the use of hyperthermia as cancer therapy by these early clinical workers can, at best, be described as intuitive.

During the past two decades, however, a considerable data base, including both laboratory and clinical studies, has been accumulated, which provides a sound rationale for the continued exploration of the role of hyperthermia in cancer therapy. The effect of elevated temperatures on cell viability has been well documented [1, 4–12]. Hyperthermia has also been shown to potentiate the cytotoxic effect of ionizing radiation and certain drugs on malignant neoplasms [1, 4–12]. It is less certain whether cancer cells are inherently more sensitive than normal cells to the damaging effects of hyperthermia, although examples of such differential sensitivity have been reported [13–22]. Although there may not be a universal increased sensitivity of all types of cancer to heat, in comparison with normal cells, leukemias and lymphomas may represent a general group of neoplasms which is unusually heat sensitive [10]. The biological basis for this is not clear; nevertheless, anecdotal response data from clinical experience, as well as an informal survey of animal data, suggest that the role of hyperthermia in the treatment of the leukopoietic neoplasms deserves special attention [10, 16–22].

Although temperatures in excess of 41°C will kill cells exponentially as a function of time and temperature—with S phase cells being particularly sensitive [1, 7, 8, 11, 18, 23]—the direct killing effects of heat may have limited clinical utility, and hyperthermia is unlikely to play a significant role in cancer therapy when

* American Cancer Society Fellow, supported in part by USPHS Grant R01-CA35361, awarded by the National Cancer Institute, DHHS.

used as a sole treatment modality [1, 7, 24]. Hyperthermia alone has produced disappointingly poor response rates, as well as short response durations [1, 24–27]. The possible biological basis for these observations is discussed in an insightful review by Oleson and Dewhirst [1]. The value of hyperthermia in the future is therefore more likely to reside in its use as an adjunct to other forms of therapy [24].

It has become obvious that the cell heterogeneity of various neoplasms limits the effectiveness of any given form of therapy, including radiation, chemotherapy, hyperthermia, or immunotherapy [24, 28–30]. A combined modality approach diminishes the chances that a subpopulation of tumor cells may be, or may become, resistant to therapy. Thus, the observation that hyperthermia, which is not intrinsically myelosuppressive, can potentiate the tumoricidal effects of radiation, chemotherapy, and immunotherapy [1, 5,7, 8, 11, 24] makes its use as part of a multimodality treatment approach attractive [24, 31]. In addition to potentiating the cytotoxic effect of conventional therapeutic modalities, hyperthermia can also alter the effects of certain noncytotoxic drugs on tumor cells [24]. Such drugs, known as *labilizers*, have no activity against neoplastic cells at normothermic temperatures but promote antineoplastic cell kill in the setting of hyperthermia. Anesthetic agents represent one class of such drugs [22, 32–34]. It is of interest that some labilizers, e.g., lidocaine and thiopental, seem to exhibit selective neoplastic cell kill at drug levels which are clinically acceptable [22].

Systems developed for clinical hyperthermia fall into three major categories: (a) local, (b) regional, and (c) systemic, or whole body.

Local Hyperthermia

Local hyperthermia can be accomplished with several different technologies (e.g., capacitive and inductive, radio frequency, ultrasound, and microwave) [1, 7, 11, 35, 36]. Most early clinical reports are anecdotal in nature, due in part to problems relating to thermometry. Further, study populations frequently included only patients with solitary lesions; hence, comparative data on response rates in matched tumors were not provided. In a controlled study with paired lesions, the effect of radiation alone can be compared with that of hyperthermia plus radiation. Controlled studies of this type, which support the use of local hyperthermia in conjunction with radiotherapy, have recently been reported [25–27, 37–40] (Table 1).

Two problem areas in local hyperthermia studies which must be addressed are invasive thermometry (i.e., the measurement of intratumor temperature) and uneven tumor heating. The uneven heating produced by current local hyperthermia technologies is particularly significant since the work of Oleson and Dewhirst supports the conclusion that it is the lowest temperature achieved in a tumor mass that is the best predictor of response [1, 40–42].

Table 1. Local hyperthermia—controlled clinical trials

Heat source	Number of lesions	Treated lesions with complete response %		Reference
		Radiation alone	Radiation plus heat	
Ultrasound	>30[a]	46% of patients had a superior response in the heated lesion		[26]
Radio frequency	33	50	65	[37]
Radio frequency	86	33	80	[25]
Microwave or radio frequency	123	39	76	[38]
Microwave	48	58	79	[39]

[a] This study contained patients with multiple lesions. Similar lesions in a given patient were matched, and data were reported in terms of the number of patients (7/15) having a superior response to heat plus radiation.

As cancers which are refractory to standard therapy tend to be disseminated, local hyperthermia has been currently relegated to a palliative role. As technology develops, however, it may have curative potential in the treatment of some primary cancers, e.g., primary head and neck, cervical, and CNS cancers, particularly when used in combination with other modalities.

Regional Hyperthermia

Deep regional hyperthermia has been somewhat hampered by the same technological limitations described for local hyperthermia; invasive thermometry is accordingly beset with even more difficulties. Several different methods of generating heat have been developed, including electromagnetic induction heating by circumferential coil, microwave, and ultrasound [1, 43–48]. Several reports by Storm et al. [43, 44] describing regional hyperthermia with or without radiation or chemotherapy indicate that this approach is feasible. However, as heating sessions (time-temperature profiles) are not reproducible for a given patient, and even less reproducible between patients, it is extremely difficult to carry out valid, controlled, randomized trials of regional hyperthermia. The development of appropriate instrumentation for specific anatomical sites, e.g., the pelvis, which can assure the reproducible delivery of a given thermal dose is a major challenge for workers in this area.

Limb perfusion hyperthermia for the treatment of sarcomas and melanomas was first reported in 1967 by Cavaliere et al. [8, 49], and later by Stehlin et al. [50]. Impressive response rates were obtained when hyperthermia was combined with chemotherapy. These studies were retrospective and relied on historical controls, so that they must be interpreted with caution. Some observers consider that these nonrandomized studies represent the most impressive historical argu-

87

ment for clinical hyperthermia. A recently published prospective randomized trial done by Ghussen et al. [51] in Germany demonstrates the efficacy of perfusional hyperthermia. Additional controlled multiinstitutional clinical trials of regional hyperthermia are currently in progress in Italy and Sweden.

Whole-Body Hyperthermia

As whole-body hyperthermia (WBH) addresses the issue of systemic disease, it offers perhaps the greatest potential for hyperthermia to be used as an adjunct to other therapies, with curative intent.

In published reports of phase I trials of WBH in humans, core temperatures have been maintained at 41°C–42°C for several hours with variable morbidity and occasional mortality [3, 9–12, 52–59]. The variety of WBH methods currently available reflects a lack of consensus as to the best application of physiological and physical principles to systemic hyperthermia. Most technologies for WBH include a requirement for general anesthesia with endotracheal intubation, as well as complex equipment to regulate patient temperature [4, 9, 10–12]. Worldwide, the system most used has been the extracorporeal approach developed by Parks et al. [8, 54]. Studies to date have demonstrated the feasibility of extracorporeal heating in combination with both radiation and chemotherapy, and significant response rates have been reported in nonrandomized studies. Similarly, the hot-water suit system, developed by Bull et al. [8, 55], has undergone extensive clinical trials [12]. This system has been modified and now includes mechanical ventilation [59].

Englehart et al. initiated the first randomized study, which compares 40.5°C WBH plus chemotherapy with chemotherapy alone in patients with small-cell lung cancer [60]. This study utilizes a diathermy hot-air system, in which the peak core temperature achieved is significantly below the 41.8°C obtained with other methods. Preliminary results of this study favor the WBH arm [61].

In spite of its potential, many workers have not been enthusiastic about WBH due to concerns relating to toxicity, the need for mechanical ventilation, the complexity of instrumentation and monitoring during treatment, and the lack of ability to deliver multiple treatments to a single patient in a given week [11, 12]. In this regard, Robins et al. have recently reported on a radiant heat system for 41.8°C WBH [62], which is safe, simple in operation, does not require general anesthesia with endotracheal intubation, allows for multiple treatment sessions per week, and lends itself to a multimodality approach. A phase I clinical trial of WBH (which incorporates the labilizers—lidocaine and thiopental—discussed above) has been completed, and second-generation studies, based on preclinical murine studies, have been initiated at the Wisconsin Clinical Cancer Center [10, 24, 62]. These studies include chemotherapy and WBH, total-body irradiation (TBI) and WBH, interferon and WBH, local radiotherapy and WBH, and WBH combined with supralethal chemotherapy and ablative TBI as part of a bone marrow transplant proconditioning regimen.

As of December 1987, the Wisconsin group has incurred no significant hyperthermia toxicity in more than 500 treatments. Responses observed have been encouraging, and plans are now being made to begin randomized prospective multiinstitutional trials with this system.

Hyperthermia in Combined Modality Therapy

As innovative technological research has improved the future potential of hyperthermia, similarly exciting pharmacological developments have kept pace. A class of chemotherapeutic drugs which have activity as single agents, are nonmyelosuppressive, and are both hyperthermia and radiation sensitizers would be ideal for use in the multimodality approach considered earlier. Lonidamine is an example of such a drug [24, 63]. Clinical trials involving lonidamine combined with radiation and/or hyperthermia are in progress [24]. Kubota et al. (using the drug bleomycin) have recently reported on such a trimodality approach in patients with bladder cancer [31].

Although use of hyperthermia in patients with metastatic disease may, in the future, prove to be both palliative and even curative, WBH may play its most significant role in the adjuvant setting (i.e., to sterilize micrometastases in patients rendered free of gross or detectable disease by surgery, but at risk for relapse, e.g., stage II breast cancer or Duke's C colon cancer). The hypothetical rationale for the use of systemic hyperthermia in combination with chemotherapeutic agents as adjuvant therapy has recently been outlined [24].

Although the scientific rationale for hyperthermia is unequivocal, its fulfillment as a cancer therapy requires further basic research and controlled clinical trials. Five thousand years have passed since the first record of a patient being treated with hyperthermia; its promise as a therapy remains.

References

1. Oleson JR, Dewhirst MW (1983) Hyperthermia: an overview of current progress and problems. Curr Probl Cancer 8: 1
2. Coley WR (1983) The treatment of malignant tumors by repeated inoculations of erysipelas: with a report of ten original cases. Am J Sci 105: 487
3. Warren SL (1935) Preliminary study of the effect of artificial fever upon hopeless tumor cases. Am J Roentgenol 33: 75
4. Milder JW (ed) (1979) Conference on hyperthermia in cancer treatment. Cancer Res 39: 2232
5. Dethlefsen LA (ed) (1982) Third international symposium: cancer therapy by hyperthermia, drugs and radiation. Natl Cancer Inst Monogr 61

6. Jain RK, Gullino PM (ed) (1980) Thermal characteristics of tumors: applications in detection and treatment. Ann NY Acad Sci 335: 1
7. Hahn GM (1982) Hyperthermia and cancer. Plenum, New York
8. Storm FK (ed) (1983) Hyperthermia in cancer therapy. Hall, Boston
9. Lowenthal JP (ed) (1984) Conference on hyperthermia in cancer treatment. Cancer Res 44: 4703
10. Robins HI, Dennis WH, Steeves RA, Sondel PM (1984) A proposal for the use of hyperthermia in treatment regimens of acute and chronic leukaemia. J Clin Oncol 2: 1050
11. Stewart JR, Gibbs FA (1984) Hyperthermia in the treatment of cancer, perspectives on its promise and its problems. Cancer 54: 2823
12. Robins HI, Neville AJ (1985) Biology and methodology of whole body hyperthermia. In: Angheleri LV, Robert J (eds) Hyperthermia in cancer treatment. CRC Press, Boca Raton
13. Giovanella BD, Morgan AC Stehilin JS, Williams LJ (1973) Selective lethal effect of supranormal temperatures on mouse sarcoma cells. Cancer Res 33: 2568
14. Kase KR, Hahn GM (1976) Comparison of some response to hyperthermia by normal human diploid cells and neoplastic cells from the same origin. Eur J Cancer 12: 481
15. Levine EM, Robbins EB (1970) Differential temperature sensitivity of normal and cancer cells in culture. J Cell Physiol 76: 373
16. Schrek R (1966) Sensitivity of normal and leukemic lymphocytes and leukemic myeloblasts to heat. J Natl Cancer Inst 37: 649
17. Symonds RP, Wheldon TE, Clarke B, Bailey G (1981) A comparison of the response to hyperthermia of murine haemopoietic stem cells (CFU-S) and L1210 leukaemia cells: enhanced killing of leukaemic cells in presence of normal marrow cells. Br J Cancer 44: 682
18. Robins HI, Steeves RA, Martin PA, Miller K, Clark AW, Dennis WH (1983). Differential sensitivity of AKR murine leukemia and normal bone marrow cells to hyperthermia. Cancer Res 43: 4951
19. Giovanella BC, Lohman WA, Heidelberger C (1970) Effects of elevated temperatures and drugs on viability of L1210 leukemia cells. Cancer Res 30: 1623
20. Flentije M, Flentje D, Sapareto SA (1984) The differential effect of hyperthermia on murine bone marrow CFU-S and AKR and L1210 leukemic stem cells. Cancer Res 44: 1761
21. Wheldon TE (1976) Exploiting heat sensitivity of leukaemic cells. Lancet 2: 1363
22. Robins HI, Steeves RA, Martin PA, Sondel PM, Yatvin MB, Dennis WH (1985) Potentiation of differential hyperthermic sensitivity of AKR leukemia and normal bone marrow cells by lidocaine or thiopental. Cancer 54: 2831
23. Henle KJ, Dethlefsen LA (1980) Time-temperature relationships for heat-induced killing of mammalian cells. Ann NY Acad Sci 335: 234
24. Robins HI (1984) The role of whole body hyperthermia in the treatment of neoplastic disease, its current status and future prospects. Cancer Res 44: 48785
25. Kim JH, Hahn EW, Ahmed S (1982) Combined hyperthermia and radiation therapy for malignant melanoma. Cancer 50: 478
26. Marmor JB, Hahn GM (1980) Combined radiation and hyperthermia in superficial human tumors. Cancer 46: 1986
27. Dewhirst MW, Connor WG, Sim DA (1982) Preliminary results of a phase III trial of spontaneous animal tumors to heat and/or radiation: early normal tissue response and tumor volume influence on initial response. Int J Radiat Oncol Biol Phys 8: 1951
28. Fidler IJ, Hart IR (1982) Biological diversity in metastatic neoplasms: origins and implications. Science 217: 998
29. Leith JT, DeWyngaert JK, Dexter DL, Calabresi P, Glicksman AS (1982) Differential sensitivity of three human colon adenocarcinoma lines to hyperthermic cell killing. Natl Cancer Inst Monogr 61: 381
30. Calabresi P, Dexter D, Heppner G (1979) Clinical and pharmacological implications of cancer cell differentiation and heterogeneity. Biochem Pharmacol 28: 1933
31. Kubota Y, Shein T, Mura T, Nishimura R, Fukushima S, Takai S (1984) Treatment of bladder cancer with a combination of hyperthermia, radiation and bleomycin. Cancer 53: 199
32. Yatvin MB, Clifton KH, Dennis WH (1979) Hyperthermia and local anesthetics: potentiation of survival in tumor-bearing mice. Science 205: 195

33. Robins HI, Dennis WH, Slattery JS, Lange TA, Yatvin MB (1983) Systemic lidocaine enhancement of hyperthermia-induced tumor regression in transplantable murine models. Cancer Res 43: 3187
34. Yau TM (1979) Procaine-mediated modification of membranes and the response to x-irradiation and hyperthermia in mammalian cells. Radiat Res 80: 523
35. LeVeen HH, Wapnick S, Piccone V, Falk G, Ahmed N (1976) Tumor eradication by radio-frequency therapy. J Am Med Assoc 235: 2198
36. Hill CR (ed) (1982) Ultrasound, microwave, and radiofrequency radiations: the basis for their potential in cancer therapy. Br J Cancer 45: 1
37. Overgaard J (1981) Fractionated radiation and hyperthermia. Experimental and clinical studies. Cancer 48: 1116
38. Arcangeli G, Cevidalli A, Nervi C, Creton G (1983) Tumor control and therapeutic gain with different schedules of combined radiotherapy and local external hyperthermia in human cancer. Int J Radiat Oncol Biol Phys 9: 1125
39. Scott RS, Johnson RJR, Kowal H, Frishnamsetty RM, Story K, Clay L (1983) Hyperthermia in combination with radiotherapy: a review of five years experience in the treatment of superficial tumors. Int J Radiat Oncol Biol Phys 9: 1327
40. Dewhirst MW, Sim DA, Sapareto S, Connor WG (1984) The importance of minimum tumor temperature in determining early and long-term responses of spontaneous canine and feline tumors to heat and radiation. Cancer Res 44: 43
41. Oleson J, Sim D, Manning M (1984) Analysis of prognostic variables in hyperthermia treatment of 163 patients. Int J Radiat Oncol Biol Phys 10: 2231–2239
42. Oleson JR, Manning MR, Sim DA, Heusinkveld RS, Aristizabal SA, Cetas TC, Hevezi JM, Connor WG (1984) A review of the University of Arizona human clinical hyperthermia experience. Front RAdiat Ther Oncol 18: 136
43. Storm FK, Harrison WH, Elliott RS, Hatgetheofilous C, Morton DL (1979) Human hyperthermia therapy: relationship between tumor type and capacity to induce hyperthermia by radiofrequency. Am J Surg 138: 170
44. Storm FK, Elliott RS, Harrison WH, Kaiser LR, Morton DL (1981) Radiofrequency hyperthermia of advanced human sarcomas. J Surg Oncol 17: 91
45. Olesen JR, Heusinkveld RS, Manning MR (1983) Hyperthermia by magnetic induction II. Clinical experience with concentric electrodes. Int J Radiat Oncol Biol Phys 9: 549
46. Sapozink MD, Gibbs FA Jr, Gates KS, Stewart JR (1984) Regional hyperthermia in the treatment of clinically advanced deep seated malignancy: results of a study employing an annular array applicator. Int J Radiat Oncol Biol Phys 10: 775
47. Lele PP, Parker KJ (1982) Temperature distributions in tissues during local hyperthermia by stationary or steered beams of unfocused and focused ultrasound. Br J Cancer 45: 108
48. Marmor JB (1983) Cancer therapy by ultrasound. Adv Radiat Biol 10: 105
49. Cavaliere R, Moricca G, DiFilippo F, Caputo A (1980) Heat transfer problems during local perfusion in cancer treatment. Ann NY Acad Sci 335: 311
50. Stehlin JS, Giovanelli BC, deIpolyi PD et al. (1975) Results of hyperthermic perfusion for melanoma of the extemities. Surg Gynecol Obstet 140: 338
51. Ghussen F, Nagel K, Groth W, Muller JM, Stutzer H (1984) A propsective randomized study of regional extremity perfusion in patients with malignant melanoma. Ann Surg 200: 764
52. Larkin JM (1979) A clinical investigation of total body hyperthermia as cancer therapy. Cancer Res 39: 2252
53. Pettigrew RT, Galt JM, Ludgate CM, Smith AN (1984) Clinical effects of whole-body hyperthermia in advanced malignancy. Br Med J 4: 679
54. Parks LC, Minaberry D, Smith DP, Neeley WA (1979) Treatment of far-advanced bronchogenic carcinoma by extracorporeally induced systemic hyperthermia. J Thorac Cardiovasc Surg 78: 883
55. Bull JM, Leed D, Schuette W, Whang-Peng J, Smith R, Byrnum G, Atkinson R, Gottdiener J, Gralnick HR, Shawker TH, DeVita VT (1979) Whole body hyperthermia: a phase I trial of potential adjuvant chemotherapy. Ann Int Med 90: 317

56. Van der Zee J, Van Rhoon GC, Wike-Hooley JL, Faithfull NS Reinhold HS (1983) Whole-body hyperthermia in cancer therapy: A report of a Phase I–II study. Eur J Cancer Clin Oncol 19: 1189

57. Barlogie B, Corry PM, Yip E, Lippman L, Johnston DA, Khalil K, Tenczynski TF, Reilly E Lawson R, Dosik G, Rijor B, Hankenson R, Frierech EJ (1979) Total body hyperthermia with and without chemotherapy for advanced human neoplasms. Cancer Res 39: 1481

58. Wiernik PH, Aisner J (1984) Doxorubicin, cyclophosphamide, and whole body hyperthermia for treatment of advanced soft tissue sarcoma. Cancer 53: 2585

59. Cronau LH, Bourke DL, Bull JM (1984) General anesthesia for whole body hyperthermia. Cancer Res 44: 4873s

60. Engelhardt R (1983) Clinical trials on thermo-chemotherapy (TCT). TCT in small cell carcinoma of the lung. Strahlentherapie 159: 371

61. Engelhardt R (1985) Whole-body hyperthermia methods and clinical results. In: Overgaard J (ed). Hyperthermic Oncology, vol 2. Taylor and Francis, London/Philadelphia, pp 263–276

62. Robins HI, Dennis WH, Neville AJ, Shecterle L, Martin PA, Grossman J, Davis TE, Neville S, Gillis W, Rusey BF (1985) A non-toxic system for 41.8°C whole body hyperthermia: Results of a phase I study using a radiant heat device. Cancer Res 45: 3937–3944

63. Silvestrini B, Band PR, Caputo A, Young CW (1984) Lonidamine. Proc Second Symp Oncol 41: 1–124

5. Photodynamic Therapy

T.F. DeLaney

The ideal in cancer treatment is selective destruction of tumor without disruption of normal cell and tissue function. An interesting recent development in oncology has been experimental in vitro, in vivo, and clinical work with light-activated photosensitizers causing impressive cytotoxic effects that are expressed differentially in tumor and normal tissue because of preferential localization of the sensitizers in neoplastic tissue and the ability to shield most normal tissue from light exposure. This therapeutic strategy is generally referred to as *photodynamic therapy* (PDT), but it has also been termed *photoradiation, phototherapy*, or *photochemotherapy*. To assess the potential application of PDT in oncologic management, the principles of photodynamic action and relevant laboratory and clinical work to date will be reviewed.

Historical Observations

The earliest report of the action of light-activated chemicals in biologic systems was in 1900 by Raab, who described the lethal effect of light on paramecium treated with an acridine dye [1]. His work showed that neither light nor dye alone had any apparent lethal effect on the cells, but that together they were effectively cytotoxic, with a dose-dependent response demonstrable for each. Numerous other reports on sensitized photochemical processes in living systems have subsequently appeared [2], but the majority of attention in the clinic has been focused on the porphyrins. Policard [3] reported in 1924 on reddish fluorescence in experimental rat sarcomas illuminated by a Wood's lamp. He attributed the fluorescence to excitation of endogenous porphyrins accumulating in the tumor site because of secondary infection by hemolytic bacteria. Lipson et al. [4] reported on the use of hematoporphyrin derivative (HpD) for fluorescence detection of tumor tissue in 1961, and subsequently on the treatment of a patient with recurrent breast cancer using HpD and localized exposure of the tumor to light in 1966 [5]. Diamond et al. [6] reported in 1972 on destruction of glioma cells in tissue culture and subcutaneously transplanted gliomas in rats with hematoporphyrin and visible light. Dougherty et al. [7] at Roswell Park reported in 1975 on the eradication of nearly 50% of subcutaneously transplanted tumors in mice and rats using intraperitoneally administered HpD and red light directed to the tumor. This was achieved without excessive damage to surrounding uninvolved skin in the light field.

Kelly and Snell [8] reported in 1976 on preferential HpD fluorescence in malignant and premalignant lesions in the urinary bladder. They included observations from treatment of a single case of human bladder cancer with HpD activated by light from a mercury lamp directed into the bladder with a glass light guide. They observed treatment effects only in those areas which had been illuminated.

These encouraging early reports on the potential utility of HpD for tumor localization and treatment, as well as the recent development of appropriate high-output laser and fiber-optic systems for light delivery, have provided the impetus for the current interest in this field. Indeed, numerous clinical and experimental investigations with HpD PDT have been pursued to examine possible efficacy in a variety of tumor sites. Before reviewing these studies, it would be helpful to examine the photochemistry and photobiology involved in photodynamic destruction of malignant tissue.

Basic Principles

PDT involves the interaction of sensitizer, light, and oxygen (Fig. 1). The ground state sensitizer is excited by the absorption of light. Sensitizer which has been excited by light can subsequently react or de-excite in several ways, as illustrated in Fig. 2. Excited sensitizer can react (Fig. 1) through a type 1 free radical mechanism or alternatively via a type 2 reaction involving reactive singlet oxygen ($^1O_2$) [2]. Oxygen has been shown to be critical for HpD photodynamic action in vitro. Both pathways result in potentially cytotoxic oxy-products. Type 2 processes are thought to predominate in PDT. Excited singlet sensitizer can undergo an intersystem crossover, a spin inversion yielding the excited triplet state, which can interact in a spin-conserving manner with ground state oxygen ($^3O_2$) to produce reactive singlet oxygen.

De-excitation of activated sensitizer can occur in several ways, as illustrated in Fig. 2. Excited singlet sensitizer can return to the singlet ground state with either liberation of heat or emission of a photon; the latter process is called fluorescence. Excited singlet sensitizer can also undergo the intersystem crossover to yield the excited triplet sensitizer. Sensitizer in this state can either react with oxygen or undergo de-excitation with liberation of a photon; light emission in this manner is termed phosphorescence. In the case of HpD, fluorescence and phosphorescence yield light in the visible red range with a peak between 600 and 700 nm. This is the photochemical basis for the fluorescence detection of tumors. Excitation with blue-green light results in pinkish-red fluorescence in tissue which has localized photosensitizer. The first recent clinical use of HpD by Lipson et al. [4] in 1961 was in fact for fluorescence detection of tumors via endoscopy in the trachea, esophagus, stomach, and bronchial tree. Fluorescence

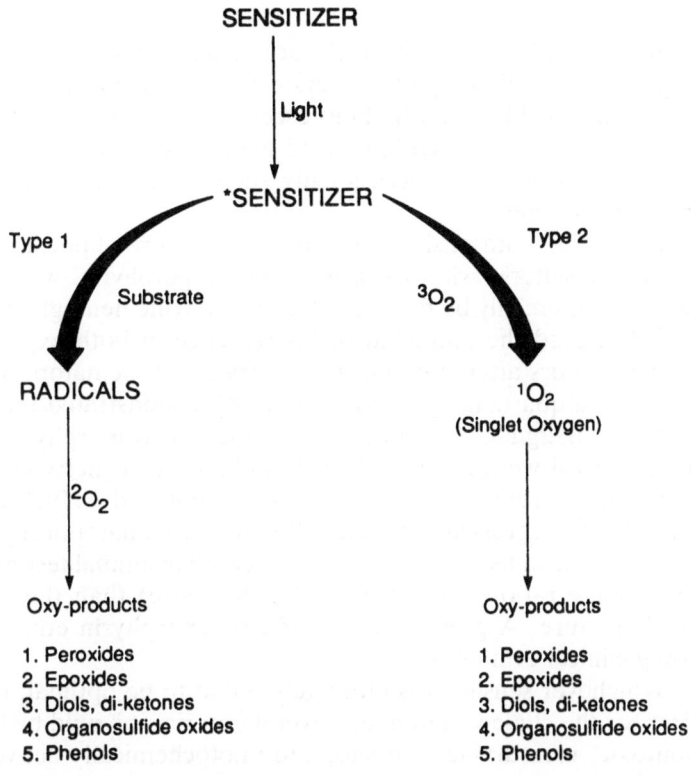

Fig. 1. Light-activated photosensitizer (*sensitizer) can interact with ground state molecular oxygen via a *type 1* (free radical) or a *type 2* (singlet oxygen) oxidative pathway to yield reactive oxygen species

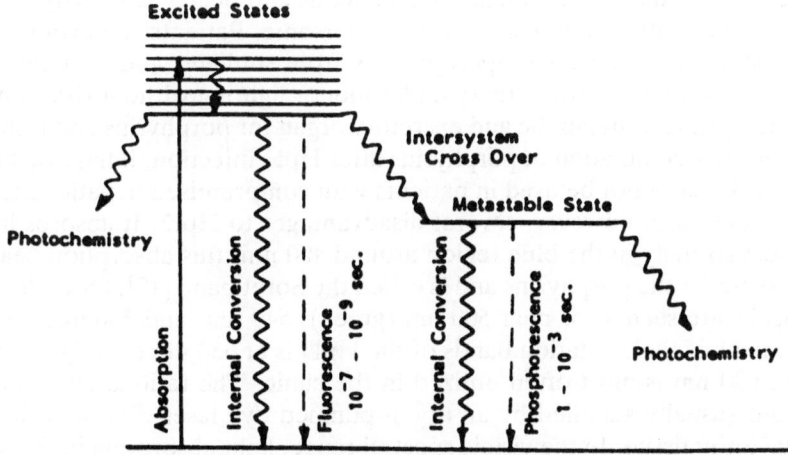

Fig. 2. Photosensitizer light absorption and possible modes of de-excitation (courtesy of D. Doiron [14])

localization of transitional cell carcinoma and carcinoma in situ, with subsequent histologic mapping of cystectomy specimens has been performed for lesions in the bladder [9]. Fluorescent areas were shown to represent either carcinoma or severe dysplasia in 15 patients studied after cystectomy, although faint flourescence was occasionally seen in regenerating mucosa surrounding fresh biopsy sites.

The HpD photosensitizer is a complex mixture of porphyrins produced by the acetic acid-sulfuric acid treatment of hematoporphyrin, which in turn is manufactured commercially by the degradation of bovine hemoglobin. Auler and Banzer [10] described the induction of fluorescence in both experimental animal and human tumors after systemic administration of hematoporphyrin and illumination with a quartz lamp. Lipson et al. [4] demonstrated that the HpD localized better in malignant tissue than the crude hematoporphyrin. Consequently, the initial clinical work in PDT utilized the HpD. Dougherty et al. [11] later purified and characterized the most active component in the HpD as an ether, although Kessel [12] suggests an ester bond linking the hematoporphyrin units. This material, whether in fact ester or ether, appeared in animal testing to provide a higher therapeutic ratio (tumor versus skin response) than the previously employed HpD mixture. A preparation of dihematoporphyrin ethers is currently undergoing clinical evaluation.

Whichever sensitizer is ultimately found to be optimal, the ideal photosensitizer for the clinic would fulfill several criteria: it would be localizable in tumor; nontoxic; measurable in tissue; and photochemically active, preferably over a relatively narrow frequency range at a wavelength with clinically applicable tissue penetration. The HpD (or the more active dihematoporphyrin compound) fulfills some but not all of these criteria. It is photochemically activated to cause unequivocal destruction of tumor, is preferentially retained by tumor compared with certain normal tissues, and is relatively nontoxic when administered systemically, although the cutaneous and ocular sensitivity to sunlight for 6–8 weeks after administration is bothersome. Patients can avoid phototoxicity by shielding themselves appropriately from sunlight, and in doing so they can carry on normal daily activity under indoor lighting without risk. Since the liver is the primary metabolic and excretory organ for porphyrins and is the site of the highest accumulation of porphyrins after HpD injection, it has also been advised that the drug not be used in patients with compromised hepatic function.

There are, however, several disadvantages to HpD. It absorbs light (Fig. 3) most strongly in the blue region around 400 nm; this absorption peak is characteristic for the porphyrins and is called the Soret band [13]. Other less prominent peaks are seen at or near 500 nm (green), 540 nm, and 580 nm. The least prominent of the excitation bands of the HpD is at 630 nm (red light); paradoxically, 630 nm is most often utilized in the clinic. The rationale for the use of red light (usually supplied by an argon-pumped dye laser; Fig. 4) is its optical behavior in tissue. In the visible spectral range, light absorption in tissue is generally inversely proportional to wavelength. Red light penetrates tissue better than green or blue light, which, although far more readily absorbed by the photosen-

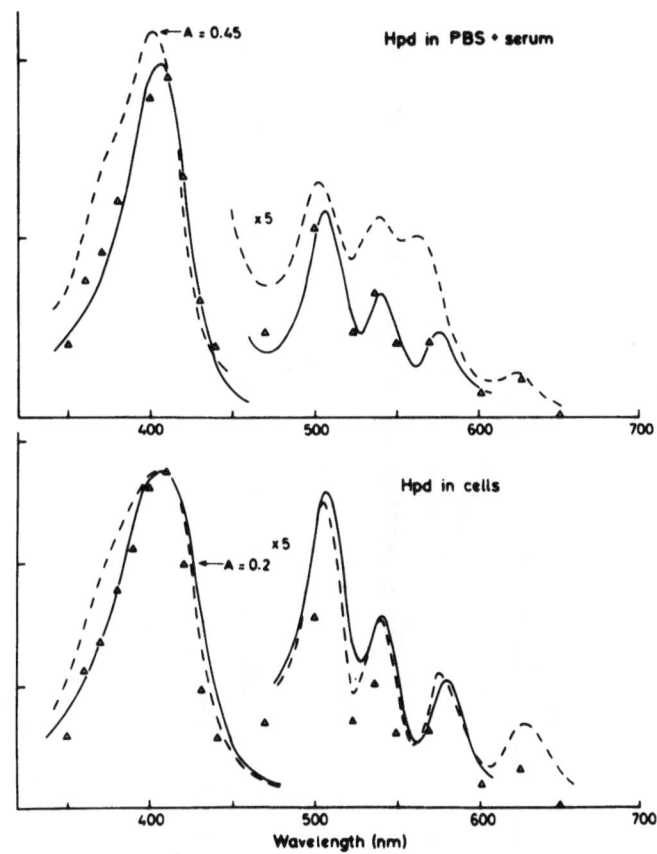

Fig. 3. HpD absorption spectra (*broken lines*), fluorescence excitation spectra (*continuous lines*), and action HpD (*triangles* cells incubated for 18 h with HpD 12.5 μg/ml in Puck's medium E2a with 3% serum). The *upper* part shows the spectra of 2.5 μg/ml HpD in phosphate buffered saline and 10% human serum, while the *lower* part shows the spectra of HpD bound to NHIK 3025 cells; the same action spectrum is shown in both parts. The cells for absorption and fluorescence were incubated for 18 h at 37°C with 50μg/ml HpD in Puck's medium E2a with 3% serum. A = absorbance. Fluorescence, excitation, and action values beyond 450 nm have been multiplied by 5. (Courtesy of J. Moan [13])

sitizing HpD, are also strongly absorbed by melanin and hemoglobin and hence have a very short range in tissue.

The penetration of red light in tissue is a complex phenomenon, dependent upon tissue density, pigmentation, blood flow, surface geometry, and tissue interfaces. As a rough approximation, incident intensity falls off exponentially by a factor of 1/e or 37% every 2 mm [14, 15]. PDT with 630 nm light produces tumor necrosis to a depth of 3–10 mm, depending on sensitizer concentration, light energy delivered, and the tissue treated. Although certain tumors such as carcinomas in situ, certain early-stage invasive lesions, some dermal malignancies,

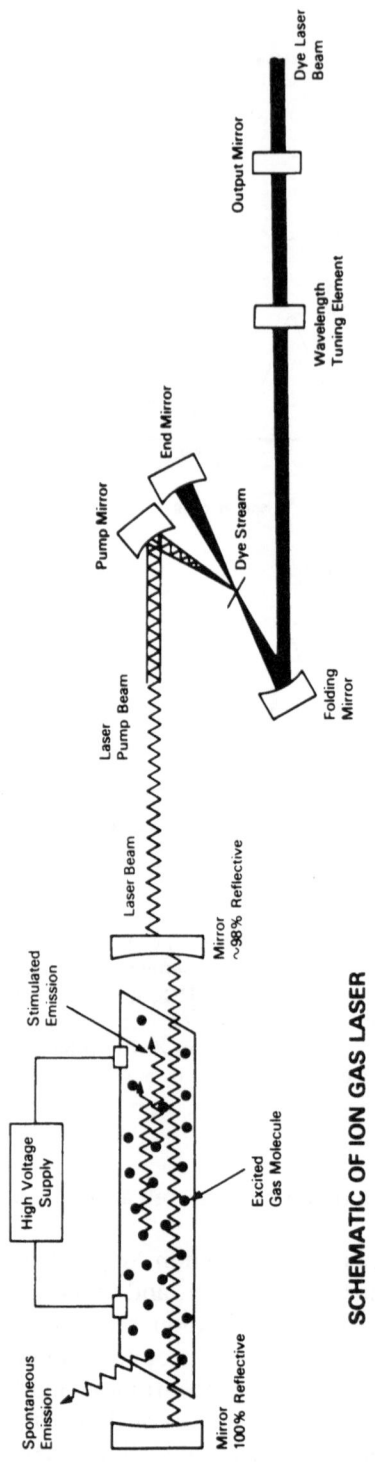

SCHEMATIC OF ION GAS LASER

SCHEMATIC OF A TYPICAL THREE MIRROR DYE LASER CAVITY

Fig. 4. The principle of the argon-pumped dye laser (modified from D. Doiron [75])

and some intraperitoneal carcinomatoses may be confined to these dimensions, light penetration with externally directed red light will not be sufficient to sterilize most tumors with a single treatment. Hence, effective use of HpD PDT with red light in the clinic will require several external treatments; placement within the tumor of interstital optical fibers; or combined modality therapy using surgery, radiotherapy, or chemotherapy to debulk tumor followed by PDT to sterilize residual tumor.

Another disadvantage of the hematoporphyrin preparation currently in use is that it in fact represents a mixture of porphyrin compounds. This makes it very difficult to study drug pharmacology, to optimize light delivery, and to predict effects on normal tissue within the light field.

In order to address some of these troubling issues, research efforts are currently directed at characterizing the active component(s) in HpD. Ongoing work has been directed as well at measuring singlet oxygen levels in order to correlate dose with response [16]. Singlet oxygen, the presumed final common mediator of photodynamic cytotoxicity, should reflect the combined effects of photosensitizer concentration and activity, light dose delivered, and tissue concentration of oxygen. In addition, research to develop other photosensitizers that satisfy the above constraints—in particular absorption at longer wavelengths with deeper tissue penetration—is in progress. The most promising of the compounds under study are the phthalocyanines [17].

PDT requires sufficient light delivery to produce effective photosensitization. The amount of light energy delivered to a particular lesion is generally expressed in joules (J) or in joules per surface area treated (i.e., joules per square centimeter). It represents the product of light output or power (in watts, i.e., joules per second) and the time of irradiation (in seconds). The energy and wavelength used are dictated by the photochemical properties of the photosensitizer, the biologic and physical characteristics of the tumor, and the mode of light delivery employed. Initial efforts with PDT employed conventional wavelength-filtered lamps, which, although generally inexpensive and reliable, were hampered by relatively low output and the inability to couple them to optical fibers, thereby making most deep lesions inaccessible.

The subsequent combination of lasers and single-strand optical fibers had a significant impact on the clinical development of PDT by permitting the effective delivery of light to deep-seated tumors, using endoscopic, interstitial (placement of optical fibers within the tumor), or intracavitary (i.e., within the bladder) techniques. Significantly higher power densities could also be achieved. The use of the laser (Light Amplification by Stimulated Emission of Radiation) in PDT differs somewhat from its use in other forms of medical therapy (Table 1). The CO_2 laser (Fig. 5) is emitted in the middle of the infrared spectrum at 10 600 nm and is efficiently absorbed by water in tissue [18]. It can cut tissue like a knife or ablate tissue by vaporization [19]. The neodymium YAG laser (Fig. 5), operating in the near infrared range at 1060 nm, is used for its thermal and coagulative properties [18] in such settings as endoscopic coagulation of bleeding varices or for management of endobronchial obstructions [19]. The primary use of the laser in PDT is to provide high-power densities of light at a desired wavelength in

Table 1. Lasers commonly used in medicine and surgery

Type	Wavelength (nm)	Tissue interaction	Application
CO_2	10 600 (infrared)	Vaporization	Cutting, ablation
Neodymium YAG	1 060 (near infrared)	Thermal	Coagulation
Argon/dye	454–514 (blue/green)	Photosensitization	Photodynamic therapy
	630 (red)		

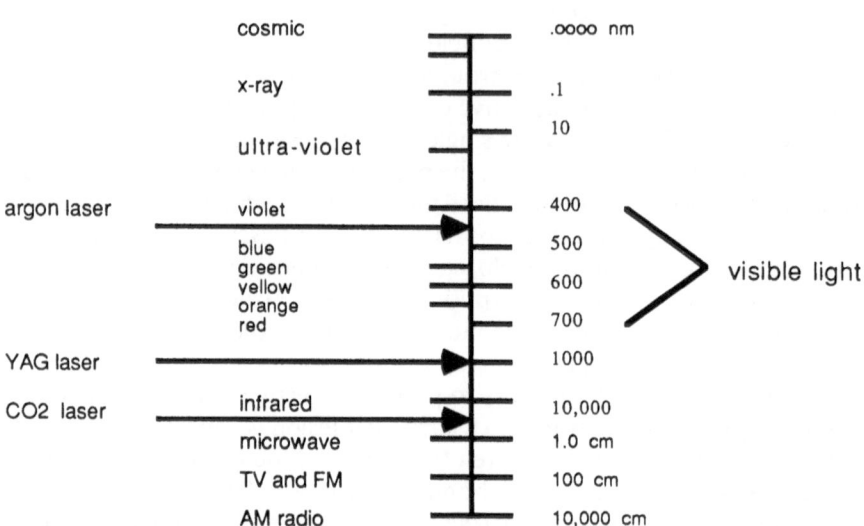

Fig. 5. The electromagnetic spectrum. (Courtesy of M. Manyak)

order to efficiently excite the photosensitizer present in tumor [20]. Thermal effect—although potentially present in varying degrees, depending on the technique of light delivery—are not necessary to effect treatment [21], as HpD activated by light alone will produce marked cytotoxicity [22].

The laser systems in use for clinical PDT are the argon-pumped dye and the pulsed metal vapor lasers, which can deliver 4–5 watts of light. A description of these systems is available in the literature [20].

The mechanism of preferential localization of HpD in tumors is not understood. There is little doubt that differential fluorescence and cytotoxicity appears between tumor and certain normal tissues in vivo; this has been reported by many independent investigators [4, 7–9]. Attempts to study the phenomenon have been hindered by the fact that HpD represents a number of porphyrin compounds with differing fluorescence quantum yields and biologic activities. Gomer et al. [23] examined the distribution of [³H] HpD and [¹⁴C] HpD in malignant and normal tissue in the mouse at various times after intraperitoneal injection. Interestingly, label counts were higher in tumor than in skin or muscle at all times sampled from 1 to 72 h after injection. However, counts in liver, spleen, and kidney were consistently higher than those in the tumor. Hence, the concentration of this mixture of porphyrins in tumor is not necessarily higher than that found in certain normal organ systems. Conversely, these investigators noted fluorescence only in tumor tissue and not in any other organ system, including liver or spleen. It was not clear whether this represented a difference in optical properties of these organs because of darker pigmentation or whether they retained different, nonfluorigenic porphyrin moieties or catabolized porphyrin products than the tumor.

Bugelski et al. [24] examined the distribution of isotopically labeled HpD in murine normal and tumor tissue using autoradiography. Tumor stroma contained more labeled HpD than did the tumor cells. They postulated that higher vascular permeability and inefficient lymphatic clearance seen in tumors might account for this distribution and the differential uptake between tumor and normal tissue. Kessel and Chou [25] used gel exclusion and reverse-phase chromatography to study the localization of HpD in tumors and concluded that the most hydrophobic of the components are involved in tumor localization.

Preclinical Studies

Although an early report by Moosman et al. [27] suggested potential differences in HpD cellular uptake between normal and tumor tissue-derived cell lines, the majority of work with in vitro cell lines indicates no such clearly reproducible difference. The major differences in localization between tumor and normal tissue appear to occur at the tissue rather than the cellular level. Henderson et al. [27] looked at both established and primary normal and tumor lines in vitro and found no difference in their ability to bind HpD, using scintillation counting of [^{3}H]HpD.

Christensen et al. [28] examined photodynamic effects on human, Chinese hamster, and murine cell lines that varied in their capacity to induce tumors in syngeneic, immunosuppressed mice. The found no evidence that cells with differing tumor-induction capacities showed any differences in relative sensitivity to photodynamic treatment in vitro. Henderson et al. [29] found that RIF mouse tumor cells were more sensitive than EMT-6 tumor cells to photodynamic treatment in vitro; paradoxically, the reverse appeared to hold for PDT in vivo.

The association between the loss of cellular viability and inhibition of membrane transport, as well as the localization of HpD fluorescence in a membrane fraction, suggests that membrane targets are likely sites of cellular inactivation by the combination of HpD and light [30]. The actual target or site of inactivation, however, has not been identified. Many types of cellular injury have been reported, but plasma membrane [31, 32] or mitochondrial injury [33] appear to be the most critical for cellular destruction. Sandberg and Romslo [33] demonstrated photodynamic damage in isolated rat liver mitochondria, with uncoupling of oxidative phosphorylation, energy dissipation, inhibition of respiration, and swelling and disruption of the mitochondria. These effects could not be elicited in the absence of any one of the photodynamic components—porphyrin, light, or oxygen—again suggesting that activated oxygen products are mediating the observed cytotoxicity.

Studies by Gomer et al. [34] of HpD photoradiation effects on Chinese hamster ovary (CHO) cells showed no mutagenic activity above backround levels. This suggests that nuclear damage after HpD PDT might be relatively less pronounced than cytotoxic effects occurring elsewhere in the cell.

The site of photodynamic destruction of tumor in vivo has been ascribed to both direct cytotoxicity on tumor cells and indirect effects, possibly resulting from damage to vessels supplying the tumor. Tochner et al. [35] sterilized an ascitic murine ovarian carcinoma implanted in the peritoneal cavity of mice, using HpD and light introduced into the peritoneal cavity. As the tumor cells in this model were essentially in a suspension of ascites fluid and not vascularized, the cytotoxic effects of PDT appear to have been directly upon tumor cells themselves.

Data from Henderson et al. [29] with both EMT-6 and RIF murine tumors in vivo and in vitro suggested that mechanisms other than direct effects on tumor cells might be responsible for the cytotoxicity seen with PDT. Their work included a number of interesting observations. The RIF line was more sensitive to PDT in vitro than was the EMT-6 line. In vivo, however, a light dose of 200 J/cm^2 controlled 100% of subcutaneously implanted EMT-6 tumors in contrast to 13% of the RIF tumors. When tumors were treated with the same light dose in vivo and then immediately explanted, tumor cell clonogenicity in vitro was surprisingly found to be nearly the same as in untreated controls. If explantation and plating were delayed for varying lengths of time from 1 to 24 h, tumor cell death occurred rapidly and progressively, indicating that tumor cell damage was expressed only if the cells remained exposed to the in situ environment after treatment. This suggested that other host-related factors, such as photodynamic effects on vasculature, are involved in tumor cell death in vivo.

Work by Star et al [36] with tumors sandwiched in transparent observation chambers showed that blood vessels in the tumor began to empty, with blanching of the tumor, about 10–15 min after PDT. Blood flow returned if the initial PDT was not too extensive; however, in cases where illumination was continued for long periods, circulation would slow, ultimately stop, and be followed by diffuse hemorrhage.

Skin lesions in patients treated with PDT show pronounced vascular changes [37]. Treated lesions manifest a predictable series of visible changes and wheal formation within the 1st h after therapy. Lesions will then go on to display a purplish discoloration within the next few hours, which gives the tissue a contused or purpuric appearance. Necrosis and eschar formation in areas of treated tumor will then appear over a period of several days to weeks, depending on the dose delivered and the size of the area treated. Laser Doppler blood flow measurements show dramatic increases in blood flow in the region of treated tumor during therapy, with subsequent decreases in blood flow over the next 1–24 h to a level usually below that seen in tumor and approximating that seen in normal tissue. Residual pulsatile tumor blood flow has been demonstrated in all of the cases measured, even in tissues where subsequent necrosis has occurred. The light doses employed in the treatment of patients have been generally three to fivefold lower than those used in experimental work with murine tumors, which may account for some of the differences observed in vascular responses to PDT. Laser Doppler blood flow measurements with subcutaneously implanted RIF tumors in the mouse are currently in progress to compare vascular responses with those observed in patients. Interestingly, blood flow will increase in nonilluminated areas adjacent to treatment fields, suggesting the release and diffusion of vasoactive mediators from the treated areas of these patients [37].

Preclinical trials of PDT in animal models included work in several anatomic sites. Jocham et al. [38] looked at the effects of PDT on the Brown-Pearce carcinoma transplanted into the urinary bladder of rabbits. They noted that HpD was preferentially taken up and retained by the tumor. In additon, they were able to destroy tumor without excessive damage to normal urothelium.

Hayata et al. [39] studied methylcholanthrene-induced tumors in canine bronchi. Six of seven animals showed fluorescence of HpD at the tumor sites. Three animals were treated with HpD activated by red light delivered fiber-optically through the bronchoscope; cytologic or pathologic complete responses were seen in all of the animals at follow-up times to 6 months. Normal tissue showed no macroscopic changes; histologically, only slight degeneration and exfoliation of columnar cells were observed. Light alone, without HpD, showed no effect on the tumors.

Increased fluorescence has been seen after intravenous injection of HpD in amelanotic melanoma transplanted in the rabbit choroid compared with uninvolved choroid [40]. Gomer et al. [41] evaluated acute normal ocular tissue toxicity following single photodynamic treatments with HpD and red light directed through the pupil and onto 1 cm^2 of the retina. They were able to demonstrate ocular damage in the form of retinal edema, detachment, and necrosis at clinically relevant doses of HpD and light. The damage, while limited to the illuminated area in all but the highest doses of light and HpD, nevertheless underscores the need for careful light delivery in this setting.

Douglass et al. [42] looked at intra-abdominal treatment of rabbits in whom the Brown-Pearce tumor had been implanted into bowel, liver, pancreas, or bladder. Upon illumination of the peritoneal cavity with ultraviolet light after HpD injection, fluorescence was generally seen only in the tumor implants. Tumor necrosis was seen after treatment of the tumors with red light at doses of 30 J/cm^2 or greater. Illumination with red light below energies of 144 J/cm^2 produced little normal tissue damage.

The toxicity of the intravenous HpD alone, without light, has been assessed in Swiss HalCR (White albino) mice, with LD_{50} values of 275 mg/kg at 24 h and 230 mg/kg (male) or 180 mg/kg (female) at 14 days [43]. HpD at these doses produced degenerative changes in hepatic, renal, splenic, and thymic tissue. These doses are well above the 10 mg/kg often used in experimental mice work examining the efficacy of PDT. The dose used for human trials has been up to 5 mg/kg HpD or up to 2.5 mg/kg of the more active dihematoporphyrin ethers preparation.

The LD_{50} of these porphyrins in mice was considerably lower when the animals were also treated with full-spectrum xenon light at relatively high energies (108 J/cm^2) to the entire dorsal surface [43]. The LD$_{50}$ was 7.5 mg/kg for the HpD and 4 mg/kg for the dihematoporphyrin ethers. Death was considered secondary to a shock syndrome. When similar studies were performed in rats with hematoporphyrin doses of 20 mg/kg, no deaths occurred, suggesting a relationship to relative surface area exposure.

Clinical Experience with PDT

The clinical experience to date with PDT has been accumulated using either the HpD or the more active preparation, the dihematoporphyrin ethers (DHE). HpD is no longer commercially available in the United States, while the DHE preparation is currently available only as an investigational drug. The first systematic use of PDT in the clinic was at Roswell Park beginning in 1976 by the group led by Dougherty [44]. Their initial efforts were with cutaneous and subcutaneous malignancies. Since that time, several thousand patients have been treated worldwide for a variety of malignancies involving various sites. The majority of these patients had relapsed after or refused conventional treatment.

When reviewing the treatment reports available in the literature, it must be remembered that PDT is a local treatment modality. As such, its impact on the overall disease process will be most important when only localized disease is present. In patients with systemic disease or disease not encompassed in the phototherapy field, PDT can only be expected to yield local palliation. For patients with localized disease, PDT will only have potential curative results if the photosensitizer concentration and light energy are sufficient to sterilize tumor. Light delivery can be optimized in lesions of minimal thickness or lesions which can be interstitially implanted with light-diffusing needles. It is not surprising that investigators have shown particular interest in PDT for lesions involving skin, carcinoma in situ of the urinary bladder, endobronchial tumors, and tumors of the head and neck.

The greatest number of patients reported on have had malignancies involving the skin—primarily recurrent metastatic breast carcinoma—but patients with basal cell carcinomas, squamous cell carcinomas, malignant melanomas, mycosis fungoides, and Kaposi's sarcomas have also been treated [44–47]. Patients have received HpD by intravenous injection and have then been treated with red light, generally 72–96 h after injection. Patients have been treated with external surface illumination, interstitial implantation for larger lesions, or some combination thereof. Most patients had disease that had not been controlled by prior surgery, chemotherapy, and/or ionizing radiation. As many patients had advanced disease in other sites as well, the aim of treatment was generally control of a local disease problem.

Although investigators have used different criteria to judge response, it is clear that complete responses have been obtained even in heavily pretreated areas. All reporting investigators have remarked upon the differential response seen between tumor and adjacent normal tissue within the light field. At light doses from 20–72 J/cm^2 that may produce necrosis and control of tumor, normal skill will become erythematous and might later show some transient hyperpigmentation, but it will otherwise tolerate therapy. Treatment appears to be effective to a depth ranging from 0.2 to 1.0 cm, depending on the dose delivered, concentration of sensitizer injected, and mode of light delivery. Investigators report complete response rates generally greater than 20% and up to 80% [43].

Several factors are important, however, in determining acute tolerance of treatment, anticipated response rate, and cosmetic outcome. Treatment of small nodules is generally well tolerated, with minimal or no patient discomfort unless high-power intensities are employed and thermal effects occur. Treatment of large, ulcerated areas of tumor even at relatively low doses (e.g., 20 J/cm^2) and moderate-power intensities can result in moderate to severe discomfort requiring narcotics for control; furthermore, thick eschars may form in such fields. While such eschars can be managed with dressing changes and enzymatic debridement, they may require weeks before granulation and healing is completed.

The skin of patients with inflammatory breast carcinomas recurring diffusely in dermal lymphatics is quite sensitive to photoradiation. Although the depth of tumor in such cases may not be great, ulceration and breakdown will occur in the often extensive areas infiltrated by tumor. Unfortunately, this may occur at doses insufficient for tumor control. With tumor extensively permeating lymphatics, tumor outside the treatment field or too deep for the range of light penetration may also reseed the treated area. The literature suggests that patients who have received doxorubicin and prior irradiation to a given area may show increased normal tissue sensitivity to photoradiation [43].

In the primary skin tumors, PDT appears most effective with basal cell carcinomas, yielding good cosmetic results and durable complete responses in over 80% of cases [45, 46]. Complete responses have been seen for up to 4 years [45]. Squamous cell lesions, either skin primaries of head and neck lesions recurring in the skin, appear less responsive [46]. Pigmented melanomas are almost completely unresponsive to PDT because of extremely efficient light absorption by melanin. Unpigmented lesions, however, can be effectively controlled by photoradiation. Control of Kaposi's sarcomas up to 3 cm in diameter has been reported [47].

The best results for cutaneous and subcutaneous lesions will be seen in relatively small (less than 2 cm), discrete lesions. For primary nonmelanotic skin cancers, PDT may prove to be curative in appropriately selected cases. Most cutaneous or subcutaneous lesions thicker than 0.5 cm will probably need several external treatments or treatment by interstitial technique. In most patients with extensive, recurrent disease for which other therapy has failed, photoradiation alone will not likely prove to be curative. It may, however, be of significant palliative benefit, particularly if some reduction in tumor volume can be achieved with surgery, radiation, or chemotherapy.

Wile et al. [48] reported on 21 patients with head and neck tumors recurrent in the primary site who were treated with HpD and red light. The majority had squamous cell carcinomas that had been refractory to conventional therapy. Complete responses were seen in 6 patients (29%), and partial responses were sen in 11 patients (52%). The complete responses were durable in four of the six cases at follow-up times from 8 to 18 months. They occurred in two patients with tongue lesions, one with a soft palate lesion, and one with a nasopharyngeal lesion. In ten patients with regional head and neck cancer recurrences in soft tissues, results were less favorable: two complete responses and three partial responses were seen. In these patients, however, tumor would often recur at the margins of the treated field; the overall course of the patients' disease did not appear substantially altered by PDT.

Takata and Imakiire [49] reported on six cases of squamous carcinomas involving larynx, oropharynx, or tongue treated with PDT. They noted significant necrosis of tumor in each of the cases, but pathologic examination of biopsy and surgical specimens revealed nests of viable tumor deep beneath the mucosal surface, suggesting inadequate light delivery and dose inhomogeneity. They noted no deleterious effects on surrounding normal tissues, although localized edema was seen after the procedure, suggesting that tracheostomy for airway protection might be indicated in the case of laryngeal lesions.

One potential use of phototherapy in the head and neck might be for detection and treatment of carcinoma in situ. In such a setting, one is able to obtain optimal light distribution because of the minimal thickness of disease. One could hope to deliver effective local therapy with minimal normal tissue side effects.

In view of the grim prognosis with high-grade gliomas, there has been some interest in PDT for these tumors, Diamond et al. [6] reported on the inactivation of glioma cells in tissue culture with hematoporphyrin and light, as well as significant destruction of gliomas transplanted subcutaneously in rats. HpD, which is protein bound in serum, does not cross the normal blood-brain barrier [6]. Laws et al [50] from the Mayo Clinic reported a phase I feasibility study with photoradiation for the treatment of malignant brain tumors. All patients were felt to be surgically incurable, and conventional therapy had failed. Patients had gross recurrent tumor at the time of treatment. Five patients were studied, four of whom had primary brain tumors and one of whom had a metastatic lesion. After HpD administration, they inserted a single quartz fiber into the tumor, using stereotactic technique, and delivered 810 J of 630 nm red light. The patients appeared to tolerate treatment well. Computerized tomography (CT) scans in two of the patients demonstrated a transient decrease in either the size of the mass or resultant mass effect after the procedure. Needle aspiration specimens of tumor showed fluorescence under blue light; normal brain in the biopsy specimens did not fluoresce.

Preliminary results with treatment of brain tumors have also been reported by McCulloch et al. [51] Patients received HpD 48 h prior to radical excision of tumor. Examination of frozen section specimens under blue light ·showed fluorescence in four of nine glioblastomas and three of three metastases examined. Red light was delivered at operation to the surgical bed. Postoperatively, patients with high-grade glioblastomas also received whole-brain irradiation. Definitive conclusions about results of treatment are difficult. Three of the nine glioblastoma patients were alive after treatment, two without evidence of disease at 35 and 42 months. The investigators did note more prominent cerebral edema following PDT and hence preferred to resect tumor to leave a cavity into which swollen brain could expand. They also noted no apparent effect on the efficacy or side effects of the subsequent radiotherapy.

PDT for malignant intracranial lesions is thus under study. Clearly, to be effective, adequate light will need to be delivered to malignant tissue in which HpD is localized. The HpD does appear to reach central nervous system lesions. The more challenging problem appears to be homogeneous delivery of light to the volume of tissue infiltrated by tumor, which often extends beyond the limits of grossly evident tumor. The combination of resection with subsequent delivery of light to the tumor bed and the use of an interstitial array of light sources are both potential approaches to this problem which require further investigation.

Another potential central nervous system application for PDT might be for the treatment of meningeal disease. Generally, such disease presents as thin plaques of tumor on the meninges that could be effectively treated by red, or even less penetrating green light, which also activates the HpD. Light delivery in this setting would represent a technical challenge that would need to be addressed in appropriate animal models. The optimum mode for photosensitizer delivery—in particular, whether intrathecal administration is possible and whether it offers any advantage compared with intravenous administration— would also need to be studied.

Photoradiation has been attempted for control of choroidal malignant melanoma, a tumor managed traditionally by enucleation but treated on an investigational basis in recent years by laser photocoagulation, trans-scleral diathermy, local radiation with scleral plaques, and external proton beam irradiation. Bruce [52] reported on 11 patients treated after intravenous administration of HpD with red light delivered transcorneally, trans-sclerally, or via a combination of these approaches. Changes in the appearance of tumor masses were noted within minutes of exposure to light. In particular, there was blanching of the tumor, with the concomitant development of edema and pinpoint hemorrhages in overlying retina. The adjacent uninvolved retina did not appear to be affected by these changes. Post-treatment fluorescein angiograms showed dramatic reductions in the vascular supply to tumor. A reduction in tumor size was seen in all patients who were 5 months or longer post-treatment, with volume decreases initially identified at 10–12 weeks after therapy. The final appearance of the tumor was that of a large chorioretinal scar. Follow-up times in this series were still under a year, so long-term results are pending. Post-treatment complications included some degree of transient chemosis, iritis, and lid swelling in all patients. Exudative retinal detachment worsened or developed in 9 of the 11 patients, appearing usually within 3 days of treatment. Detachments were more extensive in patients with larger tumors. The detachment resolved within 6 weeks in six of the nine cases. Other changes noted included choroidal detachment, cataract, vitreous hemorrhage, vitreous inflammatory reaction, and reduced visual acuity. The reduction in visual acuity occurred where tumor or retinal detachment involved the macula.

Bruce [52] used high-energy densities, generally above 1500 J/cm^2 and ranging from 293 to 6800 J/cm^2 for treatment. There is no comment about the relative degree of pigmentation in the lesions treated. Melanin is an efficient absorber of red light, so that high-energy densities must be used if sufficient light is to reach the deepest portions of tumor. These light doses will, however, increase the risk of damage to uninvolved normal tissue. Indeed, Murphree and Gomer [53] concluded after treatment of eight choroidal melanomas with PDT that pigmented melanomas of even modest height would not be adequately treated by conventional PDT alone. Hence, careful follow-up reports on patients treated in this fashion will need to be seen.

Photodynamic destruction of retinoblastoma cells in vitro has also been reported [54]. Moreover, eyes of athymic mice containing human retinoblastoma have been shown to retain higher concentrations of [^{3}H] HpD that control eyes [55]. In vivo work has demonstrated regression of human retinoblastoma in the nude mouse after PDT [56] Murphree and Gomer [53] noted favorable response of individual nodules of retinoblastoma to PDT, but continued vitreous spread of disease was limiting the effectiveness of this modality in their initial group of pediatric patients.

The earliest reported clinical use of HpD was for fluorescence detection of endobronchial tumor [57]. Several groups have more recently reported on the effective use of PDT for either palliative or potentially curative treatment of endobronchial tumors. Balchum [58] reported on palliative PDT for 35 patients with obstructive tumors of the tracheobronchial tree. HpD was administered intravenously, and then red light was delivered to the lesions via the brochoscope, using either surface illumination or insertion of an optical fiber into the lesion. Patients would undergo a "clean-up" bronchoscopy within 2–3 days of treatment in order to remove tumor debris. The majority of lesions treated were primary bronchogenic tumors, but several endobronchial metastases from other sites and one benign fibrous mass were also treated. Of the 34 patients with endobronchial cancer, 33 had a complete opening-up of the bronchial lumen to its full extent, with no visible residual endobronchial tumor remaining after one or two photodynamic treatments. Reaeration of the lung on chest X-rays was seen 1–3 days following the clean-up bronchoscopy in the four patients having atelectasis of a lung or lobe. Bronchial inflammation after PDT was minimal, and mucosal edema seldom occurred.

Complications included pneumothorax in two patients within 5 days of treatment. Pulmonary hemorrhage led to death in four patients at 4–5 weeks after phototherapy. All had large necrotic tumors in the main stem bronchus. In two of these patients, autopsy was performed, revealing necrosis of tumor in the medial aspect of the main stem bronchus and of tumor in the adjacent mediastnum. As tumor necrosis was seen on bronchoscopy in these patients prior to phototherapy, it is not clear whether the treatment or the extent of tumor was responsible for the subsequent hemorrhage.

The group at the Mayo Clinic reported on treatment results in 38 patients with 40 tumors involving the tracheobronchial tree [59] All patients had undergone previous pulmonary resection for another lung cancer or were considered inoperable for medical or technical reasons. In addition, these patients had been rejected for or had failed to respond to conventional therapy with irradiation and chemotherapy. Patients were treated with 630-nm red light by either surface or interstitial illumination. They were followed with bronchoscopies at 3- to 6-month intervals after treatment for at least 2 years after documentation of a complete response, classified as no evident tumor on a chest roentgenogram, bronchoscopy, and bronchoscopic biopsies and washings. Complete responses were seen in 14 lesions in 13 patients, requiring one treatment in nine cases and two treatments in five cases. Eleven of the complete responses were maintained at follow-up periods ranging from 3 to 53 months, with a median of 29 months. Three of the lesions recurred at 9, 12, and 35 months. Of note, all of the tumors that showed a complete response were less than 2 cm^2 in surface area and radiographically occult, having been discovered on bronchoscopy. This indicates that use of this modality for curative treatment of lung lesions may be limited to carefully selected cases.

The Mayo Clinic group also noted massive hemoptysis in three patients with large obstructing tumors within weeks of phototherapy. Pulmonary compromise was also seen in two patients unable to clear necrotic debris after PDT; bronchoscopy was required to ultimately do so.

Hayata et al. [60] reported on the treatment of eight cases of early, centrally located squamous carcinomas of the lung with phototherapy. These cases were all diagnosed by bronchoscopy. Five cases were treated with PDT alone, while in the three remaining patients, surgical resection was performed after phototherapy. A complete response endoscopically and histologically/cytological was obtained in the five nonresected cases. These patients remained disease free at 11–36 months after treatment. Of the three patients in whom resection was performed, one had a complete histologic response. The other two had complete disappearance of their lesion by endoscopic examination, but residual microscopic tumor was seen in the pathologic specimen, thought to be secondary to inadequate light delivery to the deepest portions of the tumor. These results again suggest possible benefit for the treatment of early or superificial lesions in the bronchus.

PDT has been attempted for both cure and palliation of esophageal malignancies. In the United States, where the disease most often presents in the advanced stages with both bulky tumor and adjacent involvement, investigators have reported palliation of esophageal obstruction by locally advanced lesions. In Japan and China, where mass screening clinics have been able to detect early esophageal carcinomas, PDT has been attempted with curative intent.

McCaughan et al. [61] reported on the treatment of seven patients with severe or complete obstruction of the esophagus by squamous carcinoma, adenocarcinoma, or melanoma. Patients received intravenously administered HpD, followed by the delivery of red light from an argon/dye laser coupled to an optical fiber passed through a flexible esophagoscope. All of the tumors responded, and swallowing was improved for up to 11 months. Side effects of treatment were relatively minimal and included cutaneous photosensitivity; esophagitis, which was controllable with antacids and codeine, for several days; expectoration of necrotic tumor for approximately 1 week; and edema that could require esophagoscopy and dilatation 1–2 weeks after treatment. Because of the advanced nature of their cases, survival was not affected.

Aida and Hirashima [62] treated four patients with superficial carcinomas of the esophagus and five patients with more advanced disease. Of the five patients with early lesions, two had endoscopically complete responses and remained disease free at 1 and 2 years after treatment. The other two patients went on to surgical resection and were found to have residual tumor cells in portions of the tumor felt to have been inadequately illuminated. Their advanced cases showed partial responses.

Hayata et al. [63] in Japan have also treated 16 cases of early-stage gastric carcinoma. Four patients were treated by PDT alone because of medical inoperability or refusal of surgery, while the other 12 went on to resection after PDT. Complete disappearance with endoscopic visualization was obtained in all four patients treated with PDT alone. One patient remained disease free at 30 months, disease recurred in one patient at 27 months and was retreated, and two of the patients died with recurrence of disease at 5 and 13 months respectively. Of the 12 patients who went on to resection after PDT, there was no evidence of tumor in the operative specimen in five. The seven patients with residual disease in the resected specimen, however, remained disease free at 8–43 months after surgery. Complications included epigastric pain and ulcer formation that was amenable to medical management.

PDT may thus have some applicability in early-stage gastric cancer for patients who cannot undergo curative surgery. Because of the difficulty in diagnosing early-stage cases and the propensity of gastric carcinomas to metastasize to adjacent lymph nodes, however, PDT for most gastric cancers will probably be limited to palliation of medically inoperable cases.

Photodynamic treatment of 11 patients with colorectal tumors recurring in the pelvis has been reported by Herrera et al. [64] Control of recurrence was obtained in only one patient, although control of chronic pelvic pain was achieved in five patients.

One frequent recurrence pattern in patients with gastric cancers, pancreatic carcinomas, and retroperitoneal sarcomas who have undergone intraoperative radiation therapy at the National Cancer Institute (NCI) as a component of their oncologic management has been diffuse intraperitoneal dissemination of tumor (T.J. Kinsella, W. Sindelar, and E.G. Glatstein, personal communication). For such patients, PDT at the time of operation, with light delivery via a diffusing medium instilled into the peritoneal cavity, may be technically possible. If such treatment can be accomplished with acceptable morbidity, it might offer an improvement in disease control in the abdomen.

The first reported PDT in a patient was in 1976 for transitional cell carcinoma of the bladder. Kelly and Snell [8] described destruction of tumor in the subsequent cystectomy specimen only in sites that had been illuminated. Subsequent reports on treatment of urothelial malignancies have appeared, and active investigation in this area continues.

Benson et al. [65] from the Mayo Clinic were able to demonstrate localization of HpD in transitional cell carcinoma in situ and severely dysplastic epithelium in the urinary bladder after intravenous administration and subsequent illumination of the bladder with violet light. Their observations were confirmed at histologic examination after cystectomy. The only false-positive uptake appeared in healing biopsy sites.

The Mayo Clinic group [66] initially reported biposy-proven complete tumor responses in four patients with recurrent, previously treated transitional cell carcinomas of the bladder that were focally illuminated using optical fibers introduced through the cystoscope after intravenous HpD injection. Disease did, however, later recur in other sites in the bladder which had not been illuminated. Hence, the group switched to using a modified optical fiber with a spherical diffusing bulb in order to illuminate the entire bladder [67]. They have recently reported on treatment in this fashion of 14 patients with diffuse, recurrent carcinoma in situ who had refused cystectomy. Initially using a dose of 50 J/cm^2 to the entire bladder for the first five patients, they noted severe bladder irritability. After scaling the dose back to 20 J/cm^2, treatment was better tolerated. In ten patients with carcinoma in situ alone, biopsy and urinary cytology at follow-up examination 3 months after treatment showed complete disappearance of tumor. Two patients with both carcinoma in situ and papillary noninvasive lesions were noted to have disappearance of the former but persistence of the later. Of these 12 patients, 3 subsequently developed focal disease at 6–9 months after treatment. Two patients who had focal invasive carcinoma in addition to their in situ disease had persistent invasive disease after PDT, although their in situ disease was controlled. They went on to receive cystectomy.

Experience with treatment of transitional cell carcinoma of the bladder has also been reported by two groups from Japan [68, 69]. These patients had superficial bladder tumors (primarily papillary noninvasive or with invasion limited to the lamina propria), which had generally recurred after previous surgery or radiotherapy. They were able to achieve complete responses in 50%–75% of the lesions treated, with the highest complete remission rate in tumors smaller than 1 cm.

PDT has been attempted in cases of gynecologic cancer recurring in the vagina or skin after conventional treatment. Rettenmaier et al. [70] reported treating nine lesions in six patients with HpD and red light. They were able to obtain complete responses in two lesions and partial responses in four others. The only toxicity noted was cutaneous photosensitivity.

Corti et al. [71] treated seven patients with vaginal recurrences of carcinoma of the cervix, endometrium, or rectum. They achieved five complete responses and two partial responses. They reported no treatment-related morbidity.

Tochner et al. [35] were able to control an experimental murine ovarian ascites tumor in 17 of 20 animals using intraperitoneally administered HpD and four intraperitoneal light treatments. On the basis of these experimental findings, several groups have proposed trying to treat patients with minimal-thickness intraperitoneal tumor using PDT [35, 72]. Patients presenting with advanced ovarian carcinoma (stages III and IV) are recognized to have an unfavorable prognosis, with one recent series reporting a 5-year survival rate of only 15 % after surgery and combination chemotherapy [74]. The only patient who were long-term survivors were those in whom therapy was able to produce a complete clinical response or a complete pathologic response at the time of a second-look laparotomy. Patients who have residual disease in the abdomen at the time of second-look laparotomy might benefit from intraperitoneal PDT, if adequate light delivery with acceptable morbidity can be achieved.

Summary

PDT represents another potential modality in the treatment of human malignancy. Photoactivated hematoporphyrins have definite antitumor activity in both in vitro and in vivo experimental systems. Much of the early clinical work has involved treatment of patients with advanced, recurrent disease who have not responded to conventional therapy. Because encouraging responses with acceptable toxicity have been obtained in these patients, active investigation continues and is aimed at defining the most appropriate sites and applications for the technique. Because of the limited depth of light penetration in tissue, the most promising sites may be those where there is limited thickness of tumor, such as in superficial skin lesions or carcinomas in situ involving the aerodigestive tract, bronchial tree, or genitourinary tract. Other potential uses include those where PDT could be combined with surgical or chemotherapeutic debulking, such as pleural mesothelioma or advanced-stage ovarian cancer. Whether PDT can be of benefit in surgical cases where the margins of resection are close is an interesting but speculative notion at the present time.

Clinical trials with hematoporphyrin PDT in the above-mentioned sites are in progress. Laboratory work to better understand the hematoporphyrin photosensitizer and its mechanism of action also continues, as well as investigation into alternative photosensitizers with potentially improved tumor localization, less cutaneous photosensitivity, and absorption peaks at deeper-penetrating wavelengths of light. Attempts at measurement of singlet oxygen, if successful, will permit the development of more meaningful dosimetry in order to correlate tumor and normal tissue response with measured levels of the purported cytotoxic agent. These and other developments in the fields of PDT will hopefully improve therapy for patients with cancer.

References

1. Raab O (1900) Über die Wirkung fluorescierender Stoffe auf Infusorien. Z Biol 39: 524
2. Spikes JD, Straight R (1967) Sensitized photochemical processes in biologic systems. Ann Rev Phys Chem 18: 409

3. Policard A (1924) Etude sur les aspects offerts par des tumeurs expérimentales examinées à la lumière de Wood, CR Soc Biol 91: 1423
4. Lipson RL, Baldes EJ, Olsen EM (1961) The use of a derivative of hematoporphyrin in tumor detection. J Natl Cancer Inst 26: 1
5. Lipson RL, Baldes EJ, Olsen EM (1966) Hematoporphyrin derivative for detection and management of cancer. Proc IX Internal Cancer Congr 393
6. Diamond I, Granelli SG, McDonough AF et al. (1972) Photodynamic therapy of malignant tumours. Lancet 2: 1175
7. Dougherty TJ Grindley GB, Fiel R et al. (1975) Photoradiation therapy II. Cure of animal tumors with hematoporphyrin and light. J Natl Cancer Inst 55: 115
8. Kelly JF, Snell ME (1976) Hematoporphyrin derivative: A possible aid in the diagnosis and therapy of carcinoma of the bladder. J Urol. 115: 150
9. Benson RC (1984) The use of hematoporphyrin derivative (HpD) in the localization and treatment of transitional cell carcinoma (TCC) of the bladder. In: Doiron DR, Gomer CJ (eds.) Porphyrin localization and treatment of tumors. Alan R. Liss, New York, p 795
10. Auler H, Banzer G (1942) Untersuchungen über die Rolle der Porphyrine bei geschwulstkranken Menschen und Tieren. Z Krebsforsch 53: 65
11. Dougherty TJ, Boyle DG, Weishaupt KR, Henderson BA, Potter WR, Bellnier DA, Wityk KE (1983) Photoradiation therapy—Clinical and drug advances. In: Kessel D, Dougherty TJ (eds) Porphyrin Photosensitization. Plenum Press, New York, p 3
12. Kessel D (1987) Tumor localization and photosensitization by DHE and TPPS (abstract). Presented at the Clayton Foundation Conference on Photodynamic Therapy, Los Angeles
13. Moan J, Sommer S (1984) Action spectra for hematoporphyrin derivative and Photofrin II with respect to sensitization of human cells in vitro to photoinactivation. Photochem Photobiol 40: 631
14. Svaasand LO (1984) Optical dosimetry for direct and interstitial photoradiation therapy of malignant tumors. In: Doiron DR, Gomer CJ (eds) (1984) Porphyrin localization and treatment of tumors. Alan R. Liss, New York, p 91
15. Wilson BC, Jeeves WP, Lowe DM, Adam G. (1984) Light propagation in animal tissues in the wavelength range 375–825 nanometers. In: Doiron DR, Gomer CJ (eds) Porphyrin localization and treatment of tumors. Alan R. Liss, New York, p 115
16. Parker JG (1987) Optical detection of singlet oxygen produced during the photodynamic treatment of subcutaneous murine tumors (abstract). Presented at the Clayton Foundation Conference on Photodynamic Therapy, Los Angeles
17. Ben-Hur E, Rosenthal I (1985) The phthalocyanines: A new class of mammalian cell photosensitizers with a potential for cancer phototherapy. Int J Rad Biol 47: 145
18. Fuller TA (1983) Fundamental of lasers in surgery and medicine. In: Dixon JA (ed) Surgical application of lasers. Year Book Medical Publishers, Chicago, p 11
19. Dixon JA (1983) General surgical and endoscopic applications of lasers. In: Dixon JA (ed) Surgical application of lasers, Year Book Medical Publishers, Chicago, p 72
20. Wilson BC, Patterson MS (1986) The physics of photodynamic therapy. Phys Med Biol 31: 327
21. Dougherty TJ (1984) An overview of the status of photoradiation therapy. In: Doiron DR, Gomer CJ (eds) Porphyrin localization and treatment of tumors. Alan R. Liss, New York. p 75
22. Mitchell JB, McPherson S. DeGraff W, Gamson J, Zabell A, Russo A (1985) Oxygen dependence of hematoporphyrin derivative-induced photoinaction of Chinese hamster cells. Cancer Res 45: 2008
23. Gomer CJ, Dougherty TJ (1979) Determination of [^{3}H] and [^{14}C] hematoporphyrin derivative distribution in malignant and normal tissue. Cancer Res 39: 146
24. Bugelski PJ, Porter CW, Dougherty TJ (1981) Autoradiographic distribution of hematoporphyrin in derivative normal and tumor tissue of the mouse. Cancer Res 41: 4606
25. Kessel D, Chou T (1983) Tumor-localizing components of the porphyrin preparation hematoporphyrin derivative. Cancer Res 43: 1994
26. Mossman BT, Gray MJ, Silberman L, Lipson RL (1974) Identification of neoplastic versus normal cells in human cervical cell culture. J Obstet Gynecol 42: 635
27. Henderson BW, Bellnier DA, Ziring G, Dougherty TJ (1983) Aspects of the cellular uptake and

retention of hematoporphyrin derivative and their correlation with the biological response to PRT in vitro. In: Kessel D, Dougherty TJ (eds) Porphyrin photosensitization. Plenum Press, New York, p 129

28. Christensen T, Feren K, Moan J, Pettersen E (1981) Photodynamic effects of haematoporphyrin derivative on synchronized and asynchronous cells of different origin. Br J Cancer 44: 717
29. Hendersen BW, Waldow SM, Mang TS, Potter WR, Malone PB, Dougherty TJ (1985) Tumor destruction and kinetics of tumor cell death in two experimental mouse tumors following photodynamic therapy. Cancer Res 45: 572
30. Kessel D (1981) Transport and binding of hematoporphyrin derivative and related porphyrins by murine leukemia L1210 cells. Cancer Res 41: 1318
31. Dubbelman TMAW, DeGoeji AFPM, van Steveninck J (1978) Photodynamic effects of protoporphyrin on human erythrocytes. Biochim Biophys Acta 511: 141
32. Kessel D (1977) Effects if photoactivated porphyrins at the cell surface of leukemia L-1210 cells. Biochemistry 16: 3443
33. Sandberg S, Romslo I (1980) Porphyrin-sensitized photodynamic damage of isolated rat liver mitochondria. Biochim Biophys Acta 593: 187
34. Gomer CJ, Rucker N, Banerjee A, Benedict WF (1983) Comparison of mutagenicity and induction of sister chromatid exchange in Chinese hamster cells exposed to hematoporphyrin derivative photoradiation, ionizing radiation, or ultraviolet radiation. Cancer Res 43: 2622
35. Tochner Z, Mitchell JB, Smith P, Harrington F, Glatstein E, Russo D, Russo A (1986) Photodynamic therapy of ascites tumours within the peritoneal cavity. Br J Cancer 53: 733
36. Star WM, Marijnissen JPA, van den Berg-Blok, Reinhold HS (1984) Destructive effect of photoradiation on the microcirculation of a rat mammary tumor growing in "sandwich" observation chambers. In-Doiron DR, Gomer CJ (eds) Porphyrin localization and treatment of tumors. Alan R. Liss, New York, p 637
37. DeLaney TF, Bonner R, Smith P, Travis W (1987) Photodynamic therapy for surface malignancies: Clinical results and correlation with blood flow effects secondary to photoradiation (abstract). Presented at Clayton Foundation Conference on Photodynamic Therapy, Los Angeles
38. Jocham D, Staehler G, Chaussy Ch, Hammer C, Löhrs U (1981) Laserbehandlung von Blasentumoren nach Photosensibilisierung mit Hämatoporphyrin-Derivat. Urologe A 20: 340
39. Hayata Y, Kato H, Konaka C, Hayashi N, Tahara M, Saito T, Ono J (1983) Fiberoptic bronchoscopic photoradiation in experimentally induced canine lung cancer. Cancer 51: 50
40. Krohn DL, Jacobs R, Morris DA (1974) Diagnosis of model choroid malignant melanoma by hematoporphyrin derivative fluorescence in rabbits. Invest Ophthalmol 13: 244
41. Gomer C, Doiron D, Jester J, Szirth B, Murphree A (1983) Hematoporphyrin derivative photoradiation therapy for the treatment of intraocular tumors: Examination of acute normal ocular tissue toxicity. Cancer Res 43: 721
42. Douglass HO Jr, Nava HR, Weishaupt KR, Boyle D, Sugerman MG, Halpern E, Dougherty TJ (1983) Intra-abdominal application of hematoporphyrin photoradiation therapy. In: Kessel D, Dougherty TJ (eds) Porphyrin Photosensitization. Plenum Press, New York, p 129
43. Dougherty TJ (1986) Photosensitization of malignant tumors. Sem Surg Oncol 2: 24
44. Dougherty TJ, Kaufman JE, Goldfarb A, Weishaupt KR, Boyle D, Mittleman A (1978) Photoradiation therapy for the treatment of malignant tumors. Cancer Res 38: 2628
45. Dougherty TJ (1981) Photoradiation therapy for cutaneous and subcutaneous malignancies. J Inv Derm 77: 122
46. Kennedy J (1983) HPD photoradiation therapy for cancer at Kingston and Hamilton. In: Kessel D, Dougherty TJ (eds) Porphyrin photosensitization. Plenum Press, New York, p 53
47. Tomlo L, Calzavara F, Zorat PL, Corti L, Polico C, Reddi E, Jori G, Mandoliti G (1984) Photoradiation therapy for cutaneous and subcutaneous malignant tumors using hematoporphyrin. In: Doiron DR, Gomer CJ (eds) Porphyrin localization and treatment of tumors, Alan R. Liss, New York, p 829
48. Wile AG, Novotny J, Mason GR, Passy V, Berns MW (1984) Photoradiation therapy of head and neck cancer. In: Doiron DR, Gomer CJ (eds) Porphyrin localization and treatment of tumors. Alan R. Liss, New York, p 681
49. Takata C, Imakiire M (1983) Cancer of the ear, nose and throat. In: Hayata Y, Dougherty TJ

(eds) Lasers and hematoporphyrin derivative in Cancer. Igaku-Shoin, Tokyo New York, p 70

50. Laws ER, Cortese DA, Kinsey JH, Eagan RT, Anderson RE (1981) Photoradiation therapy in the treatment of malignant brain tumors: A phase I (feasibility) study. Neurosurgery 9: 672
51. McCulloch GAJ, Forbes IJ, See KL, Cowled PA, Jacka FJ, Ward AD (1984) Phototherapy in malignant brain tumors. In: Doiron DR, Gomer CJ (eds) Porphyrin localization and treatment of tumors. Alan R. Liss, New York, p 709
52. Bruce RA (1984) Photoradiation of choroidal malignant melanoma. In: Doiron DR, Gomer CJ (eds) Porphyrin localization and treatment of tumors. Alan R. Liss, New York, p 777
53. Murphree AL, Gomer CJ (1987) Treatment of ocular tumors with photodynamic therapy (abstract). Presented at Clayton Foundation Conference on Photodynamic Therapy, Los Angeles
54. Sery TW (1979) Photodynamic killing of retinoblastoma cells with hematorporphyrin and light. Cancer Res 39: 96
55. Gomer CJ, Rucker N, Mark C, Benedict WF, Murphree AL (1982) Tissue distribution of ^{3}H-Hematoporphyrin derivative in athymic nude mice heterotransplanted with human retinoblastoma. Invest Ophthmol Visual Sci 22: 118
56. Benedict WF, Lingua RW, Doiron DR, Dawson JA, Murphree AL (1980) Tumor regression of human retinoblastoma in the nude mouse model following photoradiation therapy: A preliminary report. Med Pediatr Oncol 8: 397
57. Lipson RL, Baldes EJ, Olsen AM (1961) Hematoporphyrin derivative: A new aid for endoscopic detection of malignant disease. J Thoracic Cardiovasc Surg 42: 623
58. Balchun OJ, Doiron DR, Huth GD (1984) Photoradiation therapy of endobronchial lung cancers employing the photodynamic action of hematoporphyrin derivative. Lasers Surg Med 4: 13
59. Edell ES, Cortese DA (1987) Bronchoscopic phototherapy with hematoporphyrin derivative for treatment of localized bronchogenic carcinoma. A 5-year experience. Mayo Clin Proc 62: 8
60. Hayata Y, Kato H, Amemiya R, Ono J (1984) Indications of photoradiation therapy in early stage lung cancer on the basis of post-PRT histologic findings. In: Doiron DR, Gomer CJ (eds) Porphyrin localization and treatment of tumors, Alan R. Liss, New York, p 747
61. McCaughan JS, Hicks W, Laufman L, May E, Roach R (1984) Palliation of esophageal malignancy with photoradiation therapy. Cancer 54: 2905
62. Aida M, Hirashima T (1983) Cancer of the esophagus. In: Hayata Y, Dougherty TJ (eds) Lasers and hematoporphyrin derivative in Cancer. Igaku-Shoin, Tokyo New York, p 57
63. Hayata Y, Kato H, Okitsu H, Kawaguchi M, Konaka C (1985) Photodynamic therapy with hematoporphyrin derivative in cancer of the upper gastrointestinal tract. Sem Surg Onc 1: 1
64. Herrara L, Petrelli N, Mittleman A, Dougherty TJ (1984) Photoradiation therapy in patients with colorectal cancer. Presented at Porphyrin Photosensitization Workshop, Philadelphia
65. Benson RC, Farrow GM, Kinsey JH, Cortese DA, Zincke H, Utz DC (1982) Detection and localization of in situ carcinoma of the bladder with hematoporphyrin derviative. Mayo Clin Proc 57: 548
66. Benson RC, Kinsey JH, Cortese DA, Farrow GM, Utz DC (1983) Treatment of transitional cell carcinoma of the bladder with hematoporphyrin derivative phototherapy. J Urol 130: 1090
67. Benson RC (1986) Laser photodynamic therapy for bladder cancer. Mayo Clin Proc 61: 859
68. Tsuchiya A, Obara N, Miwa M, Ohi T, Kato H, Hayata Y (1983) Hematoporphyrin derivative and laser photoradiation in the diagnosis and treatment of bladder cancer. J Urol 130: 79
69. Hisazumi H, Misaki T, Miyoshi N (1983) Photoradiation therapy of bladder tumors. J Urol 130: 685
70. Rettenmaier MA, Berman ML, Disaia PJ, Burns RG, Weinstein GD, McCullough JL, Berns MW (1984) Gynecologic uses of photoradiation therapy. In: Doiron DR Gomer CJ (eds) Porphyrin localization and treatment of tumors. Alan R. Liss, New York, p 767
71. Corti L, Tomio L, Maluta, Minucci D, Fontana M, Calzavara F (1987) The recurrence in gynaecological field treated by PDT (abstract). Clayton Foundation Conference on Photodynamic Therapy, February 1987
72. Morstyn G, Kaye A, Thomas RJ, MacRae F (1987) High dose photoirradiation therapy using the gold metal vapor laser (abstract). Clayton Foundation Conference on Photodynamic Therapy, February 1987
73. Louie KG, Ozols RF, Myers CF, Ostchega Y, Jenkins J, Howser D, Young RC (1987) Long-

term results of a cisplatin-containing combination chemotherapy regimen for the treatment of advanced ovarian carcinoma. J Clin Onc 4: 1579

74. Doiron DR (1984) Photophysics of and instrumentation for porphyrin detection and activation. In: Doiron DR, Gomer CJ (eds) Porphyrin localization and treatment of tumors. Alan R. Liss, New York, p 41

Chemotherapy

6. Very High Dose Therapy in Lymphomas and Solid Tumors

T. Philip and R. Pinkerton

Introduction

Allogenic bone marrow transplantation is now a major treatment in hematology both for severe aplastic anemia and following intensive chemoradiotherapy regimens for chronic myeloid leukemia, high-risk acute lymphoblastic leukemia, and acute myeloid leukemia. It is also the sole therapy available in some severe combined immunodeficiencies and genetic defects. In the leukemias—with the exception of the graft-versus-leukemia effect, and unlike the other conditions mentioned—the use of marrow transplantation is not therapeutic per se, but simply a method by which high-dose, often curative therapy can be given without regard to marrow toxicity. Applying the same principle to lymphoma and solid tumors has allowed the selection of the most active agents for use in combinations, at doses limited only by extramedullary toxicity. However, the availability of HLA- and DR-matched allograft is limited by the lack of a matched sibling marrow for three-quarters of all patients, and there is a high incidence of lethal graft-versus-host disease in patients aged over 35 years. Other options are to use either autologous grafts or mismatched allografts. At present, autologous bone marrow transplantation (ABMT) is clearly the alternative of choice. ABMT is currently used either to shorten the period of aplasia after nonablative high-dose chemotherapy or as a rescue after massive, presumptively lethal myeloablative chemotherapy, often with total body irradiation (TBI). The successful use of ABMT in adults was first described by McFarland [1] in 1959, and in children by Clifford in 1961 [2].

Because of clear success in leukemias—with a reported 50% cure rate for patients receiving grafts in first remission [3]—the use of very high dose therapy in lymphoma and solid tumors has been studied by several teams since 1970 [4]. The use of the dose-effect relationship rather than bone marrow transplantation is the major objective of these studies, which have been undertaken in a wide variety of tumors [5] and therefore have potential application to a large number of patients. Some of the currently published studies of very high dose therapy for malignant lymphoma or neuroblastoma are very promising, whereas others— mainly in drug-resistant solid tumors—are associated with substantial morbidity and mortality, leaving open many questions about the appropriateness of these forms of therapy [4]. In this contribution, we will review and summarize clinical studies involving very high dose chemotherapy, emphasizing future directions of research in this area.

Dose-Response Relationship of Tumor with Chemoradiotherapy

Size of dose, frequency of administration, and combination with other agents are important contributory factors for drug efficacy. The theories postulated by Goldie and Coldman in the past decade have contributed largely to a rational explanation for many of the phenomena seen in clinical practice, and to possible strategies to optimize the effectiveness of chemotherapy. They suggest that the probability of a tumor developing a drug-resistant clone follows Poisson's law and is an inherent feature of any cell population capable of spontaneous mutation. The appearance of resistance is therefore independent of prior drug exposure and relates simply to the nature of the population dynamics [6–8]. Thus, a large tumor with a high growth fraction and rapid cell turnover is statistically more likely to develop subpopulations that are drug resistant; moreover, as the tumor grows, this likelihood increases. This is consistent with the observation that, in general, tumor bulk is a prognostic feature, and despite an often initially impressive clinical response, disease progression occurs even while the tumor is still under treatment. These observations could be used as an argument for early debulking surgery, although it must be emphasized that the log reduction in tumor cell mass with surgery is generally minimal. The Goldie-Coldman arguments are consistent with the curability of some tumors by delayed surgery, where the residual, chemoresistant mass is excised. Moreover, they provide strong support for a multimodality approach in most tumors, with combinations of chemotherapy, radiotherapy, and surgery. Very high dose therapy, according to this theory, should be applied in a situation of minimal residual disease [7]; this finding is in agreement with other theories of the dose-effect relationship, such as those of Norton and Simon [9, 10].

The Goldie-Coldman hypothesis has recently led to the application of alternating noncross-resistant drug regimens, with the aim of maximizing tumor cell kill by the introduction of regimens directed against different subpopulations within the tumor. Inherent in this strategy is also the minimization of delay between courses of therapy to prevent either reemergence of a partially treated population or the development of new resistant clones [8]. The excellent review by Frei and Canellos provides a basis for the development of this concept of the dose-effect relationship [11]. It must be emphasized that in most cases the doses used in clinical practice reflect the limitations imposed by toxicity rather than the maximum antitumor activity of the drugs. Animal studies must, therefore, be viewed with some caution when considering the extrapolation of dose-effect observations to humans. With this proviso, it is clear that many useful and stimulating data have come from animal studies, which have been extensively reviewed by Brock and Schneider [12]. Schabel has also demonstrated the linear dose-effect relationship with several agents using the Ridgway sarcoma model in dogs and with this model has illustrated the supraadditive effect of some drug combinations [13]. The problem of converting response into cure in these models has also been addressed, and again, the application of dose escalation with either single agents or combinations of drugs has been shown to make this possible [14].

Fresh human tumor xenograft studies have similarly been used to demonstrate a clear dose-effect relationship [15]: melphalan, for example, has been studied using a rhabdomyosarcoma xenograft. These studies provide useful models to compare with experience in clinical practice [15]. The additional major limitation to effectiveness with dose escalation is the heterogeneity of response within tumors and between individuals [13]. The latter may be explicable to some extent by differences in the pharmacokinetic or metabolic handling of the drug, and where possible, this must be taken into consideration for each patient. However, heterogeneity within the tumor population, as demonstrated by the variable response to the same therapy in xenografts in syngeneic animals, remains an important factor [13].

Autologous bone marrow rescue following intensive cytoreductive regimens has eliminated the primary dose-limiting toxicity of most antineoplastic drugs, namely myelosuppression. This has permitted drug doses to be increased three- to ten fold above those used without marrow rescue [16]. There are, however, several theoretical problems still to be resolved in devising massive therapy protocols. These include determining the effects of extending the time of exposure to a given drug after increasing its absolute concentration [4, 16], and investigating the possible interaction of drugs and irradiation. The choice of agents at high doses has been based either on the known responsiveness of particular tumors at conventional doses of on theoretical considerations. To date, it has not proved possible to use in vitro clonogenic assays to select drug combinations, although specific resistance in vivo may in some cases be accurately predicted from these studies [17]. Recent data from the laboratory of van Hoff are of considerable interest in this regard [18], and such laboratory investigations in vitro will continue to play an important role in indicating the potential value of new drug combinations [17].

In addition to marrow toxicity, the drugs used in high-dose regimens frequently produce toxicities in other organs, particularly the oral mucosa and gastrointestinal tract, which share with the bone marrow a rapid cellular proliferation on rate [4]. Also of note are cardiomyopathy (cyclophosphamide and doxorubicin); pneumonitis [carmustine (BCNU), lomustine, and melphalan]; liver toxicity, predominantly venooclusive disease (carmustine, cyclophosphamide, lomustine, thioguanine, and busulfan); urological toxicity and acute renal failure (cyclophosphamide and melphalan) and hemorrhagic cystitis (cyclophosphamide); and encephalic complications such as leukoencephalopathy (carmustine, lomustine, methotrexate, and TBI), lethargy (all of the drugs mentioned), and seizures (melphalan and BCNU). Other toxic syndromes observed include hemolytic-uremic syndrome and Moschcowitz's disease [4]. The problems of age and of other preexisting diseases are obviously also very important in practice. More pertinently, the extent of initial disease and the nature and complications of previous chemotherapy must be taken into account in anticipating treatment-related complications after massive therapy. This has been exemplified by the observation that when one moves from phase II studies in patients who have received prior intensive and prolonged therapy to phase III studies of patients in first complete remission (CR), a marked reduction in morbidity occurs [4].

Table 1. Phase I/II dose escalation studies with or without autologous bone marrow transplantation (ABMT) in solid tumors and lymphomas

| Drug | Usual dose (mg/m²) | Maximum tolerated dose | | Dose effect[a] at maximum tolerated dose |
		Without ABMT (mg/m²)	With ABMT (mg/m²)	
Cyclophosphamide	500	8 000	8 000	15
Etoposide (VP16)	300	2 100	3 000	10
BCNU	200	600	1 250	6
Melphalan	40	100	200	5
Cis-platinum	100	250	250	>2.5
Carboplatinum	400	1 000	2 000	5
Mitomycin C	10	40	90	9
Thiotepa	30	240	1 100	38
Aziridinyl-benzoquinone	20	—	150	7
Methotrexate	500	20 000	—	40
Cytosine arabinoside	500	20 000	—	40

[a] Times the usual dose.

Phase I/II Studies of Very High Dose Chemotherapy

As shown in Table 1, a linear dose-effect relationship has been demonstrated without bone marrow support for methotrexate (40 times the usual dose) [19], cytosine arabinoside (40 times the usual dose) [20], and *cis*-platinum [21]. The real significance (in terms of a dose effect) of doubling the dose is not always clear because of the binding of the metabolites to serum protein [21]. With bone marrow support, a clear dose effect was reported for cyclophosphamide, etoposide, mitomycin C, melphalan, aziridinylbenzoquinone (AZQ), BCNU, and amsacrine (AMSA), as extensively reviewed recently by Appelbaum and Buckner [22]. It has to be noted that for cyclophosphamide, etoposide, and mitomycin C, autologous marrow reinfusion has little to contribute, at least when the single drug is used [22], whereas with agents such as melphalan, AZQ, and BCNU, ABMT limits the period of marrow suppression [22]. The multiagent regimen phase II studies have been reviewed by Appelbaum and Buckner [22] and Pinkerton et al. [4].

Conditioning regimens such as BACT (BCNU, aracytosine, cyclophosphamide, thioguanine), BEAM (BCNU, etoposide, aracytosine, melphalan), and CBV [cyclophosphamide, BCNU, etoposide (VP16)] are very extensively used with ABMT to reduce the duration of aplasia [4]. One of the major achievements with lymphomas was to show that even in progressive disease, clear responses were observed with these protocols using the dose-effect relationship. As with the animal experiments, this dose-related response was usually insufficient to produce cure in advanced disease, whereas in relapsed patients with less aggressive disease, response and cure may be observed [4, 14]. In heavily pretreated patients, recent studies from Boston have shown rapid and complete responses resembling those of lymphomas and solid tumors [5, 23]. These studies, considered together with the animal and human lymphoma models, suggest that cure may be possible if high-dose therapy is applied earlier in the course of evolution of solid tumors.

Role of Total Body Irradiation

The feasibility of TBI was first demonstrated when it was used for marrow ablation in conditioning regimens for leukemia. Many conventional treatment regimens which utilize local irradiation take advantage of the radiosensitivity of most solid tumors and lymphomas, and it is a logical step, therefore, to study the efficacy of this treatment modality as systemic therapy. Early studies with either hemicorporeal irradiation or low-dose, hyperfractionated TBI evaluated its effectiveness in high-risk patients [24]. The necessity of TBI in massive therapy regimens for solid tumors remains an area of debate. There is an understandable reluctance to use such therapy in young childen because of the considerable early, and as yet ill-defined long-term, toxicity. Similary, the advantages of fractionated TBI remain controversial: although pulmonary toxicity is reduced [25], the relative cytotoxic effect in tumors with shouldered response curves remains to be clarified. Alternative strategies to TBI are further intensification of multiple chemotherapy and the use of double autografts [26, 27]. Although the long-term consequences of high-dose alkylating agents should also be taken into account [28], these treatment regimens are being used in cases where the likelihood of cure with conventional treatment is minimal, and choice is thus limited. Such considerations are, however, of considerable importance if the indications for massive therapy are broadened to include its use as a consolidation treatment in first CR.

Definition of Patients' Status at Autologous Bone Marrow Transplantation

Most of the time, previous therapy is not clearly reported in the world literature; however, this is obviously a major problem when comparing the results of different series. Confusion is also frequent between first CR and subsequent CR, and between first partial remission (PR, primarily refractory patients) and subsequent PR (patients with sensitive relapses). The relevant information should be clearly stated if possible in future reports in this area.

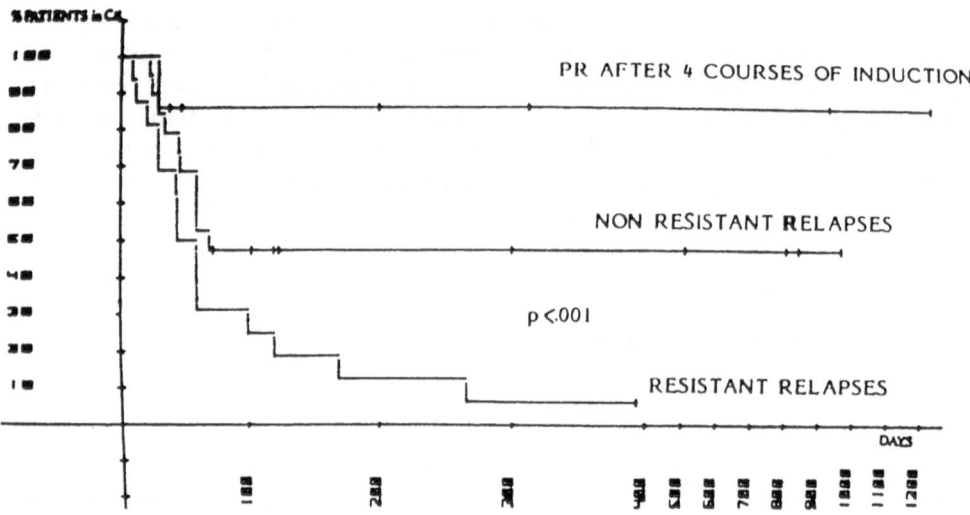

Fig. 1. Disease-free survival rate for 42 patients with non-Hodgkin malignant lymphoma. (From Philip et al., Lancet 1984)

Very High Dose Therapy in Lymphomas

A retrospective study of data from the France Autogreffe study group and investigators in London was performed in July 1983 [29–31], and reviews of the world literature were published by Appelbaum et al. in 1985 [32] and by Singer and Goldstone in 1986 [33]. From these data—as shown, for example, in Fig. 1— several conclusions can be drawn. Patients with true resistant relapses (i.e., patients whose disease is still progressing at the time of the ABMT) will usually not be cured by massive therapy. Responses were observed in 73% of the cases in Lyon, but as shown in Fig. 1, only 1 of 16 patients is still alive 4 years post-ABMT (i.e., 6%). In patients with nonresistant relapses (i.e., all other patients, excluding those with stable disease and those with a minor response on a rescue protocol), long-term survival appeared to be achieved in approximately half of the cases. Our initial data, for example, concerned 15 of 19 patients in the group with nonresistant relapses who had relapsed *on therapy* (i.e., clearly a group with a very bad prognosis). These data showed that there is no difference in outcome between patients who achieved PR or CR prior to ABMT if CR is obtained after ABMT (Fig. 1). We concluded that patients in relapse have to be separated into two groups: those with resistant relapses (patients with progressive or stable disease or a minor response on salvage chemotherapy) and those with nonresistant or sensitive relapses (patients achieving a partial or complete response within the first two courses of salvage chemotherapy). Two major criticisms have been levelled at this retrospective study: the inclusion of both adults (two-thirds) and children (one-third) and the analysis of the mixture of histologies

124

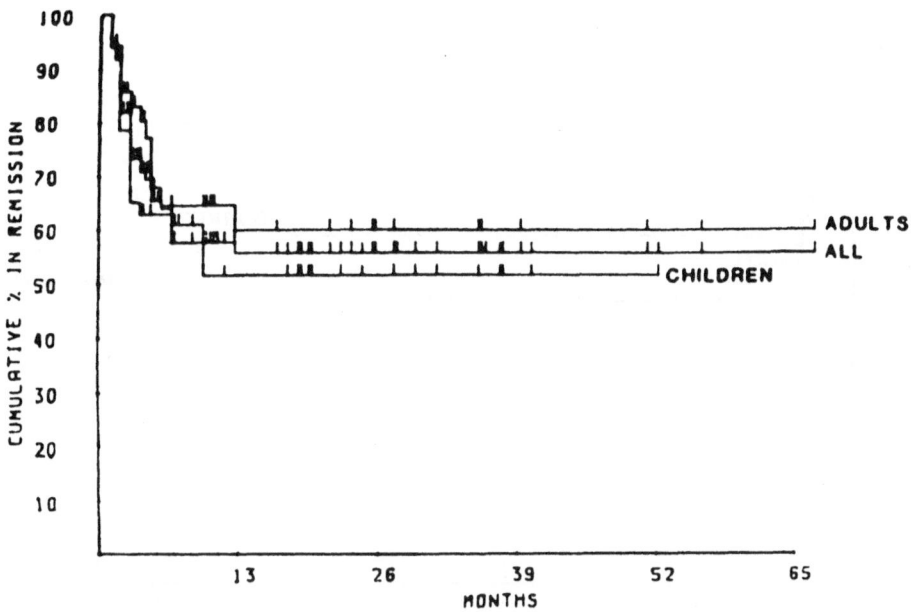

Fig. 2. Disease-free survival rate for children ($n = 60$) and adults ($n = 52$), all of whom had non-Hodgkin lymphoma and underwent autologous bone marrow transplantation in European Bone Marrow Transplantation Group trials (data compiled January 1984). (From [34])

as a single group. Our series included a high proportion of childhood non-Hodgkin lymphoma (NHL) of the Burkitt (BL) type (of 42 cases, 12 were BL, 15 intermediate-, and 15 high-grade non-BL).

As shown in Figs. 2, 3, a European study by Goldstone [34] later concluded that no statistical difference was observed either between adults and children (Fig. 2) or between BL and non-BL (Fig. 3). The concept of resistant (RR) and sensitive relapse (SR) has been subsequently confirmed in a review of 42 cases of BL in France [35], a review of 42 cases of adult diffuse lymphoma from France and England [29], and a review of 39 cases of NHL from Houston and Omaha [36].

In 1986, data from bone marrow transplant centers in Europe and America were pooled to determine the outcome of ABMT in adult patients with relapsed diffuse intermediate- or high-grade NHL (excluding BL), and to identify the prognostic significance of response to therapy preceding the bone marrow transplant procedure [37]. The patients were treated with either high-dose chemotherapy alone (61 patients) or high-dose chemotherapy plus TBI (39 patients). The median age was 35 years, and the median Karnofsky performance score was 80%. Of these patients, 34 had progressive disease that was primarily refractory to chemotherapy (i.e., they never achieved CR), while 66 achieved CR with primary chemotherapy but later relapsed. After receiving further chemotherapy (salvage) at traditional doses, 22 patients had no response or disease

125

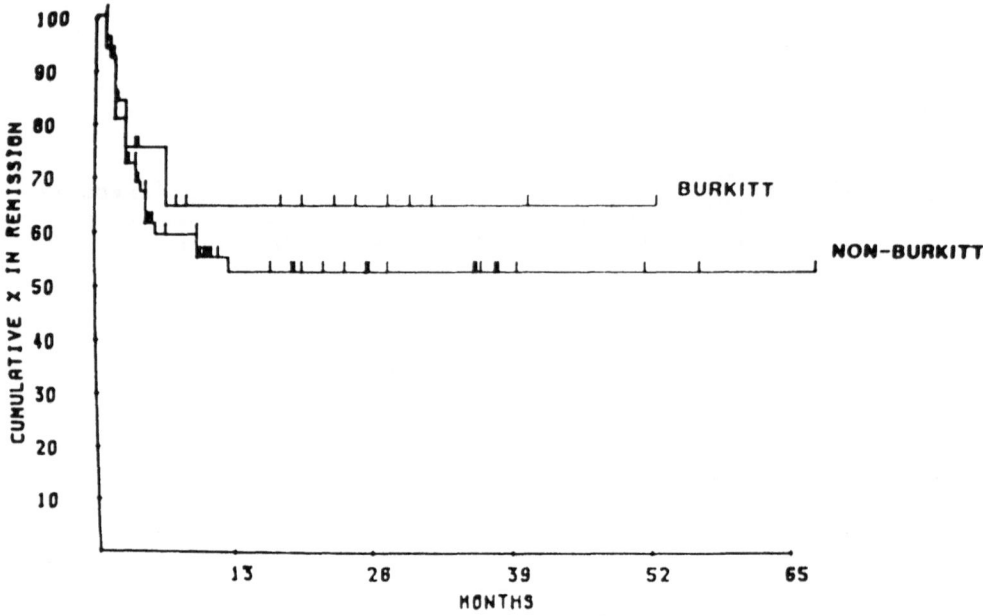

Fig. 3. Results of autologous bone marrow transplantation in patients with Burkitt's ($n = 28$) and non-Burkitt lymphoma ($n = 84$), as reported by the European Bone Marrow Transplantation Group. $P = 0.4341$

progression (i.e., RR), and 44 patients responded partially or completely (i.e., SR).

The actuarial 2-year disease-free survival rate for the entire group was 20%, with the last death at 31 months and a median observation time of 33 months (Fig. 4). Disease-free survival was significantly related to previous response to chemotherapy. The two-year disease-free survival rate was 0% in the no-CR group, 14% in the RR group, and 38% in the SR group (Fig. 5). In patients who had achieved CR with initial chemotherapy, the disease-free survival rate after ABMT was superior to that in patients never achieving CR (Fig. 6). Patients with SR had a better disease-free survival rate than patients with RR. Outcome was not affected by treatment regimen and histologic grade. Whether relapse occurred on or off therapy was not of significance to survival either, but the probability of responding to salvage therapy was significantly higher for those patients who relapsed off therapy. In conclusion, it appears that prior response to chemotherapy is an important prognostic variable in patients with intermediate- or high-grade NHL undergoing ABMT [37].

There remains the question of whether cures can be obtained with conventional salvage regimens without ABMT, as there are reports of occasional long-term survivors after relapses treated with MIME (methyl gag, ifosfamide, methotrexate, etoposide) or DHAP (dexamethasone, aracytosine, platinum) [38–

126

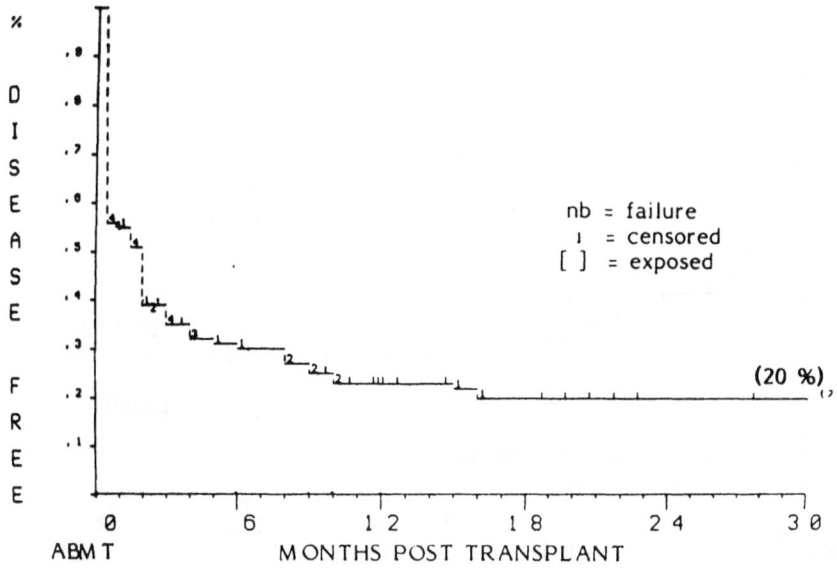

Fig. 4. Actuarial 2-year disease-free survival rate for 100 ABMT patients. (From [37])

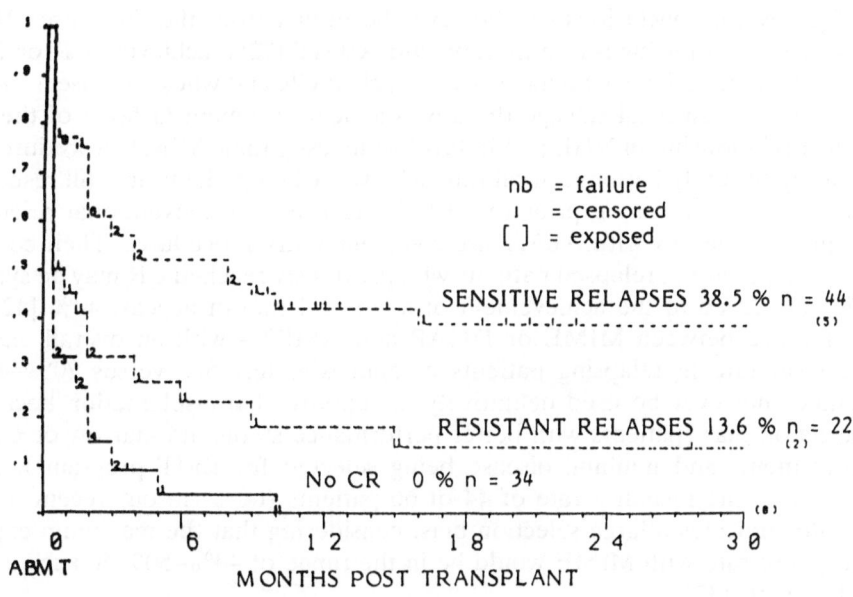

Fig. 5. Actuarial 2-year disease-free survival rate for the same patients as in Fig. 4 according to their response to salvage chemotherapy. (From [37])

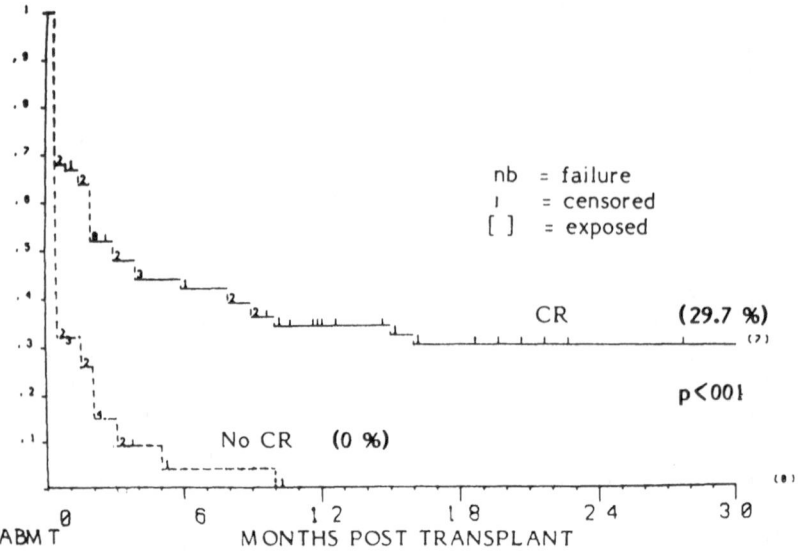

Fig. 6. Actuarial 2-year disease-free survival rate for the same patients as in Fig. 4 according to whether they had reached complete remission (*CR*) with initial therapy. (From [37])

41] (W.S. Velasquez 1986, personal communication). A randomized study is now in progress to compare conventional and high-dose treatment modalities [42]. Several conclusions can however be drawn from the literature. The response rate after high-dose therapy and ABMT (72% achieving CR or PR) in the group of patients who have never reached CR and whose disease is progressing on conventional salvage therapy is a clear argument in favor of the dose-effect relationship in NHL and in favor of investigating ABMT procedures [37]. The significantly better survival rate achieved when patients are still responding to conventional rescue prior to ABMT suggests that conventional rescue and high-dose therapy with ABMT are complementary procedures. Their combination in a group of relapsed patients who previously reached CR may be synergistic, and it led to the achievement of a survival rate of at least 40% [42]. The difference between MIME or DHAP and AMBT—with an overall expected survival rate in relapsing patients of approximately 5% versus 20%–40%—cannot however be used definitively in support of transplantation because of selection bias (patients with better performance status, no marrow or CNS involvement, and minimal disease being selected for BMT programs). As an example, the response rate of 44 of 66 patients (66%) in our recent data for adults indicates a large selection bias, considering that the maximum expected response rate with MIME would be in the range of 40%–50% in such a group of patients [37].

Several questions are still unclear and cannot be answered on the basis of the world literature review [33]. These concern the role of TBI, the role of involved field radiotherapy before or after ABMT, the indication for purging procedures (see M.C. Favrot, this volume), and whether allogenic marrow should be used if available (despite no difference being observed in the Seattle experience [32]). In our study of ABMT in adult lymphoma [37], 39 patients received a TBI-containing regimen, whereas the other 61 did not. The two groups are comparable for the number of primarily refractory cases, histology, and bulk disease. The actuarial survival rate at 2 years is 20% in both groups. In the group with primarily refractory disease (no CR) and resistant relapses, response rates are identical with and without TBI (68% versus 72%). Also, 75% of the relapses were isolated and occurred primarily at the site of initial lymphoma involvement prior to the salvage therapy, indicating that local control is a major factor. Involved field radiotherapy (15–20 G) has been advocated by Phillips et al. [43, 44], following a nonrandomized comparative study favoring this strategy.

In all the published series with ABMT, patients with marrow involvement were excluded, and marrow relapses were not a major problem following ABMT. It is impossible to distinguish relapse due to failure to eradicate the tumor and relapse due to reinfused tumor cells. However, experience with allogenic marrow transplantation suggests that failure of the preparative regimen is at present responsible for the majority of relapses [32, 23]. Encouraging results have been reported with marrow purging in adult patients with B-cell NHL (see Favrot, this volume), and we would advocate that this issue be evaluated in a comparative study [42]. (If non-TBI-containing regimens are used, it is possible that spontaneous marrow recovery could occur, and intensification therapy without ABMT is thus also a possible alternative.)

The current status of ABMT as used in the treatment of pediatric lymphomas has been extensively reviewed [4, 45], and the general conclusions are comparable to those for adults, as pointed out in an early report by our group [29]. The indications for very high dose therapy in BL are in our opinion restricted in 1987 to 20% of patients and should be divided in to two groups:

1. Massive therapy and ABMT are currently the best treatment for BL in PR after initial induction therapy or in relapse where patients are still responding to rescue protocols. The only question which remains unclear is whether the high efficacy of second-line rescue protocols will still be observed when relapses follow more aggressive initial therapy [45].
2. Massive therapy and ABMT is still an experimental treatment for BL with initial CNS involvement, a group for which results remain disappointing with conventional regimens. Preliminary results, however, are quite promising (10 of 15 patients are currently free of disease in the Lyon experience; T. Philip etal. unpublished data).

Massive therapy regimens such as BACT or BEAM are clearly not able to cure patients with progressive disease. For this group of patients, new phase II studies are urgently needed and should be carried out through a multicenter cooperative trial. These studies could be based on conventional chemotherapy regimens tested without ABMT to determine whether a dose-effect relationship can improve the results. New massive therapy combinations—including high-dose cisdichloroaminoplatinum (CDDP), melphalan, ifosfamide, BCNU, aracytosine, and high-dose methotrexate—should be explored. Combinations of various alkylating agents, as proposed by the Baltimore group, may also be a useful avenue to explore [46]. The role of TBI remains unclear in BL despite results reported in other lymphomas [47]. However, it is clear that such phase II studies will be the basis of any future progress in BL with either conventional or massive therapy regimens.

The role of very high dose therapy in lymphoblastic lymphoma in children and young adults is less clear than in BL. However, results in relapsed patients with cyclophosphamide and TBI appear to be superior to those with non-TBI-containing regimens [33]. This kind of therapy is indicated most clearly in the groups of patients who relapse with tumors still sensitive to rescue protocols. However, patients with initial CNS disease and leukemic presentations with a very high number of circulating blast cells are also good candidates for these programs.

The role of very high dose therapy in Hodgkin's disease was recently extensively reviewed by Canellos [48] and Phillips and Reece [49], and it appears that in approximately half of all patients with advanced Hodgkin's disease resistant to conventional chemotherapy, remission can be achieved with existing intensive therapy regimens and ABMT. It also appears that regimens including TBI are not better than non-TBI-containing regimens. The best results reported are with the CBV programs initially described by Spitzer et al. from M.D. Anderson Hospital [50, 51]. These results are similar to those in early studies in NHLs, and this area is probably one of the most promising for the future.

Very High Dose Therapy in Pediatric Solid Tumors

We will mainly summarize the current status of the very high dose therapy programs in rhabdomyosarcoma, Ewing's sarcoma, and neuroblastoma and describe the preliminary results in other tumors.

Rhabdomyosarcoma

Phase II studies of children with relapsed or resistant rhabdomyosarcoma have demonstrated a high response rate to high-dose melphalan with autologous marrow rescue (greater than 90%), confirming data obtained from an animal xenograft model system [15]. The duration of response was, however, almost invariably brief, with few long-term survivors (V. Postmus, personal communication; J. Jacobsen, personal communication). Therefore, it seemed appropriate to build on the basis of melphalan, and we elected to study the value of TBI in such patients [4]. In addition, because the long-term survival rate in children with stage IV disease remains poor, massive therapy might be considered for use as consolidation treatment once CR has been achieved. To date, nine patients have been treated in Lyon: six patients, all of whom were in first CR at the time of massive therapy, remain disease free. Follow-up in these cases is, however, short (median 20 months). There was one therapy-related death, but apart from infection and one case of hepatic dysfunction, the massive therapy was, in general, well tolerated. Clearly, it is too early to draw any firm conclusions about the value of such a procedure or the need to purge the marrow (five of the nine patients were purged with Asta-Z). It would appear that, as in most other tumors, one course of massive therapy, even including TBI, is unlikely to salvage patients with progressive or ressistant disease [4, 16, 52]; however, its role in the consolidation of remission in patients unlikely to be cured by conventional therapy is worthy of further evaluation on a multicenter basis.

The use of double procedures in rhabdomyosarcoma is also being studied in the current International Society of Paediatric Oncology (SIOP) trial. Stage IV patients who achieve CR after chemotherapy alone are randomized (in certain major centers) to receive vincristine, BCNU, and melphalan with ABMT (purged with the drug Asta-Z), followed after 3–4 months by procarbazine, VP16, and cyclophosphamide. A similar approach is taken for patients less than 5 years old with stage II/III parameningeal disease, who do not receive high-dose cranial irradiation. Interesting results have also come from the current National Cancer Institute (NCI) program [53], which includes selected cases with very bad prognosis (relapses, initial stage IV). A combination of vincristine, actinomycin, cyclophosphamide, and doxorubicin (Adriamycin) (VACA) followed by TBI (8 Gy, two fractions) has produced a 45% long-term survival rate (1 year median follow-up). The response rate in evaluable patients for this study was 93%. In other soft tissue sarcomas, results are less encouraging [54, 55].

Ewing's Sarcoma

Promising preliminary results were obtained by Cornbleet et al. [56] using melphalan as a single agent for Ewing's sarcoma. In a review of 35 cases, the European Bone Marrow Transplant (EBMT) group in 1984 achieved a similar response rate of 66% in evaluable patients [57]. However, as shown in Fig. 7, the general pattern of outcome seen in patients after massive therapy for lymphoma is also observed with this solid tumor [57]. The results are good for patients receiving grafts in CR (80% survival at 12 months), reasonably good for relapsed patients still responding to a rescue protocol, and very poor—despite a high response rate—for patients receiving grafts with progressive disease. The NCI's experience is again probably one of the largest at this time: using the VACA massive therapy regimen and TBI (8 Gy, two fractions), Miser has reported 26 of 57 selected very bad prognosis patients to be in continuous remission at 2 years of follow-up [53].

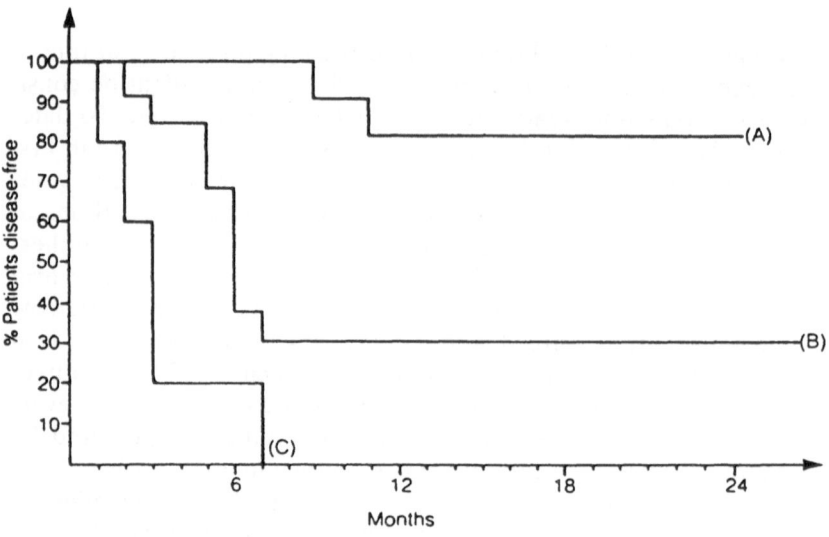

Fig. 7. Results of autologous bone marrow transplantation performed in 34 patients with Ewing's sarcoma in Europe: bad-risk patients (*A*), treated in complete remission (*n* = 11); patients with nonresistant partial remission or relapses (*B*; *n* = 13); and patients with resistant relapses (*C*; *n* = 10). (European Bone Marrow Transplantation Group review 1984, unpublished data)

Other Tumors

Using a prolonged (21-day) massive therapy regimen (including high-dose methotrexate, vincristine, cyclophosphamide, doxorubicin, dacarbazine, melphalan, and high-dose *cis*-platinum), Miser [53] reported 12 of 24 relapsed osteosarcoma patients to have no evidence of disease (NED) with a median follow-up of 6.5 years. Only fifteen patients, however, had received chemotherapy prior to the rescue protocol [53].

Because of the high cure rate in Wilms' tumour, massive therapy is rarely considered. There remain, however, those with stage IV disease or those with unfavorable histology in whom survival is less assured with conventional regimens. Early results from the Royal Marsden group, using high-dose melphalan alone, demonstrated responses in each of 6 patients with relapsed disease and two long-term survivors A. Barrett, personal communication). Such an approach may thus be of value as a consolidation procedure in high-risk patients.

Using high-dose melphalan and VP16 in malignant germ cell tumors (MGCT), responses have been described in patients resistant to *cis*-platinum–containing regimens [58]. Baumgartner et al. [59] have reported the use of vincristine, doxorubicin, high-dose cyclophosphamide, and single-fraction TBI in 3 patients with stage IV MGCT. Although responses were seen in the 2 cases resistant to conventional chemotherapy, the only survivor (27 months) received a graft in CR.

ABMT has also been used in stage IV retinoblastoma, although there are insufficient data to comment on its value [60].

Neuroblastoma

Because of the limited availability of matched related donors in this very young group of patients, experience with autologous marrow is greater than with allogenic transplanation. Moreover, unlike leukemia, neuroblastoma only involves the bone marrow secondarily, and the marrow may be cleared of tumor by effective chemotherapy prior to marrow harvest. Various purging techniques have been developed which, in vitro, are capable of removing residual tumor cells from marrow. The need for such purging procedures in practice remains a contentious issue, as the clonogenic potential of reinfused neuroblastoma cells is difficult to demonstrate (see M.C. Favrot and T. Philip, this volume). The main limiting effect in the use of megatherapy procedures remains the ability of such therapy to ablate the malignant cell population completely. It is difficult to summarize the state of the art due to the lack of published data; however, at the recent Houston Autologous Bone Marrow Transplantation meeting, all the major groups working in this area reported current results [61–64].

In relapsed, highly selected patients, a 20% progression-free survival rate at 2 years was reported when TBI was used in the conditioning regimen; no progression-free survivors were reported when a non-TBI-containing regimen was used [61, 62]. With or without TBI, with single- or double-graft procedures, a 35%–40% progression-free survival rate at 2 years was reported in patients receiving grafts in first CR [61–64]. No advantage was shown in this group for the TBI-containing regimen; indeed, the mortality is higher (20% versus 10%). Of the patients treated by the Lyon-Marseille-Curie group with grafts in first PR and a TBI-containing regimen, 20% are alive and progression free at 2 years. It is clear that in all studies, no plateau has yet been reached on the curves after 2 years.

The timing of relapse post-BMT (i.e., between 3 and 12 months postgraft for the majority of the cases) has kindled interest in the concept of a double-graft procedure in this disease. Selected patients in PR after induction therapy received a double graft without TBI; there were no survivors at 2 years (O. Hartmann, personal communication). The Lyon-Marseille-Curie group have early data for relapsed patients using a double graft, with TBI being included in the second conditioning regimen; there were some survivors at 2 years [61].

Phase II studies with these high-dose regimens have been encouraging, although their construction has to a large extent been empirical. An exception to this is high-dose melphalan. The European Neuroblastoma Study Group (ENSG) has carried out a prospective randomized study in stage III and IV patients who achieved at least partial remission after a standardized, cis-platinum–containing induction regimen. There was a significant advantage for the melphalan group in terms of both median survival and the duration of progression-free survival. This provides a rational basis for the inclusion of this agent at high doses in future protocols [65]. TBI is still included in many schedules because of in vitro radiosensitivity data and early clinical experience [66]. However, because of concern about the contribution of this modality to both short- and long-term morbidity, its inclusion requires prospective evaluation. It is possible that the substitution of other drugs at high doses might provide a higher therapeutic index [67].

Very High Dose Therapy for Solid Tumors in Adults

A number of phase II studies of high-dose single-agent therapy with ABMT have been carried out or are in progress in patients with solid tumors. From the extensive review by Appelbaum and Buckner [22], some facts are clear. BCNU at doses of approximately 800–1500 mg/m^2 produces a good response rate in melanoma (45% response, 16% CR), lung cancer (46% response, no CR), brain cancer (44% response, 7% CR), and sarcoma (75% response, no CR) [22]. Melphalan at doses of 140–200 mg/m^2 has also been reported to produce good response rates in melanoma (74% response, 31% CR), neuroblastoma (70% response, 50% CR), Ewing's sarcoma (80% response, 20% CR), germ cell tumor (67% response, 17% CR), ovarian carcinoma (56% response, 14% CR), breast cancer (67% response, mostly CR), and colon carcinoma (56% response, 14% CR) [22]. VP16 at doses of 1500–2100 mg/m^2 also showed good response rates in germ cell cancer (83% response, 16% CR), small-cell lung cancer (85% response, 31% CR), and brain cancer (50% response, no CR). Cyclophosphamide at 1 500–2 000 mg/m^2 was also shown to be effective in small-cell lung cancer (84% response, 56% CR), ovarian carcinoma (75% response, mostly CR), and testicular cancer (60% response, no CR) [22].

Studies of high-dose combinations have been reviewed by Antman et al. [5] but are still in their early days and are a direct continuation of the phase I dose escalation studies. These schedules mainly use combinations of alkylating agents [23], as first proposed in leukemia by the Baltimore group [46]. The STAMP 1 and 2 programs (Solid Tumor Autologous Marrow Program) from Boston are very encouraging because rapid CR was observed; this result is similar to the early experience in lymphomas with very high dose therapy in resistant patients. These protocols, the first to achieve such rapid CR in advanced solid tumors, are very promising in spite of the short duration of the responses [5, 23, 68]. Although most of these regimens have no proven clinical benefit in end-stage disease, the high response rate may provide important leads for the development of new combinations to be used in a setting of minimal residual disease [68].

Small-Cell Lung Cancer

The study by Humblet et al. from the Ludwig Institute in Brussels is of particular note because after standard induction treatment, patients with small-cell lung cancer were randomized to a further course of chemotherapy at conventional dosage versus late intensification with autologous marrow support [69]. In the ABMT arm, the CR rate increased from 39% before randomization to 79%. Median relapse-free survival after randomization was 68 versus 55 weeks in favor of consolidation. The conclusion is that very high dose therapy results in a significant increase in the CR rate and a significant increase in the relapse-free survival, but with no major improvement in the overal survival [69]. In another study by Farha et al. [70] at M.D. Anderson Hospital in Texas, untreated patients initially received high-dose therapy followed by marrow rescue. Patients then received prophylactic cranial irradiation and four courses of the same drugs at standard dosage, followed by radiotherapy to the primary tumor. All patients responded (54% completely), with a median time to treatment failure and a median survival of 41 and 56 weeks, respectively.

Souhami et al. at the University College Hospital in London treated 25 newly diagnosed patients with high-dose cyclophosphamide and radiotherapy to the primary site [71]. Of these patients, 56% attained CR, with a median duration of 43 weeks and a median survival of 69 weeks. These results are comparable to those of a standard regimen for small-cell lung cancer but were obtained with a single treatment.

Spitzer et al. at M.D. Anderson Hospital have studied 32 patients with untreated, limited small-cell lung cancer. The patients received three cycles of induction therapy, followed by two courses of intensification with ABMT [72]. Of the 13 patients who were in CR at the time of transplant, 5 remain disease free at 4 or more years, whereas only one of nine partial responders before transplant remains disease free. Contrasts between reports are found in the relapse pattern. In Humblet's patients, relapse occurred mainly in the primary site, while relapses were mainly systemic in Spitzer's patients. This difference may stem from the absence of thoracic irradiation in Humblet's study.

Melanoma

The relatively promising results in small-cell lung cancer contrast with those for the chemotherapy-resistant tumor melanoma. A significant CR rate for high-dose melphalan is first seen at doses of 180 mg/m^2. There appears to be a dose-response relationship in the study by Lazarus et al. [73] of doses of 180 and 225 mg/m^2; however, in a larger study by Cornbleet et al., patients treated with 260mg/m^2 melphalan achieved only an 8% CR rate, with a 43% response rate overall [74]. Melphalan or BCNU at standard doses produces responses in 10%–20% of patients. When these drugs are given at high doses with ABMT, response rates of 40%–65% occur, and a significant percentage of CRs is observed. High-dose chemotherapy without BMT in melanoma was also recently reported by the Baltimore group [75].

Germ Cell Tumor

Most patients with newly diagnosed metastatic testicular cancer respond readily to curative standard-dose regimens. The few in whom multiple regimens fail, and who are therefore eligible for ABMT studies, represent an extensively treated group with refractory tumors. Of 13 patients treated at M.D. Anderson

Hospital with 4500 mg/m^2 CPA and 600 mg/m^2 VP16, 7 responded (4 completely); however, the responses were quite short, with the time to treatment failure ranging from 1 to 5 months [76]. Of ten patients treated at the University of California at Los Angeles with high dose cyclophosphamide, VP16, and melphalan, five died of toxicity. One patient obtained CR and is alive at 6 years [77]. Wolff reported on 11 patients treated with high-dose VP16 (2400 mg/m^2), with a 90% response rate (10%CR), including 4 of 5 patients in whom standard-dose VP16 had failed [78]. However, the median time to treatment failure was again short—2 months. Biron from Lyon also reported on 15 cases of refractory tumors treated with VP16 and melphalan followed by ABMT [58]. Responses were observed in 9 of 15 patients (60%), but only 2 achieved CR, and there were no disease-free survivors at 2 years. Similar results in refractory tumors were reported by O. Postmus and J. Pico (personal communication).

Better regimens will have to be developed for testicular cancer, where patients at high risk should be identified sufficiently early to evaluate high-dose therapy when drug resistance is less likely and tumor burden is lower. In Lyon, for example, five patients were selected because they had not achieved CR after four courses of vinblastine, actimomycin D, bleomycin cisplatinum (VABCDDP). They all received a combination of VP16, CDDP, and ifosfamide with ABMT. Of these 5 patients, 4 are alive disease free 6–18 months post-ABMT (unpublished data). Comparable results have been obtained in Villejuif, France, with a very similar approach (J. Pico, personal communication). Very recently, data for 64 ABMT recipients with germ cell tumors were collected by the participants of the EBMTG. Of these patients, 35 had refractory disease after *cis*-platinum therapy, 21 responded to the conditioning regimen, and 3 are alive disease free at 2 years. Eight patients with sensitive relapses and 21 in first PR or CR were also selected according to classical bad-prognosis criteria. Of these 29, 15 are still alive disease free with more than 12 months' follow-up (EBMTG, unpublished results collected by J. Pico).

Breast Cancer

Eder et al. [23] have reported on a total of 18 patients treated with the STAMP 1 protocol at both the phase I and phase II protocol doses. There were six complete and eight partial responses, and the median time to treatment failure was 4.7 months. In a review of the ABMT literature on breast cancer, Stewart [79] reported on the first 5 patients treated with a Seattle protocol, consisting of high dose cyclophosphamide and TBI, for patients in whom standard treatment had failed. Two of the five patients responded completely, but the follow-up was too short for comment. At M.D. Anderson Hospital, 16 patients have been treated with 750 mg/m^2 AMSA. Two partial responses were obtained, and mucositis was dose limiting [79]. Gisselbrecht also reported on ten cases of inflammatory breast cancer in first CR (six cases) or after relapse (four cases). He observed three complete and seven partial responses. Six patients are still disease free, with a median follow-up of 8 months [80]. There is general agreement on the following indications for early intensification with ABMT in breast cancer: estrogen-receptor-negative, inflammatory, metastatic cases at diagnosis and more than ten involved lymph nodes at surgery, including positive internal mammary nodes.

Brain Tumors

Virtually all of the larger series of ABMT for brain tumors have included high-dose BCNU. Hilderbrand et al. from Brussels reported on the first group of seven patients treated with lomustine (CCNU) but observed no responses by computed tomography of the brain [81]. Of 20 patients treated with 1050 mg/m^2 BCNU and 60 Gy whole-brain radiotherapy, 85% were still alive between 1 and 28 months later [82]. In a study reported by Phillips et al., in which a dose of 1200 mg/m^2 BCNU was used, 2 of 27 patients who previously failed to respond were disease free at >3.5 years, but 6 of 12 patients treated adjuvantly were disease free between 7 and 59 months later [83, 84]. Perren et al. [85] also reported very promising results in highgrade gliomas, using high-dose BCNU prior to radiotherapy and very early after surgery. Perren reported that 11 of 67 patients with grade IV gliomas were alive disease free 26–84 months postdiagnosis. In Biron's report on 45 patients, the results are similar, but the follow-up is short (12 months). These studies are at least a promising start; however, toxicity was substantial, with the development of BCNU-associated pulmonary fibrosis and hepatic necrosis [83, 84]. The role of high-dose BCNU and whole-brain radiotherapy has been incompletely assessed but seems promising.

Ovarian Carcinoma

There is agreement to explore very high dose therapy in patients with residual disease at second-look surgery. Using melphalan alone or in combination, D. Maraninchi reported 5 complete responses in 11 patients, with a median duration of 6 months (personal communication). Using high dose cyclophosphamide and TBI, N. Marty reported 7 of 13 patients to be disease free, but none of the survivors had been followed up for 2 years (personal communication). Using high dose cyclophosphamide and VP16, V. Mulmer also reported 3 of 4 patients to be disease free with a short follow-up. The American experience, recently reviewed by Antman, is comparable [5].

Future Prospects for Very High Dose Therapy in Lymphomas and Solid Tumors

Studies of experimental tumor systems in vitro and in vivo have demonstrated clearly that the ability to kill tumor cells is directly related to the dose of radio- or chemotherapeutic agents [11]. Goldie and Coldmann [6, 8] and Norton and

Simon [9, 10] have also shown, with others [4], that minimal residual disease provides the best opportunity for the dose-effect relationship to be explored. Results obtained in human models of very high dose therapy, with or without ABMT, for leukemia are consistent with these theoretical assumptions [4]. Because of the success of BMT in the treatment of leukemia, there has been increased interest in the possible application of marrow transplantation in NHL; here, too, definite success can be found in the literature. Lymphoma is on the borderline between leukemia and solid tumors, and this model is thus encouraging for oncologists.

However, several questions still remain with regard to solid tumors. In the majority of phase II studies, impressive response rates are observed in progressive disease resistant to conventional drug doses; thus, there is clinical confirmation of a dose-effect relationship in the solid tumors. However, the majority of these responses are incomplete, whereas for leukemia and lymphoma they are usually complete, even in resistant disease. It appears that the best combinations of drugs for solid tumors have yet to be found. In this context, the recent report from Boston of rapid achievement of CR in breast cancer with the STAMP program may provide a significant lead [5].

Because of the contamination of autologous marrow by malignant cells (see M.C. Favrot, this volume), the question whether these regimens can be explored without ABMT is open [4]. If TBI is not included in a conditioning regimen, this question is a realistic one because there is clear evidence that many protocols of this kind are not completely ablative [4].

A final question was well summarized by Hryniuk in a recent review [52]:

Dose the single treatment of A mg which requires marrow rescue really have an advantage over A/2 mg (half the dose intensity) administered twice (to give the equivalent amount of drug) with the two treatments separated by the minimum number of weeks required for spontaneous unassisted marrow recovery? Or any advantage over A/3 mg (one third the dose intensity) administered three times but separated by the same time intervals as A/2 mg? Or over A/4 mg administered four times etc. . . . Is more better? Probably. But does it have to be administered all at once?

These questions still leave room for the use of very high dose therapy in future solid tumor therapy, but the place and role of ABMT, which is merely a means of lessening severe marrow toxicity, will be dependent upon the answers to these questions.

References

1. McFarland W, Granville NB, Damesheck W (1959) Autologous bone marrow infusion as an adjunct in therapy of malignant disease. Blood 14: 503–521
2. Clifford P, Clift RA, Duff JK (1961) Nitrogen mustard therapy combined with autologous marrow infusion. Lancet i: 687
3. Thomas ED, Buckner CD, Banaji M (1977) One hundred patients with acute leukemia treated by chemotherapy, total body irradiation and allogeneic marrow transplantation. Blood 49: 511

4. Pinkerton R, Philip T, Bouffet E, Lashford L, Kemshead J (1986) Autologous bone marrow transplantation in paediatric solid tumours. Clin Haematol 15: 187
5. Antman K, Eder JP, Frei E (1987) High dose chemotherapy with bone marrow support for solid tumors. In: De Vita H (ed) Important advances in oncology. (in press)
6. Goldie JH, Coldman AJ (1979) A mathematical model for relating the drug sensitivity of tumors to their spontaneous mutation rate. Cancer Treat Rep 63: 1727
7. Goldie JH, Coldman AJ (1983) Quantitative model for multiple levels of drug resistance in clinical tumors. Cancer Treat Rep 67: 923
8. Goldie JH, Coldman AJ (1985) Genetic instability in the development of drug resistance. Semin Oncol 12: 222
9. Norton L, Simon R (1977) Tumor size, sensitivity to therapy and design of treatment schedules. Cancer Treat Rep 61: 1307
10. Norton L (1985) Implications of kinetic heterogeneity in clincal oncology. Semin Oncol 12: 231
11. Frei E, Canellos GP (1980) Dose: a critical factor in cancer chemotherapy. Am J Med 69: 585
12. Brock N, Schneider B (1984) Models in cytostatic chemotherapy. Cancer 54: 1229
13. Shabel F, Griswold D, Thomas H, Laster R (1984) Increasing the therapeutic response rate to anticancer drugs by applying the basic principles of pharmacology. Cancer 54: 1160
14. Gehan E (1984) Dose-response relationship in clinical oncology. Cancer 54: 1204
15. Houghton JA, Cook RL, Lutz PJ, Hougthon PJ (1985) Melphalan: a potential new agent in the treatment for childhood rhabdomyosarcoma. Cancer Treat Rep 69: 91
16. De Vita V (1986) Dose response is alive and well. J Clin Oncol 4: 1157
17. Salmon SE, Trent JM (1984) Human tumor cloning, Grune and Stratton, Orlando, p 700
18. Van Huff D, Clark GM, Weiss G, Marshall M, Buchok JB, Knight W, Lemaistre CF (1986) Use of in vitro dose response effects to select antineoplastics for high dose or regional administration regimens. J Clin Oncol 4: 1827
19. Djerassi I (1975) High dose methotrexate and citrovorum factor rescue. Background and rationale. Cancer Chemother Rep 6: 3
20. Duff Y (1985) How much is too much high dose cytosine arabinoside? J Clin Oncol 5: 601
21. Hayes DM, Cvitkovic E, Golbey R, Schneider E, Helson L, Krakoff R (1977) High dose cis platinum diaminedichloride. Cancer 39: 1372
22. Appelbaum FR, Buckner CD (1986) Overview of the clinical relevance of autologous bone marrow transplanation. Clin Haematol 1: 1
23. Eder JP, Antman K, Peters W, Henner WD, Ellias A, Shea T, Schryber S, Andersen J, Come S, Schnipper L, Frei E (1986) HIgh dose combination alkylating agent chemotherapy with autologous bone marrow support for metastatic breast cancer. J Clin Oncol 4: 1592
24. D'Angio GJ, Evans AE (1983) Cyclic low dose total body irradiation for metastatic neuroblastoma. Int J Radiat Oncol Biol Phys 9: 1961
25. Pino Y, Torres JL, Bross DS (1982) Risk factors in interstitial penumonitis following allogeneic bone marrow transplantation. Int J Radiat Oncol Biol Phys 8: 1301
26. Goldstone AH, Souhami RL, Lynch DC (1984) Intensive chemotherapy and autologous bone marrow transplantation for relapsed lymphoma. Exp Hematol 12 [Suppl 15]: 137
27. Hartmann O, Kalifa C, Beaujean F, Patte C, Lemerle J (1985) Treatment of advanced neuroblastoma with two consecutive high dose chemotherapy regimens and ABMT. In: Evans AE, D'Angio GJ, Seeger RC (eds) Advances in Neuroblastoma research. Alan R. Liss, New York, p 565
28. Hartmann O, Oberlin O, Lemerle J (1984) Acute leukaemia in two patients treated with high dose melphalan and autologous marrow transplantation for malignant solid tumours. J Clin Oncol 2: 1424
29. Philip T, Biron P, Maraninchi D, Goldstone AH, Hervé P, Souillet G, Gastaut JL, Plouvier E, Flesh Y, Philip I, Harousseau JL, Le Mevel A, Rebattu P, Linch DC, Freycon F, Milan JJ, Souhami RL (1985) Massive chemotherapy with ABMT in 50 cases of bad prognosis non Hodgkin's lymphoma. Br J Haematol 60: 599
30. Philip T, Bernard JL, Zucker JM, Souillet G, Favrot MC, Philip I, Bordigoni P, Lutz JP, Plouvier E, Carton P, Robert A, Kemshead J (1985) Purging autologous bone marrow transplantation in 25 cases of advanced neuroblastoma. Lancet ii: 576

139

31. Rebattu P, Philip T, Maraninchi D, Hartmann O, Cahn JY, Bordigoni P, Colombat JP, Le Mevel A, Laporte JP, Biron P (1985) Indications et résultats de l'autogreffe de moelle dans les lymphomes malins non Hodgkiniens (étude de 92 cas). Nouv Rev Fr Hématol 27 [Suppl 2]: 252

32. Appelbaum FR, Sullivan KM, Thomas ED, Buckner CD, Clift RA, Deeg HJ, Fefer A, Hill R, Sanders J, Steward P, Storb R (1985) Marrow transplantation as treatment for patients with recurrent malignant lymphoma. Int J Cell Cloning 4: 216

33. Singer CR, Goldstone AH (1986) Non Hodgkin's lymphomas. Clin Haematol 15: 105

34. Goldstone AH (1985) Autologous bone marrow transplantation for non Hodgkin's lymphoma. In: Dicke KA, Spitzer G, Zander AR (eds) Autologous bone marrow transplantation. Proceedings of the 1st international symposium. University of Texas M.D. Anderson Hospital and Tumor Institute Houston, p 67

35. Philip T, Hartmann O, Pinkerton R, Patte C, Biron P, Souillet G, Bernard JL, Freycon F, Bordigoni P, Laporte JP, Marguerite G, Le Mevel A, Plouvier E, Favrot MC, Philip I, Lemerle J (1985) Massive chemotherapy with autologous bone marrow transplantation in Burkitt's lymphoma (a review of 50 patients treated in France). Blood Transfus Immunohaematol 5: 521

36. Armitage JO, Gingrich RD, Foley JF, Kessinger MA, Klassen LW, Kumar PO, Tempero MA, Vaughan WP (1985) which patients with lymphoma can be salvaged with high-dose cytoreduction and autologous marrow rescue? In: Dicke KA, Spitzer G. Zander AR (eds) Autologous bone marrow transplantation Proceedings of the 1st international symposium. University of Texas M.D. Anderson Hospital and Tumor Institute Houston, p 57

37. Philip T, Armitage JO, Spitzer G, Chauvin F, Jagannath S, Cahn JY, Colombat P, Goldstone AH, Gorin NC, Flesh M, Laporte JP, Maraninchi D, Pico JL, Bosly A, Anderson C, Shots R, Biron P, Cabanillas F, Dicke K (1987) High dose therapy and ABMT in 100 adults with intermediate or high grade non Hodgkin's lymphoma. N Engl J Med 316: 1493–1497

38. Cabanillas F, Hagemeister FB, Bodey GP, Freireich EJ (1982) IMVP-16: an effective regimen for patients with lymphoma who have relapsed after initial combination chemotherapy. Blood 60: 693

39. Cabanillas F, Hagemeister FB, McLaughlin P, Salvador P, Velasquez WS, Riggs S, Freireich EJ (1984) Mime combination chemotherapy or refractory or recurrent lymphomas. Proc Ame Soc Clin Oncol 3: 250

40. Cabanillas F, Hagemeister FB, Bodey GP (1984) M.D. Anderson experience with VP16 for therapy of refractory or recurrent lymphoma. In: Issel BF, Muggia FM, Carter SK (eds) Etoposide (VP-16): current status and new developments. Academic Press, New York, p 313

41. Cabanillas F, Hagemeister FB, Riggs S, Salvador P, Velasquez WS, McLaughlin P, Smith T (1985) Results of ifosfamide-etoposide combinations for patients with recurrent or refractory aggressive lymphoma. In: Cavalli F (ed) Malignant lymphomas and Hodgkin's disease: experimental and therapeutic advances. Martinus Nijhoff, Boston, p 485

42. Philip T, Armitage J, Spitzer G, Cabanillas F, Velasquez W, Hagenbeck T, Jagannath S (1988) Background for an international randomized study on relapsed diffuse intermediate and high grade lymphoma in adults. In: Dicke K, Spitzer G, Jagannath S (eds) Proceedings of the 3rd International symposium on autologous bone marrow transplantation. Houston, pp 313–333

43. Phillips GL (1983) Current clinical trial with intensive therapy and autologous bone marrow transplantation for lymphomas and solid tumors. In: Gale RP (ed) Recent advances in bone marrow transplantation. UCLA symposia new series, vol 7. Alan R. Liss, New York, p 43

44. Phillips GL, Herzig RH, Lazarus HM, Fay JW, Wolff SN, Mill WB, Lin H, Thomas PRM, Glasgow GP, Shina DC, Herzig GP (1984) Treatment of resistant malignant lymphoma with cyclophosphamide total body irradiation and transplantation of cryopreserved autologous marrow. N Engl J Med 31: 1557

45. Philip T, Biron P, Philip I, Frappaz D, Pinkerton R, Souillet G, Bernard JL, Laporte JP, Philippe N, De Terlizzi M, Demeocq F, Dufillot JF, Kremens B, Bonetti F, Favrot MC (1988) Autologous bone marrow transplantation in Burkitt's lymphoma (50 cases in the Lyon protocol). In: Dicke K, Spitzer G, Jagannath S (eds) 3rd international symposium on autologous bone marrow transplantation. Houston, pp 249–261

46. Santos GW, Tutschka PJ, Brookmeyer R (1983) Marrow transplantation for acute non lym-

140

phocytic leukemia after treatment with busulfan and cyclophosphamide. N Engl J Med 309: 1347

47. Philip T, Pinkerton R, Hartmann O, Patte C, Philip I, Biron P, Favrot MC (1986) The role of massive therapy with autologous bone marrow transplantation in Burkitt's lymphoma. Clin Haematol 15: 205

48. Canellos P (1985) Bone marrow transplantation as salvage therapy in advanced Hodgkin disease: allogenic or autologous? J Clin Oncol 11: 1451

49. Phillips GL, Reece DE (1986) Clinical studies of autologous bone marrow transplantation in Hodgkin's disease. Clin Haematol 15: 151

50. Spitzer G, Dicke KA, Litam J, Verma DS, Zander AR, Lanzotti V, Valdivieso M, McCredie KB, Samules ML (1980) High dose combination chemotherapy with autologous bone marrow transplantation in adult solid tumors. Cancer 45: 3075

51. Carella AM, Santini G, Girodano D, Frassoni F, Nati S, Congiu A, Occhini D, Rossi E, Martinengo M, Damasio E, Lercari G, Marmont AM (1984) High dose chemotherapy and nonfrozen ABMT in resistant or relapsed malignant lymphomas. Cancer 54: 2836

52. Hryniuk W (1986) Is more better? J Clin Oncol 5: 621

53. Miser J (1987) High dose therapy and ABMT in pediatric solid tumors. In: De Bernardi B (ed) Novel therapeutic approaches in pediatric oncology. Martinus Nijhoff, Boston, (in press)

54. Philip T, Hervé P, Racadot E (1982) Intensive cytoreductive regimen and autologous bone marrow transplantation in leukaemias and solid tumours (a review). Transplant Clin Immunol 14: 86

55. Philip T (1985) Chimiothérapie massive et autogreffe de moelle dans les tumeurs des parties molles (15 cas). Bull Cancer (Paris) 72: 62

56. Cornbleet M, Corringham R, Prentice H, Boesen E, McElwain TJ (1981) Treatment of Ewing sarcoma with high dose melphalan and autologous bone marrow transplantation. Cancer Treat Rep 63: 241

57. Philip T (1984) Status of the role of ABMT in solid tumours in Europe. Proceedings of the European Bone Marrow Transplant Group, Granada, 1984

58. Biron P, Philip T, Maraninchi D (1985) Massive chemotherapy and ABMT in progressive disease of non-seminomatous testicular cancer. In: Dicke K, Spitzer G, Zander AR (eds) Autologous bone marrow transplantation. University of Texas, M.D. Anderson Hospital and Tumor Institute Houston, p 203

59. Baumgartner C, Bleher EA, Brun Del Re G (1984) Autologous bone marrow transplantation in the treatment of children and adolescents with advanced malignant tumors. Med Pediatr Oncol 12: 104

60. Ekert H, Ellis WM, Waters KD, Tauro GP (1982) Autologous bone marrow rescue in the treatment of advanced tumours of childhood. Cancer 49: 603

61. Philip T, Zucker JM, Bernard JL, Biron P, Kremens B, Quintana E, Gentet JC, Bordigoni P, Frappaz D, Souillet G, Philip I, Chauvin F, Favrot MC (1987) Bone marrow transplantation in an unselected group of 65 stage IV neuroblastoma patients. In: Dicke K, Spitzer G, Jagannath S (eds) Proceedings of the 3rd international symposium on autologous bone marrow transplantation. Houston, pp 407–417

62. Hartmann O (1987) Institut Gustave Roussy experience in neuroblastoma. In: Dicke K, Spitzer G, Jagannath S (eds) Proceedings of the 3rd international autologous bone marrow transplantation. Houston

63. Seeger B (1987) The UCLA experience in neuroblastoma. In: Dicke K, Spitzer G, Jagannath S (eds) Proceedings of the 3rd international symposium on autologous bone marrow transplantation. Houston

64. August CA (1987) The Philadelphia experience in neuroblastoma. In: Dicke K, Spitzer G, Jagannath S (eds) Proceedings of the 3rd international symposium on autologous bone marrow transplantation. Houston

65. Pinkerton R (1987) The ENSG experience in neuroblastoma. In: Dicke K, Spitzer G, Jagannath S (eds) Proceedings of the 3rd International symposium on autologous bone marrow transplantation. Houston, pp 401–405

66. Deacon JM, Wilson PA, Peckham MJ (1985) The radiobiology of human neuroblastoma. Radiother Oncol 3: 201

67. Hartmann O, Benhamou E, Beaujean F, Pico JL, Kalifa C, Patte C, flamant F, Lemerle J (1986) High dose busulfan and cyclophosphamide with autologous bone marrow transplantation support in advanced malignancies in children: a phase II study. J Clin Oncol 4: 1804

68. Antman K, Eder JP, Elias A, Shea T, Peters WP, Andersen J, Schryber S, Henner WD, Finberg R, Wilmore D, Kaplan W, Lew M, Kruskall MS, Anderson K, Gorgone B, Bast R, Schnipper L, Frei E (1987) A high dose combination alkylating agent preparative regimen with autologous bone marrow support: the DFCI/BIN experience. Cancer Treat Rep 71: 19–25

69. Humblet Y, Symann M, Bosly A, Delaunois L, Francis C, Machiels J, Beauduin M, Doyen C, Prignot J (1987) Transplantation in selected small cell carcinoma of the lung: a randomized study. J Clin Oncol 12: 1921–1930

70. Farha P, Spitzer G, Valdivieso M (1983) High dose chemotherapy and autologous bone marrow transplantation for the treatment of small cell lung carcinoma. Cancer 52: 1351

71. Souhami RL, Harper PG, Linch D (1983) High dose cyclophosphamide with autologous marrow support for treatment of small cell carcinoma of the bronchus. Cancer Chemother Pharmacol 10: 205

72. Spitzer G, Dicke K, Zander AR, Farha P, Valdivieso M (1986) High dose intensification therapy with autologous bone marrow support for limited small cell bronchogenic carcinoma. J Clin Oncol 4: 4

73. Lazarus H, Herzig R, Wolff S (1985) Treatment of metastatic malignant melanoma with intensive melphalan and autologous bone marrow transplantation. Cancer Treat Rep 69: 473

74. Cornbleet MA, McElwain TJ, Kumar PJ (1983) Treatment of advanced malignant melanoma with high dose melphalan and autologous bone marrow transplantation. Br J Cancer 48: 329

75. Tchekmedyian JS, Tait N, Van Echo D, Aisner J (1986) High dose chemotherapy without bone marrow transplantation in melanoma. J Clin Oncol 4: 1811

76. Blijham G, Spitzer G, Litam J (1981) The treatment of advanced testicular carcinoma with high dose chemotherapy and autologous marrow support. Eur J Cancer 17: 443

77. Champlin R (1985) Autologous bone marrow transplantation of testicular carcinoma. Int J Cell Cloning 3: 260

78. Wolff S (1983) Intensive VP16-213 chemotherapy for advanced refractory germinal cell tumors. J Cell Biol [Suppl] 2: 125

79. Stewart P (1982) Autologous bone marrow transplantation in metastatic breast cancer. Breast Cancer Res Treat 2: 85

80. Gisselbrecht J (1986) The St Louis experience with ABMT in breast carcinoma. European Organisation for Research and Treatment of Cancer Meeting, Bruxelles, 1986

81. Hildebrand J, Badjou R, Collard-Ronge E (1980) Treatment of brain gliomas with high dose of CCNU and autologous bone marrow transplantation. Biomedicine 32: 71

82. Takvorian T, Parker LM, Hockberg FH (1983) Autologous bone marrow transplantation: host effects of high dose BCNU. J Clin Oncol 1: 610

83. Phillips G, Fay J, Herzig G (1985) Autologous bone marrow transplantation in malignant glioma. Int J Cell Cloning 3: 257

84. Phillips GL, Wolff SN, Fay JW, Herzig RH, Lazarus HM, Schold C, Herzing GP (1986) Intensive 1, 3, bis-(2 chloroethyl)1-nitrosourea (BCNU) monochemotherapy and autologous marrow transplantation for malignant glioma. J Clin Oncol 4: 639

85. Perren TJ, Mbidde E, Selby P, Workman P, Whitton A, MacElwan TJ (1987) High dose BCNU with ABMT and full dose radiotherapy for grade IV astrocytoma. In: EBMT Meeting Switzerland, Interlaken, March 1987 (in press)

86. Biron P, Mornex F, Vial C, Chauvin F, Veyssere M, Philip I, Philip T (1987) Pilot study of high dose carmustine, transplantation, radiotherapy and surgery for patients with glioma. In: Dicke K, Spitzer G, Jagannath S (eds) Proceeding of the 3rd international symposium on autologous bone marrow transplantation. Houston

142

7. Allogeneic Marrow Transplantation for Malignancy —Current Problems and Prospects for Improvement*

F.R. Appelbaum

Introduction

For many patients with hematologic malignancies, allogeneic marrow transplantation offers either the best or the only chance for cure, and for this reason it has become a widely used form of therapy. However, the procedure as currently employed has only limited effectiveness: many patients die from complications of the procedure, and in many others the disease recurs, despite transplantation. Further, a considerable number of patients for whom transplantation would be indicated cannot receive the treatment because they lack an appropriate donor. In this chapter, the current role of allogeneic marrow transplantation in the treatment of malignant disease and the major problems which limit the effectiveness of this procedure are reviewed. Major emphasis will be given to ways in which these problems are being addressed or might be addressed in the future.

Role of Allogeneic Marrow Transplantation for Malignancy

The following represents a brief review of the current role of allogeneic marrow transplantation for malignant disease, based primarily on data obtained in Seattle over the last decade. In these studies, we have generally used a transplant-preparative regiment consisting of 60 mg/kg cyclophosphamide (CY) per day for 2 days, followed by total body irradiation (TBI) delivered as either 10 Gy in a single fraction or 12–15.75 Gy fractionated over 6 or 7 days. Most of the results, unless otherwise stated, refer to the use of human leukocyte antigen (HLA)-matched family member donors and the use posttransplant of methotrexate (MTX), cyclosporine, or a combination of the two as graft-versus-host disease (GVHD) prophylaxis. Several other reviews of marrow transplantation have recently been published [1–4].

*This investigation was supported by PHS Grant Numbers CA 18029, CA 15704, CA 18105, awarded by the National Cancer Institute, Department of Health and Human Services.

Clinical Results in Acute Nonlymphocytic Leukemia

Recurrent Form

Between 1970 and 1975, 54 patients with end-stage refractory acute nonlymphocytic leukemia (ANL) received transplants from HLA-identical siblings, and six are living and well 11–15 years after grafting, with no further antileukemic therapy [5]. The actual relapse rate was approximately 65%. Since publication of this result, a substantial number of patients with recurrent ANL (132) have received transplants in first resistant relapse, second remission, or untreated first relapse [6]. At 3 years, the survival rate was equally good for those transplanted in untreated first relapse (34%) and those transplanted in second remission (34%). That these two are equal argues that patients should not necessarily be reinduced prior to transplantation since getting the patient into second remission is of no apparent advantage, and since some patients may die during the attempt. The results of treatment both at untreated first relapse and in second remission are better than those of treatment in resistant first relapse (24%). Taken together, these results argue that the best time for transplantation, if not in first remission, is as soon as possible after first relapse. This observation in turn provides a strong rationale for the development of sensitive markers—either cytogenetic, immunologic, or biochemical—to detect early relapse.

First Remission

Based on the premise that patients in first remission are healthier and therefore better able to withstand transplantation—and that they should have a decreased tumor burden, which is perhaps less drug resistant—19 patients received transplants in first remission. Of these patients, 10 remain alive and well now more than 7 years after transplantation [7]. By 1986, 231 patients with ANL in first remission had been transplanted in Seattle, and 49% ± 3% were alive at 3 years after transplantation [6]. Age was a predictor of success, with approximately 70% of patients aged under 20 years surviving, as opposed to 40%–45% of those aged over 20; there was little difference in those aged 20–30, 30–40, and 40–50.

Role of Allogeneic Marrow Transplantation in the Treatment of ANL

A major clinical question is whether patients with ANL in first remission should receive transplants straightaway or whether one should follow them closely and perform transplantation at the first moment of relapse. A number of chemotherapy regimens can cure a proportion of adults with ANL. Our experience in 74 patients with ANL given high-dose cytosine arabinoside consolidation is that 34% will be alive 3 years from treatment [8]. Among the 66% in whom such therapy is predicated to fail, it may be possible to cure 30% with transplantation at first relapse. The combined rate of cure of 34% with chemotherapy and an additional 30% of the remainder (19.8%) would be close to 50%, and therefore similar to that for transplantation in first remission. This argument does not take into account the fact that the chemotherapy curve has yet to show a clear

144

plateau, and that past rates of cure with conventional chemotherapy have been in the range of 20%–25%. Further, transplantation will not be feasible in those patients who die during chemotherapy or acquire medical problems which prohibit transplantation, such as chronic liver disease or deep-seated fungal infections. To determine which approach is superior—transplantation in first remission or transplantation at first relapse—a prospective comparative trial would be required.

There have been a number of prospective studies comparing the outcome of conventional chemotherapy with that of allogeneic marrow transplantation. In each of these studies, transplantation showed either a statistically significant advantage or an advantage that did not quite reach statistical significance [9–11]. These studies did not answer (nor were they intended to) the question whether transplantation should be performed in first remission rather than at first relapse since the chemotherapy group was composed of patients without matched donors, in whom, therefore, transplantation could not be performed at first relapse. Rather, these studies were designed to compare in a prospective manner the outcome of chemotherapy and that of transplantation in like groups of patients, taking care to remove, as much as possible, any selection bias in each treatment group. Since transplantation showed an advantage, the stage has been set for attempting to answer the second question, i.e., whether there is an advantage to transplantation in first remission versus transplantation at first relapse.

Allogeneic Versus Autologous Transplantation

Recent results of autologous transplantation for ANL in both first and second remission demonstrate remarkably good outcomes; up to 45% of patients were alive and in remission 2 years after autologous transplantation in first remission, and up to 40% were alive and in remission in a small group of patients who received autologous marrow transplants for ANL in second remission [12, 13]. These results have been obtained both with marrow treated in vitro with agents designed to remove clonogenic tumor cells and with untreated marrow. As unlikely as it might seem, current results support the proposition that, at least in some cases, either the marrow in a patient who is in remission but destined to relapse without transplantation must contain insufficient tumor cells to lead to disease recurrence or, after the transplant, some active phenomenon (perhaps autoimmune-like) must lead to the elimination of residual tumor. No matter what the mechanism of action may be, these results—albeit obtained in relatively small, possibly highly selected patient populations—are sufficiently encouraging to raise the question whether autologous or allogeneic transplantation for ANL is superior. Autologous transplantation has the obvious advantage of avoiding GVHD and its complications. Allogeneic transplantation has the advantage of almost certainly having a lower relapse rate post-transplant, both because autologous marrow must lead to relapse in some cases and because autologous marrow lacks a graft-versus-tumor effect. This latter effect, based on the results of twin and T-cell-depleted marrow transplant studies, may be substantial.

In view of these considerations, we and others have begun a three-arm prospective study of allogeneic transplantation versus autologous transplantation versus continued chemotherapy for patients with ANL in first remission. Those randomized to conventional chemotherapy will have the option of transplantation at first relapse. Within the setting of autologous transplantation, there remain a number of important questions concerning different methods of in vitro marrow treatment, including their relative safety and effectiveness.

Clinical Results in Acute Lymphocytic Leukemia

Outcome of Transplantation

The results of marrow transplantation for acute lymphocytic leukemia (ALL) are similar to those in ANL: a small but definite percentage of patients with end-stage disease can be cured, and the percentage increases when transplantation is carried out earlier in the patient's course. The results obtained in Seattle and those reported by the International Bone Marrow Transplant Registry (IBMTR) show that survival at 3 years post-transplant is approximately 15%–20% for patients with advanced disease, 30%–35% for patients in second remission, and 35%–45% for patients in first remission [3, 5, 14–16]. The actuarial chance of relapse is high for all three groups, being approximately 70%, 50% and 35% respectively.

Role of Marrow Transplantation in the Treatment of ALL

Since marrow transplantation is the only form of therapy that can cure patients with drug-resistant disease, there is little argument that it should be performed in such patients if at all possible. A prospective study of marrow transplantation versus continued chemotherapy for patients with ALL in second remission demonstrated a clear advantage to transplantation [17]. Possible exceptions to this conclusion are patients who relapse off therapy after a long disease-free interval: such patients may do as well with subsequent chemotherapy as with transplantation [18]. There has not been a prospective study comparing the outcome of marrow transplantation for ALL in first remission with that of either chemotherapy alone or chemotherapy plus transplantation at first relapse. In fact, the improved outcome of contemporary chemotherapy programs for normal-risk children, and more recently for adults as well, makes it difficult to justify such a trial [19, 20]. There are, however, patients will ALL at high risk for relapse following conventional chemotherapy (such as those with Philadelphia chromosome-positive ALL). That such patients would benefit from transplantation in first remission is an (as yet) unproven but testable hypothesis.

Allogeneic Versus Autologous Transplantation

Many reports document long-term disease-free survival in a proportion of patients treated for ALL in second or subsequent remission with high-dose chemoradiotherapy followed by autologous marrow transplantation [20]. The arguments about which form of therapy (allogeneic or autologous) is superior

146

for patients with ALL parallel those already raised for ANL: autologous transplantation is safer, but allogeneic transplantation will result in fewer post-transplant relapses. There has not yet been a direct comparison of these two approaches in a prospective controlled trial.

Clinical Results in Chronic Myelogenous Leukemia

Outcome of Transplantation

Results in Seattle and those reported by the IBMTR and others demonstrate long-term survival in 49%–56% of transplant patients treated during chronic phase chronic myelogenous leukemia (CML), 15%–28% of those treated during accelerated phase, and 14%–16% of those treated in blast crisis [3, 21, 22]. The actuarial probability of relapse was 12%–20% for transplant patients treated in chronic phase, 40%–56% for those treated in accelerated phase, and 50%–75% for those treated in blast crisis.

Role of Transplantation in the Treatment of CML

There is no other curative approach for CML at this time; therefore, in any patient aged less than 50 with CML and an available donor, transplantation should probably be performed. The major question is one of timing: marrow transplantation during chronic phase offers the greatest possibility of cure but carries a risk of early death from transplant-related complications. Delaying transplantation may result in disease progression and therefore a poorer outcome of transplantation. Even if the disease does not progress, data from the Seattle series suggest that transplant results are best if carried out within 1 year of diagnosis [21]. In the end, the timing of transplantation for patients with CML is both a medical and a philosophical decision.

Marrow Transplantation for Malignant Lymphoma

Between July 1970 and January 1985, 100 patients with recurrent malignant lymphoma were treated in Seattle with CY, TBI, and marrow transplantation [23]. The actuarial disease-free survival rate at 5 years was 22%, with a 60% probability of relapse. In this initial experience and in subsequent studies, transplant patients treated in either first relapse or second remission did significantly better, with a 2-year disease-free survival rule of 42% and a probability of relapse of 41% [24]. Disease histology (Hodgkin's disease, high-grade non-Hodgkin's lymphoma, or intermediate-grade non-Hodgkin's lymphoma) has so far not been predictive of outcome, nor has source of marrow (autologous, allogeneic, or syngeneic). There has not yet been a formal comparison of marrow transplantation with other forms of salvage therapy. However, the results obtained with marrow transplantation for recurrent malignant lymphoma, especially those in early relapse, are better than the reported results of almost any salvage chemotherapy program [25].

147

Transplantation for Preleukemia

Although occasional patients with preleukemic syndromes respond to low-dose cytosine arabinoside or other interventions, there is no therapy with curative potential for this group of diseases except for marrow transplantation [26]. Recent reports suggest that more than 50% of patients with de novo preleukemia can achieve long-term disease-free survival following allogeneic marrow transplantation [27, 28]. Results in secondary preleukemia, although very preliminary, are not as encouraging, but some long-term disease-free survivors have been reported [28].

Other Hematologic Malignancies

Although published series so far consist of only a few case reports or very small series, so that accurate statistics are lacking, long-term disease-free survival has been seen following marrow transplantation for a number of other hematologic malignancies, indicating a possible role for this approach in myeloma, myelosclerosis, hairy-cell leukemia, and histiocytic medullary retriculosis [29–32].

Solid Tumors

In the case of hematologic malignancies, the results of allogeneic marrow transplantation set the stage for experiments using autologous marrow. In the treatment of solid tumors, where marrow involvement is less common, the situation is reversed. Thus, most transplants for solid tumors have been performed with autologous marrow, and allogeneic marrow transplantation would only be explored in the event that these results become encouraging; so far, unfortunately, this has not been the case. Although substantial response rates have been seen in tumors generally considered to be unresponsive or minimally responsive to conventional therapy, these responses have generally been short and incomplete, and their extent does not yet justify the toxicities expected with allogeneic transplantation. An important exception is the case of metastatic neuroblastoma, where long-term disease-free survival and probable cure has been achieved in a definite proportion of patients with otherwise incurable disease following either autologous or allogeneic marrow transplantation [33].

The Problem of Disease Recurrence

Definition

For almost every category of disease mentioned in the above review, the major reason for failure of the transplant procedure is disease recurrence. The term "disease recurrence" means the reappearance of the original malignant cell population as determined by DNA markers, and it implies that the transplant regimen was unable to eradicate the original malignant clone [34]. While probably more than 95% of cases of relapse following transplantation are of this type, recurrence of malignancy which appears morphologically identical to the original leukemia has occasionally been seen in cells of donor rather than host origin [35, 36]. The mechanism accounting for this phenomenon is unknow, but its existence suggests that the immediate cellular milieu is important. The process could involve transfection of DNA between cells. Further investigation of these unusual relapses is likely to yield important insights concerning leukemic causation. Also, occasional cases of immunoblastic lymphosarcoma in cells of donor origin have been seen [37]. These cases have been associated with Epstein-Barr viral genomes within the tumor cell DNA and have generally occurred in very immunosuppressed patients with advanced GVHD [36]. Again, investigation of these cases will probably provide important information concerning the sequence of events involved in viral oncogenesis. The vast majority of disease recurrences, however, are due to regrowth of the original malignant clone, and it is this form of recurrence which must be diminished if substantial progress is to be made in the utility of allogeneic marrow transplantation.

Methods to Lessen Post-Transplant Relapse Rates

Earlier Transplantation

As noted in each of the diseases reviewed above, transplantation earlier in the disease course results in less post-transplant relapse. However, early transplantation is not always the answer. Some patients have refractory disease at diagnosis. For others (ALL and many categories of lymphoma), transplantation in first remission is not indicated or chosen by the physican and patient. Even with transplantation in first remission, the post-transplant relapse rates remain unacceptably high. Therefore, other methods of lessening post-transplant relapse rates are needed.

Better Chemotherapy

The preparative regimen most commonly used until now has been a combination of CY and TBI. There is no reason to believe that CY is the best single agent to combine with TBI, and several phase II studies of other single agents combined with TBI have been published, including VP-16 and high-dose cytosine arabinoside [K Blume 1987, personal communication; 38, 39] The results to date have suggested a possible advantage with these newer regimens. Since combination chemotherapy is, in general, more effective than single-agent chemotherapy in conventional treatment trials, combination chemotherapy with TBI may well be more effective than single-agent therapy with TBI as a transplant-preparative regimen; several studies addressing this hypothesis are under way.

Better External Beam Irradiation

The initial form of TBI used for marrow transplantation was single-dose TBI delivered by dual cobalt sources at around 0.07 cGy/min. In 1982, Thomas et al. [40] published the results of a prospective randomized trial for patients with ANL in first remission, which demonstrated that the survival rate in patients given TBI in six daily fractions of 2 cGy each was superior to that in patients given a single dose of 10 Gy TBI. Fractionated TBI was better tolerated and resulted in fewer long-term complications than single-dose TBI, but it did not alter the post-transplant relapse rate. Surprisingly, this study remains the only prospective randomized trial comparing two different TBI regimens. Investigators at the Memorial Sloan Kettering Cancer Center have treated patients with ALL in second and subsequent remission using hyperfractionated TBI followed by CY and have published results which appear superior to those achieved in Seattle [41]. Whether this possible improvement is due to the use of hyperfractionated TBI as opposed to daily fractionation or to the ordering of TBI and CY is unknown, but both possibilities deserve attention. Some patients who relapse following marrow transplantation do so at sites of previous bulk disease. This type of relapse is most commonly seen in transplant patients treated for malignant lymphoma and suggests that the addition of local boost radiotherapy to the preparative regimen might be of benefit for these patients. Whether boost radiotherapy is best given before or after transplant and whether it can contribute to improved survival is as yet unknown. Studies by Phillips et al. [42] suggest that pretransplant boost radiotherapy can be given with relative safety and may contribute to improved survival for patients with Hodgkin's disease, but that it does not clearly benefit patients with other diagnoses. An idea similar in concept to boost radiotherapy is to shield organs where lethal toxicities are most commonly seen; for example, in patients with a low risk of relapse post-transplant (e.g., preleukemia), where the most common reason for failure is interstitial pneumonia, a small amount of lung shielding might prove to be of benefit.

Antibody-Isotope Conjugates

The use of either boost radiotherapy or shielding is designed to increase the dose of radiotherapy to the tumor and limit the dose to potential sites of toxicity. A possibly more effective way of achieving the goal of directed radiotherapy is to link radioisotopes to monoclonal antibodies and use the antibodies to target radiotherapy to the tumor site. Unlabelled monoclonal antibodies reactive with tumor-associated antigens have been shown to concentrate on tumor cells following in vivo administration [43–46]. However, the use of unlabelled antibodies as a treatment for malignancy has met with only limited therapeutic success for two major reasons: some tumor cells lack the target antigen and are therefore unaffected by the antibody, and further, even when coated with antibody, many tumor cells persist because the host lacks effector mechanisms for eliminating the antibody-coated tumor cell [47]. Attaching a radioisotope to the antibody should overcome these limitations since the cytotoxic effects of

150

radiation do not depend on host effector mechanism, and antigen-negative cells in proximity to antibody-coated targets may also be killed.

The use of antibody-isotope conjugates as a transplant-preparative regimen has just begun to be explored. We have shown in a canine model that marrow is very accessible to antibody targeting: within 1 h of the administration of a radiolabelled antibody directed toward marrow progenitor cells, the amount of isotope in the marrow compared with that in any other organ achieves a ratio of 5:1 or more [48]. We have further shown that antibody-isotope conjugates can be used in dogs to ablate marrow prior to autologous transplantation without adversely affecting subsequent engraftment. These experiments have set the stage for the application of this technique as part of the treatment regimen for patients with ALL, ANL, CML, or diseases originating in the marrow. We have also shown that lymph nodes can be targeted, albeit not as easily as marrow [49]. An initial patient with nodular, poorly differentiated lymphocytic lymphoma resistant to standard chemotherapy—whose tumor also failed to respond to an infusion of unlabelled anti-idiotype antibody—has recently been treated in Seattle with the same anti-idiotype antibody labelled with ^{131}I followed by autologous marrow transplantation. This patient achieved a complete response and remains disease free at 6 months [50].

A large number of questions pertain to this sort of approach. For example, the optimal kind of target antigen is unknown. Is it better to target a true tumor-specific antigen (if such, apart from idiotype, exist) or to target a differentiation antigen which includes not only the tumor but surrounding normal tissue in the area of the tumor (marrow for leukemia and lymph nodes for lymphoma)? Are whole antibodies or antibody fragments better? What antibody dose and infusion schedule is optimal? Which, among the many available isotopes, will prove best, and how can these isotopes be best linked to the antibody? The list of additional unanswered important questions is long, but the available animal data and preliminary results in patients are sufficiently encouraging to suggest that this general approach of using antibody-isotope conjugates as part of the marrow transplant regimen will be increasingly investigated over the next several years.

Bone-Seeking Isotopes

A unique feature of marrow is its close proximity to bone. Microscopy of bone marrow biopsy samples shows that marrow cells are rarely if ever more than a millimeter or two away from bony trabeculae. There exist substances which have an enormous capacity to target bone and which are therefore used as bone-scanning agents. By attaching a β-emitting (i.e., radiation of low penetration) isotope to such substances, it should be possible to deliver very localized radio-therapy to the marrow space, thereby increasing the dose to the tumor cells in ANL, ALL, CML, or preleukemia, without significantly radiating any other organ. An ideal isotope for this purpose would deposit the majority of its energy locally (within 1 or 2 mm) and would have a weak γ component to allow for accurate scanning. In addition, the isotope should have a short half-life to permit subsequent marrow engraftment. We have begun animal studies with such a compound [153]samarium EDTMP), and the early results are very encouraging; ratios of radioactivity in marrow to that in any other organ of at least 20:1 can be achieved, and marrow ablation accomplished without toxicity to any other organ. The ultimate application of this approach will probably be in combination with other systemic therapies (such as combination chemotherapy with or without additional TBI) in order to achieve adequate immunosuppression and treat extremeduallary disease.

Adoptive Immunotherapy

Several observations demonstrate that there is almost certainly a graft-versus-tumor effect following allogeneic transplantation for hematologic malignancies. Relapse rates following syngeneic transplants are higher than those following allogeneic transplants [1, 51]. Among allogeneic transplant recipients, those who developed clinically significant GVHD have a lower incidence of relapse than those without GVHD [52–4]. Further, recipients of T-cell-depleted marrow have a higher incidence of disease recurrence than recipients of unmanipulated marrow [55]. All of these observations demonstrate that in addition to immunologically reacting against its new host, the transplanted marrow also reacts against the host's tumor. Moreover, the tumor may be the most sensitive target of all.

To date, it has been difficult to take advantage of the lesser incidence of recurrent leukemia in patients with GVHD since this advantage has been offset by a greater probability of other causes of death. However, evidence from studies in rodent transplant models suggest that the allogeneic graft-versus-leukemia effect can be distinguished in some cases from GVHD [56, 57]. These effects (graft-versus-leukemia and GVHD) may be distinguishable in two ways; either by differences in target antigens or by differences in the type of effector cells. The graft-versus-host reaction is probably directed against many different antigens, some of which are relatively tissue specific; hence, GVHD may involve isolated organs. This implies that there is a population of donor effector cells with relative specificity either for the tumor itself or for the host tissue in which the tumor arose. If those cells with relative specificity for tumor or the tissue from which the tumor developed could be isolated, cloned, and expanded in vitro, these cells could be administered to the patient after transplantation in an attempt to augment the antitumor effects of the transplant procedure. Alternatively, it may be possible to separate those cells responsible for tumor eradication from those contributing to GVHD simply on the basis of T-cell phenotype. Rodent experiments suggest that class I-restricted cytotoxic T cells contribute to GVHD, but not to tumor eradication, while the reverse is true for class II-restricted T cells.

While the technique of specific adoptive immunotherapy has only just begun to be applied clinically in humans, the observation of a graft-versus-tumor effect following allogeneic marrow transplantation supports the approach. Further, murine studies show that with interleukin-2 (IL-2), T cells sensitized to tumor antigens can be expanded in vitro and then infused, resulting in eradication of established tumor [58, 59]. Thus, the requirements for the application of this approach already exist.

Establishment of Stable Chimerism

Inherent in the concept of successful allogeneic transplantation is the requirement for stable engraftment without the development of clinically significant GVHD.

Stable Engraftment

Problem of Graft Rejection

Over the last decade, most allogeneic transplants for malignancy were performed using HLA-matched donors, preparative regimens employing TBI, and unmanipulated marrow. In this situation, stable engraftment was almost always achieved, and graft rejection was very uncommon, occuring in less than 1% of cases. Two developments have changed this circumstance. First, the use of donors who are not completely matched has increased the incidence of graft rejection. In Seattle, we have seen failure of stable engraftment in less than 1% of matched donor-recipient pairs, in approximately 5% of donor-recipient pairs mismatched for a single antigen (A, B, or D), and in 15%–20% of two-antigen mismatched pairs [60]. A second development which has led to more graft rejection is the use of marrow depleted of T cells. While T-cell depletion has convincingly resulted in less GVHD, this has been at the cost of an increase in graft rejection in most studies [61]. Presumably, one target of donor T cells are cells of host origin responsible for residual host immunity. Without T cells in the marrow inoculum, there is, in some cases, sufficient recovery of host immunity to reject the transplanted marrow. This immunologic recovery would not occur were T cells left in the transplanted marrow to react with host cells. Some have suggested that graft failure following T-cell depletion results because T cells are required for stem-cell growth. This is unlikely since graft failure has not been seen following autologous transplantation for T-cell lymphoma, where T-cell depletion has been used in an effort to remove possible tumor cells.

The population of host cells responsible for graft rejection may depend upon the particular clinical situation. For example, canine studies suggest that in the situation of untransfused mismatched donor-recipient pairs, a non-T-cell Ia-positive population of host cells is responsible [62]. On the other hand, in the situation of matched recipients specifically sensitized to their donor via previous transfusions, host T cells are at least partly responsible for graft rejection [63]. Understanding the mechanisms of graft rejection is of obvious importance in designing ways to overcome the problem.

Methods to Prevent Graft Rejection

One obvious way to overcome the problem of graft rejection is to increase the immunosuppressive effects of the preparative regimen in order to remove the population of host cells responsible for rejection. Initial attempts have involved either additional chemotherapy (such as cytosine arabinoside) or more TBI in the preparative regimen. The results to date suggest that these modifications result in a decrease in the incidence of graft rejection but an increase in transplant-related toxicities and no obvious survival advantage [64]. Adding relatively small doses of total lymphoid irradiation (TLI) to the preparative regimen is being explored and again has decreased, but has not totally eliminated, the problem of graft rejection with either T-cell-depleted or mismatched marrow [65].

Several investigators are now studying the effects of adding to the preparative regimen antibodies directed against those cells thought to be responsible for graft rejection. In a canine model, we showed that the addition to the preparative regimen of either an anti-Ia antibody or an antibody raised against radiation-resistant marrow cells allowed engraftment in mismatched dogs in a setting where, without antibody, graft rejection was virtually always seen [62, 66]. Similarly, in dogs, anti-T-cell antibodies were partially successful in facilitating engraftment in sensitized matched marrow recipients [63]. However, even in carefully constructed animal models, unmodified antibodies have only limited effectiveness. Methods to increase the effectiveness of these agents may involve labelling antibodies with either toxins or isotopes. In this regard, the issues already alluded to in "Antibody-isotope conjugates" will pertain.

It may also be possible to decrease the incidence of graft rejection by specific manipulations of donor marrow. It is as yet unknown if those cells within donor marrow responsible for promoting engraftment are identical to those responsible for the development of GVHD. If not, it may be possible to deplete marrow of only certain populations of T cells to prevent GVHD and to leave behind or even enrich for other populations to promote engraftment. Another approach being explored is to incubate marrow with growth factors in vitro before transplantation in order to promote engraftment. Preliminary work in rodent models reported by Blazar et al. [67] suggests that incubation of T-cell-depleted marrow with granulocyte/macrophage colony-stimulating factor (GM-CSF) prior to transplant allowed engraftment across an MHC barrier, where unincubated marrow failed to engraft. Similarly, it may be possible to use such growth factors in vivo post transplant to promote proliferation of the donor graft without encouraging the proliferation of host immune cells.

Graft-Versus-Host Disease

Along with the problem of disease recurrence, GVHD is the major limitation of allogeneic marrow transplantation. Although the mortality due directly to GVHD in many studies is low (often around 5%–10% for matched donor-recipient pairs), the impact of GVHD is far greater than is implied by this figure since it contributes to death ascribed to other causes, such as infection, inter-

154

stitial pneumonia, or liver disease. Among 231 transplant patients with ANL treated in first remission in Seattle, the diagnosis of clinically significant GVHD was associated with a 250% increase in mortality [6].

GVHD is thought to be the result of the reaction of alloreactive T cells transferred with the marrow, or developing from it, against target cells of the genetically different host. Clinically, GVHD can be separated into two distinct syndromes, acute GVHD and chronic GVHD, the manifestations of which have been the subject of several reviews [68–70]. The incidence of acute GVHD is dependent upon many factors, the most obvious of which are the age of the patient, the degree of histocompatibility between donor and recipient, and the form of GVHD prophylaxis used. Among HLA-matched donor-recipient pairs given standard methotrexate (MTX) or cyclosporine post-transplant, the incidence of clinically significant GVHD has been approximately 40% [71, 72].

A number of approaches have been taken to reduce the impact of GVHD on the outcome of marrow transplantation. Many studies have addressed the use of immunosuppressive drugs post-transplant. The combination of MTX and cyclosporine or cyclosporine and prednisone is superior to either MTX or cyclosporine used alone [73–75]. Whether triple therapy (MTX cyclosporine, and prednisone) will further improve outcome is currently being tested. New immunosuppressive agents are currently undergoing testing in animal models [76]. Carrying out transplantation within laminar airflow isolation is another technique which appears able to reduce the incidence of acute GVHD [77].

A method to avoid GVHD, already alluded to, which holds great promise is T-cell depletion of donor marrow. A number of techniques to remove T cells have been developed, including the use of antibodies plus complement, antibody-toxin conjugates, antibodies coupled to magnetic beads, and lectin agglutinins [61, 78, 79]. There is no convincing evidence that any one of these techniques is superior to the others. To date, available evidence suggests that all of the techniques are capable of removing the large majority of T cells from donor marrow (usually in excess of 99%), but until it is known exactly how many, and which, T cells should be removed, it will remain difficult to choose among these methods since they may vary in efficiency and in the particular populations of T cells removed. Importantly, all these techniques appear capable of substantially reducing the incidence of GVHD. However, all are also associated with a substantial increase in the incidence of graft rejection, even in the setting of HLA-matched donor-recipient pairs. The problem is even worse in the setting of mismatched transplants, where graft rejection rates of 30%–50% have been seen following the use of T-cell-depleted marrow. Since most graft rejections result in death, there are no studies which yet demonstrate improved survival with the use of T-cell-depleted marrow grafts. However, the markedly decreased incidence of GVHD seen with T-cell depletion suggests that the technique has great promise in eliminating the problem of GVHD if the problem of graft rejection can be overcome. As already discussed in "Methods to prevent graft rejection," this will probably require the development of preparative regimens with greater and more specific immunosuppressive effects but without increased toxicity. In this regard, the use of antibody-isotope or antibody-toxin conjugates holds great promise.

Expansion of the Donor Pool

Only 35%–40% of patients have HLA-identical family members available to serve as donors, a fact which obviously limits the applicability of allogeneic marrow transplantation. It may be possible to expand the donor pool in a variety of ways, including the use of mismatched family member donors, or matched (or mismatched) unrelated donors. Available data show that with currently available techniques for GVHD prophylaxis, the use of mismatched donors is associated with an increase is GVHD [60]. This increase is not necessarily prohibitive, however. Patients receiving transplants from family member donors mismatched at a single antigen have more GVHD than matched patients but survive equally well. Patients mismatched for two or more antigens have both more GVHD and poorer survival than matched patients. It may be possible to improve the results of mismatched transplants by selecting only certain mismatches. Experience gained in platelet transfusions, for example, suggests that there are certain antigen pairs which resemble each other more closely than other antigen pairs and are therefore said to be cross-reactive. It is possible that mismatched transplants between such cross-reactive groups may fare better than other mismatched transplants. The ability to predict the extent of GVHD prior to transplantation should also allow for more effective selection of mismatched donors. Certain donor-associated factors have been shown to be predictive of the development of GVHD in matched donor-recipient pairs (donor sex and the presence of certain HLA alleles in the donor), and recently an in vitro test possibly predictive of GVHD has been described by Vogelsang et al. [80]. However, even in the best of circumstances, the use of mismatched marrow carries with it a high risk of clinically significant GVHD, and the routine use of mismatched marrow will require the development of better techniques of GVHD prevention.

Some patients have received transplants from matched unrelated donors and have achieved prolonged disease-free survival. However, the number is as yet too small to allow conclusions about how much GVHD will be seen in this circumstance and how it will influence survival. Almost certainly, the results will not be as good as with matched family members. However, as methods of GVHD prophylaxis improve, the use of unrelated donors will almost certainly increase. In anticipation of this increased use, the federal government is supporting the development of a national marrow donor registry involving more than 50 centers and including 50 000–80 000 potential donors. The establishment of such a pool has raised many questions. Are we really ready to rush headlong into this venture until more preliminary work is done? Should the government pay for the registry or should the charge go to those who use it? What degree of donor risk is acceptable? How will potential donors be protected from coercion? Should cadaveric marrow be routinely harvested and cryo-preserved? All of these questions will doubtless demand answers in the near future. At present, the results of transplants using unrelated donors are probably not encouraging enough to recommend this approach as standard therapy, but as GVHD prophylaxis measures improve,the increased use of unrelated donors is inevitable.

Alternative Sources of Hematopoietic Stem Cells

The vast majority of allogeneic transplants have used hematopoietic stem cells harvested from marrow. At least two other sources of hematopoietic stem cells exist: the peripheral blood and fetal liver. Animal and now human studies have shown that autologous peripheral blood stem cells can be used to restore hematopoiesis following otherwise lethal TBI. However, peripheral blood stem cells have not, so far, been used for human allogeneic transplantation because peripheral blood has a far higher concentration of mature T cells and far fewer stem cells than marrow, a situation which favors the development of GVHD while, at the same time, making complete engraftment more difficult. Recently, Chang et al. [81] reported successful engraftment using autologous marrow cultured in vitro for 10 days. As our understanding of cell separation techniques and growth factors increases, one can imagine the day when only a small amount of marrow or purified peripheral blood will suffice to establish cultures in which the desired cells can be expanded in preparation for hematopoietic cell transplantation.

Another source of hematopoietic stem cells is fetal liver. In mammalian ontogeny, the liver is the primary hematopoietic organ for some time. Fetal liver cells are rich in hematopoietic stem cells while containing few T cells, and in animal studies they have been used to restore hematopoiesis without severe GVHD [82]. Some children with severe combined immunodeficiency have apparently been cured by fetal liver-cell infusions [83]. However, there is as yet scanty evidence that enduring complete chimerism can be achieved in adults treated for either aplastic anemia or leukemia with standard transplant-preparative regimens followed by fetal liver-cell infusions [84].

Other Transplant-Related Toxicities

While the two major problems of allogeneic marrow transplantation are establishment of stable chimerism and eradication of the malignant disease, other substantial problems exist. These can generally be divided into those toxicities due to the preparative regimen and those secondary to infectious complications.

Preparative Regimen-Related Toxicities

A number of patients die due to toxicities directly related to the preparative regimen, such as severe mucositis, veno-occlusive disease of the liver, acute myocarditis, and idiopathic interstitial pneumonia. As more intensive preparative regimens are explored in efforts to eradicate resistant disease or provide greater immunosuppression to prevent rejection of T-cell-depleted marrow, it is likely that the incidence of these toxicities will, if anything, increase. The precise incidence, at present, of life-threatening and fatal toxicities in each organ system, which can be directly related to the preparative regimen, is difficult to judge by reviewing published literature, in part because no consistent grading system for regimen-related toxicity has been applied. Recently, we have published such a grading system and have used it to retrospectively analyze the results of more than 100 HLA-matched allogeneic transplants following a preparative regimen of CY and 12 Gy fractionated TBI [85, 86]. A 10% incidence of grade III (life-threatening) or grade IV (fatal) toxicity directly related to the preparative regimen was seen.

The precise mechanisms leading to these toxicities are not, for the most part, understood, nor is it understood why severe or fatal toxicities are seen in one patient and minimal toxicity is seen in another. Understanding the mechanisms of specific organ toxicity might allow for the development of specific protective measures, as, for example, the use of mesna to protect the bladder from the toxicity of high-dose CY without interfering with its antitumor or immunosuppressive effects. Understanding the differences in individual patient sensitivities is important since these differences presumably reflect genetically determined or acquired differences in drug metabolism, target cell sensitivity, or repair mechanisms, which might be measurable pretransplant. This would allow for the development of more individualized preparative regimens.

Infectious Complications

Nearly all patients develop granulocytopenia and fever during the first 2 or 3 weeks post-transplant, and in about one-third of the patients positive blood cultures are found. Gram-positive organisms predominate (about 20% of cases), but gram-negative organisms (10%) and fungi (2%–5%) are also seen. Based on this spectrum of organisms, patients with fever and granulocytopenia have in the past been treated in Seattle with an empiric regimen consisting of an aminoglycoside, an antipseudomonal penicillin, and vancomycin. More recently, renal dysfunction has become a more common problem because of the use of cyclosporine and amphotericin, and therefore a double β-lactam regimen has been employed. Granulocytopenic patients who after 6 or 7 days do not respond to antibiotics are treated with amphotericin B, especially if they have two or more surveillance sites positive for fungus. Prophylactic granulocyte transfusions can prevent early infections but have not been shown to affect survival. Similarly, laminar airflow isolation reduces the incidence of infection but has been shown to improve survival only in transplant patients treated for aplastic anemia, but not for leukemia. For patients receiving transplants from HLA-matched donors, the risk of death due to infection during the early granulocytopenic period using current methods of supportive care is low—approximately 5%. This incidence is probably higher when mismatched donor-recipient pairs are considered.

The most important infections occurring in the interval between successful engraftment and day 100 post-transplant are viral or protozoan. Approximately 75% of patients with detectable antibody to cytomegalovirus (CMV) pretransplant have some evidence of CMV activation post-transplant. Often activation is asymptomatic and manifested only by a rise in antibody titer or viral excretion in the urine. Sometimes, CMV can cause hepatitis, fever with marrow suppression, or a gastrointestinal syndrome associated with nausea, vomiting, and abdominal pain. The most serious result of CMV activation is CMV pneumonia, which occurs in roughly 15% of patients and has a case mortality of about 85%. Primary CMV infection can be prevented in CMV-seronegative patients by the exclusive use of CMV-screened seronegative blood products. In this regard, it may be important to consider using CMV-negative blood products for CMV-negative patients during initial chemotherapy so that they may remain CMV negative when referred for transplantation. Immunoprophylaxis using CMV-immune globulin has also been reported to be of use in CMV-negative patients. There is, however, no proven effective therapy for established CMV infection, although trials with a new antiviral agent, dihydroxymethylethoxymethylguanine (DHPG), are encouraging [87, 88]. If these studies continue to show activity, the prophylactic use of DHPG against CMV activation should be considered. We have recently found that moderate doses of DHPG are tolerable in the immediate post-transplant period (F.R. Appelbaum, unpublished work). Another approach to the prevention of CMV infection may prove to be the use of adoptive immunotherapy. If one can isolate and expand T cells from the donor which are specific for CMV-infected targets, it might be possible to infuse these cells during the post-transplant period to provide the patient with specific immunity to CMV infection.

Many other infectious complications—such as herpes simplex infection, *Pneumocystis carinii* pneumonia, or late infections with herpes zoster—are less of a problem now that specific forms of therapy have been applied. The use of systemic acyclovir early in the post-transplant period prevents herpes simplex. Similarly, the use of prophylactic trimethoprim sulfamethoxazole can prevent the development of *Pneumocystis carinii*. Early treatment of herpes zoster after the transplant with acyclovir or vidarabine can usually limit this complication.

Further reduction in the incidence of bacterial, fungal, and viral infections post-transplant might be possible if more rapid myeloid and lymphoid recovery were achieved. The isolation and now production of various proteins which stimulate cell growth both in vitro and in vivo—such as GM-CSF, G-CSF, and IL-3—may provide a way to speed lymphohematopoietic recovery post-transplant.

It is not the purpose of this chapter to review the large area of infectious complications in the immunosuppressed patient since many other excellent reviews have recently been prepared, and the reader is referred to these [89, 90].

Integration of Marrow Transplantation into the Therapeutic Plan

Unfortunately, little has been done to integrate marrow transplantation into the overall treatment plan for most patients with hematologic malignancies. Rather, patients are usually treated with standard chemotherapeutic regimens, and at some moment the physician or the patient decides that transplantation is warranted, and the patient is referred for the procedure. This approach ignores at least two considerations which may prove to be of importance to the patient: first, there is the issue of timing, and second, there is the question of how initial chemotherapy or radiotherapy may influence subsequent salvage transplant approaches.

Consider, for example, the situation of a 40-year-old man with a newly diagnosed high-grade lymphoma. If one decides that the best time to perform transplantation in this patient is at first relapse and that chemotherapy should be used initially in the hope of achieving an enduring remission, then at the very least, while the patient is being treated with chemotherapy, either an HLA-identical family member should be identified or the patient's marrow should be stored, so that transplantation could be carried out without delay in the event of a relapse. Further consideration should be given to the type of initial therapy the patient is given. For example, adding chest radiotherapy to his initial treatment regimen might increase his chance of cure by a few percentage points but recude his chance of being successfully treated with transplantation, were he to relapse, since a higher incidence of fatal interstitial pneumonia has been observed post-transplant in patients with a history of prior chest radiotherapy [23]. With the availability of marrow transplant regimens with curative potential both for patients in first remission and for those at first relapse, the question how best to integrate transplantation into the patient's treatment plan requires more attention. In this way, the best overall strategy, with the highest chance for survival of the patient, can be identified.

References

1. Thomas ED (1983) Marrow transplantation for malignant diseases (Karnofsky Memorial Lecture). J Clin Oncol 1: 517–531
2. O'Reilly RJ (1983) Allogeneic bone marrow transplantation: Current status and future directions. Blood 62: 941–964
3. Bortin MM, Gale RP (1986) Current status of allogeneic bone marrow transplantation: A report from the international bone marrow transplant registry. In: Terasaki PI (ed) Clinical transplants. (In press)
4. Appelbaum FR, Thomas ED (1985) The role of marrow transplantation in the treatment of leukemia. In: Bloomfield CD (ed) Chronic and acute leukemias in adults. Martinus Nijhoff, Boston,
   pp 229–262
5. Thomas ED, Buckner CD, Banaji M, Clift RA, Fefer A, Flournoy N, Goodell BW, Hickman RO, Lerner KG, Neiman PE, Sale GE, Sanders JE, Singer J, Stevens M, Storb R, Weiden PL (1977) One hundred patients with acute leukemia treated by chemotherapy, total body irradiation, and allogeneic marrow tansplantation. Blood 49: 511–533
6. Clift RA et al. (1987) The treatment of acute non-lymphoblastic leukemia by allogeneic marrow transplantation. Bone Marrow Transplantation 2: 243–258
7. Thomas ED, Buckner CD, Clift RA, Fefer A, Johnson FL, Neiman PE, Sale GE, Sanders JE, Singer JW, Shulman H, Storb R, Weiden PL (1979) Marrow transplantation for acute nonlymphoblastic leukemia in first remission. N Engl J Med 301: 597–599

8. Tallman MS, Appelbaum FR, Amos D, Goldberg RS, Livingston RB, Mortimer J, Weiden PL, Thomas ED (1987) Evaluation of intensive post-remission chemotherapy for adults with acute nonlymphocytic leukemia using high-dose cytosine arabinoside with L-asparaginase and amsacrine with etoposide. J Clin Oncol 5: 918–926

9. Appelbaum FR, Dahlberg S, Thomas ED, Buckner CD, Cheever MA, Clift RA, Crowley J, Deeg HJ, Fefer A, Greenberg PD, Kadin M, Smith W, Stewart P, Sullivan K, Storb R, Weiden P (1984) Bone marrow transplantation or chemotherapy after remission induction for adults with acute nonlymphoblastic leukemia—A prospective comparison. Ann Intern Med 101: 581–588

10. Champlin RE, Ho WG, Winston GH, Gale RP, Winston D, Selch M, Mitsuyasu R, Lenarsky C, Elashoff R, Zighelboim J, Feig SA (1985) Treatment of acute myelogenous leukemia: A prospective controlled trial of bone marrow transplantation versus consolidation chemotherapy. Ann Intern Med 102: 285–291

11. Powles RL, Morgenstern G, Clink HM (1980) The place of bone-marrow transplantation in acute myelogenous leukaemia. Lancet 1: 1047–50

12. Linch DC, Burnett AK (1986) Clinical studies of ABMT in acute myeloid leukaemia. Clin Haematol (Autologous Bone Marrow Transplantation) 151: 167–186

13. Yeager AM, Kaizer H, Santos GW, Saral R, Colvin OM, Stuart RK, Brainey HG, Burke PJ, Ambinder RF, Burns WH, Fuller DJ, Davis JM, Karp JE, May WS, Rowley SD, Sensenbrenner LL, Vogelsang GB, Wingard JR (1986) Autologous bone marrow transplantation in patients with acute nonlymphocytic leukemia, using ex vivo marrow treatment with 4-hydroperoxycyclophosphamide. N Engl J Med 315: 141–148

14. Clift RA, Buckner, Thomas ED, Sanders JE, Stewart PS, McGuffin R, Hersman J, Sullivan KM, Sale GE, Storb R (1982) Allogeneic marrow transplantation for acute lymphoblastic leukemia in remission using fractionated total body irradiation. Leuk Res 6: 409–412

15. Clift RA, Buckner CD, Thomas ED, Sanders JE, Stewart PS, Sullivan KM, McGuffin R, Hersman J, Sale GE, Storb R (1982) Allogeneic marrow transplantation using fractionated total body irradiation in patients with acute lymphoblastic leukemia in relapse. Leuk Res 6: 401–407

16. Sanders JE, Flournoy N, Thomas ED, Buckner CD, Lum LG, Clift RA, Appelbaum FR, Sullivan KM, Stewart P, Deeg HJ, Doney K, Storb R (1985) Marrow transplant experience in children with acute lymphoblastic leukemia: An analysis of factors associated with survival, relapse and graft-versus-host disease. Med Pediatr Oncol 13: 165–172

17. Johnson FL, Thomas ED, Clark BS, Chard RL, Hartmann JR, Storb R (1981) A comparison of marrow transplantation with chemotherapy for children with acute lymphoblastic leukemia in second or subsequent remission. N Engl J Med 305: 846–851

18. Rivera GK, Buchanan G, Boyett JM, Camitta B, Ochs J, Kalwinsky D, Amylon M, Vietti TJ, Crist WM (1986) Intensive retreatment of childhood acute lymphoblastic leukemia in first bone marrow relapse: A pediatric oncology group study. N Engl J Med 315: 273–278

19. Hoelzer D, Thiel E, Loffler H, Bodenstein H, Plaumann L, Buchner T, Urbanitz D, Koch P, Heimpel H, Engelhardt R, Muller U, Wendt F-C, Sodomann H, Ruhl H, Herrmann F, Kaboth W, Dietzfelbinger H, Pralle H, Lunscken Ch, Hellriegel K-P, Spors S, Nowrousian RM, Fischer J, Fulle H, Mitrou PS, Pfreundschuh M, Gorg Ch, Emmerich B, Queisser W, Meyer P, Labedzki L, Essers U, Konig H, Mainzer K, Herrmann R, Messerer D, Zwingers T (1984) Intensified therapy in acute lymphoblastic and acute undifferentiated leukemia in adults. Blood 64: 38–47

20. Schauer P, Arlin ZA, Mertelsmann R, Cirrincione C, Friedman A, Gee TS, Dowling M, Kempin S, Straus DJ, Koziner B, McKenzie S Thaler HT, Dufour P, Little C, Dellaquila C, Ellis S, Clarkson B (1983) Treatment of acute lymphoblastic leukemia in adults: Results of the L-10 and L-10M protocols. J Clin Oncol 1: 462–470

20a. Ritz J, Sallan SE, Bast RC, Lipton JM, Clavell LA, Feeney M, Hercend T, Nathan D, Schlossman SF (1982) Autologous bone-marrow transplantation in Calla-positive acute lymphoblastic leukemia after in vitro treatment with J5 monoclonal antibody and complement. Lancet 2: 60–63

20b. Kersey JH, Weisdorf D, Nesbit ME, LeBien TW, Woods WG, McGlave PB, Kim T, Vallera DA, Goldman A, Bostrom B, Hund D, Ramsey NKG (1987) Comparison of autologous and allogeneic bone marrow transplantation for treatment of high-risk refractory acute lymphoblastic leukemia. N Engl J Med 317: 416–467

21. Thomas ED, Clift RA, Fefer A, Appelbaum FR, Beatty P, Bensinger WI, Buckner CD, Cheever MA, Deeg HJ, Doney K, Flournoy N, Greenberg P, Hansen JA, Martin P, McGuffin R, Ramberg R, Sanders JE, Singer J, Stewart P, Storb R, Sullivan K, Weiden PL, Witherspoon R (1986) Marrow transplantation for the treatment of chronic myelogenous leukemia. Ann Intern Med 104: 155–163

22. Goldman JM, Apperley JF, Jones L, Marcus R, Goolden AWG, Batchelor R, Hale G, Waldmann H, Reid CD, Hows J, Gordon-Smith E, Catovsky D, Galton DAG (1986) Bone marrow transplantation for patients with chronic myeloid leukemia. N Engl J Med 314: 202–208

23. Appelbaum FR, Sullivan K, Thomas ED (1985) Treatment of malignant lymphoma in 100 patients with chemoradiotherapy and marrow transplantation. Exp Hematol 13: 321 (abstract)

24. Appelbaum FR, Sullivan KM, Buckner CD, Clift R, Hill R, Sanders JE, Storb R, Thomas ED (1986) Treatment of malignant lymphoma at first relapse or second remission with marrow transplantation. In: Proceedings of Third International Symposium on Autologous Transplantation, Houston, TX, December 1986 (In press)

25. Cabanillas F, Hagemeister FB, Bodey GP (1982) IMVP-16: an effective regimen for patients with lymphoma who have relapsed after initial combination chemotherapy. Blood 60: 693–697

26. Appelbaum FR, Storb R, Ramberg RE, Shulman HM, Buckner CD, Clift RA, Deeg HJ, Fofar A, Sanders J, Stewart P, Sullivan K, Witherspoon R, Thomas ED (1984) Allogeneic marrow transplantation in the treatment of preleukemia. Ann Intern Med 100: 689–693

27. Appelbaum FR, Storb R, Ramberg RE, Shulman HM, Buckner CD, Clift RA, Deeg HJ, Fefer A, Sanders J, Self S, Singer J, Stewart P, Sullivan K, Witherspoon R, Thomas ED (1987) Treatment of preleukemic syndromes with marrow transplantation. Blood 69: 92–96

28. Appelbaum FR, Storb R, Buckner CD, Ramberg RE, Shulman HM, Sargur M, Clift RA, Deeg HJ, Fefer A, Sanders J, Singer J, Stewart P, Sullivan K, Witherspoon R, Thomas ED (1987) The role of marrow transplantation in the treatment of preleukemia, therapy-related preleukemia, and acute leukemia evolving from preleukemia. In: Gale RP, Champlin R (eds) Progress in bone marrow transplantation. UCLA symposia on molecular and cellular biology, new series, vol 53. Alan R. Liss, New York, pp 103–111

29. Navari RM, Sharma P, Deeg HJ, McDonald GB, Thomas ED (1983) Pneumatosis cystoides intestinalis following allogeneic marrow transplantation. Transplant Proc 15: 1720–1724

30. Smith JW, Shulman HM, Thomas Ed, Fefer A, Buckner CD (1981) Bone marrow transplantation for acute myelosclerosis. Cancer 48: 2198–2203

31. Phillips GL, Herzig RH, Lazarus HM (1984) Treatment of resistant malignant lymphoma with cyclophosphamide, total body irradiation, and transplantation of cryopreserved autologous marrow. N Engl J Med 310: 1557–1561

32. Osserman EF, Dire LB, Dire J, Sherman WH, Hersman JA, Storb R (1982) Identical twin marrow transplantation in multiple myeloma. Acta Haematol 68: 215–223

33. August CS, Serota FT, Koch PA (1984) Treatment of advanced neuroblastoma with supralethal chemotherapy, radiation, and allogeneic or autologous marrow reconstitution. J Clin Oncol 2: 609–616

34. Boyd CN, Ramberg RC, Thomas ED (1982) The incidence of recurrence of leukemia in donor cells after allogeneic bone marrow transplantation. Leuk Res 6: 833–837

35. Fialkow PJ, Thomas ED, Bryant JI, Neiman PE (1971) Leukaemic transformation of engrafted human marrow cells in vivo. Lancet i: 251–255

36. Thomas ED, Bryant JI, Buckner CD, Clift RA, Fefer A, Johnson FL, Neiman P, Ramberg RE, Storb R (1972) Leukaemic transformation of engrafted human marrow cells in vivo. Lancet i: 1310–1313

37. Schubach WH, Miller G, Thomas ED (1985) Epstein-Barr virus genomes are restricted to secondary neoplastic cells following bone marrow transplantation. Blood 65: 535–538

38. Herzig HR, Coccia PF, Lazarus HM (1985) Bone marrow transplantation for acute leukemia and lymphoma with high-dose cytosine arabinoside and total body irradiation. Semin Oncol XII/2 [Suppl 3]: 185–186

39. Champlin R, Jacobs A, Gale RP (1985) High dose cytarabine in consolidation chemotherapy or with bone marrow transplantation for patients with acute leukemia: Preliminary results. Semin Oncol XII/2 [Suppl 3]: 190–195

40. Thomas ED, Clift RA, Hersman J, Sanders JE, Stewart P, Buckner CD, Fefer A, McGuffin R, Smith JW, Storb R (1982) Marrow transplantation for acute nonlymphoblastic leukemia in first remission. Int J Radiat Oncol Biol Phys 8: 817–821

41. Shank B, Hopfan S, Kim JH, Chu FCH, Grossbard E, Kapoor N, Kirkpatrick D, Dinsmore R, Simpson L, Reid A, Chui C, Mohan R, Finegan D, O'Reilly RJ (1981) Hyperfractionated total body irradiation for bone marrow transplantation: I. Early results in leukemia patients. Int J Radiat Oncol Biol Phys 7: 1109–1115

42. Phillips G, Wolff S, Herzig G (1983a) Local (L) radiotherapy (RT) followed by cyclophospha-mide (CY), fractionated (F) total body irradiation (TBI) and autologous marrow transplantation (AMT) for refractory malignant lymphoma (ML). Blood 62 [Suppl 1]: 228a

43. Bernstein ID, Nowinski RC (1982) Monoclonal antibody treatment of transplanted and spon-taneous murine leukemia. In: Oettgen H, Mitchell M (eds) Hybridomas in the diagnosis and treatment of cancer. Raven Press, New York, pp. 97–112

44. Badger CC, Shulman H, Peterson AV, Bernstein ID (1986) Monoclonal antibody therapy of spontaneous AKR T-cell leukemia. Cancer Res 46: 4058–4063

45. Meeker TC, Lowder J, Maloney DG, Miller RA, Thielemans K, Warnke R, Levy R (1985) A clinical trial of anti-idiotype therapy for B cell malignancy. Blood 65: 1349–1363

46. Press OW, Appelbaum F, Ledbetter JA, Martin PJ, Zarling J, Kidd P, Thomas ED (1987) Monoclonal antibody 1F5 (anti-CD20) serotherapy of human B cell lymphomas. Blood 69: 584–591

47. Badger CC, Bernstein ID (1983) Monoclonal antibody therapy of murine leukemia. J Exp Med 157: 828–842

48. Appelbaum FR, Badger C, Nelp WB, Brown P, Deeg HJ, Schuning F Storb R (1986) ^{131}I-labeled monoclonal antibodies as a preparative regimen for marrow transplantation: Initial dosimetry. Exp Hematol 14: 241(abstract)

49. Appelbaum FR, Badger C, Deeg HJ, Nelp WB, Storb R (1987) Use of ^{131}iodine-labelled anti-immune response-associated monoclonal antibody as a preparative regimen prior to bone mar-row transplantation: Initial dosimetry. Natl Cancer Inst Mongors 3: 67–71

50. Badger CC, Eary J, Brown S, Press O, Davis J, Appelbaum FR, Nelp W, Krohn K, Miller R, Levy R, Bernstein ID (1987) Therapy of lymphoma with I-131-labeled anti-idiotype antibodies (Anti-Id). Abstract for Seventy-Eighth Annual Meeting of the American Association for Cancer Research, Atlanta, GA, May 20–23, 1987

51. Bortin MM (1974) Graft versus leukemia. In: Bach FH, Good RA (eds) Clinical immunobiology 2. Academic Press, New York, pp 287–306

52. Weiden PL, Flournoy N, Thomas ED, Prentice R, Fefer A, Buckner CD, Storb R (1979) Anti-leukemic effect of graft-versus-host disease in human recipients of allogeneic-marrow grafts. N Engl J Med 300: 1068–1073

53. Weiden PL, Flournoy N, Sanders JE, Sullivan KM, Thomas ED (1981) Antileukemic effect of graft-versus-host disease contributes to improved survival after allogeneic marrow transplanta-tion. Transplant Proc 13: 248–251

54. Weiden PL, Sullivan KM, Flournoy N, Storb R, Thomas ED, the Seattle Marrow Transplant Team (1981) Antileukemic effect of chronic graft-versus-host disease. Contribution to improved survival after allogeneic marrow transplantation. N Engl J Med 304: 1529–1533

55. Appelley JF, Jones L, Arthur C, Guo AP, Rassool F, Hale G, Waldmann H, Goldman JM (1986) Incidence of relapse after T-cell depleted marrow transplant for chronic granulocytic leukaemia (CGL) in 1st chronic phase (CP). Blood 68: 270a (abstract)

56. Truitt RL, Rose WC, Rimm AA, Bortin MM (1978) Graft versus leukemia. VIII. Selective reduction in anti-host reactivity without loss of antileukemia reactivity by treatment of donor mice with lipopolysaccharide. Exp Hematol 6: 488

57. Okunewick JP, Meredith RF, Brozovich BJ, Seeman PR, Schieb AL (1979) Rauscher leukemia as a model for studies of marrow transplantation therapy. Results using syngeneic, allogeneic and hybrid donors. Int J Cancer 24: 438

58. Cheever MA, Greenberg PD, Fefer A (1981) Specific adoptive therapy of established leukemia with syngeneic lymphocytes sequentially immunized in vivo and in vitro and non-specifically expanded by culture with Interleukin 2. J Immunol 126: 1318–1322

59. Greenberg PD, Cheever MA, Fefer A (1981) Eradication of disseminated murine leukemia by chemoimmunotherapy with cyclophosphamide and adoptively transferred immune syngeneic Lyt 1$^+$2$^-$ T lymphocytes. J Exp Med

60. Beatty PG, Clift RA, Mickelson EM, Nisperos B, Flournoy N, Martin PJ, Sanders JE, Stewart P, Buckner CD, Storb R, Thomas ED, Hansen JA (1985) Marrow transplantation from related donors other than HLA-identical siblings. N Engl J Med 313: 765–771

61. Martin PJ, Hansen JA, Buckner CD, Sanders JE, Deeg HJ, Stewart P, Appelbaum FR, Clift R, Fefer A, Witherspoon RP, Kennedy MS, Sullivan KM, Flournoy N, Storb R, Thomas ED (1985) Effects of in vitro depletion of T cells in HLA-identical allogeneic marrow grafts. Blood 66: 664–672

62. Deeg HJ, Storb R, Szer J, Appelbaum FR, Hackman RC, Thomas ED (1985) Facilitation of engraftment of DLA nonidentical marrow by treatment of the recipient with monoclonal anti-Ia antibody. Transplant Proc 17: 493–494

63. Storb R, Weiden PL, Graham TC, Lerner KG, Nelson N, Thomas ED (1977) Hemopoietic grafts between DLA identical canine litter-mates following dimethyl myleran. Evidence for resistance to grafts not associated with DLA and abrogated by antithymocyte serum. Transplantation 24: 349–357

64. Hale G, Waldmann H (1986) Depletion of T-cells with Campath-1 and human complement. Analysis of GVHD and graft failure in a multi-centre study. Bone Marrow Transplantation 1[Suppl 1]: 93 (abstract)

65. Slavin S, Or R, Weshler Z, Hale G, Waldmann H (1986) The use of total lymphoid irradiation for abrogation of host resistance to T-cell depleted marrow allografts. Bone Marrow Transplantation 1[Suppl 1]: 98 (abstract)

66. Schuening F, Storb R, Deeg HJ, Appelbaum F, Loughran T, Graf L (1986) Facilitation of engraftment of DLA-nonidentical marrow by treatment of recipients with monoclonal antibody directed against radioresistant marrow cells. Exp Hematol 14: 562 (abstract)

67. Blazar BR, Widmer MB, Soderling CCB Vallera DA (1986) Granulocyte/macrophage colony-stimulating factor (GM-CSF) induced facilitation of T-cell depleted allogeneic bone marrow grafts across the MHC barrier in mice. Blood 68[Suppl 1]: 518

68. Storb R, Thomas ED (1985) Graft-versus-host disease in dog and man. The Seattle Experience. Immunol Rev 88: 215–238

69. Sullivan KM, Witherspoon R, Deeg HJ, Doney K, Appelbaum F, Sanders J, Lum L, Loughran T, Hill R, Anasetti C, Shields A, Nims J, Shulman H, Storb R, Thomas ED (1987) Chronic graft-versus-host disease in man. In: Gale RP, Champlin R (eds) Progress in bone marrow transplantation. UCLA symposia on molecular and cellular biology, new series, vol 53. Alan R. Liss, New York, pp 473–487

70. Santos GW, Hess AD, Vogelsang GB (1985) Graft-versus-host reactions and disease. Immunol Rev 88: 169–192

71. Storb R, Deeg HJ, Thomas ED, Applebaum FR, Buckner CD, Cheever MA, Clift RA, Doney KC, Flournoy N, Kennedy MS, Loughran TP, McGuffin RW, Sale GE, Sanders JE, Singer JW, Stewart PS, Sullivan KM, Witherspoon RP (1985) Marrow transplantation for chronic myelocytic leukemia: A controlled trial of cyclosporine versus methotrexate for prophylaxis of graft-versus-host disease. Blood 66: 698–702

72. Deeg HJ, Storb R, Thomas ED, Flournoy N, Kennedy MS, Banaji M, Appelbaum FR, Bensinger WI, Buckner CD, Clift RA, Doney K, Fefer A, McGuffin R, Sanders JE, Singer J, Stewart P, Sullivan KM, Witherspoon RP (1985) Cyclosporine as prophylaxis for graft-versus-host disease: A randomized study in patients undergoing marrow transplantation for acute nonlymphoblastic leukemia. Blood 65: 1325–1334

73. Storb R, Deeg HJ, Whitehead J, Appelbaum F, Beatty P, Bensinger W, Buckner CD, Clift R, Doney K, Farewell V, Hansen J, Hill R, Lum L, Martin P, McGuffin R, Sanders J, Stewart P, Sullivan K, Witherspoon R, Yee G, Thomas ED (1986) Methotrexate and cyclosporine compared with cyclosporine alone for prophylaxis of acute graft versus host disease after marrow transplantation for leukemia. N Engl J Med 314: 729–735

74. Storb R, Deeg HJ, Farewell V, Doney K, Appelbaum F, Beatty P, Bensinger W, Buckner CD, Clift R, Hansen J, Hill R, Longton G, Lum L, Martin P, McGuffin R, Sanders J, Singer J,

Stewart P, Sullivan K, Witherspoon R, Thomas ED (1986) Marrow transplantation for severe aplastic anemia: Methotrexate alone compared to a combination of methotrexate and cyclosporine for prevention of acute graft-versus-host disease. Blood 68: 119–125

75. Forman SJ, Blume KG, Krance RA, Miner PJ, O'Donnel MR, Nademanee AP, Snyder DS, Metter GE, Hill LR (1986) A prospective randomized study on acute graft-versus-host disease (GVHD) in 107 patients with leukamia: Methotrexate/prednisone (CSA/PSE). Blood 68[Suppl 1]: 1004 (abstract)

76. Storb R, Kolb HJ, Deeg HJ, Weiden PL, Appelbaum F, Graham TC, Thomas ED (1986) Prevention of graft-versus-host disease by immunosuppressive agents after transplantaton of DLA-nonidentical canine marrow. Bone Marrow Transplantation 1: 167–177

77. Storb R, Prentice RL, Buckner CD, Clift RA, Appelbaum F, Deeg J, Doney K, Hansen JA, Mason M, Sanders JE, Singer J, Sullivan KM, Witherspoon RP, Thomas ED (1983) Graft-versus-host disease and survival in patients with aplastic anemia treated by marrow grafts from HLA-identical siblings. Beneficial effect of a protective environment. N Engl J Med 308: 302–307

78. Reisner Y, Kirkpatrick D, Dupont B, Kapoor N, Pollack MS, Good RA, O'Reilly RJ (1981) Transplantation for acute leukaemia with HLA-A and B nonidentical parental marrow cells fractionated with soybean agglutinin and sheep red blood cells. Lancet 2: 327–331

79. Filipovich AH, Vallera D, Youle R, Quinones RA, Neville D, Kersey JH (1984) Ex vivo treatment of donor bone marrow with anti-T cell immunotoxins for the prevention of graft vs. host disease. Lancet 1: 469

80. Vogelsang GB, Hess AD, Berkman AW, Tutschka PJ, Farmer ER, Converse PJ, Santos GW (1985) An in vitro predictive test for graft versus host disease in patients with genotypic HLA-identical bone marrow transplants. N Engl J Med 313: 645–650

81. Chang J, Morgenstern G, Deakin D, Testa NG, Coutinho L, Scarffee JH, Harrison C, Dexter TM (1986) Reconstitution of haemopoietic system with autologous marrow taken during relapse of acute myelobalstic leukaemia and grown in long-term culture. Lancet 1: 294–295

82. Uphoff DE (1958) Preclusions of secondary phase of irradiation syndrome by inoculation of fetal hematopoietic tissue following lethal total body x irradiation JNCI 20: 625–632

83. O'Reilly RJ, Padlack MS, Kapoor N, Kirkpatrick D, Dupont B (1983) Fetal liver transplantation in man and animals. In: Gale RP (ed) Recent advances in bone marrow transplantation. Alan R. Liss, New York, 799–830

84. Prummer O, Fliedner TM (1986) The fetal liver as an alternative stem cell source for hemolymphopoietic reconstitution. Int J Cell Cloning 4: 237–249

85. Appelbaum FR (1987) Hammering away at solid tumors. Cancer Treat Rep 71: 115–117

86. Bearman SI, Appelbaum FR, Buckner CD, Petersen FB, Clift RA, Thomas ED (1986) Toxicity associated with preparative regimens in patients undergoing bone marrow transplantation. Blood 68 [Suppl 1] 997 (abstract)

87. Shepp DH, Dandliker RN, de Miranda P, Burnette TC, Cederberg DM, Kirk LE, Meyers JD (1985) Activity of 9-[2-hydroxyl-1-(hydroxymethyl)ethoxymethyl]guanine in the treatment of cytomegalovirus pneumonia. Ann Intern Med 103: 368–373

88. Collaborative DHPG Study Group (1986) Treatment of serious cytomegalovirus infections with 9-(1,3-dihydroxy-2-proipoxymethyl)guanine in patients with AIDS and other immunodeficiencies. N Engl J Med 314: 801–805

89. Meyers JD, Thomas ED (in press) Infection complicating bone marrow transplantation. In: Rubin RH, Young LS (eds) Clinical approach to infection in the immunocompromised host. Plenum Press, New York

90. Winston DJ, Gale RP, Meyer DV, Young LS and UCLA Bone Marrow Transplantation Group (1979) Infectious complications of human bone marrow transplantation. Medicine 58: 1–31

8. Regional Therapies

A. Surbone and C.E. Myers

Introduction

Regional drug delivery represents an approach to increase the selectivity of anti-neoplastic drugs for tumor versus normal tissues. The rationale is to increase the drug concentration at the target site and to reduce it at sites where toxicity occurs. Moreover, some tumors grow in specific body compartments which are not always easily penetrated by drugs administered systemically, e.g., the cerebro-spinal fluid (CSF) in meningeal carcinomatosis and the peritoneal cavity in ovarian and gastrointestinal (GI) malignancies. Regional delivery has appeared promising in several clinical situations, and we will review here the results of clinical trials for the main methods of regional drug administration: intra-arterial (IA), intraperitoneal (IP), intrathecal (IT), and intravesical. We will also briefly discuss the local approach to third-space accumulations.

As the aim of this book is to describe new directions in cancer treatment, we will focus on the recent advances in regional drug delivery, including the use of biological response modifiers and of monoclonal antibodies, and we will speculate on future prospects. We believe that major improvements in cancer treatment will be the result of the rational design of new drugs and optimization of their administration. For this reason, we will stress the principles behind regional drug delivery that enable us to increase our ability to both predict and achieve positive clinical results.

Several factors have to be taken into consideration: anatomical (the degree of drug penetration is based on the actual tissue exposure to the drug, which varies with different routes of administration and with different tumor types), technical (feasibility and complications of regional delivery), and pharmacological. While we will consider the anatomical and technical variables for each regional delivery mode, we will treat separately those pharmacological concepts that appear relevant to a better understanding and design of regional drug therapy in general. It will become clear from the analysis of the clinical data that major consideration should be given to appropriate patient selection, in order to improve the results and to avoid the administration of complex treatments to patients who are not likely to benefit from them.

Essential Pharmacological Concepts

For regional chemotherapy to be effective, it is necessary that a) the drug is active against the particular tumor type; b) systemic toxicity rather than local toxicity is considered the limiting factor to clinical efficacy; c) the drug has a high total body clearance relative to the clearance of drug from the local region to the systemic circulation; d) the drug does not require metabolic activation at a site different from the target tissue; and e) preferably, the drug should be inactivated at the target site or by intervening tissue, so that a very low systemic dose is delivered.

The main pharmacological concepts relevant to regional drug therapy are:

1. *Pharmacokinetics and pharmacodynamics.* Once a drug enters the body, it is distributed and eliminated, so that different concentrations are reached in different body compartments. Pharmacokinetics is the study of the distribution-elimination phase and deals with concentrations and time. The study of drug effects is the subject of pharmacodynamics, which therefore deals with efficacy and toxicity.

2. *Dose-response.* Both efficacy and toxicity are related to the concentrations achieved at different sites, which in turn depend on the dose administered. It is often assumed that an increase in dose (and therefore in concentration at the target site) invariably leads to an increase in efficacy. However, the relationship between dose and response is not linear: this means that on the concentration-response curve there is a critical level where the maximum drug effect has been reached, and beyond which even major increases in drug concentration will produce only minimal differences in efficacy. In cancer chemotherapy, we most often deal with situations where we expect to achieve substantial improvements in tumor cell kill by increasing the dose. However, due to the lack of selectivity and of rescue methods available, dose increments invariably lead to systemic toxicity, which becomes dose limiting. The rationale for regional drug delivery is to increase the concentration at the target site, while minimizing increases in systemic drug concentrations. A knowledge of the dose-response curve for the drug selected would be extremely useful in predicting the efficacy of regional delivery.

3. *Basic pharmacokinetic considerations.* Systemic and tissue drug exposure are inversely proportional to the total body clearance. Total body clearance occurs through three different mechanisms: metabolism, excretion, and irreversible binding. With the regional delivery mode, the regional exchange rate is the other determinant of target tissue exposure. For conventional chemotherapeutic agents, it can be estimated as 1 ml/min for the IT route, 10 ml/min for the IP route, and 100–1500 ml/min for the IA route. The ratio of the target site concentration to the systemic concentration gives the selectivity for regional delivery. To increase this ratio, it would be necessary to slow the regional exchange rate and to reduce the systemic delivery. The latter could be achieved in the case of a drug metabolized or eliminated by the

tissue that receives it locally, so that a first-pass effect would prevent it from reaching the systemic circulation, e.g., 5-fluorouracial (5FU) and fluorodeoxyuridine (FUDR) given via the hepatic artery. It is clear that once the drug has left its target tissue and has entered the systemic circulation, it then behaves as an IV administered drug.

4. *Basic drug characteristics.* Theoretically, the entire advantage of regional drug delivery should be obtained at the first encounter of drug with its target. Therefore, in the IA route, the selection of a phase-specific drug would be suboptimal due to the short treatment time. A non-phase-specific drug, such as an alkylating agent, would be preferable. Phase-specific drugs could be used when continuous infusion is technically feasible. As previously mentioned, the local tissue toxicity must be minimal, and the drug must not require any metabolic activation outside the site of administration.

Clinical Applications

From the previous paragraphs, it would appear very easy to predict the clinical outcome of each regional drug delivery protocol. Unfortunately, many other factors (anatomical, technical, and host-tumor interactions) need to be evaluated; moreover, the principles stated above cannot be considered separately. We will give here two examples of clinical situations:

1. *Doxorubicin.* There is evidence of a dose-response curve for this drug, and before undertaking a phase I IP trial [1], we calculated that the IP route should convert an incurable tumor into a tumor with an appreciable cure rate. The clinical phase I trial confirmed the expected concentration advantage. It also showed that this could indeed translate into better therapeutic efficacy, as there is a much higher doxorubicin concentration in tumor cells after IP administration, than after administration of the same dose IV. However, doxorubicin produced severe chemical peritonitis even at low doses, and it therefore proved not to be of clinical value as a drug for IP use.

2. *5FU.* Most of the time, we assume linear pharmacokinetics for every drug, but this is not always true. In fact, when a saturable process takes place (enzymatic degradation, binding, etc.), the relationship between drug concentration and regional clearance cases to be linear. This is the case with IP administration of 5FU because of its enzymatic degradation in the liver. The result is that as the drug dose increases, the liver clearance and total body clearance of the drug drop. The effect of this nonlinear pharmacokinetics is that if the total body clearance drops, the ratio of total body to peritoneal clearance diminishes. This, in turn, leads to a decrease in the pharmacological advantage for IP chemotherapy.

These two examples are not meant to discourage regional delivery. However, increased efforts should be made to carry out both careful preclinical evaluation and careful monitoring of pharmacokinetics during the clinical trial.

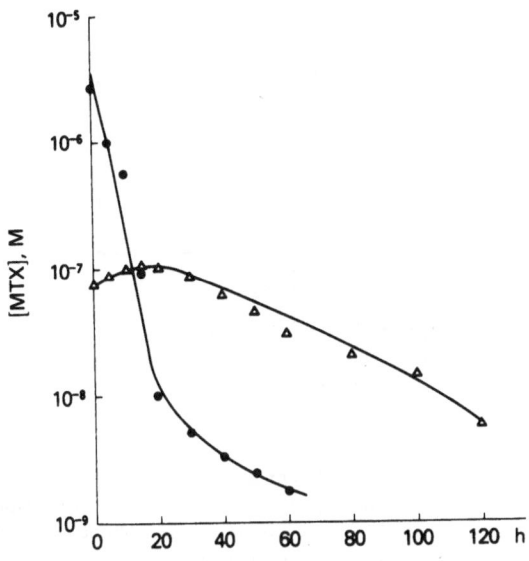

Fig. 1. Methotrexate (*MTX*) levels in plasma (●) and peritoneal fluid (△) in a patient with ovarian cancer following IV treatment with 20 mg/kg methotrexate

Malignant Effusions

Direct instillation of cytotoxic agents has been used initially to control malignant effusions. We will not describe here in detail the experience in this field, as it is already part of the standard management of cancer at this site. Both cytotoxic agents (bleomycin, thiotepa, mechlorethamine, 5FU, doxorubicin, and *cis*-platinum) and radioactive isotopes ([198]Au and ^{32}P) have been utilized, after an attempt to drain the third-space fluid collection, for pleural, peritoneal, and pericardial malignant effusions. The response rate varies from 30% to 60%.

The problem of third-space fluid accumulation has been one of the conceptual bases for the development of regional drug delivery. In fact, the rationale behind intracavitary therapy arose as a consequence of research on the impact of large peritoneal fluid accumulations on the pharmacokinetics of IV administered drugs. Chabner and Young [2] showed that when methotrexate (MTX) is administered IV to patients with a large amount of ascites, the blood levels are sustained for much longer than usual. MTX penetrates the peritoneal cavity, and then the large volume of drug-containing fluid acts as a reservoir, metering drug to the plasma during the terminal phase of drug clearance (Fig. 1). The analysis of this phenomenon revealed that the peritoneum acted as a diffusion barrier, and that the peritoneal clearance of a drug was much lower than its plasma clearance (5 ml/min vs 120 ml/min for MTX). This immediately suggested that if a drug was directly instilled into the peritoneal cavity, the peritoneal drug concentrations should be much higher than those in plasma.

169

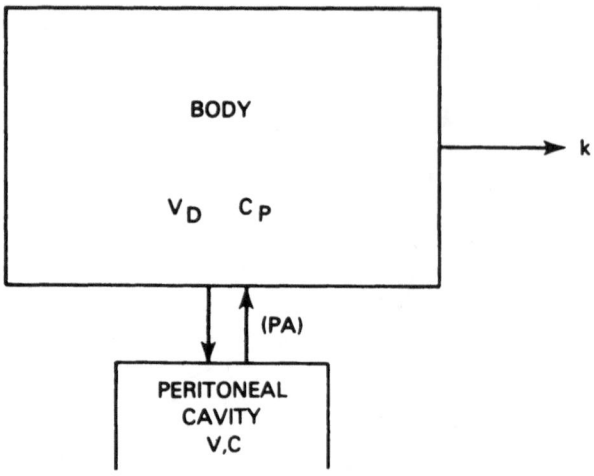

Fig. 2. A two-compartment model of the relationship between intraperitoneal drug and systemic drug levels. V_D and C_p represent the volume of distribution and the plasma concentration of the drug, respectively, V and C represent the volume and drug concentration in the peritoneal fluid; PA, peritoneal clearance; k, total-body clearance

IP Therapy

Two very common malignancies, ovarian and colon carcinoma, tend to remain confined to or to recur in the abdominal cavity. Other GI tumors and occasionally breast cancer also spread to the peritoneum and to the intra-abdominal organs. Ovarian cancer is the most frequent cause of death from gynecologic malignancy and represents the fourth most frequent cause of death in women in the United States of America. Colon cancer represents the second most frequent cause of death from cancer in the United States, affecting both sexes, and having an incidence in the USA of approximately 120000 new cases a year. The results of systemic therapy in these diseases are still not satisfactory, and therefore a major attempt has been made to improve drug efficacy through regional delivery. The basic pharmacokinetic model for IP therapy will be described here in detail; this model also applies to all other routes of regional drug delivery (Fig. 2).

Pharmacokinetics

The peritoneal fluid is a compartment which can be characterized by its volume and the contained drug. The whole-body compartment is also characterized by a volume and a concentration [3]. The exchange between these two compartments is defined by the product of the permeability between them and their area of contact. Since neither the area of contact nor the permeability can be determined in a clinical situation, the process of exchange must be expressed as a

170

clearance value in milliliters per minute. The total-body clearance represents the rate (k) at which the drug is removed from this two-compartment system. From this model, it is possible to derive a series of equations. The two-compartment model can be expressed as follows:

$$C_p/C_{tb} = [R(PA) + k]/PA, \qquad (1)$$

where C_p and C_{tb} are drug concentrations in peritoneal fluid and total body (plasma), respectively; PA is the peritoneal clearance (in milliliters per minute); k is the total-body clearance; and R is a factor required to account for protein binding. The equation applies also to the area under the concentration curve (AUC). In the case of IP administration—where, for anticancer drugs, k is much higher than PA, and protein binding is geneally not important—Eq. 1 can be further simplified to Eq. 2:

$$C_p/C_{tb} = Cl_{tb}/Cl_p, \qquad (2)$$

where C_p and C_{tb} are the concentrations in the peritoneum and in the body, and Cl_{tb} and Cl_p are the clearances in the total body and in the peritoneum, respectively. This explains why an ideal drug should have rapid total-body clearance and very slow regional clearance, as previously mentioned. Also, the total-body clearance of the ideal drug should not be affected by the dose (e.g., the drug clearance should not decrease as a result of saturable enzymatic degradation). If this were so, the pharmacological advantage of IP therapy would also decline as a function of the dose.

In order to make use of Eq. 2, the values of drug clearance from the body and from the peritoneum should be known. Generally, the total-body clearance is determined during phase I and phase II studies for all drugs. Determination of the peritoneal clearance is based mostly on the molecular weight and on the lipid solubility of the drug. In fact, the passage of drugs across the peritoneum occurs either through intercellular or through intracellular pores. The first is dependent upon the size or molecular weight, while the second depends on the lipid solubility (Fig. 3, Table 1). Initially, this relationship had been established in the peritoneal dialysis literature for naturally occurring substances such as glucose, creatinine, and urea. Now, extensive data also exist for the antineoplastic drugs, due to the fact that the results obtained for them in animal models can be reliably applied to humans.

As can be appreciated from Table 1, lipid-soluble drugs cross the peritoneum at a much more rapid rate than would be estimated from their molecular weight (e.g., hexamethylmelamine); clearly, these lipid-soluble drugs would not be ideal for IP delivery, as they would leave the cavity at too fast a rate.

Table 2 shows that the pharmacokinetic model proposed here has been used successfully to predict the behavior of MTX, 5-FU, cytosine arabinoside (Ara-C), and *cis*-platinum given IP. As an example, we will show how calculations were done in the case of MTX, taking into account that for this drug, saturable clearance and protein binding do not represent a significant problem. MTX total-body clearance is 113 ml/min, and its peritoneal clearance is 5.1 ml/min. The pharmacological advantage for IP administration, or ratio of IP to IV drug

171

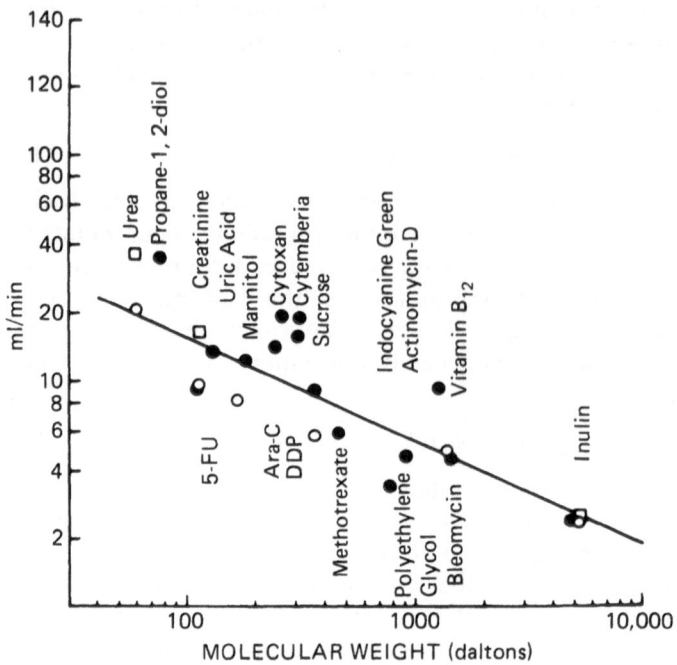

Fig. 3. The relationship between molecular weight and peritoneal clearance for a range of natural compounds and drugs in humans ($\bigcirc\square$) and rats ($\bullet$). Rat data scaled according to (body weight)$^{0.7}$

concentration after regional administration, would be $(5.1 + 113)/5.1 = 23$ (or, simplified, $113/5.1 = 22$). This calculation is an excellent estimate of the actual results published after clinical trials [4]. Generally, the peritoneal clearance of most antineoplastic drugs is below 30 ml/min, as they are commonly water-soluble and with molecular weights between 100 and 1000. For these same reasons, their total-body clearances are usually equal to or greater than the glomerular clearance (higher than 100 ml/min). From this is follows that the pharmacological advantage for most cancer drugs after IP administration is at least three fold, and it can be several thousandfold for a drug such as cytosine arabinoside.

For most drugs used in the treatment of ovarian cancer, as previously mentioned, the ratio of the AUC (ratio of total drug exposure for the peritoneal cavity to that for the plasma) is now known: 6 for carboplatinum (CBDCA), 12 for *cis*-platinum, 65 for melphalan and Etoposide (VP-16), 92 for MTX, and 400–2500 for 5FU. This pharmacology gives the clinician considerable flexibility in the clinical use of IP therapy. Peak drug levels that would never be tolerated systemically can be achieved by single bolus infusions, while high IP drug levels can be maintained for prolonged periods using repeated exchange dialysis (very high MTX levels have been maintained for more than 100 h, with systemic leucovorin rescue).

Once an advantage in the AUC ratio has been established for the peritoneal

Table 1. Absorption of drug from rat peritoneum over a 1 h period

Drug	Absorption (%)	Molecular weight (daltons)	K(Heptane)
Asparaginase	9.0	133 000	0.19
Bleomycin	12.7	1 400	0.002
Actinomycin D	21.0	1 256	0.23
Doxorubicin	10.9	544	–
Dichloromethotrexate	25.6	540	0.002
Methotrexate	15.0	472	0.001
Phenylalanine mustard	25.0	323	0.1
Chlorambucil	69.2	304	0.01
Cis-diammine-dichloroplatinum	24.6	300	<0.001
Cyclophosphamide	37.0	261	0.2
Cytosine Arabinoside	29.5	243	0.006
Hexamethylmelamine	91.7	210	11.2
Thiotepa	74.4	188	0.2
5-Fluorouracil	28.4	130	0.09

Table 2. The pharmacological advantage of IP drug administration

Reference	Drug	Advantage[a]
Speyer et al. [14]	5FU	111–898
Gyves et al.	5FU	550–7852
Demicheli et al.	5FU	120–1350
Ozols et al. [1]	Doxorubicin	474
Howell et al. [19]	Cis-DDP	21
Casper et al. [20]	Cis-DDP	30
Jones et al. [4]	Methotrexate	18–36
Howell et al. [13]	Methotrexate	92

[a] Ratio of AUC or peak drug levels, range or mean.
5FU, 5-fluorouracil

cavity for a given drug, it is necessary to consider the distribution of the drug within the peritoneal cavity, for ideally there should be an even exposure of the entire peritoneal surface to the drug-containing fluid. Then, the degree of drug penetration into the tumor mass has to be considered, and finally, one must examine the factors that govern drug egress from the peritoneum.

IP Drug Distribution

Peritoneography [5] has proven that intra-abdominal seeding of cancer cells depends on the flow of ascitic fluid and is determined by peritoneal reflections and recesses, by gravity, and by subdiaphragmatic pressure. The commonest sites of metastatic implants are the pouch of Douglas at the rectosigmoid level, the right lower quadrant at the end of the small mesentery, the left lower quadrant along the superior border of the sigmoid mesocolon and colon, and the right paracolic gutter lateral to the cecum and ascending colon. The success of IP therapy requires that the entire peritoneal surface be bathed in the drug-containing fluid. This is often very difficult in a clinical situation, where patients have generally had multiple surgery and have tumor deposits, as previously described, which plaster bowel, mesentery, and abdominal wall together. There is experimental evidence that the IP pressures affect the plasma-peritoneum exchanges, and that a large IP volume of fluid would permit the maintenance of higher concentrations in the cavity [6]. Based on the above considerations, several authors [7, 8] have studied the distribution of the fluid in order to determine the amount of drug-containing fluid which is necessary to achieve an adequate drug distribution. The use of 40–80 ml meglumine diatrizoate (Hypaque) in 2 liters of dialysis fluid allowed a good and almost complete visualization of the distribution of the fluid in the peritoneal cavity and of the tumor masses. Thus, 1.8–2.0 liters is the volume now accepted as sufficient to distend the abdominal cavity and obtain an even fluid distribution. Such an amount of fluid is also well tolerated by most patients.

The mechanisms of drug egress from the peritoneal cavity can be summarized as follows. The visceral peritoneum drains into the portal vein, and therefore from 30% to 70% of the instilled drug goes to the liver, while the parietal peritoneum drains into the inferior vena cava. In addition, there is direct binding to tissues, IP metabolism, and absorption via lymphatics.

Tumor Penetration

The penetration of the tumor mass is affected by distribution within the peritoneum, by diffusion into the tumor mass, and by drug removal via the tumor capillaries. The diffusivity of a drug is a function of its molecular weight, and so is the capillary permeability. However, the capillary permeability falls off more rapidly than the diffusion as a function of molecular weight. As a result, capillary removal is the major factor limiting the depth of penetration, and in the molecular weight range of most conventional antineoplastic drugs, the penetration is constant.

The depth of penetration has been estimated in experimental [9] and clinical trials [10]. As an example, the human data on doxorubicin confirmed the experimental evidence that this drug does not penetrate for more than six to eight cell layers. Other studies [11] have shown that *cis*-platinum tissue levels are higher for the first 3 mm from the peritoneal surface when the drug is given IP instead of IV. It therefore becomes extremely important to clearly define the subsets of patients who will benefit from IP drug therapy, and it will be evident from the review of clinical trials that absence of bulky disease is an advantage. On the other hand, it also becomes necessary to explore new agents, selecting those which are more likely to penetrate deeper, such as protein-sized agents of molecular weight higher than 15 000 daltons. It should also be borne in mind that the tumor is exposed not only to the IP drug but also the IV drug concentration, and this could result in a therapeutic benefit. An additional factor is that most carcinomatous tumor masses lack lymphatic drainage. While this removes the lymphatics as a potential route of drug egress from the tumor, it also means that proteins such as albumin, which leak from the capillaries into the tumor, will tend to accumulate. As a result, the pressure within the tumor mass will increase. This is one of the major forces which decrease tumor blood flow. One consequence of this increased pressure gradient across the tumor mass is that there will be bulk flow from the tumor center towards its exterior. This bulk flow will tend to lessen the ability of drugs and proteins administered IP to penetrate the tumor mass.

Drug Delivery

Before reviewing the clinical results, we will briefly consider some of the technical aspects of IP delivery. The vast bulk of experience comes from peritoneal dialysis, and the problems encountered in cancer chemotherapy are not substantially different. In the rare instances of protocols requiring only a single instillation every few weeks, it might be sufficient to insert an 18-gauge needle percutaneously. However, most of the clinical trials now use repeated instillations, and under these circumstances, the percutaneous approach carries too high a risk of bowel perforation and infection. Therefore, it is necessary to consider indwelling catheters. The two main types are the Tenckhoff and the Port-a-cath, with several variants. The Tenckhoff catheter system has been widely applied in the treatment of renal failure, and its efficacy has also been repeatedly proven in cancer chemotherapy. It can be inserted blindly or surgically (during peritoneoscopy or laparotomy).

When considering the oncological experience, the most significant complications have been (a) pain associated with fluid instillation, (b) bacterial infections of the catheter and/or the peritoneum and, (c) failure to drain. The pain during fluid instillation is most often the result of stretching of adhesions, while the failure to drain is often due to fibrin plugs in the catheter and/or twisting of the catheter. The frequency of infections depends mostly on the skills of the medical and nursing staff and on appropriate patient training. All these problems have been encountered in the renal failure literature too, and information is available on how to manage these complications. It is generally true that early failures are due to lack of proper patient selection and surgical skills, while long-term failures are mostly due to infectious events and are heavily influenced by nursing care and patient instruction [12]. The same applies to oncological situations, but here the concept of proper patient selection becomes less clearly defined since often there are few remaining alternatives. Also, due to the immunosuppression consequent upon both the neoplasm and antineoplastic therapies, cancer patients are at higher risk of infections and of severe complications from infectious events.

For these reasons, various catheters have been tried. Howell et al. [13] have used the Port-a-cath system, which is a subcutaneously implantable drug deliv-

175

ery system. It offers the major advantage to the patient of not having a foreign object protruding from the abdomen and of not requiring any care during the intervals between therapies. This leads to a reduced risk of infections and simplifies the issues of nursing care and patient education. However, drainage problems become magnified, and for protocols requiring repeated exchange dialysis, the Tenckhoff system is still preferred. Unfortunately, neither appears optimal, and better catheters need to be designed in order to decrease the complication rate.

Clinical Studies

Several phase I and phase II trials of IP therapy have been published for ovarian and colon cancer. In reviewing them, both the efficacy and the type of toxicity will be considered. The phase I trials of IP MTX [4, 13] showed dose-limiting toxicity to be bone marrow suppression, which could be controlled by the use of leucovorin rescue. For 5FU [14–16], the dose-limiting toxicities are bone marrow suppression and chemical peritonitis. For doxorubicin [1, 17], the dose-limiting toxicity proved to be a form of serious and prolonged chemical peritonitis. *Cis*-platinum [18–20] was limited by the systemic dose absorbed, which caused renal toxicity, nausea and vomiting, and neurotoxicity, but peritoneal irritation was not a significant problem. Various methods have been used to reduce the systemic toxicity of *cis*-platinum, and thiosulfate and hypertonic saline both appeared effective in reducing the degree of nephrotoxicity and allowing higher doses to be administered [19, 20]. Melphalan also was proven to have dose-limiting systemic rather than local toxicity [21]. CBDCA has dose-limiting systemic toxicity, in the form of myelosuppression [22]. Vinblastine sulfate (Velban) had to be abandoned by the IP route because of the frequency of induction of paralytic ileus [23]. Ara-C was minimally toxic, both systemically and locally [24].

All the early clinical trials were done in cancer patients in whom numerous other therapies had already failed, but in spite of this, responses were observed. Of the ten patients treated with doxorubicin, three obtained an objective response and two had reduction in ascites formation. 5FU produced only one response (7%), but it was a complete remission which lasted for more than 3 years. The response rate to melphalan was similarly low (7%). No major activity was seen for MTX and Ara-C. The drug that appears most promising for IP therapy is *cis*-platinum. In a fairly large phase II trial, a 30% complete response rate has been reported in ovarian cancer patients previously treated with systemic *cis*-platinum [25]. Pilot studies [26] are now being conducted to investigate the role of IP *cis*-platinum both as a first-line therapy in advanced disease and as adjuvant chemotherapy for early stages. The latter patients particularly could benefit from regional *cis*-platinum, as both the early trials and the phase II study have shown that the subset of patients most likely to benefit from IP therapy is the one with small-volume disease [27]. IP chemotherapy could

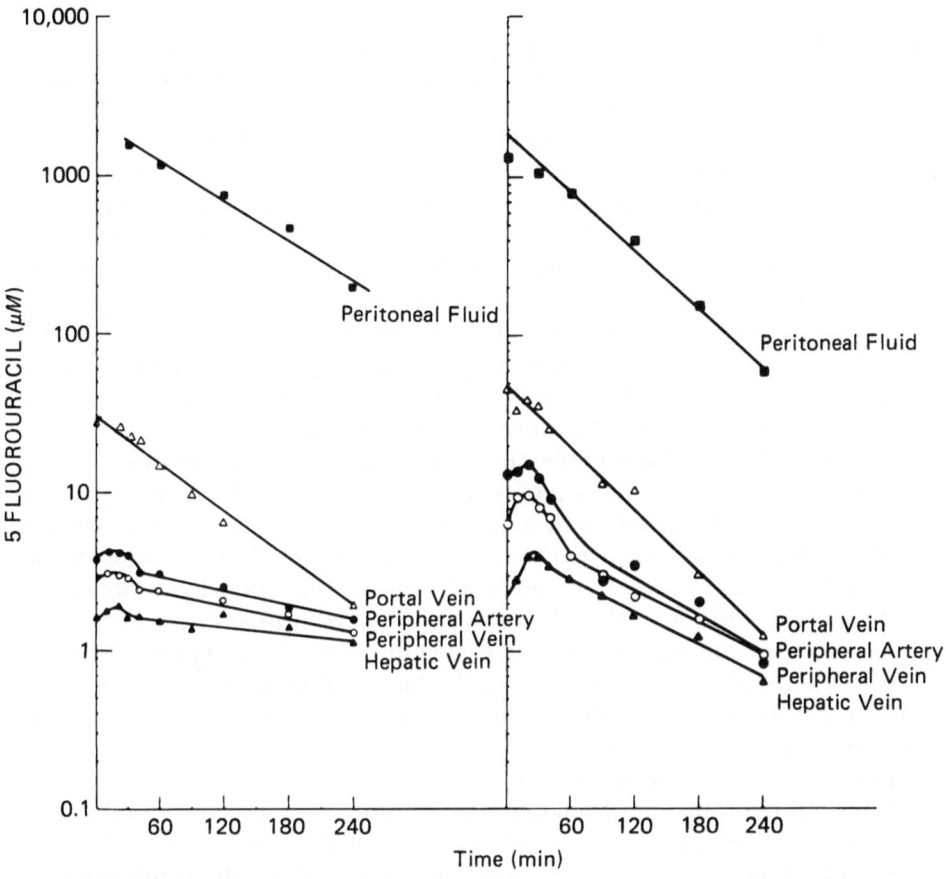

Fig. 4. Portal, systemic, and intraperitoneal drug levels in a patient treated with intraperitoneal 5FU (4mM) measured at the start of a week of treatment (*left*) and at the end of treatment (*right*). The difference between the two sets of curves probably represents the effect of drug-induced peritonitis on peritoneal clearance

therefore be used as a substitute for IP radioisotopes in early ovarian cancer, or after surgical debulking of advanced disease, or as a consolidation after systemic chemotherapy or abdominal radiotherapy [28].

In GI malignancies, IP 5FU has been used to achieve high IP and portal vein concentrations and could for this reason be considered as an alternative to hepatic artery infusion for the control of liver metastasis [14, 29]. On the basis of the demonstration that high portal drug concentrations can be achieved (Fig. 4) and of the results of a subsequent randomized trial of IV versus IP 5-FU [30], which demonstrated that greater amounts of drug could be delivered by the IP route, it might be appropriate to investigate the role of IP 5-FU in patients at high risk of developing hepatic metastasis [31].

New Developments

The use of IP delivery to treat bulky disease is not irrational, but it should be done using different agents, with deeper penetration into the tumor mass. Biological response modifiers and monoclonal antibodies have been tried, and part of the rationale behind their use is their high molecular weight [32–34]. In fact, protein-sized molecules (>15000 daltons) leave the peritoneal cavity only through the lymphatics [35], and it is known that very often, tumors have no internal lymphatic drainage. As a consequence, the depth of penetration of protein-sized agents should not be as limited as for conventional chemotherapeutic agents. For this to be true, sufficient time should be allowed for penetration. In fact, diffusion is a function of the square root of time (e.g., if a drug diffuses 1x in 1 h, it will diffuse 12x in 144 h), and a drug could take weeks to completely cross a 5- to 10-cm mass. As described above, this process will be slowed by bulk flow from the tumor center to its periphery.

Radiolabeled monoclonal antibodies have been successfully used to localize tumor masses [36], after both IV and IP administration. The IP route appears to give better tumor detection, with more than 95% of the lesions identified in patients with pseudomyxoma peritonei [37], as confirmed by subsequent histological evaluation. Several radiolabeled antiovarian monoclonal antibodies have been used with some clinical activity in stage III ovarian cancer, and those studies are at present ongoing. We can expect in the future to improve the selection of the antibody [higher affinity for the target antigen; human rather than mouse origin; conjugation with different therapeutic isotopes; use of antibody fragments, e.g., lacking crystallizable fragment (Fc) regions which increase nonspecific binding and hepatosplenic uptake].

The use of liposome-encapsulated drugs could give pharmacological advantages when administered IP, as the release from the peritoneum would be slower, and the systemic concentrations reduced. In the future, the combination of such a form of drug therapy with monoclonal antibodies could possibly lead to increased therapeutic efficacy with minimal toxicity.

Immunotherapy with both α- and γ-interferon [38, 39] has been used in advanced ovarian cancer, and the pharmacokinetics resulted in high IP concentrations after regional administration. Previous trials with *Corynebacterium parvum* [40] had documented some responses in patients with minimal residual disease.

Recently, IP interleukin-2 and lymphokine-activated killer (LAK) cells have been studied in peritoneal carcinomatosis [41]. Toxicity has been observed both systemically and locally, but three partial responses have been obtained in patients with disease greater than 2 cm. This approach deserves further investigation.

Other future possibilities are the development and use of systemic neutralizing agents to be administered concurrently with the IP therapy (such as IV leucovorin and IP MTX, IV thiosulfate and IP *cis*-platinum) [42]; the use of agents that could enhance the uptake and the cytotoxicity of antineoplastic drugs (such as glutaminase in combination with melphalan) [43]; and finally, the design of IP combination chemotherapy [44, 45]. Other attempts (such as hypo- and/or hyperthermia [46, 47]) have been made without major clinical impact. Again, new approaches should be designed on the basis of solid pharmacological and experimental rationale, rather than on continuing in the tradition of empirical clinical trials.

IA Therapy

The goal of IA infusion is the same as that of IP delivery: to increase the therapeutic index of antineoplastic agents. The pharmacological principles are not different from those already discussed for the IP route [48], except for the fact that the blood flow becomes a major determinant of the AUC ratio. A blood flow of 100 ml/min is what we can expect in a small artery, while a large artery will probably have a flow of approximately 1000–1500 ml/min [49]. If we repeat, for IA delivery, the same basic calculations we used for IP MTX, we will see that with an approximate total-body clearance of 200 ml/min and a carotid flow of 300 ml/min, the ratio would be only 1.67. We can therefore say that the ideal drug for IA infusion should have a high clearance rate, e.g., carmustine (BCNU), and should be administered through a low-flow artery; this would result in the highest delivery advantage.

For the IA route, possibly even more than for the IP route, the role of first-pass effect is extemely important, as is the time when it occurs in relation to the tumor exposure. Drug metabolized in the site of administration will give a high pharmacological advantage (e.g., 5FU and FUDR in hepatic delivery). Another determinant is the anatomy of the tumor blood supply, which is variable, depending on the histology, size, and location of the neoplastic mass. Mostly, IA therapy has been used for head and neck tumors, for sarcomas and melanomas of the extremities, and for liver perfusion.

Drug Delivery

The artery chosen for drug delivery can be reached in several ways (direct injection through a needle, direct catheterization, or indirect retrograde catheterization through collaterals or distant vessels). The ideal situation would be to be able to drain all the drug from the vein, to avoid systemic exposure. This is the purpose of isolation-perfusion techniques [50], but a complete isolation of the target tissue is possible only in particular anatomical areas (e.g., limbs). In all other situations, there may be an advantage in the fact that the dilution in the systemic blood will lead to recirculation through the tumor vessels, but the systemic toxicity of the drug must also be considered.

IA drugs should always be given at reduced doses, based not on the usual body surface, but on the volume of tissues supplied by the catheterized vessel. The local concentration should be maintained at a high level, and, during continuous infusions, it appears better to reduce the infusion duration rather than the dose. The administration of 5FU and/or FUDR by intrahepatic infusion is a separate case, as these drugs are metabolized in the liver, and therefore the dose that reaches the systemic circulation is very low.

All IA delivery techniques present some technical difficulties which can be summarized as follows: (a) those related to the catheter insertion (bleeding, perforation, and infections); (b) those related to the indwelling catheter (occlusion, vessel wall trauma, breaking, dislocation, and infections); (c) those related to the drug (arteritis, cerebral complications from drugs infused into the common carotid during head and neck perfusion, chemical peritonitis in case of catheter dislocation during hepatic infusion); and (d) those related to possible associated procedures (bullous edema and functional impairment of the extremities due to hyperthermia during hyperthermic limb perfusion, and nerve paralysis due to compression during the use of a tourniquet for extremity perfusion). Overall, these complications and technical problems amount to not more than 10%–15% of cases and can be reduced if well-trained physicians and nurses are familiar with their early signs. Unlike what has been described for IP therapy, IA therapy generally utilizes drug combinations. Moreover, drugs are often given IA in preparation for local treatments (surgery and/or radiation therapy), and the radiosensitizer properties of some of them are used to enhance radiation efficacy.

Clinical Studies

As a general rule, IA delivery is mostly used (a) to obtain rapid regression of a tumor mass in order to convert an inoperable into a resectable tumor, (b) for analgesia and palliation of locally intractable pain, (c) as a preparation for local treatment in a combined modality approach, and (d) for control of liver metastases.

More recently, portal vein infusion of 5FU, as a postsurgical adjuvant chemotherapy for colon cancer, has been pioneered by a British group [51] with encouraging results. Further studies are continuing.

In head and neck tumors, the results have been encouraging, showing improved survival and disease-free survival in patients with advanced disease treated with IA combination chemotherapy prior to surgery [52–54].

In sarcomas and melanomas of the extremities, combination chemotherapy has been used together with hyperthermia. As recently reported [55, 56], hyperthermic perfusion has shown activity both preoperatively in stage I melanoma and postoperatively in stage I–III, with increases in both survival and disease-free survival. The results in sarcoma treatment [57–59] have been encouraging both in the multimodality approach to early stages and as an accepted palliation for advanced stages when pain cannot be controlled otherwise. Hyperthermia leads to the appearance of different toxicities (bullous edema and functional impairment), which can be severe but are generally transient.

180

Hepatic Infusion

In the field of hepatic infusion, only 5-FU and FUDR have shown efficacy for the control of metastasis from colon cancer. The rationale behind the use of these two drugs is that (a) both have shown efficacy in GI malignancies; (b) both are inactivated by the liver, and therefore the systemic dose can be maintained at a very low level, while achieving high local concentrations; (c) different approaches can be utilized (intrahepatic artery or portal vein infusion) according to the size of the metastasis to be treated, as micro- or small metastases depend on the portal vein flow, while the bigger metastases are supplied by the hepatic artery; and (d) both could be useful as adjuvant therapy for patients at high risk of developing liver metastases.

5-FU infusion through the portal vein as adjuvant therapy has been studied, as previously mentioned [51], in a large, randomized, placebo-controlled trial. There was a statistically significant survival advantage ($p < 0.002$) for the treated arm. The results of the Northern Californian Oncology Group randomized trial of IA versus IV FUDR treatment of established liver metastases have recently been reported [60]: responses were significantly higher and longer-lived in the IA arm. The main toxicity observed was biliary sclerosis, due to excessively high FUDR concentration. This was limited by subsequent dose reduction. In the IA arm, the dose-limiting toxicity was elevation of liver enzymes, while no systemic toxicity was observed. Some groups [61] have tried adjuvant constant arterial infusion of FUDR via a hepatic arterial infusion pump for treatment of completely resected colonic liver metastasis; in that small group of patients, no impact on survival was seen, and significant morbidity was observed. As mentioned in the section on IP therapy, IP 5FU seems to produce hepatic artery concentrations similar to those achieved by catheterization, and this approach could be used as a substitute for IA therapy in the future.

Other Studies

The use of IA therapy with degradable microspheres [62, 63] could increase drug levels in the region of capillaries, without a concomitant increment in overall liver drug levels; this could improve the therapeutic index. Another related experimental possibility is the use of combination chemotherapy together with gelfoam [64] to induce chemoembolization and tumor infarction; such studies are at present ongoing.

IA therapy has also been used in other clinical situations—such as cervical and uterine carcinomas; kidney, bladder, and vesical tumors; nonoat-cell carcinomas of the lung; and brain neoplasia—with controversial results. The difficulty of the problem can be appreciated if one focuses on the IA therapy for brain malignancies. A large phase III study [65] of malignant gliomas has been undertaken, comparing IV with intracarotid BCNU in 283 randomized patients. A lack of therapeutic advantage was observed together with serious toxicity, such as irreversible encephalopathy and visual loss ipsilateral to the infused carotid artery. Even if the toxic events could be decreased by reducing the drug dose, the analysis of the results led to discontinuation of the randomization. Also, studies have ben conducted to analyze the role of opening the blood-brain barrier (BBB) with intracarotid mannitol, but the animal data indicate that the opening effect was almost totally restricted to the cortex, while no change was observed in the "blood-tumor barrier" [66]. We will discuss this concept further, but it is clear that such an attempt is unlikely to have any therapeutic efficacy.

In conclusion, IA delivery appears promising for certain tumor types and patient subsets, and it needs to be investigated, together with other strategies, as a potential means of improving the therapeutic index [67].

IT Therapy

The same compartment model as was described for IP and IA delivery can be applied to the administration of drugs into the CSF. When tumors spread to the leptomeninges or metastasize to the brain, the survival of untreated patients is less than 6 weeks. Chemotherapy is effective, alone or in combination with radiation therapy, but needs to be delivered regionally because of the presence of the BBB.

Before discussing the technical aspects and the clinical results, it is important to briefly summarize what is known about the BBB. First, this terminology has been introduced because of the evidence that (a) water-soluble, ionized molecules do not easily penetrate into the CSF after systemic administration and (b) the brain extracellular fluid is similar to the CSF rather than to that of the other tissues (e.g., it appears more like an ultrafiltrate than a transudate). There is an anatomical explanation for these phenomena: the endothelial cells of the brain capillaries are joined together by tight junctions and do not have the usual fenestrae; therefore, the BBB behaves as a lipid bilayer. There are two methods of predicting whether a drug will penetrate the BBB, which are respectively based on (a) the partition coefficient and (b) the diffusion coefficient. Also, the possibility of carrier-mediated systems through the capillary membrane needs to be considered. When dealing with a lipid-soluble drug, its entry into the BBB will depend on the blood flow. It has been recently demonstrated by quantitative autoradiography that the blood flow is generally decreased in brain tumors, and that the possible disruption of the BBB (which in the past has been considered as a characteristic of brain tumors) is variable both in different tumors and in different areas of the same neoplasia. This is to say that we should start thinking in terms of blood-*tumor* barrier rather than blood-*brain* barrier; this will probably help the development of more effective treatments.

The first therapeutic success in this field was obtained with IT MTX in 1958 [68], and it was followed by sporadic observations until a large study was conducted on 59 leukemic children [69, 70]. Since then, the survival of acute leukemic children has dramatically improved due to the control of meningeal leukemia.

Meningeal carcinomatosis is seen more and more frequently in solid tumors due to the improvement in survival that has been achieved with systemic therapy. IT therapy has also proven its efficacy in meningeal involvement from solid tumors, and there are now some long-term survivors. Moreover, patients who die after treatment for meningeal carcinomatosis are usually seen to have minimal CNS disease at autopsy, death being due to disseminated disease outside the meninges. This situation differs from that of meningeal involvement accompanied by parenchymal metastasis because in the latter case the achievement of a complete response is much more difficult. The drug that has been most often studied and used by the IT route is MTX, and we will not review in detail the extensive literature on this subject, as it is now part of the standard oncological armamentarium [70–74]. However, we shall focus on some of the technical and pharmacokinetic aspects of IT MTX delivery, as their analysis can give important insights relevant to the development of new strategies.

First, MTX is known to have neurotoxicity due to its penetration across the BBB (almost 3% of a concomitant plasma level). Its neurotoxicity is enhanced when MTX is given IT. Indeed, when drugs are administered IT, adverse local effects represent the most worrisome toxicity.

The obtainment of an even and adequate distribution also represents an important problem. Two routes of IT administration are available: by lumbar puncture (LP) and by ventricular reservoir (Ommaya). With the LP route, several factors contribute to the development of local toxicity and also to the failure to achieve an even distribution: (a) after an LP, the MTX concentrations in the ventricular CSF are variable and do not generally exceed 10% of the spinal CSF concentration [75]; (b) the concentration peak at the injection site is in the range 10^{-4}–$10^{-3}M$, which is elevated and can lead to arachnoiditis [76]; and (c) LPs are complicated in 10% of cases by CSF leakage from the subarachnoid space due to inappropriate needle positioning [77, 78], which predisposes to elevated local concentrations with possible unexpected toxicity, and to suboptimal MTX concentration at the ventricular level. On the other hand, the intraventricular route allows for stable concentrations to be achieved, and the difference between the concentrations obtained by the two routes has been compared to the difference in plasma levels after an oral versus and IV dose of a drug [79]. However, Ommaya reservoir placement, if certainly advised for treatment and prophylaxis of meningeal leukemias in children, is not devoid of complications [80, 81] and represents a surgical intervention often refused by the patients. Despite the pharmacokinetic data, there is not yet definitive evidence of the superiority of the intraventricular route in terms of clinical results in solid tumors with leptomeningeal metastasis.

These considerations make the choice between the two routes of administration very difficult when dealing with meningeal carcinomatosis in adults with solid tumors; in deciding, the clinician must weight the overall prognosis of the patient, taking into account other sites of disease. Practical considerations, such as the availability and expertise of a neurosurgical team, will also have to be considered. From a theoretical point of view, the major advantages of the intraventricular route would be to allow a more uniform distribution and to reduce the peak concentration of a drug; in fact, it has been proven that toxicity is related to the concentration peak. Intraventricular reservoirs would allow the administration of a lower total dose (concentration x time theory [82] or of continuous infusions [83].

It should be borne in mind that (a) meningeal infiltration at the level of the arachnoid granulations may reduce CSF reabsorption and therefore enhances the risk of toxic phenomena due to an increased CSF drug concentration (this explains why IT administration of drugs results in more toxicity when used to treat established disease rather than for prophylaxis); (b) drugs such as MTX are reintroduced into the CSF by retograde diffusion from the brain tissue, and their clearance curve is biphasic [84]; (c) after CSF instillation of a drug, the penetration into the brain tissue does not exceed a few millimeters in depth [85–87]; (d) the concentration in the parenchyma relates to both space and time factors due to the presence of concentration gradients (in fact, the drug introduced by IT delivery is removed by the capillaries, and their distribution will greatly affect the depth of penetration into the parenchyma); and (e) the concomitant use of radiation therapy affects drug pharmacokinetics through damage to endothelial cells and in particular to the chorioid plexus (which leads to altered CSF turnover and decreased drug clearance) [88–91]. This last aspect needs further consideration. In fact, almost all studies have shown the superiority of clinical results obtained with combined modality rather than with either chemotherapy or radiotherapy alone. However, the combined modality approach invariably leads to CNS sequelae in the long-term survivors (e.g., leukoencephalopathy) [92–96]. The decision whether to use combined modality or to attempt single-modality therapy, therefore, depends on the risk-benefit ratio and must also take into account the long-term prognosis. However, it must be stressed that the increase in delayed toxicity directly reflects the improvement in survival, and that the prognosis of untreated meningeal carcinomatosis is less than 6 weeks. Finally, all efforts should be made to design new therapies and less toxic prophylaxis [97].

The CNS toxic effects are not very different when agents other than MTX are used, even though the follow-up is still too limited in time to allow for definitive conclusions [98]. Clinical trials have been conducted with IT Ara-C [99, 100], thiotepa [101], and sequential drug combinations [102, 103].

Given the lack of lymphatic drainage in the CNS and the presence of the BBB, a possible pharmacological and therapeutic advantage may be expected, as in the case of IP delivery, by the use of protein-sized agents. We would anticipate deeper penetration in the brain tissue, if enough time is allowed (see section on IP therapy). An immunotoxin (WT1-Ricin A chain) has been reported not to be toxic in rhesus monkeys [104]. It was administered via Ommaya reservoir, and cytocidal levels were achieved in both ventricular and lumbar CSF, while a significant level was not detected in serum. A CSF concentration exceeding the ID_{50} was maintained for more than 24 h. ^{131}I monoclonal antibodies have undergone a phase I trial]105], with evidence of minimal toxicity and of clinical efficacy in that small group of patients. The antibody was injected via LP, after scintigraphic evidence of an even spinal and ventricular distribution. The use of interleukin-2 and LAK cells is also under investigation [106].

In conclusion, the most important aspects to be considered in IT therapy are the local toxicity and the drug distribution; all efforts should be made to improve the present results and techniques. The use of monoclonal antibody, which allows for better definition of the target and possibly limits the toxicity, could be very promising.

Intravesical Therapy

For completeness, intravesical delivery should be mentioned, as it is a legitimate regional therapy. Its use has become standard, both for treatment of superficial bladder cancer and as an adjuvant to surgery. Chemotherapy (thiotepa, Mitomycin C, and doxorubicin) has been used, with responses ranging from 30% to 60% in different studies [107]. Immunotherapy has been tried with bacille Calmette-Guérin (BCG), which prevents the development of invasive carcinomas but has local toxicity [108], and also with α-interferon [109]. Monoclonal antibodies could be used in the future, possibly conjugated with highly potent toxins [110].

Conclusions

Among the new approaches to cancer treatment, we believe that regional delivery is and will remain an important form of therapy. The rationale upon which regional therapy is based appears to be solid, namely to improve the therapeutic index of antitumor agents. We think that both drug sensitivity and drug resistance have to be considered first when approaching the design of a new form of cancer treatment. Then, pharmacokinetic data need to be collected and properly interpreted, in order to avoid wasting resources. Finally, the technical aspects of regional delivery still warrant a major improvement. Just as for any other kind of therapy, the major goals must be a true improvement in patient survival and relapse-free survival and the minimization of toxicity.

References

1. Ozols RF, Young RC, Speyer JL et al. (1982) Phase I and pharmacological studies of adriamycin administered intraperitoneally to patients with ovarian cancer. Cancer Res 42: 4265–4269
2. Chabner BA, Young RC (1973) Threshold methotrexate concentration for in vivo inhibition of DNA synthesis in normal and tumorous target tissues. J Clin Invest 52: 1804–1811

3. Dedrick RL, Myers CE, Bungay PM et al. (1978) Pharmacokinetic rationale for peritoneal drug administration in the treatment of ovarian cancer. Cancer Treat Rep 62 (1): 1–11
4. Jones RB, Collins JM, Myers CE et al. (1981) High volume intraperitoneal chemotherapy with methotrexate in patients with cancer. Cancer Res 41: 55–59
5. Myers MA (1973) Peritoneography. Normal and pathologic anatomy. Am J Roentgenol Rad Ther Nucl Med 117: 353–365
6. Flessner MF, Dedrick RL, Schultz JS (1985) A distributed model of peritoneal-plasma transport: tissue concentration gradients. Am J Physiol 248: F413–F424
7. Rosenheim N, Blake D, McIntyre P et al. (1978) The effect of volume on the distribution of substances instilled into the peritoneal cavity. Gynecol Oncol 6: 106–110
8. Dunnick N, Jones R, Doppman J et al. (1979) Intraperitoneal contrast infusion for assessment of intraperitoneal fluid dynamics. Am J Radiol 133: 221–223
9. Collins JM, Dedrick RL, Flessner MF et al. (1982) Concentration-dependent disappearance of fluorouracil from peritoneal fluid in the rat: Experimental observations and distributed modeling. J Pharm Sci 71: 735–738
10. Ozols RF, Locker GY, Doroshow JH et al. (1979) Pharmacokinetics of adriamycin and tissue penetration in murine ovarian cancer. Cancer Res 39: 3209–3214
11. McVie JG, Dikhoff T, Van der Heide J et al. (1985) Tissue concentration of platinum after intraperitoneal cisplatin administration in patients. Proc AACR 26: 162
12. Flanigan MJ, Dai D Ngheim, Schulak JA et al. (1987) The use and complications of three peritoneal dialysis catheter designs. Trans Am Soc Artif Intern Organs XXXIII: 33–38
13. Howell SB, Chu BCF, Wung WE et al. (1981) Long duration intracavitary infusion of methotrexate with systemic leucovorin protection in patients with malignant effusions. J Clin Invest 67: 1161–1169
14. Speyer JL, Sugarbaker PH, Collins JM et al. (1981) Portal levels and hepatic clearance of 5-fluorouracil after intraperitoneal administration in humans. Cancer Res 41: 1916–1922
15. Speyer JL, Collins JM, Dedrick RL et al. (1980) Phase I and pharmacological studies of 5-fluorouracil administered intraperitoneally. Cancer Res 40: 567–572
16. Ozols RF, Speyer JL, Jenkins J et al. (1984) Phase II of 5-fluorouracil administered intraperitoneally to patients with refractory ovarian cancer. Cancer Treat Rep 68: 1229–1232
17. Ozols RF, Grotzinger KR, Fisher RI et al. (1979) Kinetic characterization and response to chemotherapy in a transplantable murine ovarian cancer. Cancer Res 39: 3202–3208
18. Pretorius RG, Hacker NF, Berek JS et al. (1983) Pharmacokinetics of ip cisplatin in refractory ovarian carcinoma. Cancer Treat Rep 67: 1085–1092
19. Howell SB, Pfeifle CE, Wung WE et al. (1982) Intraperitoneal cisplatin with systemic thiosulfate protection. Ann Intern Med 97: 1085–1092
20. Casper ES, Kelsen DP, Alcock NW et al. (1983) Ip cisplatin in patients with malignant ascites: pharmacokinetic evaluation and comparison with the iv route. Cancer Treat Rep 67: 235–238
21. Howell SB, Pfeifle CE, Olshen RA et al. (1984) Intraperitoneal chemotherapy with melphalan. Ann Intern Med 101: 14–18
22. Colombo N, Speyer J, Wernz J et al. (1987) Phase I–II study of intraperitoneal CBDCA in patients with advanced ovarian cancer. Proc ASCO 6: 444
23. Alberts DS, Chen HSG, Chang SY et al. (1979) The disposition of intraperitoneal bleomycin, melphalan and vinblastine in cancer patients. Clin Pharmacol Ther 26: 73–80
24. King ME, Pfeifle CE, Howell SB (1984) Intraperitoneal cytosine arabinoside therapy in ovarian carcinoma. J Clin Oncol 4: 662–669
25. ten Bokkel-Huinink WW, Dubbelman R, Aartsen E et al. (1985) Experimental and clinical results with intraperitoneal cisplatin. Semin Oncol 12(3)[Suppl 4]: 43–46
26. Speyer J, Beller U, Colombo N et al. (1987) First line intraperitoneal chemotherapy in advanced ovarian adenocarcinoma. A pilot study. Proc ASCO 6: 443
27. Ozols R (1985) Intraperitoneal chemotherapy in the management of ovarian cancer. Semin Oncol 3 [Suppl 4]: 75–80
28. Myers CE, Collins JM (1983) Pharmacology of intraperitoneal chemotherapy. Cancer Invest 1 (5): 395–407
29. Myers CE (1984) The use of intraperitoneal chemotherapy in the treatment of ovarian cancer. Semin Oncol 11 (3): 275–284

30. Suarbaker PH, Gianola FJ, Speyer JC et al. (1985) Prospective randomized trial of intravenous versus intraperitoneal 5-Fluorouracil in patients with advanced primary colon or rectal cancer. Surgery 98 (3): 414–421
31. Speyer JL (1985) The rationale behind intraperitoneal chemotherapy in gastrointestinal malignancies. Semin Oncol 12(3) [Suppl 4]
32. Flessner MF, Fenstermacher JD, Blasberg RG et al. (1985) Peritoneal absorption of macromolecules studied by quantitiative autoradiography. Am J Physiol 248: H26–H32
33. Flessner MF, Dedrick RL, Schultz JS (1985) Exchange of macromolecules between peritoneal cavity and plasma. Am J Physiol 248: H15–H25
34. Parker RJ, Hartman KD, Sieber SM (1981) Lymphatic absorption and tissue disposition of liposome-entrapped C-adriamycin following intraperitoneal administration to rats. Cancer Res 41: 1311–1317
35. Dedrick RL, Myers CE, Bungay PM et al. (1978) Pharmacokinetic rationale for peritoneal drug administration in the treatment of ovarian cancer. Cancer Treat Rep 62: 1–11
36. Colcher D, Esteban J, Carrasquillo JA et al. (1986) Comparison of route of administration of radiolabeled monoclonal antibodies in patients with colorectal cancer. J Nucl Med 27: 902
37. Larson SM, Carrasqillo JA, Sugarbaker P et al. (1986) Considerations for radiotherapy of pseudomyxoma peritonei with IP [131]I B72.3, a monoclonal antibody. J Nucl Med 27: 1021
38. Berek JS, Hacker NF, Lichtenstein A et al. (1985) Intraperitoneal recombinant alpha-interferon for "salvage" immunotherapy in stage III epithelial ovarian cancer: a Gynecologic Oncology Group study. Cancer Res 45: 4447–4453
39. D'Acquisto R, Markaman M, Hakes T et al. (1987) Phase I trial of intraperitoneal recombinant gamma-interferon in advanced ovarian carcinoma. Proc ASCO 6: 471
40. Bast RC, Berek JS, Obrist R et al. (1983) Intraperitoneal immunotherapy of human ovarian carcinoma with *Corynebacterium parvum*. Cancer Res 43: 1395–1401
41. Steis R, Bookman M, Clark J et al. (1987) Intraperitoneal lymphokine activated killer (LAK) cells and Interleukin-2 (IL-2) therapy for peritoneal carinomatosis: Toxicity, efficacy and laboratory results. Proc ASCO 6: 984
42. Howell SB (1985) Intraperitoneal chemotherapy: The use of concurrent systemic neutralizing agents. Semin Oncol 12(3) [Suppl 4]: 17–22
43. Holcenberg J, Anderson T, Ritch P et al. (1983) Intraperitoneal chemotherapy with melphalan plus glutaminase. Cancer Res 43: 1381–1388
44. Muggia FM (1985) Colorectal cancer: Speculations on the role of intraperitoneal therapy. Semin Oncol 12(3) [Suppl 4]: 112–115
45. Myers CE (1985) The clinical setting and pharmacology of intraperitoneal chemotherapy: an overview. Semin Oncol 11 (3): 12(3) [Suppl. 4]: 12–16
46. Shingleton WW, Parker RT, Mahaley S (1961) Abdominal perfusion for cancer chemotherapy with hypothermia and hyperthermia. Surgery 50: 260–265
47. Spratt JS, Adcock RA, Sherrill W et al. (1980) Hyperthermic peritoneal perfusion system in canines. Cancer Res 40: 253–255
48. Collins JM (1984) Pharmacologic rationale for regional drug delivery. J Clin Oncol 2(5): 498–504
49. Collins JM (1984) Pharmacokinetic rationale for intraarterial therapy. In: Howell (ed) Proceedings of the Conference on Inta-arterial and Intracavitary Chemotherapy.
50. Mulcare RJ, Solis A, Fortner JG (1973) Isolation and perfusion of the liver for cancer chemotherapy. J Surg Res 15: 87–95
51. Taylor I, Machin D, Mullee M et al. (1985) A randomized controlled trial of adjuvant portal vein cytotoxic perfusion in colorectal cancer. Br J Surg 72: 359–363
52. Carter SK (1977) The chemotherapy of head and neck cancer. Semin Oncol 4: 413–424
53. Archangeli G, Neri C, Righini R et al. (1983) Combined radiation and drugs: The effect of intraarterial chemotherapy followed by radiotherapy in the head and neck cancer. Radiother Oncol 1: 101–107
54. Molinari R (1982) Present role of intraarterial regional chemotherapy in head and neck cancer. Chemioterapia 1: 263–274
55. Ghussen F, Anderson S, Smalley R et al. (1987) Hyperthermic perfusion with alkeran in patients with melanoma: four year follow-up. Proc ASCO 6: 829

56. Rege V, Leone L, Soderberg C et al. (1987) Hyperthermic perfusion for stage I malignant melanoma of the extremity. Proc ASCO 6: 832
57. Weisenburger TH, Eilber FR, Grant TT et al. (1981) Multidisciplinary "limb salvage" treatment of soft tissue and skeletal sarcomas. Int J Radiat Oncol Biol Phys 7: 1495–1499
58. Jaffe N, Knapp J, Chung VP et al. (1983) Osteosarcoma: Intraarterial treatment of the primary tumor with *cis*-diammine-dichloroplatinum II (CDP). Cancer 51: 402–407
59. Sears HF (1982) Soft tissue sarcomas. Semin Oncol 8: 129–240
60. Hohn D, Stagg R, Friedman M et al. (1987) The NCOG randomized trial of intravenous versus hepatic arterial FUDR for colorectal cancer metastatic to the liver. Proc ASCO 6: 333
61. Merrick HW, Skeel RT (1987) Constant arterial infusion adjuvant chemotherapy for completely resected colonic liver metastasis: a long term follow-up. Proc ASCO 6: 329
62. Dakhil S, Ensminger W, Cho K et al. (1982) Improved regional selectivity of hepatic arterial BCNU with degradable microspheres. Cancer 50: 631–635
63. Thom AK, Sigurdson ER, Daly JM (1987) Use of degradable starch microspheres in patients with hepatic metastasis. Proc ASCO 6: 311
64. Hohn D, Chase J, Stagg R et al. (1987) A phase I–II trial of gelfoam chemoembolization in patients with primary liver tumors. Proc ASCO 6: 332
65. Shapiro WR, Green SB, Burger PC et al. (1987) A randomized comparison of intraarterial vs. intravenous BCNU for patients with malignant glioma (study 8301): interim analysis demonstrating lack of efficacy for IA BCNU. Proc ASCO 6: 268
66. Shaprio WR, Shapiro JR (1986) Principles of brain tumor chemotherapy. Semin Oncol 13: 55–69
67. Oldfield E, Dedrick RL, Chatterji DC et al. (1983) Reduced systemic drug exposure by combining intracarotid chemotherapy with hemoperfusion of jugular drainage. Surg Forum 34: 535–537
68. Whiteside JA, Philip FS, Dargeon HW et al. (1958) Intrathecal amethopterin in neurological manifestations of leukemia. Arch Int Med 101: 279–285
69. Hyman CB (1965) Central nervous system involvement by leukemia in children. I Relationship to systemic leukemia and description of laboratory manifestations. Blood 25: 1–22
70. Hyman CB, Bogle JM, Brubaker CA et al. (1965) Central nervous system involvement by leukemia in children. II Therapy with intrathecal methotrexate. Blood 25: 13–22
71. Ongerboer de Visser BW, Somers R, Noovet WH et al (1983) Intraventricular methotrexate therapy of leptomeningeal metastasis from breast carcinoma. Neurology 33: 1565–1572
72. Wasserstrom WR, Glass JP, Posner JB (1982) Diagnosis and treatment of leptomeningeal metastasis from solid tumors: experience with 90 patients. Cancer 49: 750–754
73. Yap HY, Yap BS, Rasmussen S et al. (1982) Treatment for meningeal carcinomatosis in breast cancer. Cancer 49: 219–222
74. Bleyer WA (1977) Clinical pharmacology of methotrexate II. Improved dosage regimen derived from age-related pharmacokinetics. Cancer Treat Rep 61: 1999–2001
75. Shapiro WR, Young DF, Mehta BM (1976) Methotrexate: distribution in cerebrospinal fluid after intravenous, ventricular and lumbar puncture injections. N Engl J Med 293: 161–166
76. Bleyer WA, Poplack DG (1978) Clinical studies on central nervous system pharmacology of methotrexate. In: Pinedo HM (ed) Clinical pharmacology of anti-neoplastic drugs, pp. 115–131
77. Gagliano RG Costanzi JJ (1976) Paraplegia following intrathecal methotrexate. Cancer 37: 1663–1668
78. Larson SM, Schall GL, DiChiro G (1971) The influence of previous lumbar puncture and pneumoencephalography on the incidence of unsuccessful radioisotope cisternography. J Nucl Med 12: 494–501
79. Collins JM (1983) Pharmacokinetics of intraventricular administration. J Neurol Oncol 1: 283–291
80. Obbens EAMT, Leavens ME, Beal JM et al. (1985) Ommaya reservoir in 387 cancer patients: a 15 year experience. Neurology 35 (9): 1274–1278
81. Machado M, Salcman M, Kaplan RS et al. (1985) Expanded role of the cerebrospinal fluid reservoir in neurooncology: indications, causes of revision and complications. Neurosurgery 17: 600–603

188

82. Bleyer WA, Poplack DG, Ziegler JL et al. (1978) Concentration x time methotrexate via a subcutaneous reservoir: a less toxic regimen for intraventricular chemotherapy of cental nervous system neoplasms. Blood 51: 835–842

83. Dakhil S, Ensminger W, Kindt G et al. (1981) Implanted system for intraventricular drug infusion in central nervous system tumors. Cancer Treat Rep 65: 401–411

84. Collins JM, Dedrick RL (1983) Distributed model for drug delivery to CSF and brain tissue. Am J Physiol 245: R303–310

85. Fenstermacher JD, Blasberg RG, Patlak CS et al. (1981) Methods of quantifying the transport of drugs across brain barrier systems. Pharmacol Ther 14: 217–248

86. Blasberg R, Patlak CS, Shapiro WR (1977) Distribution of methotrexate in cerebrospinal fluid after intravenous administration. Cancer Treat Rep 61: 633–641

87. Blasberg R, Patlak Cs, Fenstermacher JD (1975) Intrathecal chemotherapy: brain tissue profiles after ventriculocisternal perfusion. J Pharmacol Exp Ther 195: 73–83

88. Kaplan RS, Wiernik PH (1982) Neurotoxicity of antineoplastic drugs. Semin Oncol 9: 103–130

89. Rubin R, Owens E, Rall D (1979) Transport of methotrexate by the choroid plexus. Cancer Res 28: 689–692

90. Veninga TS, Dankert J, Ebels EJ et al. (1984) Early transient accumulation of methotrexate in the cerebrospinal fluid of rabbits after treatment with methotrexate and roentgen X-rays. Acta Radiol Oncol 23: 69–73

91. Levin VA, Edwards MS, Byrd A (1979) Quantitative observations on the acute effects of x-irradiation on brain capillary permeability. Int J Rad Oncol Biol Phys 5: 1633–1635

92. Rubinstein LJ, Herman MM, Longo TF et al. (1975) Disseminated leukoencephalopathy: a complication of treated central nervous system in leukemia and lymphoma. Cancer 35: 291–305

93. Price RA, Jamieson PA (1975) The central nervous system in childhood leukemia. II Subacute leukoencephalopathy. Cancer 35: 306–318

94. Bresnan MD, Gilles FH, Lorenzo AV et al. (1972) Leukoencephalopathy following combined irradiation and intraventricular methotrexate therapy of brain tumours in childhood. Trans Am Neurol Assoc 97: 204–206

95. Price RA, Birdwell DA (1978) The central nervous system in childhood leukemia. III Mineralizing microangiopathy and dystrophic calcification. Cancer 42: 717–728

96. Riccardi R (1985) Abnormal computed tomography brain scans in children with acute lymphoblastic leukemia: serial long-term follow-up. J Clin Oncol 3: 12–18

97. Balis FM, Savitch JL, Bleyer WA et al. (1985) Remission induction of meningeal leukemia with high-dose intravenous methotrexate. J Clin Oncol 3: 485–489

98. Kim S, Kim JD, Geyer MA et al (1987) Multivesicular liposomes containing Ara-C for slow-release intrathecal therapy. Proc ASCO 6: 122

99. Wang JJ, Pratt CB (1970) Intrathecal arabinosyl cytosine in meningeal leukemia.Cancer 25: 531–534

100. Fulton DS, Levin VA, Gutin PH (1982) Intrathecal cytosine arabinoside for the treatment of meningeal metastasis from malignant brain tumors and systemic tumors. Cancer Chemother Pharmacol 8: 285–291

101. Gutin PH, Weiss HD, Wiernik PH et al. (1982) Treatment of malignant meningeal disease with intrathecal thiotepa: a phase II study. Cancer Treat Rep 66: 1549–1551

102. Sullivan MP, Moon TE, Trueworthy R et al., (1977) Combination intrathecal therapy for meningeal leukemia: two versus three drugs. Blood 50 (3): 471–478

103. Trump DL, Grossman SA, Thompson G et al. (1982) Treatment of neoplastic meningitis with intraventricular thiotepa and methotrexate. Cancer Treat Rep 66 (7): 1549–1551

104. Hertler A, Schlossman D, Lester C et al. (1987) Intrathecal administration of WT1-Ricin A chain immunotoxin. Prox ASCO 6: 989

105. Lashford LS, Mosely R, Davies AG et al (1987) A pilot study of ^{131}I monoclonal antibodies in the therapy of leptomeningeal tumours. Proc ASCO 6: 280

106. Okamoto Y, Shimizu K, Miyao Y et al. (1986) Clinical studies of adoptive immunotherapy of human disseminated brain tumors with LAK cells and recombinant interleukin-2. No To Shinkei 38 (6): 593–598

107. Torti FM, Lum BL (1984) The biology and treatment of superficial bladder cancer. J Clin Oncol 2 (5): 505–531
108. Camacho F, Pinsky C, Kerr D et al. (1980) Treatment of superficial bladder cancer with intravesical BCG. Proc ASCO 21: 359
109. Torti FM, Shortliffe LD, Williams RD et al. (1984) Superficial bladder cancers are responsive to Alpha-2 Interferon administered intravesically. Proc ASCO 3: 160
110. Chopin DK (1984) In vivo staining and diagnostic cytology of bladder cancer with monoclonal antibodies G4 and E7. J Urol 131: 107A (abstract 14)

9. Drug Resistance in Cancer

S.P. Ivy, R.F. Ozols, and K.H. Cowan

Introduction

The impact of cancer chemotherapy on the survival of all cancer patients has been significant, most notably in younger patients. The list of diseases curable with chemotherapy includes acute lymphocytic leukemia, adult Hodgkin's disease, non-Hodgkin's lymphomas of adults and children, pediatric solid tumors, ovarian cancer, and testicular cancer in young males [1]. Other tumors, such as adult leukemias, breast cancer, and small-cell lung cancer, are highly responsive to combination chemotherapy, but permanent remissions are achived in few of these patients. Unfortunately, these chemotherapy-responsive tumors will eventually reoccur in some patients. Although second remissions in patients with diseases such as Hodgkin's disease, acute leukemia, and testicular cancer can be achieved with salvage chemotherapy, relapses in most cancer patients are associated with development of drug resistance and lack of durable second remissions. Understanding the mechanisms involved in the development of clinical drug resistance is essential for the design of rational, effective salvage therapy.

Why do tumors initially responsive to therapy relapse and subsequently become refractory to chemotherapy? Why do some tumors, particularly those of epithelial origin, appear to be resistant de novo? Recent studies have begun to unravel the molecular changes associated with the development of resistance to a number of specific antineoplastic agents. Indeed, some studies now suggest that the process of resistance to some antineoplastic agents may be related to more fundamental patterns of cellular response to toxins such as carcinogens. These studies have led to important insights into diagnosis and therapeutic approaches to overcoming clinical drug resistance in patients.

Drug resistance is classified in three categories—inherent, acquired, and acute inducible. Tumors that are initially unresponsive to chemotherapy—such as colon cancer, nonsmall-cell lung cancer, and malignant melanoma—are inherently resistant. In contrast, recurrent tumors that are unresponsive to therapy following successful primary therapy are classified as exhibiting acquired resistance. Inducible resistance refers to biochemical changes that can be transiently induced in tumor or host cells, and which subsequently result in decreased cytotoxicity from antineoplastic agents. While inherent and acquired resistance are generally believed to be due to stable genetic changes in cells (gene deletion, mutation, and amplification), acute inducible resistance is most probably a manifestation of rapidly reversible epigenetic changes in gene expression in cells. An example of inducible resistance is found in mouse bone marrow treated with various cytotoxic agents. Adams et al. [2] found that animals treated with agents such as cyclophosphamide are able to survive supralethal doses of the same agent given 7 days after the first priming dose. The time course of increased survival paralleled the increase in the levels of glutathione and gluathione transferase, suggesting that resistance is acutely inducible.

This chapter will review some general principles involved in the development of drug resistance. Gene amplification and the phenomenon of multidrug resistance, two important aspects of drug resistance, will be discussed in more detail.

Pharmacologic Factors Associated with Resistance

Before reviewing specific genetic and biochemical changes associated with antineoplastic drug resistance, it is important to remember that there are a variety of pharmacologic factors which determine the overall clinical response to therapy:

1. Drug bioavailability
2. Drug metabolism
3. Drug elimination
4. Sanctuary sites (CNS, testes)
5. Excessive host toxicity (prior therapy, age)
6. Limited drug diffusion (mass size)
7. Altered cell kinetics
8. Increased salvage factors

Many of these factors affect the actual concentration of drug delivered to the tumor. For example, many antineoplastic drugs, including 6-mercaptopurine, are poorly and erratically abosrbed following oral administration. Zimm et al. [3] found a fivefold variation in drug exposure following oral administration of 6-mercaptopurine to patients with acute lymphoblastic leukemia. A similar wide range in bioavailability has been reported in patients receiving melphalan (LPAM) [4, 5] and hexylmethylamine [6]. Thus, lack of a therapeutic response to these agents when given orally may relate to the inability to achieve effective cytocidal concentration of drug, and not to "resistant" mechanisms at the tumor cell level.

Similarly, differences in the rate of drug metabolism or elimination in patients may markedly affect tumor cell exposure to drug and potentially limit the clinical response or the toxicity of these agents. Tumors present in sanctuary sites (CNS or testes), into which drug penetration is poor, are another example of ineffective drug delivery. Tumors in these sites may appear to be resistant to chemotherapy. Furthermore, patients who have had prior courses of chemotherapy or radiation therapy frequently develop increased toxicity during subsequent cycles of salvage therapies and consequently may receive lower doses of therapy. Ineffective therapy may not represent a lack of tumor sensitivity to chemotherapy.

In addition to the above examples, large tumor masses are often refractory to chemotherapy. There may be several reasons for this phenomenon, including limited drug diffusion into large masses, the presence of central areas of relative hypoxia (limiting the effectiveness of certain agents), increased concentrations of salvage nucleosides (bypassing the toxic mechanism of certain agents), and reduced cell fraction in more vulnerable phases of the growth cycle. Many of these factors influence the clinical response achieved by limiting the "effective" concentration of drug being delivered to tumor cells or the relative effectiveness of these agents once they have arrived at their targets. Thus, it is important to keep in mind that other factors, including pharmacokinetic considerations, are important determinants of clinical response.

However, it is also apparent that while the factors discussed above may influence the response rate of a given tumor to cytotoxic therapy, stable genetic and biochemical changes in tumor cells seem to be responsible for much of the clinical resistance to antineoplastic agents. Goldie and Coldman [7] have presented a mathematical model which attempts to describe the emergence of drug resistance in tumors. Based on classical studies of the frequently of mutations in bacteria by Luria and Delbruck [8], the Goldie-Coldman model assumes that the major reason for clinical drug resistance is the selection of tumor cells with stable genetic mutations. Furthermore, the model proposes that the frequency of these genetic mutations is thus related to the total number of tumor cells and to the spontaneous mutation rate of these populations of cells.

The Goldie-Coldman model has several important clinical implications. It supports the desirability of using combination chemotherapy regimens since the selection of multiply resistant tumor cells would be less frequent. Furthermore, early treatment of tumors with adjuvant or neoadjuvant chemotherapy would be best since the smallest tumors would have the highest probability of having the smallest number of drug-resistant cells. Noncross-resistant regimens should be given in an alternating schedule rather than sequentially to reduce the risk of selecting resistant cells. Finally, many of the cytotoxic drugs used in the treatment of cancer are themselves mutagenic and may increase the frequency of spontaneous mutations, resulting in a drug-resistant phenotype. Less effective agents which are highly mutagenic should be eliminated from combination chemotherapy regimens.

Mechanisms of Drug Resistance

As alluded to previously, numerous drug-resistant cell lines have been isolated and used to characterize specific mechanisms involved in drug resistance. Some of the mechanisms associated with resistance to cytotoxic agents are shown in

193

Table 1. When considering the different mechanisms involved in drug resistance, several basic principles are important. For any drug or class of drugs, there often exists a variety of mechanisms by which a cell may become resistant. When these changes occur as isolated defects, the level of resistance may be relatively low. However, when cells are selected for higher levels of resistance, as is frequently the case in vitro, resistant cells often develop multiple alterations. Many mechanisms of resistance are specific for an individual drug or class of drugs. Resistance to antimetabolites, for example, does not generally result in cross-resistance to other classes of antineoplastic drugs, such as anthracyclines. In contrast, cells selected for resistance to vinca alkaloids or anthracyclines frequently develop cross-resistance to a wide variety of other agents that differ markedly not only in their structures but their apparent mechanisms of action [9]. This phenomenon has been referred to as multidrug resistance (MDR) or pleiotropic drug resistance.

As shown in Table 1, changes in the rate of cellular uptake and accumulation appear to be associated with resistance to drug such as methotrexate (MTX), phenylalanine mustard, and nitrogen mustard. These defects are generally believed to involve specific changes in membrane transport systems. In the case of MTX, the decrease in drug uptake apparently involves changes in the folate transport system [10–14]. In phenylalanine mustard resistance [15], decreased uptake is believed to be due to a defect in an amino acid transport system [16]. Another class of resistant cells in which decreased drug accumulation occurs involves changes in drug efflux systems. This modification is one of the changes present in multidrug-resistant cells. Dano [17] and Skovsgaard [18] described decreased drug accumulation as a consistent finding in drug-resistant cells selected for vincristine or daunomycin resistance and provided evidence which suggested that this was the result of increased activity of an energy-dependent efflux pump. Using a colchicine-resistant Chinese hamster ovary (CHO) cell line, Juliano and Ling [19] demonstrated that enhanced efflux in these multidrug-resistant cells was associated with the overexpression of a high-molecular-weight membrane protein (P170), which will be discussed below.

Many antineoplastic drugs, particularly antimetabolites, are pro-drugs, which need to be converted to their active forms, often by phosphorylation, in tumor cells in order to exert their cytotoxicity. Resistance in vitro to pro-drugs such as cytosine arabinoside, 5-flurouracil (5-FU), 6-mercaptopurine, and 6-thioguanine is frequently associated with defects in the intracellular enzymes that activate these drugs (Table 1). Recent studies have also shown that alterations in the intracellular metabolism of MTX can also affect its cytotoxicity. In most cells, MTX undergoes conversion to a complex family of MTX polyglutamates that are formed by the addition of one to four glutamyl residues to the native drug (Fig. 1). Polyglutamation is accomplished through the same enzyme activity that converts folate cofactors to their polyglutamate forms. The importance of MTX polyglutamate formation is perhaps best illustrated by a human breast cancer cell line in which resistance to MTX was associated with diminished formation of MTX polyglutamyl derivatives [20]. This cell line is cross-resistant to other anti-folates, such as aminopterin, which also undergoes intracellular conversion to

Table 1. Mechanisms of drug resistance

	Drug	Defect
Alterations in drug uptake	Methotrexate	Defective carrier transport
	Melphalan	Defective carrier transport
	Mechlorethamine	Defective carrier transport
Alterations in intracellular drug accumulation	Doxorubicin	Increased drug efflux
	Vinca alkaloids	Increased drug efflux
	Actinomycin D	Increased drug efflux
Decreased drug activation	Cytosine arabinoside	Decreased deoxycytidine kinase
	5-Fluorouracil	Decreased oratate monophosphate (OMP) transferase
	6-Mercaptopurine	Decreased hypoxanthine phosphoribosyl-transferase (HPRT)
	6-Thioguanine	Decreased HPRT
	Methotrexate	Decreased polyglutamate formation
Increased metabolic inactivation	6-Mercaptopurine	Increased alkaline phosphatase
	6-Thioguanine	Increased alkaline phosphatase
	Cytosine arabinoside	Increased cytidine deaminase
	Alkylators	Increased glutathione, increased glutathione transferase
	Cis-platinum	Increased metallothionein
Alterations in target proteins	Methotrexate	Altered DHFR
	Steroid hormones	Altered receptors
	Vinca alkaloids	Altered tubulins
	FUDR	Altered thymidylate synthase
Alterations in cellular metabolism	Cytosine arabinoside	Increased CTP pools
	5-Fluorouracil	Increased CTP pools
	Methotrexate	Increased purine pyrimidine salvage
	6-Mercaptopurine	Increased hypoxanthine salvage
Alterations in cofactor levels	6-Thioguanine	Decreased PRPP
	FUDR	Decreased folate cofactors
Alterations in cellular repair mechanisms	Alkylators	Increased DNA repair enzymes
	Nitrosoureas	Increased DNA repair enzymes
Increased levels of target proteins	Methotrexate	Increased DHFR
	PALA	Increased CAD protein
	FUDR	Increased thymidylate synthase
	Deoxycoformycin	Increased adenosine deaminase

CTP, cytosine triphosphate; FUDR, fluorodeoxyuridine; PALA, *N*-phosphonacetyl-L-aspartic-acid; DHFR, dihydrofolate reductase; PRPP, polyribosyl pyrophosphate.

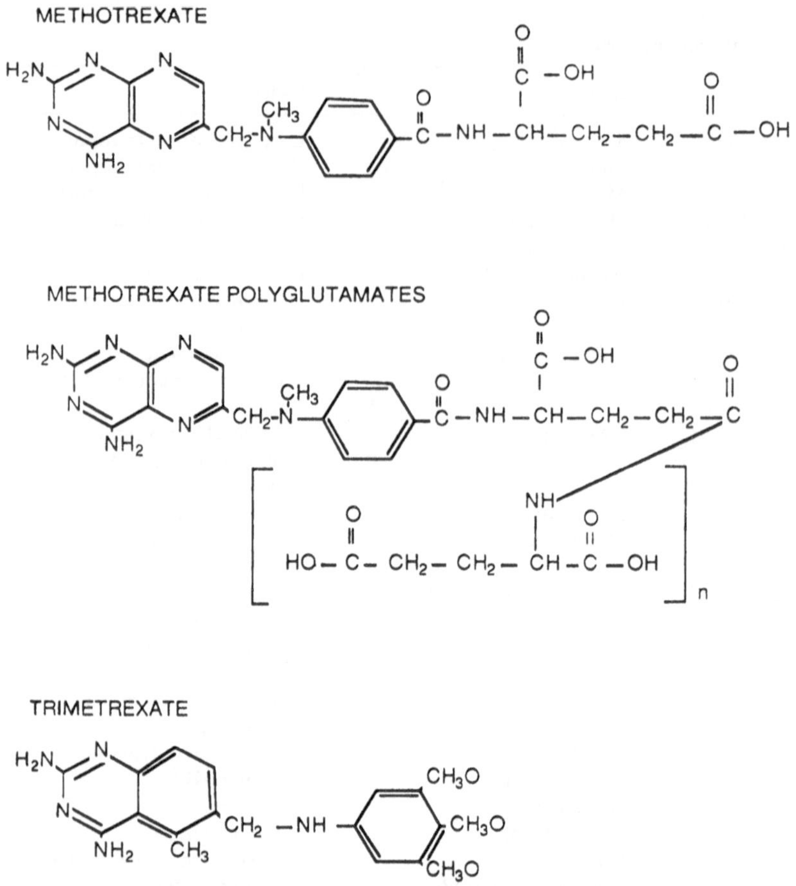

METHOTREXATE

METHOTREXATE POLYGLUTAMATES

TRIMETREXATE

Fig. 1. Structure of methotrexate, methotrexate polyglutamyl derivatives (n is a variable number of γ-glutamyl residues), and trimetrexate, a nonclassical folate analog

polyglutamates. However, these breast cancer cells were sensitive to another antifolate analog, trimetrexate, which differs structurally from MTX and does not undergo conversion to polyglutamyl derivatives. These studies suggest that there are important differences in the presumed mechanism of cytotoxicity among the antifolate analogs (Fig. 1).

Increased intracellular metabolism of cytotoxic drugs to inactive species is also associated with resistance. Resistance to both thiopurines and cytosine arabinoside has been reported to be associated with changes in the level of specific drug-metabolizing enzymes. Instead of increased enzymatic metabolism, resistance may also result from increased drug inactivation by enhanced binding to sulfhydryl-rich scavenger peptides and proteins, such as glutathione [21] and metallothionein [22].

Specific alterations in target proteins by point mutation or changed regulation can also lead to drug resistance. For example, MTX resistance can result from single amino acid substitutions in the target enzyme, dihydrofolate reductase, resulting in an enzyme with a reduced drug-binding affinity. Other examples of this type of resistance include altered or decreased steroid hormone receptors [23, 24], altered tubulin in vinca alkaloid resistance [25–27], and altered thymidylate synthase in fluorodeoxyuridine (FUDR) resistance [28].

Another example of an altered target protein which results in resistance to VP 16 and various intercalator compounds has been described in cells containing an alteration in topoisomerase II. In these studies [29, 30], modified topoisomerase II activity was related to reduced ability to form drug-induced, protein-associated DNA strand breaks in VP16-resistant CHO cells compared with wild-type cells. In general, most intercalators and epipodophyllotoxins appear to inhibit mammalian topoisomerase II by trapping the enzyme within DNA cleavage complexes, which can be detected in cells as protein-associated DNA strand breaks.

Changes in intracellular nucleotide pools or in the relative flux through salvage nucleotide pathways can also affect drug sensitivity. For example, changes in the level of polyribosyl pyrophosphate (PRPP), a cofactor involved in the activation of both thiopurines and 5FU, can alter the sensitivity of cells to these agents [31, 32]. Indeed, one of the proposed mechanisms for the synergy between MTX and 5FU when given sequentially is believed to be due to antifolate-induced increase in cellular PRPP pools. Furthermore, the binding of fluoro-deoxyuridinemonophosphate (FdUMP; one of the active forms of 5FU) to its target enzyme thymidylate synthase is dependent on the concentration of reducd folates in cells. Thus, diminished intracellular pools of reduced folates can lead to 5FU and FUDR resistance. Diminished intracellular folate pools may be particularly important in clinical resistance to 5FU. Preliminary results of several recent clinical trials in which leucovorin was given with 5FU seemed to show improved clinical responses when compared with 5FU alone [33].

Drug resistance can also result from the selection of cells which possess an increased ability to repair cellular damage. This phenomenon is noted particularly in cells resistant to alkylating agents, in which resistance is associated with an increase in DNA repair enzyme activities [34–37].

Finally, the development of increased levels of target proteins is one of the most common mechanisms associated with resistance in vitro. This type of drug resistance is of particular interest because Alt et al. [38] showed that resistance to MTX was associated with an increase in the level of dihydrofolate reductase (DHFR), which resulted from the amplification of the DNA sequences that code for this enzyme. Since this phenomenon appears to be a common genetic alteration in tumor cell lines, resulting in specific resistance to a variety of drugs, we shall discuss the mechanisms of gene amplification in more detail.

Gene Amplification and Drug Resistance

Early studies in cells selected for resistance to MTX [39] demonstrated that the resistant cells frequently develop cytogenetic abnormalities, including elongated

197

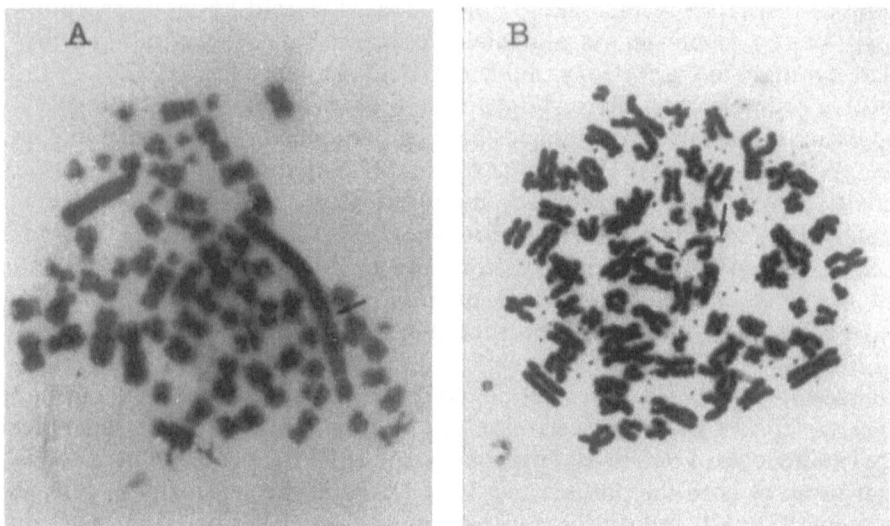

Fig. 2. A Cytogenetic analysis of a methotrexate-resistant human breast cancer cell line (MTX^R MCF-7) containing amplified DHFR genes. The *arrow* points to marker chromosomes (HSRs) not present in the parent cell line. **B** Cytogenetic analysis of a methotrexate-resistant small-cell lung cancer cell line (NCI-H249P) containing amplified DHFR genes. The *arrows* point to double minute chromosomes (DMs) not present in the parent cell lines

marker chromosomes with homogeneously staining regions (HSRs) or increased numbers of double-minute chromosomes (DMs) (Fig. 2). Subsequent studies revealed that both of these cytogenetic abnormalities are the result of a marked increase in gene copy number [40, 41]. The importance of these two cytogenetic forms of gene amplification is apparent when resistant cells are grown subsequently under nonselective conditions, i.e., in the absence of drug. Stably resistant cells maintain high levels of MTX resistance and amplified DHFR genes for long periods when grown in the absence of drug. Such cells generally contain the amplified DHFR genes as stably integrated copies in the form of HSRs. In contrast, unstably resistant cells readily lose their elevated levels of DHFR enzyme and gene copies and revert to an MTX-sensitive state when grown in the absence of drug [41]. Unstably resistant cells generally contain the amplified DHFR genes on structures called DMs (Fig. 2) [41]. DMs are small, paired, extrachromosomal structures which lack centromeres. Since they segregate unequally into replicating daughter cells, they are readily lost from cell populations during subsequent mitoses in nonselective (drug-free) conditions. The mechanisms of formation of HSRs and DMs are still not well understood. HSRs and DMs do not generally coexist in drug-resistant cell lines or individual cell lines which are continuously selected for resistance in vitro. These cell lines tend to form one type of structure or the other. These findings suggest that specific cellular factors determine which type of amplified structure is formed.

Gene amplification is a general mechanism which can result in resistance to a

Table 2. Gene amplification and drug resistance

Selection	Protein overproduced	Gene amplification demonstrated
Methotrexate	Dihydrofolate reductase	+
PALA	CAD protein	+
FUDR	Thymidylate synthase	+
Deoxycoformycin	Adenosine deaminase	+
Hydroxyurea	Ribonucleotide reductase	
Dimethylfluoro-ornithine	Ornithine decarboxylase	+
Vinca alkaloids	170 000-dalton glycoprotein	+
Actinomycin D	150 000-dalton glycoprotein	+
	19 000-dalton glycoprotein	
Compactin	Hydroxymethylglutaryl-CoA reductase	+
Methionine sulfoximine	Glutamine synthetase	+
Pyrazofurin azauridine	UMP synthetase	+

CoA, coenzyme A; UMP, uridine-5-monophosphate; PALA, N-phosphonacetyl-L-aspartic acid.

wide variety of drugs or toxins (Table 2). For example, Wahl et al. [42] demonstrated that resistance to N-phosphonacetyl-L-aspartic acid (PALA), a potent inhibitor of the second enzyme involved in the de novo synthesis of pyrimidines, was associated with the overproduction of this enzyme and the amplification of DNA sequences coding for the multifunctional protein (CAD protein or pyr 1–3) that includes the target enzyme for PALA (aspartate transcarbamylase) as well as two other enzymes involved in de novo UMP synthesis.

Cadmium resistance has also been shown to result from increased levels of metallothionein [43], a low-molecular-weight scavenger protein that is rich in sulphydryl groups, and amplification of metallothionein genes. Since this thiol-rich scavenger protein can also bind to and inactivate cis-platinum [44] and alkylating agents, cadmium-resistant cells containing increased levels of metallothionein are cross-resistant to cis-platinum [44] and chlorambucil [22].

As will be discussed below, gene amplification is also involved in the development of MDR. The P170 glycoprotein DNA sequences (also referred to as mdr) are amplified and overexpressed in many if not all multidrug-resistant hamster and human cell lines [45–51].

While gene amplification is a common mechanism of resistance in vitro, its role in clinical resistance is not well defined. Studies by Curt et al. [52] demonstrated that a small-cell lung cancer cell line established from a patient who relapsed after MTX therapy was resistant to MTX in vitro. Resistance in this cell line was associated with increased levels of DHFR enzyme and amplified DHFR gene sequences present in the form of DMs. These DMs were lost from the cell population during subsequent passage in drug-free medium for 6 months. At this time, the cells reverted to an MTX-sensitive phenotype and no longer contained increased levels of DHFR enzyme or increased DHFR gene copies. This case was the first example of gene amplification in clinical drug resistance.

Other investigators have also found that DHFR gene amplification occurs

199

clinically. Trent et al. [53] studied cells from a patient who was treated for psoriasis with MTX and later developed ovarian cancer. Ovarian tumor cells obtained at the time of diagnosis were resistant to MTX in vitro and had increased copies of DHFR gene sequences demonstrated by in situ hybridization. Additional studies by Horn et al. [54] and Cardman et al. [55] have demonstrated the presence of amplified DHFR genes in patients with acute leukemia treated with MTX. Thus, resistance to MTX in vivo can clearly involve DHFR gene amplification and is similar to resistance in vitro.

Multidrug or Pleiotropic Drug Resistance

As alluded to previously, amplification of gene sequences is also associated with the development of a resistant phenotype commonly referred to as pleiotropic resistance or MDR. Indeed, cell lines with the phenotype of MDR have been the focus of research for a number of laboratories. These studies have provided unique insight into some of the basic mechanisms of drug resistance. As alluded to earlier, cells with MDR are generally selected for resistance to a single agent, such as an anthracycline, a vinca alkaloid, an epipodophyllotoxin, or actinomycin D. Although selected for resistance to a single agent, these cells commonly, if not invariably, develop cross-resistance to other agents to which they have not been exposed. Since these agents vary widely in their structure, membrane transport, and site of action, it was at first quite perplexing that cells would simultaneously develop cross-resistance to all of these agents. Studies by Ling et al. [19] first demonstrated that multidrug-resistant cells have a defect in intracellular drug accumulation, and that this defect was associated with increases in a high-molecular-weight (130 000–170 000-daltons) membrane glycoprotein, which he referred to as P-glycoprotein.

The role of gene amplification in MDR had been suspected since many multidrug-resistant cell lines were found to contain HSRs and DMs. Using a variety of techniques several laboratories have now isolated amplified DNA sequences from multidrug-resistant hamster and human cell lines [47–51]. The complete cDNA sequence for this gene has recently been published by Gros et al. [56] and Chen et al. [57]. The gene contains two internally duplicated regions, one of which apparently codes for a transmembrane domain, the other a nucleotide (ATP?)-binding region. This gene has marked sequence homology with the genes of several bacterial transport proteins and may be part of an energy-dependent efflux pump.

Many studies indicated that the decrease in intracellular drug accumulation exhibited by multidrug-resistant cell lines was due to an increase in an energy-dependent drug efflux process. Recent experiments by Cornwell et al. [58] and Safa et al. [59] have examined the role of the P170 protein in mediating increased drug efflux. They found that a photoaffinity analog of vinblastine binds to a 170 000-dalton membrane protein which is overexpressed in multidrug-

200

resistant hamster cell lines. This binding is competed for by unlabelled vinblastine and anthracyclines. These experiments indicate that this glycoprotein recognizes antineoplastic drugs, thus supporting the role of P170 as part of a putative drug efflux pump.

The dominant genetic nature of the multidrug-resistant phenotype is suggested by studies in which transfection of the DNA from resistant CHO cells into drug-sensitive cells results in the transfer of drug resistance and an increase in the expression of P-glycoprotein in the recipient cells [60]. Moreover, transfection of mdr-1 cDNA, a gene encoding a P170 protein, was able to confer MDR on sensitive cells. While the role of this gene in multidrug-resistant cell lines is well established, there is evidence which suggests that overexpression of P170 may not be the only mechanism responsible for MDR. Each multidrug-resistant cell lines exhibits a different pattern of cross-resistance. Thus, either each cell line expresses different P170 proteins, or alternatively, there are other biochemical and genetic changes associated with MDR in addition to P170 overexpression. The latter hypothesis is supported by the finding that decreased drug transport and resistance do not correlate in all cell lines [61–63]. Moreover, studies by Sirotnak et al. [62] and Siegfried et al. [63] have shown that MDR in one cell line cannot be completely overcome by raising the intracellular drug concentration to equal that obtained in drug-sensitive cells. Both of these findings suggest that other mechanisms besides decreased drug accumulation are involved in MDR. Although other mechanisms have yet to be identified, laboratories have reported increases in various cytosolic proteins in multidrug-resistant cells [64–69]. Whether any of these proteins play a role in MDR is as yet unclear.

Associations Between MDR and a Chemical Carcinogenesis Model

Although the role of P170 in MDR has been established, the preceding discussion suggests that other mechanisms for MDR exist. Indeed, recent studies have indicated that MDR may involve biochemical changes in drug detoxification pathways. Remarkable similarity exists among the biochemical changes found in multidrug-resistant human breast cancer cells and in an in vivo model system of resistance which develops in response to chronic carcinogen exposure.

In the early 1970s, Farber [70–71] first developed a rat model for chemical carcinogenesis. In this model, animals are exposed to a carcinogen for 2–3 weeks. Subsequent to induction, liver cell proliferation is induced by partial hepatectomy. In the weeks that follow, hyperplastic liver nodules (HNs) appear, most of which spontaneously regress over a period of weeks to months. A few of the HNs progress to frank hepatocellular carcinoma. One interesting feature of these HNs is that they develop resistance to carcinogen-induced cytotoxicity. Furthermore, treatment with any one of a wide variety of structurally diverse carcinogens can produce the same morphologic and biochemical changes. In

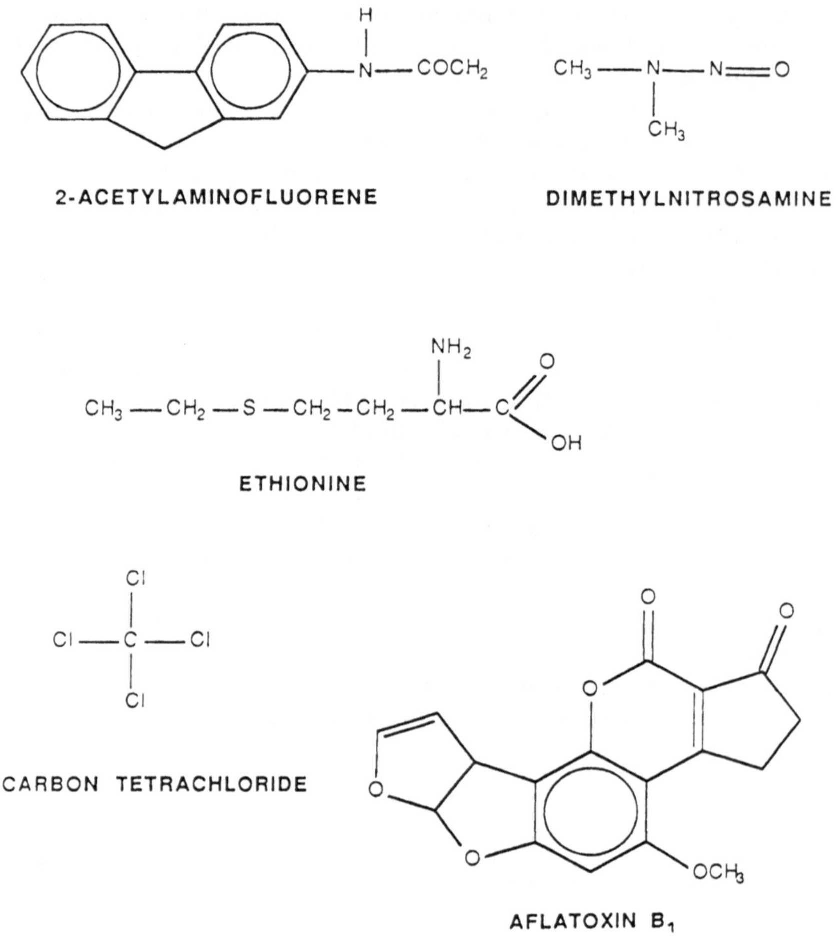

2-ACETYLAMINOFLUORENE

DIMETHYLNITROSAMINE

ETHIONINE

CARBON TETRACHLORIDE

AFLATOXIN B₁

Fig. 3. The structures of a diverse group of toxins and carcinogens associated with both resistance and cross-resistance in the rat hyperplastic nodules of the Solt-Farber model

each instance, regardless of the selecting agents, the HNs apparently develop cross-resistance to a wide range of toxic foreign compounds that differ in structure and mechanism of action (Fig. 3); in this the HNs resemble the tumor cells selected for MDR.

Resistance to carcinogens and xenobiotics can occur in a number of ways in liver cells. As shown in Table 3, resistance to a wide range of structurally unrelated agents in HNs is associated with a number of changes. Farber et al. [71] showed that resistance in HNs is associated with a decrease in 2-acetylaminofluorine (AAF) accumulation and a decrease in AAF binding to DNA. Moreover, studies by a number of groups have shown that xenobiotic resistance (XR) in HNs is also associated with specific changes in phase I and

Table 3. Comparison of biochemical changes in multidrug-resistant breast cancer cells and in xenobiotic-resistant rat hepatocytes

Biochemical change	Carcinogen resistance in rat HNs	Multidrug resistance in MCF-7 cells
↓ Toxin uptake	Yes	Yes
↑ P170 (*mdr*)	Yes	Yes
↓ P450 isozymes	Yes	Yes—aryl hydrocarbon hydroxylase
↑ Anionic glutathione transferase	Yes	Yes
↑ Pentose phosphate pathway activity	Yes	Yes
↑ UDP-glucuronyl transferase I	Yes	Yes
↑ Glutathione	Yes	No change
↑ γ-Glutamyltransferase	Yes	No change
↓ Sulfotransferase	Yes	No (increased twofold)
↑ Epoxide hydrolase	Yes	NT
↑ DT-diaphorase (quinone reductase)	Yes	Yes

↓, decreased; ↑, increased; NT, not tested; HN, hyperplastic nodule; UDP, uridine diphosphate

phase II drug-detoxifying enzymes. These changes are summarized in Table 3.

Overall there is a marked decrease in phase I drug-metabolizing enzyme activities. This includes both a decrease in total cytochrome P450 and decreases in several P450-dependent enzymes, including aryl hydrocarbon hydroxylase (AHH), aminopyrine-N-demethylase, and cytochrome b_5 [72]. This down-regulation of the phase I enzymes in rat HNs is important since these activities convert carcinogens such as benzo[a]pyrene to more potent hydroxylated species. In addition to these diverse changes in phase I enzymes, increased levels of several phase II drug-metabolizing enzymes have been noted, including uridine diphosphate (UDP)-glucuronyl transferase, glutathione S-transferase (GST), and sulfotransferases [70, 73, 74]. Glutathione (GSH) and γ-glutamyl-transferase are both increased [70]. These enzyme activities detoxify carcinogens such as benzo[a]pyrene by conjugation with polar moieties [75]. All these biochemical changes taken together provide the cell with the capacity to resist a wide variety of toxic substances.

Recent studies have shown that marked similarities exist between multidrug-resistant human breast cancer cells and xenobiotic-resistant rat hepatic HNs [76]. Although AHH is readily inducible by polycyclic hydrocarbons in the drug-sensitive wild-type (WT) MCF-7 cells, this enzyme activity is neither expressed nor inducible in the multidrug-resistant MCF-7 subline. Furthermore, expression of several drug-conjugating enzymes is increased in cells selected for MDR; in particular, an anionic GST [77, 78] is induced in the multidrug-resistant cells. Indeed, the anionic GST induced in multidrug-resistant MCF-7 cells is immuno-logically and biochemically related to the GST isozyme induced in rat HNs [77, 78].

Table 4. Modulation of drug resistance

Drugs	Antineoplastic drugs affected	Proposed mechanism of increased cytotoxicity

Calcium antagonists
  Verapamil
  Nifedipine
  Nitrendipine
  Caroverine
	VCR, DNR, DOX	Increased accumulation by blocking drug efflux

Calmodulin inhibitors
  Prenylamine
  Trifluoroperazine
  Clomipramine
	VCR, DNR, DOX	Increased accumulation by blocking drug efflux

W-13	BLEO	Inhibition of DNA repair
Amphotericin	DOX, ACTD, BCNU	Altered lipid composition of
Polysorbate 80 (Tween 80)	DOX	plasma membrane leading to
Perhexiline maleate	DOX	increased accumulation
Triparanol analogs Tamoxifen	DOX	Increased drug accumulation
Antiarrhythmics Quinidine	DOX, VCR	Increased drug accumulation
Antihypertensives Reserpine	DOX	Increased drug accumulation

Thiol depleters
  Buthionine
    sulfoximine
	LPAM, PLAT, DOX	Drug inactivation, free radical metabolism, protection/repair of DNA

VCR, vincristine; DNR, daunorubicin; DOX, doxorubicin; BLEO, bleomycin; LPAM, melphalan; PLAT, *cis*-platinum; ACTD, actinomycin D; BCNU, bis-chloroethyl nitrosourea

These initial findings prompted a more thorough comparison of the biochemical changes associated with XR in rat HNs and with MDR in MCF-7 cells. These studies have been recently reviewed [79, 80] and are shown in Table 4. Resistance in both systems is manifested by decreased toxin accumulation, increased *mdr* (P-glycoprotein) gene expression [81], decreased activity of phase I enzymes (including AHH), increased phase II conjugating enzymes (including anionic GST and UDP-glucuronyl transferase I), increased pentose phosphate shunt pathway activity [to maintain diminished levels of nicotinamide-adenine dinucleotide phosphate (NADPH)], and changes in several other drug-metabolizing enzymes (e.g., DT-diaphorase).

These similarities suggest that chronic carcinogen exposure may result in a coordinated set of responses which ultimately result in protection of the cell from the toxic effects of carcinogens. These same responses may also protect the tumor cell which ultimately emerges from the cytotoxic effects of antineoplastic agents. Perhaps this is why tumors associated with increased carinogen exposure, such as colon and nonsmall-cell lung cancer, are intrinsically resistant to chemotherapy. If so, then understanding the biochemical changes involved in specific mechanisms of resistance to antineoplastic drugs may offer insights into therapies which modulate or circumvent cellular resistance.

Reversal of Drug Resistance

By understanding the molecular mechanism associated with the development of resistance to antineoplastic agents, one could either decrease the frequency of resistance or design therapies which could bypass the resistant mechanism or take advantage of the selective biochemical changes associated with resistance. For example, it is now clear that gene amplification is associated with the development of drug resistance in vivo as well as in vitro. It is important to consider treatments that would reduce the frequency of gene amplification. In vitro studies have identified a variety of factors that can influence the frequency of gene amplification, including treatment with phorbol ester [82], ultraviolet irradiation [83], hydroxyurea [84], and N-acetoxy-N-acetylaminofluorene [83]. These factors appear to act by causing unscheduled rounds of DNA synthesis, resulting in the synthesis of extra copies of specific gene sequences. Other studies by Barsoum and Varshavsky [85] have demonstrated that the addition of growth factors and hormones such as insulin, vasopressin, and epidermal growth factor also affects the frequency of DHFR gene amplification. These studies have shown that a variety of factors can increase the frequency of gene amplification in vitro. These include agents that stimulate cell growth as well as agents that inhibit DNA synthesis. On the other hand, studies have also shown that treatment of cells containing amplified DHFR genes on DMs with hydroxyurea enhances the loss of these amplified genes from cells [86]. Thus, it appears that there are agents which may increase the frequency of gene amplification and agents that may hasten the loss of amplified sequences. Understanding the mechanisms involved in gene amplification may provide insights into therapies aimed at decreasing the development of this phenomenon.

Pharmacologic Modulation of Drug Resistance

Understanding the molecular mechanisms of MDR has improved the prospects for the development of agents that may modulate this resistance. The circumvention of MDR by modulating the accumulation of cytotoxic agents is of particular interest. Some drugs that do not themselves possess any antitumor activity have been shown to potentiate the cytotoxic effects of anticancer drugs in multidrug-resistant cells (Table 4). The calcium antagonists, calmodulin inhibitors, polyene antibiotics, triparanol analogs, and antiarrhythmic agents exert their effect, at least in part, by increasing the net accumulation of antineoplastic drugs in relatively resistant tumor cells.

Calcium antagonists are one of the newest groups of drugs that are capable of reversing drug resistance in experimental tumor systems. Tsuruo et al. [87] demonstrated in 1981 that both in vitro and in vivo resistance to vincristine in P388 leukemia was reversed with verapamil. The combination of vincristine and verapamil improved survival in mice inoculated with a vincristine-resistant P388 leukemia, while cellular accumulation of vincristine was increased by exposure of the drug-resistant cells to verapamil. Alterations in vincristine binding to tubulin were not observed.

Subsequent studies have demonstrated that the cytotoxicities of other antineoplastic drugs may be enhanced by calcium channel blockers. In studies with P388 leukemia and Ehrlich ascites cells, verapamil produced marked potentiation of daunorubicin and doxorubicin (Adriamycin) cytotoxicity [88]. Slater et al. [88] noted that the survival of mice with a daunorubicin-resistant Ehrlich ascites tumor was increased from 22 to 44 days when verapamil was administered together with daunorubicin.

Although verapamil does block calcium channels, the role of calcium in the expression of pleiotropic drug resistance and the importance of alterations in calcium fluxes in the reversal of resistance are still not clear. Tsuruo initially postulated that verapamil reversed drug resistance by inhibition of a calcium-dependent drug efflux system [87]. However, Kessel [89] was unable to demonstrate alterations in ^{45}Ca fluxes in P388 drug-sensitive and drug-resistant cells following treatment with either verapamil or nitrendipine [89]. In addition, the elimination of calcium from the media did not affect anthracycline transport.

However, other studies did demonstrate that verapamil efflux was more rapid in the drug-resistant cell line. These results suggested that verapamil may be competing for the same outward transport system as P170 and may be responsible for the decreased accumulation of anthracyclines in doxorubicin-resistant P388 cells. Indeed, using membrane vesicles from sensitive, resistant, and revertant KB cells, Cornwell et al. [90] found that vesicles from resistant cells (containing increased levels of P170) bound eightfold more [^{3}H]vinblastine than sensitive cell vesicles. The binding of [^{3}H]vinblastine was inhibited by vinblastine, vincristine, daunomycin, verapamil, nifedipine, and quinidine, but it was not affected by dexamethasone, colchicine, and actinomycin D. Thus, this assay may prove useful for screening agents that may reverse binding to or inhibition of P170 function.

Clinical Approaches to MDR

The clinical approaches to MDR are as diverse as the problem. How can gene amplification be modulated or avoided in a clinical setting? Does combination chemotherapy affect gene amplification? Can bone marrow cells be made more resistant to the cytotoxic effects of chemotherapy which limit treatment? Are agents such as verapamil useful in reversing drug resistance?

The clincial usefulness of verapamil in the reversal of MDR may depend on the plasma levels that can be achieved. Most in vitro studies with murine leukemia have shown a dependence on the concentration of the calcium channel

206

blocker and used verapamil concentrations of 1–3 μg/ml [91]. These levels are substantially higher than the peak plasma levels of verapamil (400–500 ng/ml) that have been achieved following daily doses of verapamil in cardiac patients [92]. Following a single intravenous dose, verapamil plasma levels decrease in a biexponential manner, with an initial half-life of 18–35 min. Verapamil is rapidly metabolized in the liver, with only 15% of the drug remaining unchanged in the body 1–2 h after administration [92, 93]. The maximally tolerated level of verapamil and the safe duration of infusions that can be maintained in cancer patients have yet to be determined. The major toxic effects of verapamil are hypotension, bradycardia, and congestive heart failure; these effects are usually reversed by stopping the infusion. Occasionally, the cardiac toxicities require treatment with atropine, calcium gluconate, or vasopressors. Adverse side effects are more likely to occur in patients with either poor left ventricular function, sick sinus syndrome, or atrioventricular conduction delay [93].

The use of intravenously administered verapamil in cancer patients has been studied in a phase I pharmacokinetic study of vinblastine and verapamil. In this study, verapamil was administered as a loading dose (0.02–0.1 mg/kg), followed by a maintenance infusion (0.036–0.18 mg kg $^{-1}$h^{-1}) for 5 days, with continuous cardiac monitoring [94]. Junctional cardiac arrhythmias and increased P-R interval were the dose-limiting toxicities observed in this trial. Verapamil levels of 70–200 ng/ml were achieved using this schedule.

In a trial in the National Cancer Institute (NCI) Medicine Branch [95], refractory ovarian cancer patients are being treated with a combination of verapamil and doxorubicin. Pharmacokinetic and toxicity data revealed plasma levels in the range of 2000–4000 ng/ml, higher than previously reported without dose escalation. The levels of verapamil achieved with this intensive schedule are comparable to the concentrations of verapamil that produced a dose-modifying factor of 1.5–4.3 in human ovarian cancer cell lines established from drug-refractory patients in vitro [96]. In this study, the high levels of verapamil achieved do not appear to increase the acute noncardiac toxicity of doxorubicin. Myelosuppression and gastrointestinal toxicity were similar to that reported with doxorubicin alone in this patient population [95]. However, the dose escalation on day 1 of verapamil produced significant acute cardiac toxicity. Three of the six patients developed second-degree heart block or hypotension. Two patients also had increased pulmonary capillary wedge pressure.

The use of verapamil in combination with antineoplastic agents must be carefully evaluated. In particular, the effect of verapamil on the incidence and severity of doxorubicin-induced cardiomyopathy has not yet been established. This is important since verapamil administration increased the cardiotoxic doses doxorubicin [97]. In another study done in Swiss mice, although doxorubicin cardiomyopathy was not potentiated by verapamil, nifedipine was found to exert a synergistic effect on doxorubicin cardiac toxicity [98]. Thus, the effect of calcium channel blockers on doxorubicin cardiotoxicity in patients will need to be established by careful serial cardiac evaluation during clinical trials. Verapamil may prove to be more useful in combination with agents such as vinblastine, which does not cause cardiac toxicity.

Other Drugs that Reverse Drug Resistance

Recent experimental studies suggest that pharmacologic manipulation of drug resistance is not limited to agents that alter drug accumulation in resistant cells. In fact, elevated cellular GSH levels are present in some drug-resistant lines [21]. Agents that lower GSH levels both in vivo and in vitro are being examined as potential modulators of drug resistance.

GSH, a tripeptide thiol found in all animal cells, plays a critical role in a variety of cellular functions, including drug metabolism, amino acid transport, and protection from toxic metabolites. This latter function may account for the correlation between GSH levels and the cytotoxicity of some anticancer agents. GSH may decrease the cytotoxicity of some drugs by increasing their metabolism to less active compounds or by detoxification of any drug-induced free radical species. Increased metabolism to less active compounds is catalyzed by GSTs.

Free radical detoxification occurs through the oxidation-reduction cycle of GSH and the enzymes glutathione reductase, glutathione peroxidase, and superoxide dismutase. The role of free radicals in the cytotoxicity of doxorubicin remains controversial, although free radical-induced damage is clearly a mechanism of anthracycline-induced cardiac damage. Similarly, intracellular thiols are also thought to be involved in modulating the effects of radiation by detoxification of free radicals generated by irradiation. Indeed, agents that lower levels of intracellular GSH have been shown to increase radiation sensitivity [99–101] and doxorubicin toxicity [102].

In addition to drug detoxification, GSH may also modulate the efficacy of antineoplastic drugs or irradiation by facilitating the repair of drug- or irradiation-induced damage to DNA. Human lymphoid cells in tissue culture can be protected from the effects of radiation by the addition of glutathione monoethyl ester to the medium [103]. The mechanism of this protection is not known. Since some protection can be observed even when glutathione ester is given after irradiation, the mechanism may include the enhanced repair of DNA damage.

A variety of agents have been used to decrease GSH levels, e.g., the oxidizing agent diethylmaleate. Until recently, the lack of specificity, accompanying toxicity, and the rapid resynthesis of GSH after removal of these agents have limited any potential clinical application. Depletion of GSH by selective inhibition of the enzymes involved in GSH synthesis may prove to be more clinically appropriate [104]. Buthionine sulfoximine (BSO) is a synthetic amino acid that inhibits the enzyme γ-glutamylcysteine synthetase and leads to a marked reduction in cellular GSH levels. While animal toxicity studies with BSO are limited, preliminary whole-animal toxicology indicates that mice can tolerate transient depletion of GSH in the kidney, liver, and plasma [104]. On the basis of these earlier results showing that alkylating agent resistance was accompanied by increased GSH levels, Suzukake et al. [105] studied the effect of BSO on the cytotoxicity of LPAM in LPAM-sensitive and -resistant L1210 leukemia. They found that BSO at nontoxic concentrations (50 μM) reduced the GSH level by

50% and completely restored sensitivity to LPAM in an LPAM-resistant L1210 cell line.

The levels of GSH in human ovarian cancer cell lines and the effect of BSO upon LPAM cytotoxicity have also been examined [106]. Compared with cell lines established from previously untreated patients, GSH levels were elevated two- to threefold in cell lines established from patients refractory to alkylating agent-containing combination chemotherapy regimens. In addition, an LPAM-resistant variant cell line, 1847ME, developed in vitro, was also found to have a twofold elevation in GSH content relative to its parental drug-sensitive cell line. Incubation of the tumor cells with BSO at doses that are nontoxic to tumor cells decreased GSH levels to 20% of the control value and increased the cytotoxicity of LPAM in both parental and LPAM-resistant cell lines. Although GSH may play a role in the protection of cells from alkylators such as LPAM, the mechanism of this protection is not clear.

The effect of BSO-mediated depletion of GSH on the cytotoxicity of antineoplastic drugs to normal tissues may determine the potential clinical relevance of such an approach. Since GSH depletion will likely potentiate the cardiac toxicity of anthracyclines, such a combination of doxorubicin plus BSO would not appear to be clinically useful. However, preliminary observations in mice and in human bone marrow cells suggest that BSO may selectively potentiate the toxicity of LPAM in tumor cells compared with normal tissues, although the reasons for any difference are unclear. The "rescue" of GSH depletion may be possible in normal tissues by the administration of compounds such as glutathione ester, which, in contrast to GSH, is rapidly transported and hydrolyzed intracellularly. Indeed, glutathione ester has been used to partially protect against the lethal effects of irradiation even when administered after irradiation of human lymphoid cells [107]. Any clinical trial of BSO in combination with alkylating agents or cis-platinum must await the completion of animal toxicology studies and additional pharmacologic studies in the appropriate experimental systems.

Genetic Approaches to Resistance

Advances in molecular biology have opened the way for new approaches to the treatment of drug-resistant tumors. Since myelosuppression is one of the limiting toxicities of many cytotoxic agents, insertion of drug resistance genes into bone marrow stem cells may permit the safe use of higher doses of systemic chemotherapy. Cline et al. [108] demonstrated the feasibility of this approach using a gene coding for an altered DHFR that had a reduced affinity for MTX. Following DNA-mediated transfection into mouse bone marrow cells, the recipient cells were able to render an irradiated animal less sensitive to MTX. Using improved techniques, Carr et al. [109] have demonstrated similar findings. Despite technical improvements, this approach is limited by the relatively poor efficiency of transfer of DNA into the marrow cells using standard techniques.

However, recent advances now permit the efficient transfer of genes into bone marrow cells using defective retroviral vectors [110]. The use of such vectors should make it practical to consider the transfer of drug resistance genes, such as an altered DHFR gene [111, 112], into pluripotent marrow stem cells. As progress is made regarding retrovirus receptors, it may prove possible to genetically engineer vectors that are able to penetrate specific populations of bone marrow cells, or alternatively to specifically infect tumor cells.

In particular, the use of self-inactivating (SIN) retroviral vectors may prove useful. These vectors provide a potentially effective clinical means to introduce drug resistance genes into stem cells [113]. SIN vectors lack enhancer and promoter functions in their long terminal repeats (LTRs), which should minimize the possibility of activating cellular oncogenes. When viruses derived from SIN vectors are used for infection, transcriptional inactivation of the provirus in the infected cell occurs. These vectors may provide major advantages for safer gene therapy. While the use of these vectors in the treatment of inborn errors of metabolism is being anticipated, it is also possible that such vectors will ultimately have a role in the treatment of cancer. Although the use of retroviral vectors or inducible antisense constructs for drug resistance genes is not at the level of clinical testing, the advances in recombinant DNA technology have made them realistic considerations.

Conclusions

The phenomenon of drug resistance is as diverse as the agents which are implicated in its cause. Drug resistance is mediated in a number of ways, including defective carrier transport, increased cellular activity of drug-metabolizing enzymes, increased drug efflux, altered drug accumulation, increased inactivation by conjugation, altered receptors, altered cofactor levels, altered cellular repair mechanisms, and increased or altered levels of target proteins. Although the diversity of mechanisms is striking, unique systems of multidrug-resistant cell lines exist which share common features. These cell lines exhibit decreased drug accumulation, increased drug efflux, gene amplification, unique patterns of cross-resistance to many agents which the cells have not been treated with, and expression of a 170 000-dalton membrane glycoprotein with sequence homology to bacterial membrane transport proteins.

Drug resistance is a major clinical problem. Its intricacies are just starting to be dissected. In the future, both pharmacologic and genetic approaches to overcome drug resistance may prove useful.

References

1. DeVita VT Jr (1982) Principles of chemotherapy. In: DeVita VT Jr, Hellman S, Rosenberg SA (eds) Cancer: principles and practice of oncology. JB Lippincott, Philadelphia, pp 132–155
2. Adams DJ, Carmichael J, Wolf CR (1985) Altered mouse bone marrow glutathione and glutathione transferase levels in response to cytotoxins. Cancer Res 45: 1669–1673
3. Zimm S, Collins JM, Riccard R, O'Neill D, Narang PK, Chabner BA, Poplack DG (1983) Variable bioavailability of oral mercaptopurine: In maintenance chemotherapy in acute lymphoblastic leukemia being optimally delivered. N Engl J Med 308: 1005–1009
4. Tattersall MHN, Weinberg A (1978) Pharmacokinetics of melphalan following oral or intravenous administration in patients with malignant disease. Eur J Cancer 14: 502–509
5. Alberts DS, Chang SY, Chen H-SG et al. (1980) Comparative pharmacokinetics of chlorambucil and melphalan in man. Recent Results Cancer Res 74: 124–130
6. D'Incalci M, Bolis G, Mangioni C et al. (1978) Variable absorption of hexamethylamine in man. Cancer Treat Rep 62: 2117–2119
7. Goldie JH, Coldman AJ (1979) A mathematical model formulating the drug sensitivity of tumors to their spontaneous mutation rate. Cancer Treat Rep 63: 1727–1733
8. Luria SE, Delbruck M, (1943) Mutations of bacteria from virus sensitivity to virus resistance. Genetics 28: 491–511
9. Bech-Hanson NT, Till JE, Ling V (1976) Pleiotropic phenotype of colchicine-resistant CHO cells: Cross resistance and collateral sensitivity. J Cell Physiol 88: 22–23
10. Kessel D, Hall TC, Roberts D (1965) Uptake as a determinant of methotrexate response in mouse leukemia. Science 150: 752–754
11. Harrap KR, Hill BT, Furness ME et al. (1971) Sites of action of amethopterin: intrinsic and acquired drug resistance. Ann NY Acad Sci 186: 312–324
12. Hill BT, Bailey BD, White JC et al. (1979) Characteristics of transport of 4-amino folates and folate compounds of two lines of LY178Y lymphosblasts, one with impaired transport of methotrexate. Cancer Res 39: 2440–2446
13. Ohnoshi T, Ohnuma T, Takehasi I et al. (1982) Establishment of methotrexate-resistant human acute lymphoblastic leukemia cell in culture and effects of folate antagonists. Cancer Res 42: 1655–1660
14. Sirotnak FM, Moccio DM, Kelleher LE et al. (1981) Relative frequency and kinetic properties of transport defective phenotypes among methotrexate-resistant L1210 clonal cell lines derived in vivo. Cancer Res 14, 4447–4452
15. Redwood WR, Colvin M (1980) Transport of melphalan by sensitive and resistant L1210 cells. Cancer Res 40: 1144–1149
16. Goldenberg GJ, Vanstom CL, Israels LG et al. (1970) Evidence for transport carrier of nitrogen mustard in nitrogen mustard-sensitive and -resistant L5178Y lymphoblasts. Cancer Res 30: 2285–2291
17. Dano K (1973) Active outward transport of daunomycin in resistant Ehrlich ascites tumor cells. Biochim Biophys Acta 323: 466–473
18. Skovsgaard T (1978) Mechanism of cross resistance between vincristine and daunorubicin in Ehrlich ascites tumor cells. Cancer Res 38: 4622–4727
19. Juliano RL, Ling V (1976) A surface glycoprotein modulating drug permeability in Chinese hamster ovary cell mutants. Biochims Biophys Acta. 455: 152–162
20. Cowan KH, Jolivet J (1984) A methotrexate-resistant human breast cancer cell line with multiple defects, including diminished formation of methotrexate polyglutamates. J Biol Chem 259: 10793–10800
21. Suzukake K, Vistica BP, Vistica DT (1983) Dechlorination of L-phenylalanine mustard by sensitive and resistant tumor cells and its relationship to intracellular glutathione content. Biochem Pharmacol 32: 165–167
22. Endreson L, Bakka A, Rugstad HE (1983) Increased resistance to chlorambucil in cultured cells with a high concentration of cytoplasmic metallothionein. Cancer Res 43: 2918–2926

23. Sibley CH, Thompkins GM (1974) Mechanisms of steroid resistance. Cell 2: 221–227
24. Nawata H, Bronzert D, Lippman ME (1983) Isolation and characterization of a tamoxifen-resistant cell line derived form MCF-7 human breast cancer cells. J Biol Chem 256: 5016–05021
25. Ling V, Aubin JE, Chase A et al. (1979) Mutants of Chinese hamster ovary (CHO) cells with altered colcemid-binding affinity. Cell 18: 423–430
26. Cabral F, Sobel ME, Gottesman MM (1980) CHO mutants resistant to colchicine, colcemid or griseofulvin have altered beta-tubulin. Cell 20: 29–36
27. Keates RAB, Sarangi F, Ling V (1981) Structural and functional alteration in microtubule protein from Chinese hamster ovary cell mutants. Proc Natl Acad Sci USA 78: 5638–5642
28. Heidelberger C, Kaldor G, Mukherjeek L et al. (1960) Studies on flourinated pyrimidines: XI. In vitro studies on tumor resistance. Cancer Res 20: 903–909
29. Pommier Y, Schwartz RE, Zwelling LA et al. (1986) Reduced formation of protein associated DNA strand breaks in Chinese hamster cells resistant to Topoisomerase II inhibitors. Cancer Res 46: 611–616
30. Pommier Y, Kerrigan D, Schwartz RE et al. (1986) Altered DNA Toposiomerase II activity in Chinese hamster cells resistant to Toposiomerase II inhibitors. Cancer Res 46: 3075–3081
31. Kimiko I, Sartorelli AC (1984) Altered 5-phosphoribosyl 1-pyrophosphate amidotransferase activity in 6-thioguanine resistant HL60 promyelocytic leukemia cells. Cancer Res 44: 3679–3685
32. Houghton JA, Maroda SJ, Phillips JO et al. (1982) Biochemical determinants of responsiveness to 5-fluorouracil and its derivatives in xenografts of human colorectal adenocarcinomas in mice. Cancer Res 42: 144–149
33. Bruckner HW, Rustum YM (eds) (1984) Proceedings of a symposium on the current status of 5-fluorouracil-leucovorin calcium combination. Advances in cancer chemotherapy. NY
34. Crawthorne AR, Roberts JJ (1966) Mechanisms of the cytotoxic action of alkylating agents in mammalian cells and evidence for the removal of alkylated groups from deoxyribonucleic acid. Nature 211: 150–153
35. Parsons PG, Smellie SG, Manson LE et al. (1982) Properties of human melanoma cells resistant to 5- (3', 3'-dimethyl-1-trazeno) imidazole-4-carboxamide and other methylating agents. Cancer Res 42: 1454–1461
36. Carr FJ, Fox BW (1981) DNA strand breaks and repair synthesis in Yoshida sarcoma cells with differential sensitivities to bifunctional alkylating agents and UV light. Mutat Res 83: 233–249
37. Bedford P, Fox BW (1982) Repair of DNA interstrand cross links after busulphan. A possible mode of resistance. Cancer Chemother Pharmacol 8: 3–7
38. Alt FW, Keller RE, Bertino JR, Schimke RT (1978) Multiplication of dihydrofolate reductase genes in methotrexate-resistant variants of cultured murine cells. J Biol Chem 253: 1357–1370
39. Biedler JL, Spengler BA (1976) Metaphase chromosome anomaly: association with drug resistance and cell specific products. Science 191: 185–187
40. Nuberg JH, Kaufman RJ, Schimke RT, Urlaub, Chasin L, (1978) Amplified dihydrofolate reductase genes are localized to a homogeneously staining region of a single chromosome in a methotrexate-resistant Chinese hamster ovary cell line. Proc Natl Acad Sci USA 75: 5553–5556
41. Brown PC, Beverly SM, Schimke RT (1981) Relationship of amplified dihydrofolate reductase genes to double minute chromosomes in unstably resistant cell lines. Mol Cell Biol 1: 1077–1083
42. Wahl GM, Padgett RA, Stark GR (1979) Gene amplification causes overproduction of the first three enzymes of UMP synthesis in N-(phosphoracetyl)-L-aspartate-resistant hamster cells. J Biol Chem 254: 8679–8689
43. Beach LR, Palmiter RD (1981) Amplification of the metallothionein-1 gene in cadmium-resistant mouse cells. Proc Natl Acad Sci USA 78: 2110–2114
44. Bakka A, Endresen L, Johnson ABS et al. (1981) Resistance against cis-dichlorodiammine-platinum in cultured cells with a high content of metallothionein. Toxicol Appl Pharmacol 61: 215–226
45. Riordan JR, Deuchars K, Kartner N, Alon N, Trent J, Ling V (1985) Amplification of P-glycoprotein genes in multidrug resistant cell lines by monoclonal antibodies. Nature 316: 817–819

46. Roninson IB (1983) Detection and mapping homologous, repeated, amplified DNA sequences by DNA renaturation in agarose gels. Nucleic Acid Res 11: 5413–5431
47. Gros P, Croop J, Roninson I et al. (1986) Isolation and characterization of DNA sequences amplified in multidrug-resistant hamster cells. Proc Natl Acad Sci USA 83: 337–341
48. Fojo AT, Whang-Peng J, Gottesman MM et al. (1985) Amplification of DNA sequences in human multidrug-resistant KB carcinoma cells. Proc Natl Acad Sci USA 82: 7661–7665
49. Scotto KW, Biedler JL, Melera PW (1986) Amplification and expression of genes associated with multidrug resistance in mammalian cells. Science 232: 751–755
50. Van der Bliek AM, Van der Velde-Koerts T, Ling V et al. (1986) The overexpression and amplification of five genes in a multidrug-resistant Chinese hamster ovary cell line. Mol Cell Biol 6:1671–1678
51. Fairchild CR, Ivy SP, Kao-Shan C-S, Whang-Peng J, Rosen N, Israel MA, Melera PW, Cowan KH, Goldsmith ME (1987) Isolation of amplified DNA sequences associated with pleiotropic drug resistance from human breast cancer cells. Cancer Res 47: 5141–5148
52. Curt GA, Carney DM, Cowan KH, Jolivet J, Bailey BD, Drake JC, Kao-Shan CW, Minna JD, Chabner BA (1983) Unstable methotrexate resistance in human small cell carcinoma associated with double minute chromosomes. N Engl J Med 308: 199–202
53. Trent JM, Buick RM, Olson S, Horns DC, Schimke RT (1984) Cytologic support for gene amplification in methotrexate-resistant cells obtained from a patient with ovarian adenocarcinoma. J Clin Oncol 2: 8–15
54. Horns RC, Dower WJ, Schimke RT (1984) Gene amplification in a leukemic patient treated with methotrexate. J Clin Oncol 2: 1–7
55. Cardman MD, Schornagel JH, Rivest RS, Srimatkandada S, Portlock CS, Duffy T, Bertino JR (1984) Resistance to methotrexate due to gene amplification in a patient with acute leukemia. J Clin Oncol 2: 16–20
56. Gros P, Croop J, Housman D (1986) Mammalian multidrug resistant gene: Complete cDNA sequence indicates strong homology to bacterial transport proteins. Cell 47: 371–380
57. Chen C-J, Chen JE, Ueda K, Clark DP, Pastan I, Gottesman MM, Roninson IB (1986) Internal duplication and homology with bacterial transport proteins in the mdr 1 (P glycoprotein) gene from multidrug resistant human cells. Cell 47: 381–389
58. Cornwell MM, Safa AR, Felsted RL et al. (1986) Membrane vesicles from multidrug-resistant human cancer cells contain a specific 150–170 kDa protein detected by photoaffinity labeling. Proc Natl Acad Sci USA 83: 3847–3850
59. Safa AR, Glover CJ, Meyers MB et al. (1986) Vinblastine photoaffinity labeling of a high molecular weight surface membrane glycoprotein specific for multidrug-resistant cells. J Biol Chem 261: 6137–6140
60. Gros P, Neriah YB, Croop JM et al. (1986) Isolation and expression of the complementary DNA that confers multidrug resistance. Nature 323: 728–731
61. Kessel D, Corbett T (1985) Correlation between anthracycline resistance, drug accumulation and membrane glycoprotein patterns in solid tumors of mice. Cancer Lett 28: 187–193
62. Sirotnak FM, Yang CH, Mines LS et al. (1986) Markedly altered membrane transport and intracellular binding of vincristine in multidrug-resistant Chinese hamster cells selected for resistance to vinca alkaloids. J Cell Physiol 126: 266–274
63. Siegfried JM, Tritton TR, Sartorelli AC (1983) Comparison of anthracycline concentrations in S180 cell lines of varying sensitivity. Eur J Cancer Clin Oncol 19: 1133–1137
64. Beidler JL, Peterson HF (1981) In: Molecular actions and targets for cancer chemotherapeutic agents. Academic Press, New York, pp 453–482
65. Meyers MB, Biedler JL (1981) Increased synthesis of a low molecular weight protein in vincristine-resistant cells. Biochem Biophys Res Commun 99: 228–235
66. Peterson RHF, Biedler JL (1978) Plasma membrane proteins and glycoproteins from Chinese hamster cells sensitive and resistant to Actinomycin D. J Supramol Struct 9: 289–298
67. Beck WT (1983) Vinca alkaloid-resistant phenotype in cultured human leukemia lymphoblasts. Cancer Treat Rep 67: 875–882
68. Beck WT, Mueller TJ, Tanser LR (1979) Altered surface membrane glycoproteins in vinca alkaloid resistant human leukemia lymphoblasts. Cancer Res 39: 2070–2076

69. Peterson PHF, Meyers MB, Spengler BA, Biedler JL (1983) Alteration of plasma membrane glycopeptides and gangliosides of Chinese hamster cells accompanying development of resistance to daunorubicin and vincristine. Cancer Res 43: 222–228

70. Farber E (1984) Cellular biochemistry of the stepwise development of cancer with chemicals: GHA Clowes Memorial Lecture. Cancer Res 44: 5463–5474

71. Farber E, Parker S, Gruenstein M (1976) The resistance of putative premalignant liver cell populations, hyperplastic nodules, to the acute cytotoxic effects of some hepatocarcinogens. Cancer Res 36: 3839–3887

72. Roomi MW, Ho RK, Sarma DSR, Farber E (1985) A common biochemical pattern in preneoplastic hepatocyte nodules generated in four different models in the rat. Cancer Res 45: 564–571

73. Sato K, Kitahara A, Satoh K et al. (1984) The placental form of glutathione S-transferase as a new marker protein for pre-neoplasia in rat chemical hepatocarcinogenesis. Gann 75: 199–202

74. Kitahara A, Satoh K, Nishimura K et al. (1984) Changes in molecular forms of rat hepatic glutathione S-transferase during chemical hepatocarcinogenesis. Cancer Res 44: 2698–2703

75. Burchall B: Identification and purification of multiple forms of UDP-Glucuronyl Transferase. In: Hodgson E, Bond JR, Philpot RM (eds) Reviews in biochemical toxicology, vol 3 Elsevier/North Holland, New York, pp 1–32

76. Cowan KH, Batist G, Tupule A, Sinha BK, Myers CE (1986) Similar biochemical changes associated with multidrug resistance in human breast cancer cells and carcinogen induced resistance to xenobiotics in rats. Proc Natl Acad Sci USA 83: 9328–9332

77. Batist G, Tupule A, Sinha BK et al. (1986) Overexpression of a novel anionic glutathione transferase in multidrug-resistant human breast cancer cells. J Biol Chem 261: 15544–15549

78. Batist G, deMuys J-M, Cowan KH et al. (1986) Purification of a novel gluathione-S-transferase in multidrug resistant human breast cancer cells. Proc Am Assoc Cancer Res 27: 1072

79. Myers CE, Cowan KH, Sinha BK, Chabner BA (1987) The phenomenon of pleiotropic drug resistance. In: DeVita VT, Hellman S, Rosenberg SA (eds) Important advances in oncology. J.B. Lippincott, Philadelphia, pp 27–38

80. Tupule A, Batist G, Sinha BK et al. (1986) Similar biochemical changes associated with pleiotropic drug resistance in human breast cancer cells and xenobiotic resistance induced in carcinogens. Proc Am Assoc Cancer Res 27: 1076

81. Fairchild CR, Ivy SP, Rushmore T, Farber E, Cowan KH (1987) unpublished data

82. Varshavsky A (1981) Phorbol ester dramatically increases incidence of methotrexate-resistant mouse cells; possible mechanisms and relevance to tumor promotion. Cell 25: 561–572

83. Schimke RT (1984) Gene amplification, drug resistance, and cancer. Cancer Res 44: 1735–1742

84. Tlsty TD, Brown PC, Schimke RT (1982) Enhancement of methotrexate resistance and dihydrofolate reductase gene amplification by treatment of mouse 3T6 mouse cells with hydroxyurea. Mol Cell Biol 3: 1097–1107

85. Barsoum J, Varshavsky A (1983) Mitogenic hormones and tumor promoters greatly increase the incidence of colony-forming cells bearing amplified dihydrofolate reductase genes. Proc Natl Acad Sci USA 80: 5330–5334

86. Snapka RM, Varshavsky A (1983) Loss of unstably amplified dihydrofolate reductase genes from mouse cells is greatly accelerated by hydroxyurea. Proc Natl Acad Sci USA 80: 7533–7537

87. Tsuruo T, Iida H, Tsukagoshi S, Sakarai Y (1981) Overcoming of vincristine resistance in P388 leukemia in vivo and in vitro through enhanced cytotoxicity of vincristine and vinblastine by verapamil. Cancer Res 41: 1967–1972

88. Slater LM, Murray SL, Wetzel MW (1982) Verapamil restoration of daunorubicin responsiveness in daunorubicin-resistant Enrlich ascites carcinoma. J Clin Invest 70: 1131–1134

89. Kessel D, Wilberding C (1984) Mode of action of calcium antagonists which alter anthracycline resistance. Biochem Pharmacol 33: 1157–1160

90. Cornwell MM, Gottesman MM, Pastan IH (1986) Increased vinblastine binding to membrane vesicles from multidrug resistant KB cells. J Biol Chem 261: 7921–7928

91. Tsuruo T, Iida H, Kawabata H, Bukagoshi S, Sakarai Y (1984) High calcium content of pleiotropic drug resistant P388 and K562 leukemia and Chinese hamster ovary cells. Cancer Res 44: 5095–5099

92. Frishman W, Kirsten E, Klein M, Pine M, Johnson SM, Hillis LD, Packer M, Kates R (1982) Clinical relevance of verapamil plasma levels in stable angina pectoris. Am J Cardiol 50: 1180–1184

93. McGoon MD, Vlietstra RE, Holmes DR, Osborn JE (1982) The clinical use of verapamil. Mayo Clin Proc 57: 495–510

94. Benson AB III, Koeller JM, Trump DC, Egorin M, Olman E, Witte RS, Davis TE, Tormey DC (1984) A phase I study and pharmacokinetics of vinblastine (VLB) and verapamil (VPL) given by concurrent intravenous infusion. Proc Am Assoc Cancer Res 25: 162

95. Ozols RF, Rogan AM, Hamilton TC, Klecker R, Young RC (1984) Verapamil plus adriamycin in refractory ovarian cancer: Design of a clinical trial on the basis of reversal of adriamycin resistance in human ovarian cancer cell lines. Proc Am Assoc Cancer Res 25: 300

96. Rogan AM, Hamilton TC, Young RC, Klecker RW, Ozols RF (1984) Reversal of adriamycin resistance by verapamil in human ovarian cancer. Science 224: 994–996

97. Rabkin SW, Otten M, Polimeni PT (1983) Increased mortality with cardiotoxic doses of adriamycin after verapamil pretreatment despite prevention of myocardial calcium accumulation. Can J Physiol Pharmacol 61: 1050–1056

98. Klugman S, Bartoli-Klugman F, Decorti G, Silvestri F, Camerini F (1981) Adriamycin experimental cardiomyopathy in Swiss mice: Different effects of two calcium antagonistic drugs on ADM-induction of cardiomyopathy. Pharmacol Res Commun 13: 769–776

99. Biaglow JE, Varnes ME (1983) The role of thiols in cellular response to radiation and drugs. Radiat Res 95: 437–455

100. Biaglow JE, Clark ER, Morsequadio MM, Varnes ME, Mitchell JB (1983) Non protein thiols and the radiation response of A549 human lung carcinoma cells. Int J Radiat Biol 44: 489–495

101. Bump EA, Yu NY, Brown MJ (1982) Radiosensitization of hypoxic tumor cells by depletion of intracellular glutathione. Science 217: 544–545

102. Russo A, Mitchell JB (1985) Potentiation and protection of doxorubicin cytotoxicity by cellular glutathione modulation. Cancer Treat Rep 69: 1293–1296

103. Hirano I, Kachi H, Ohashi (1962) Mechanisms of natural and acquired resistance to methyl-bis-(2-chloroethyl) amine-N-oxide in ascites tumors II. Gann 53: 73–80

104. Griffith OW, Meister A (1979) Potent and specific inhibition of glutathione synthesis by buthionine sulfoximine (s-u-butyl homocysteine sulfoximine). J Biol Chem 253: 7558–7560

105. Suzukake K, Petro BJ, Vistica DT (1982) Reduction in glutathione content of L-PAM-resistant L1210 cells confers drug sensitivity. Biochem Pharmacol 31: 121–124

106. Green TA, Vistica DT, Young RC, Hamilton TC, Rogers AM, Ozols RF (1984) Potentiation of melphalan cytotoxicity in human ovarian cancer cell lines by glutathione depletion. Cancer Res 44: 5427–5431

107. Wellner VP, Anderson ME, Puri RN, Jensen GL, Meister A (1984) Radioprotection by glutathione ester. Transport of glutathione ester into human lymphoid cells and fibroblasts. Proc Natl Acad Sci USA 81: 4732–4735

108. Cline MJ, Stand H, Mecola K, Morse RL, Ruprecht R, Brown J, Salser W (1980) Gene transfer in intact animals. Nature 284: 422–424

109. Carr F, Medina WD, Dube S, Bertino JR (1983) Genetic transformation of murine bone marrow cells to methotrexate. Blood 62: 180–186

110. Miller DW, Eckner RJ, Jolly DJ, Friedman T, Verma IM (1984) Expression of a retrovirus encoding human HPRT in mice. Science 225: 630–632

111. Miller AD, Law MF, Verma IM (1984) Generation of helper free amphotropic retroviruses that transduce a dominant acting reductase gene. Mol Cell Biol 5: 431–437

112. Ricciardone MD, Trauber DR, Matis LA, Cowan KH (1986) Retrovirus expression vectors which transfer methotrexate (MTX) resistance. Proc Am Assoc Cancer Res 41: 11

113. Sheau-Fung Y, Von Ruden T, Kantoff PW, Garber C, Seiberg M, Ruther U, Anderson WF, Wagner EF, and Gilboa E (1986) Self-inactivating retroviral vectors designed for transfer of whole genes into mammalian cells. Proc Natl Acad Sci 83: 3194–3198

10. Multidrug Resistance in Tissue Culture and Human Tissues

A. Fojo

Introduction

Resistance to chemotherapy remains a major obstacle in the treatment of many malignancies. Successful chemotherapy is likely to evolve either from a continued search for new agents or from an understanding of the basis of drug resistance, with the ultimate goal of finding ways to overcome this. A pessimist might be doubtful regarding the likelihood of finding effective new agents for tumors such as colon cancer, melanoma, and nonsmall-cell carcinoma of the lung. Although it is true that these malignancies have proven refractory to nearly all agents that have been tried, the same could have been said of many tumors we now consider curable. For this reason, the search for new agents must continue. But can we overcome drug resistance and make existing ineffective therapy successful? In the laboratory, this has already been accomplished; whether this can be achieved in a clinical setting is just beginning to be tested.

This chapter will review multidrug resistance mediated by the *mdr*-1 gene whose product is P-glycoprotein. Recent developments have led to an increased understanding of this mechanism of resistance. Although we await evaluation of its clinical importance, some practical lessons have already been learned.

Multidrug Resistance Phenotype

It is interesting that in all the human and rodent systems that have been studied, the multidrug resistance phenotype has been remarkably similar [1–8]. From work in several laboratories, our understanding of this phenomenon has increased substantially. We now recognize a set of traits that comprise the multidrug resistance phenotype, including:

1. Resistance to a variety of natural products that are structurally unrelated, including the anthracyclines, actinomycin D, colchicine, the vinca alkaloids, and the podophyllotoxins. Alkylating agents are not included, although co-resistance to these compounds is often seen in a clinical setting.
2. Increased amounts of a 170 000-dalton membrane glycoprotein (P-170 or P-

glycoprotein), originally described by Ling et al. [3]. This glycoprotein functions as an energy-dependent efflux pump, which lowers intracellular drug concentration [7, 9, 10]

3. Reversibility of the multidrug resistance phenotype by a group of diverse agents, including the calcium channel blockers, the phenothiazines, and some antiarrhythmic agents [11–13].

4. Cytogenetic evidence of gene amplification in highly resistant cell lines, including single- or double-minute chromosomes, homogeneously staining regions or abnormally banding regions [1, 14]. In some cell lines, resistance is unstable, with loss of tolerance when cells are maintained in drug-free medium, and cytogenetic analysis has demonstrated the presence of single- and double-minute chromosomes. In other cell lines, homogeneously staining regions have been identified, and in these the phenotype is more stable.

Characterization of Multidrug Resistance

The cytogenetic evidence of gene amplification has been substantiated by the isolation of genomic and cDNA probes which recognize amplified/overexpressed sequences in multidrug-resistant cell lines [14–20]. Several approaches have been utilized to isolate these molecular probes, demonstrating the options available for successful cloning. In multidrug-resistant human KB carcinoma cell lines, a modification of the technique of in-gel renaturation developed by Roninson was used to obtain cloned fragments from two independent cell lines (Fig. 1) [14]. Gene amplification in these cell lines had previously been demonstrated utilizing a DNA segment also which was cloned from multidrug-resistant hamster cells, taking advantage of the increased frequency of renaturation of amplified sequences [15, 16]. In multidrug-resistant Chinese hamster ovary cells, cDNA clones encoding part of P-glycoprotein were isolated from an expression library, utilizing an antibody against P-170 [17]. In addition, the *mdr*-1 gene and

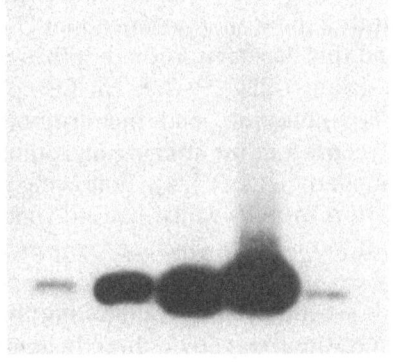

Fig. 1. Southern blot analysis of DNA from five KB (HeLa) cell lines hybridized with a probe obtained by cloning amplified sequences from a multidrug-resistant cell line. The probe was isolated using a modification of the in-gel renaturation procedure described by Roninson. The left-hand lane shows the single copy signal in the parental KB cell line, while the right-hand lane shows the same results in a revertant obtained by growing a multidrug-resistant cell line out of selection medium. The three middle lanes show amplification of the same 4.0 KB Hind III fragment in three independently selected multidrug-resistant cell lines

four other genes that are overexpressed and amplified in this same cell line were identified by differential screening of a cDNA library [18]. Finally, in Chinese hamster lung cells, amplified/overexpressed sequences were identified by cDNA screening with amplified DNA probes obtained by $C_o t$ (10–300) enrichment of DNA from a multidrug-resistant cell line [19]. Although isolated from independently selected cell lines, the probes in all cases recognize a 4.8-kb mRNA species that is the product of the *mdr*-1 gene and encodes P-glycoprotein.

A Model for the mdr-1 Gene Product (P-Glycoprotein)

The primary sequence of P-glycoprotein has been determined in human and rodent systems from sequence data obtained with full-length cDNAs [20, 21]. The results demonstrate an open reading frame for a protein of 1276–1280 amino acids. Analysis of the sequence suggests that the molecule arose as a result of an internal duplication, with both segments containing a consensus ATP binding site. In addition, inspection of the deduced sequence reveals the presence of six hydrophobic regions in each half of the molecule, fitting all criteria for transmembrane domains, and several potential glycosylation sites. Consequently, the model can be viewed as two domains, each with an ATP binding site, functioning as an energy-dependent transport system involved in active drug efflux.

Function of P-Glycoprotein/Photoaffinity Labelling

A role for P-glycoprotein as an energy-dependent efflux pump had been previously suggested from experiments in several laboratories investigating drug accumulation and drug efflux in multidrug-resistant cell lines. Increasing levels of drug resistance are associated with decreased accumulation and rapid efflux from drug-loaded cells. This reduced accumulation had been previously demonstrated to be energy dependent [7, 9, 10, 22]. Drug efflux requires initial binding, and this has been studied utilizing membrane vesicles prepared from multidrug-resistant cells [23–27]. In KB cells, these vesicles bind increased amounts of [^{3}H]vinblastine, and the drug-binding component has been identified as P-glycoprotein by utilizing an iodinated photoaffinity analog of vinblastine (^{125}I-labelled NASV) [24]. Following photoactivation, this analog labels a 170 000-dalton protein which can be specifically immunoprecipitated with monoclonal antibody C219, which recognizes P-glycoprotein. The labelling can be inhibited by excess cold vinblastine or vincristine, and to a lesser extent by daunomycin and actinomycin D, suggesting that P-glycoprotein can bind these drugs and is therefore likely to be directly involved in their efflux from cells.

This system also provides a means of studying agents which reverse multidrug resistance [25]. Both quinidine and verapamil are excellent inhibitors of ^{125}I-labelled NASV binding, whereas phenothiazines are not. These findings indicate that there is more than one mechanism for reversing drug resistance mediated by P-glycoprotein. This raises the possibility that synergism could be obtained by combining agents with different mechanisms. In a clinical setting, this may prove to be of value.

MDR-1 Gene and Drug Resistance

Before considering a possible role for the *mdr*-1 gene in clinical drug resistance, its importance in clinical cell culture had to be firmly established. The evidence that the *mdr*-1 gene plays a role in drug resistance includes the following:

1. Numerous independently selected human and rodent multidrug-resistant cell lines have amplified the *mdr*-1 gene [14–19].
2. Reversion of the multidrug-resistant phenotype following the withdrawal of selective pressure is associated with a decrease in *mdr*-1 expression and amplification [28].
3. Sensitive cells transformed with DNA from multidrug-resistant cell lines develop a pattern of multidrug resistance similar to that of the donor cell line and have increased amounts of *mdr*-1 mRNA/P-glycoprotein [29].
4. Full-length cDNAs for the *mdr*-1 gene can confer the multidrug resistance phenotype following transfection [30, 31].

Taken together, these results provide strong support for a role of the *mdr*-1 gene in multidrug resistance in tissue culture systems.

Increased Expression Can Precede Gene Amplification

In several well-studied models of drug resistance, gene amplification has been identified as the primary molecular alteration, with less emphasis given to expression [32]. With *mdr*-1, the degrees of overexpression and amplification vary widely among various resistant cell lines [28]. The KB carcinoma cell lines KB-A1 and KB-V1, the 2780 ovarian carcinoma cell line selected with doxorubicin (Adriamycin), and the CEM lymphoblastic cell line selected with vinblastine all have similar levels of *mdr*-1 expression but have amplified the gene 10–160 times. These findings suggest that at some step during the selection of these cell lines, expression and amplification were not coordinated. In addition, in one of the KB carcinoma cell lines, the early steps of incremental increases in drug resistance were characterized by increased expression without gene amplification. These early steps have levels of resistance that most likely correspond to those found in a clinical setting. This suggests that clinical drug resistance may result from increased expression without amplification. The paucity of examples of gene amplification in a clinical setting could in part be explained by this, and it argues for measuring the levels of *mdr*-1 mRNA or the protein product.

Expression of *mdr*-1 Gene in Normal Tissues and Tumors

Expression of the *mdr*-1 gene has been detected in specific normal human tissues [33] (Table 1). A survey of normal tissues shows that *mdr*-1 is expressed at low levels in most organs but at higher levels in a few. The *mdr*-1 gene is expressed at very high levels in the adrenal gland; at high levels in kidney; at intermediate

Table 1. *mdr*-1 mRNA in normal tissues [33]

Tissue or cell line[a]	mRNA level[d]
Adrenal (4)	160
Adrenal medulla	> 500
Kidney (6)	50
Kidney medulla	75
Colon (10)	31
Liver (4)	25
Lung (9)	20
Jejunum	20
Rectum	20
Brain	12
Prostate	8
Skin, subcutaneous tissue, skeletal muscle, heart, spleen (2), bone marrow (3), lymphocytes, esophagus, stomach, ovary, kidney cortex, spinal cord	1–5
KB-3-1	1
KB-8-5[b]	40
KB-V1 (Vbl)[c]	> 500

[a] Number of tissue samples studied (when > 1) is given in parentheses. Values given are means.
[b] Resistance relative to the parent KB-3-1 is 3-fold for doxorubicin and 6-fold for vinblastine.
[c] Resistance relative to the parent KB-3-1 is 420-fold for doxorubicin and 210-fold for vinblastine (Vbl).
[d] Quantitated by densitometry of slot blots of 10 μg of total RNA. Values, expressed relative to level for drug-sensitive KB-3-1 cells, were determined by comparison with KB-8-5 RNA, which gave a reproducible, easily detectable signal.

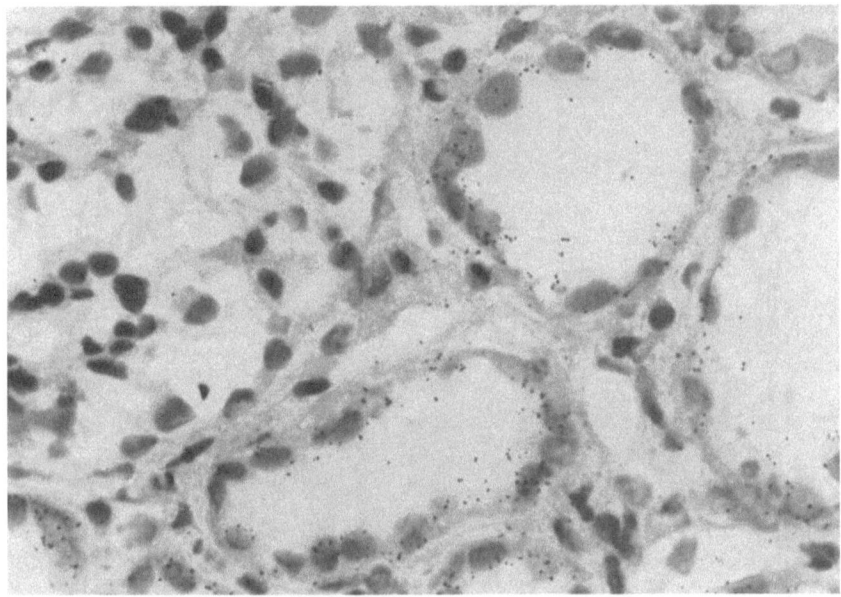

Fig. 2. Photomicrograph of a kidney cortex showing the results of an RNA in situ hybridization experiment performed utilizing a ^{35}S-labelled RNA probe encoded by the middle one-third of the *mdr*-1 mRNA. Several proximal tubules surrounding a glomerulus can be identified. The grains localize *mdr*-1 expression to the proximal tubules of the kidney

levels in lung, liver, jejunum, colon, and rectum; and at low levels in many other organs. Expression is not only organ specific but can be localized to specific areas within each organ by in situ hybridization with RNA probes. In the kidney and colon, expression is seen in the proximal tubule and surface epithelium, respectively (Fig. 2). In the liver, there is uniform distribution of message among the hepatocytes. All three layers of the adrenal cortex have readily detectable levels, which are lowest in the zona reticularis. In the adrenal medulla, expression is confined to the ganglion cells. Although *mdr*-1 was isolated from multidrug-resistant cells, the normal tissue survey suggests that P-glycoprotein has a normal function at these sites. One possibility is a role in the excretion of drugs or other organic molecules. As other genes for drug resistance are identified, it is likely that expression in some normal tissues will also be demonstrated.

To a certain extent, the normal tissue expression has been predictive of expression in untreated tumors [33] (Table 2). Elevated *mdr*-1 expression has been found in many, but not all, tumors from the adrenal gland, colon, and kidney, organs with elevated *mdr*-1 mRNA levels (Fig. 3). These findings suggest that the *mdr*-1 gene can continue to be expressed after transformation to the malignant phenotype, where it may play a role in the failure of initial chemotherapy. Examination of such expression by in situ hybridization demonstrates homogeneous expression in some tumors, but a heterogeneous pattern in many [34]. Examination of tumors in this fashion may help to provide evidence sup-

221

Table 2. *mdr*-1 mRNA in tumors [33]

Tumor	Patient no.	Treatment[b]	mRNA level[c]
Pheochromocytoma	6		> 500
	11		67
	12		64
	8		61
	9		40
	3		26
	10		19
	1	Vcr	18
	1		3
	7		15
	2		13
	4		1
	5		1
	13		1
Neuroblastoma	1	Vcr, Dox	25
	2	Vcr, Dox	24
	3	Vcr, Dox	10
Adrenocortical cancer	1		72
	2		2
Colon cancer[a]	1		20(42)
	2		23(29)
	3	5FU, Mit C	54(17)
	4		41(21)
	5		20(19)
	6		18(31)
	7		76(84)
	8		7(6)
Childhood cancers			
Neuroepithelioma	1	Vcr, Act D	8
	2	Vcr, Act D	7
Ewing's sarcoma	1	Vcr, Act D	1
	2	Vcr, Act D	7
Rhabdomyosarcoma	1	Vcr, Act D	7
	2	Vcr, Act D	74
Acute lymphoblastic leukemia	1–9		5–14
	10		68

Vcr, vincristine; Dox, doxorubicin; 5FU, 5-fluorouracil; Mit C, mitomycin C; Act D, actinomycin D
[a] Values for adjacent normal colon tissue are given in parentheses.
[b] Some samples were from patients who had relapsed following combination chemotherapy, and some of the drugs these patients had received are shown.
[c] Relative to KB-3-1 cells. Data are from densitometry of blots.

porting the preexistence of resistant populations in untreated tumors, especially if serial samples can be obtained, and conversion to a more homogeneous pattern is demonstrated.

Increased levels have also been observed in some tumors at the time of relapse following initial chemotherapy. These increased levels have been observed

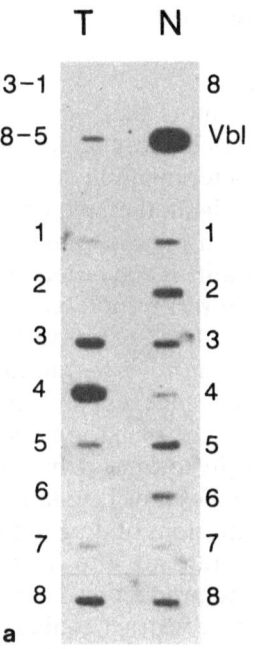

a

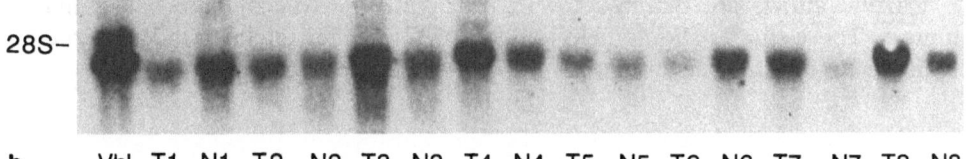

b   Vbl T1 N1 T2 N2 T3 N3 T4 N4 T5 N5 T6 N6 T7 N7 T8 N8

Fig. 3a, b. *mdr*-1 expression in normal colon (*N*) and colon tumors (*T*). Total RNA was analyzed by slot blot (10 μg, **a**) and Northern blot (6 μg, **b**) hybridization. A cDNA probe encoding the proximal one-third of the protein was used for the slot blot analysis after nick translation; a riboprobe made from the middle one-third of the full-length cDNA was used in the Northern blot analysis. 3-1 is the parent KB (HeLa) subclone from which the multidrug-resistant KB sublines were selected. 8 and 8-5 Vbl are multidrug-resistant cell lines. The resistance relative to the parent cell line for 8-5 is 3-fold for doxorubicin and 6-fold for vinblastine; for Vbl these values are 10-fold for doxorubicin and 420-fold for vinblastine. In the Northern blot analysis only 1 μg Vbl RNA was loaded, and the panel shown is a composite of three different gels, each with its own internal control

both in tumors where elevated expression is found in untreated samples, such as pheochromocytomas and neuroblastomas, and in cases where levels are low before treatment, such as acute lymphocytic leukemia. How prevalent these results are awaits further analysis; however, in combination chemotherapy, it is clear that resistance need not develop to all agents utilized for treatment to fail. Prospective clinical studies now under way will answer questions regarding the role of *mdr*-1 in primary and acquired resistance.

Clinical Applications and Future Directions

Although it seems likely that more than one mechanism is responsible for multidrug resistance, the ability to identify tumors with increased *mdr*-1 expression offers several possibilities. Determination of the levels of *mdr*-1 mRNA could be used to predict sensitivity to chemotherapy, obviating the need for cumbersome culture assays. This will become more valuable as other molecular probes of drug resistance genes are identified and tested in the clinical arena. A related use would be in the assessment of recurrent disease, to ascertain whether resistance has developed during therapy. In addition, such identification, coupled with the knowledge that some agents can reverse multidrug resistance in tissue culture, may help to increase the effectiveness of current chemotherapeutic agents. Drugs such as quinidine and verapamil are active in culture, and quinidine is effective at levels used clinically to treat arrhythmias. Judgement of their clinical value awaits the results of studies now beginning, but these agents are certain to increase intracellular concentrations of drug in tumors expressing elevated levels of *mdr*-1. Whether this will translate into increased cytotoxicity remains to be determined. Finally, since the product of the *mdr*-1 gene is a membrane glycoprotein, it may be possible to construct conjugates of antibodies with toxins or radioisotopes that can be used therapeutically against drug-resistant tumor cells expressing it.

Current efforts are directed toward clarifying the role of *mdr*-1 in human tumors. These studies should help to determine whether the knowledge accrued in tissue culture can be successfully utilized in a clinical setting.

References

1. Biedler JL, Riehm H (1970) Cellular resistance to actinomycin D in Chinese hamster cells in vitro: cross-resistance, radioautographic and cytogenetic studies. Cancer Res 30: 1174–1184
2. Ling V, Thompson L (1974) Reduced permeability in CHO cells as a mechanism of resistance to colchicine. J Cell Physiol 83: 103–116
3. Juliano RL, Ling V (1976) A surface glycoprotein modulating drug permeability in Chinese hamster ovary cell mutants. Biochem Biophys Acta 455: 152–162
4. Beck WT, Mueller TJ, Tanzer LR (1979) Altered surface membrane glycoproteins in vinca alkaloid-resistant human leukemic lymphoblasts. Cancer Res 39: 2070–2076
5. Akiyama S-I, Fojo AT, Hanover JA, Pastan I, Gottesman MM (1985) Isolation and genetic characterization of human KB cell lines resistant to multiple drugs. Somat Cell Molec Genet 11: 117–126
6. Shen D-W, Cardarelli C, Hwang J, Cornwell M, Richert N, Ishii S, Pastan I, Gottesman MM (1986) Multiple drug resistant human KB carcinoma cells independently selected for high-level resistance to colchicine, Adriamycin or vinblastine show changes in expression of specific proteins. J Biol Chem 261: 7762–7770
7. Inaba M, Kobayashi H, Sakurai Y, Johnson RK (1979) Active efflux of daunomycin and adriamycin in sensitive and resistant sublines of P388 leukemia. Cancer Res 39: 2200–2203

8. Mirski SEL, Gerlach JH, Cole SP (1987) Multidrug resistance in a human small cell lung cancer cell line selected in adriamycin. Cancer Res 47: 2594–2598
9. Carlsen SA, Till JE, Ling V (1977) Modulation of drug permeability in Chinese hamster ovary cells. Biochim Biophys Acta 467: 238–250
10. Fojo AT, Akiyama S-I, Gottesman MM, Pastan I (1985) Reduced drug accumulation in multiple drug-resistant human KB carcinoma cell lines. Cancer Res 45: 3002–3007
11. Tsuruo T, Iida H, Kitatani Y, Yokota K, Tsukagoshi S, Sakurai Y (1984) Effects of quinidine and related compounds on cytotoxicity and cellular accumulation of vincristine and adriamycin in drug-resistant tumor cells. Cancer Res 44: 4303–4307
12. Tsuruo T, Iida H, Tsukagoshi S, Sakurai Y (1986) Increased accumulation of vincristine and adriamycin in drug-resistant P-388 tumor cells following incubation with calcium antagonists and calmodulin inhibitors. Cancer Res 42: 4730–4733
13. Akiyama S-I, Shiraishi N, Kuratomi Y, Nakagawa M, Kuwano M (1986) Circumvention of multiple-drug resistance in human cancer cells by thioridazine, trifluoperazine and chlorpromazine. JNCI 76: 839–844
14. Fojo AT, Whang-Peng J, Gottesman MM, Pastan I (1985) amplification of DNA sequences in human multidrug-resistant KB carcinoma cells. Proc Natl Acad Sci USA 82: 7661–7665
15. Roninson IB, Abelson HT, Housman DE, Howell N, Varshavski A (1984) Amplification of specific DNA sequences correlates with multidrug resistance in Chinese hamster cells. Nature 309: 626–628
16. Roninson IB, Chin JE, Choi K, Gros P, Housman DE, Fojo AT, Shen D-W, Gottesman MM, Pastan I (1986) Isolation of human *mdr* DNA sequences amplified in multidrug-resistant KB carcinoma cells. Proc Natl Acad Sci USA 83: 4538–4542
17. Riordan JR, Deuchars K, Kartner N, Alon N, Trent J, Ling V (1985) Amplification of P-glycoprotein genes in multidrug-resistant mammalian cell lines. Nature 316: 817–819
18. Van der Blief AM, Van der Velde-Koerts T, Ling V, Borst P (1986) Overexpression and amplification of five genes in a multidrug-resistant Chinese hamster ovary cell line. Mol Cell Biol 6: 1671–1678
19. Scotto KW, Biedler JL, Melera PW (1986) Amplification and expression of genes associated with multidrug resistance in mammalian cells. Science 232: 751–755
20. Chen C-J, Chin JE, Ueda K, Clark DP, Pastan I, Gottesman MM, Roninson IB (1986) Internal duplication and homology with bacterial transport proteins in the *mdr*-1 (P-glycoprotein) gene from multidrug-resistant human cells. Cell 47: 381–389
21. Gros P, Croop J, Housman D (1986) Mammalian multidrug resistance gene: complete cDNA sequence indicates strong homology to bacterial transport proteins. Cell 47: 371–380
22. Willingham MC, Cornwell MM, Cardarelli CO, Gottesman MM, Pastan I (1986) Single cell analysis of daunomycin uptake and efflux in multidrug-resistant and sensitive KB cells: effect of verapamil and other drugs. Cancer Res 46: 5941–5946
23. Cornwell MM, Gottesman MM, Pastan I (1986) Increased vinblastine binding to membrane vesicles from multidrug resistant KB cells. J Biol Chem 261: 7921–7928
24. Cornwell MM, Safa AR, Felsted RL, Gottesman MM, Pastan I (1986) Membrane vesicles from multidrug-resistant human cancer cells contain a specific 150-170 kDa protein detected by photo-affinity labelling. Proc Natl Acad Sci USA 83: 3847–3850
25. Cornwell MM, Pastan I, Gottesman MM (1987) Certain calcium channel blockers bind specifically to multidrug-resistant human KB carcinoma membrane vesicles and inhibit drug binding to P-glycoprotein. J Biol Chem 262: 2166–2170
26. Safa AR, Glover CJ, Swell JL, Meyers MB, Biedler JL, Felsted RL (1987) Identification of the multidrug resistance-related membrane glycoprotein as an acceptor for calcium channel blockers. JBC 262: 7884–7888
27. Akiyama S-I, Cornwell MM, Kuwano M, Pastan I, Gottesman MM (1988) Most drugs that reverse multidrug resistance also inhibit photoaffinity labeling of P-glycoprotein by a vinblastine analog. Molec Pharm 33: 144–147
28. Shen D-W, Fojo A, Chin JE, Roninson IB, Richert N, Pastan I, Gottesman MM (1986) Human multidrug-resistant cell lines: increased *mdr*-1 expression can precede gene amplification. Science 232: 643–645

29. Shen D-W, Fojo A, Roninson IB, Chin JE, Soffir R, Pastan I, Gottesman MM (1986) Multidrug-resistance of DNA-mediated transformants is linked to transfer of the human *mdr*-1 gene. Mol Cell Biol 6: 4039–4044

30. Gros P, Ben Neriah Y, Croop JM, Housman DE (1986) Isolation and expression of a complementary DNA that confers multidrug resistance. Nature 323: 728–731

31. Ueda K, Cardarelli C, Gottesman MM, Pastan I (1987) MDR 1 gene confers resistance to colchicine, doxorubicin and vinblastine. PNAS 84: 3004–3008

32. Federspiel NA, Beverly SM, Schilling JW, Schmike RT (1984) Novel DNA rearrangements are associated with dihydrofolate reductase gene amplification. J Biol Chem 259: 9127–9140

33. Fojo AT, Ueda K, Slamon DJ, Poplack DG, Gottesman MM, Pastan I (1986) Expression of a multidrug resistance gene in human tumors and tissues. Proc Natl Acad Sci USA

34. Mickley L et al., in preparation

11. Development of New Chemotherapeutic Agents

V. Narayanan

Introduction

There is a continuing need to discover and develop new chemotherapeutic agents for the treatment of cancer. The reasons are several. Cancer chemotherapy generally cures only rare tumors such as choriocarcinoma, teratoma, hemopoietic malignancies, and childhood cancers. Very rarely, if at all, are drugs effective against major killers such as lung, colon, melanoma, and breast cancers. Even where some measure of effectiveness is achieved, this is usually due not to any single agent, but to a combination of drugs or combined modality treatment. Surgery and radiation treatments are no doubt very useful. However, these are limited by the tendency for many solid tumors to metastasize to distant sites, the metastatic event frequently occurring prior to diagnosis. Thus, chemotherapy will continue to play a vital role in the treatment of cancer. Clearly, the cornerstone of effective cancer chemotherapy is the drug molecule itself.

Challenges of New Drug Discovery

The research to discover new anticancer agents is particularly challenging because of several factors: (a) the lack of adequate knowledge of the biochemistry of tumor cell types and our inability to identify and define exploitable biochemical differences between tumor cell types and normal cells; (b) tumor heterogeneity; (c) the development of biochemical resistance to the drug or drugs used for treatment; and (d) the low predictability of animal tumor models, especially for solid tumors. Strategies for discovering new drugs involve two key steps: identification of new leads and structure-activity/toxicity fine-tuning. A small but significant number of new drug discoveries stem from "rational" drug design and analog synthesis. However, the majority of the new leads, both of synthetic and of nature product origins, are discovered through the "semirational" approach of screening.

227

Rational Drug Design

The greatest success in the rational approach to anticancer drug design has been in the area of antimetabolites; in fact, of the antitumor agents with established clinical activity, six are rationally designed antimetabolites. The early developments of antifolates and purine antagonists by functional group replacements have given major impetus to the antimetabolite area [1]. There is continued interest in the development of novel antifolates, with the goal of improving the therapeutic index and overcoming methotrexate (MTX) resistance. These new compounds include alterations in the glutamic acid moiety of MTX, lipophilic diaminopyrimidines, and quinazoline derivatives. One diaminopyrimidine (metadichlorofen, DDMP) is currently in phase II clinical trials. As predicted, DDMP rapidly enters the central nervous system (CNS) and does not require a carrier-mediated transport system for cell entry. DDMP may also be useful in the treatment of MTX-resistant tumors. Quinazoline antifolates are inhibitors of both dihydrofolate reductase and thymidylate synthetase. The compound CB-3717 is the tightest-binding thymidylate synthetase antifolate that has yet been synthesized, and its affinity for this enzyme is ten times greater than its affinity for dihydrofolate reductase. The compound has a high therapeutic index in pre-clinical animal testing and is undergoing clinical trials. A recent development in this area is the use of computer graphics to simulate the formation of effective drug-enzyme complexes.

The fact that the 5-position of uracil has to be methylated for thymidine and DNA synthesis led to the early rational design and development of 5-carbon-substituted pyrimidine antimetabolites, the most significant of which is 5-fluorouracil (5FU). Even now, 5FU continues to be the focus of attention as a model for pro-drug synthesis, as well as analog synthesis. Another example of rational design of an effective antimetabolite is arabinosylcytosine (ara-C).

In recent years, several conceptual and methodological advances have provided new approaches to the design of enzyme inhibitors. Analogs of transition state intermediates (activated complexes formed by combination of the substrates and synchronously converted into the products) would be ideal candidates to inhibit a particular enzymatic reaction because they could be tailored to fit the active site of the target enzyme. Some examples of compounds in this category are the development of tetrahydrouridine as an effective inhibitor of cytidine deaminase, 2'-deoxycoformycin as an adenosine deaminase inhibitor, and N-(phosphonacetyl)-L-aspartate (PALA) as an inhibitor of aspartic-transcarboxylase reactions. Another variation of the enzyme inhibition approach for designing anticancer agents is the concept of *suicide enzyme inhibitors*. These are compounds that possess latent reactive functional groups which are unmasked by the enzyme, which is then inactivated; thus, the enzyme's own activity leads to its inhibition. Kcat inhibitors bind tightly to the enzyme, which is thereby permanently inhibited. An excellent example is L-difluoromethyl ornithine (DFMO), which inhibits polyamine biosynthesis by blocking ornithine decarboxylation. Preliminary studies indicate that DFMO in combination with cytotoxic drugs may have value in the treatment of cancer.

228

A new and exciting avenue for rational drug design is the emerging knowledge of the processes of oncogene expression and activation. For example, it has been shown that tyrosine kinases can phosphorylate phosphotidylinositol, leading to the activation of protein kinase C and the C^{2+}/calmodulin-dependent pathways. Protein kinase C has been implicated in the tumor promotion action of phorbol esters. Mitogens such as epidermal growth factor (EGF) have also been shown to induce the phosphotidylinositol response. Therefore, synthetic drug design aimed at selective inhibition of protein kinase C would be very attractive.

Molecular Modifications

Once a promising "lead" compound, either a synthetic or natural product, is discovered, it is exploited by the medicinal chemist through molecular modifications. The goal is to synthesize a drug having greater activity or less toxicity than the parent compound. Bioisosteric replacement is the principal tool that a medicinal chemist utilizes to develop analogs of lead compounds. The parameters being changed are molecular size, steric shape, bond angles, hybridization, electron distribution, lipid solubility, water solubility, pKa, chemical reactivity to cell components and metabolizing enzymes, and capacity to undergo receptor interactions through hydrogen bonding. Two examples will illustrate the scope of analog synthesis. Currently, there is a great deal of preclinical and clinical work going on in the design and development of "second-generation" anthracyclines. Doxorubicin hydrochloride (Adriamycin) analogs that do not appear to have the dose-limiting cardiotoxicity of doxorubicin and do not induce alopecia are under investigation, e.g., aclacinomycin, 4-demethoxydaunorubicin, and 4'-epidoxorubicin. With regard to the platinum derivatives, the high clinical utility of cisplatin is restricted by the onset of limiting toxicities, the most important of which are nausea and vomiting, neurotoxicity, and myelosuppression. In an effort to improve the therapeutic index of cisplatin, there has been a strong interest in the development of second-generation analogs. It is only recently that clinical trials of several of the most promising analogs have been undertaken. The most important one to date is cyclobutanedicarboxylatoplatinum (CBDCA). In animal experiments and in early clinical trials, CBDCA shows comparable anticancer activity, with reduced nephrotoxicity and reduced acute gastrointestinal toxicity.

Computer Models

Computer graphics and nonbonded energy calculations are being increasingly used to model the intercalative binding of compounds such as doxorubicin, nogalamycin, distamycin, anthraquinone, and acridine derivatives to double-stranded DNA. These compounds have actual or potential antitumor properties, which relate to their DNA-binding abilities. Computer simulation may thus be useful in drug design [2].

Another development is the application of computer simulation to understanding the effects of antimetabolites on metabolic pathways, e.g., models of antifolate action and of deoxyribonucleoside triphosphate and purine ribonucleotide biosynthesis. Kinetic modeling of anticancer drug effects has been used to examine the dependence of drug sensitivity upon enzyme kinetic parameters and metabolic pool sizes, and to develop optimal ways to combine multiple drugs.

Natural Products as Sources of New Leads

Both natural products and compounds of synthetic origin are good sources of new anticancer leads. The natural products area encompasses fermentation, plant, and animal (especially marine) products. Anthracyclines, bleomycins, and mitomycins have emerged from fermentation broths. The higher plants have provided a few antitumor agents in current use—the Vinca alkaloids vinblastine and vincristine, and the podophyllotoxins, VP-16 and VM-26. The marine product area is a relatively new one that is being explored.

The Natural Products Branch of the National Cancer Institute (NCI) has recently initiated a new program for the acquisition of unusual natural products. Novel techniques and unusual substrates are utilized to generate new leads. In vitro prescreens are also constantly improved or changed to increase the efficiency of the program. Currently used screens include enzyme inhibition, tubulin binding, phage induction, DNA binding, and cytotoxicity against various murine and human cell lines. Active fractions from the in vitro prescreens are then tested against the in vivo systems in a drug development flow, which will be described later. Once the bioactive substance has been isolated and is free from contaminants, structure determination follows, a task that has been greatly accelerated through the use of modern high-resolution spectroscopic tools.

Screening for New Leads

The rest of the chapter will be devoted to discussing the screening approach to the discovery of new anticancer leads. Screening and unexpected (serendipitous) observations are, and always have been, responsible for the vast majority of new lead discoveries. Screening has the advantage over other more efficient procedures of revealing unexpected chemical structural types to be agents active under the test conditions. These lead compounds can then serve as starting points for further elaboration of suitable drugs.

For several years, the NCI of the United States of America has supported and even now continues to engage in a major collaborative anticancer screening program [3]. The strategy for the discovery and development of new anticancer agents currently in place in the Drug Development Program at NCI is based on the acquisition and screening of a large number of widely varying compounds of both synthetic and natural product origins.

A multidisciplinary systems approach for new drug discovery and development has been adopted, based on continuous interactions and feedback between medicinal chemists, biologists, pharmacists, and clinicians. The various stages of drug development and the logic which guides the program are called the Linear Array. It delineates the steps which must take place to assure the flow of compounds through the experimental systems and into the clinic: (a) acquisition of new compounds, (b) screening, (c) production and formulation, (d) toxicology, (e) phase I clinical trials, (f) phase II clinical trials, and (g) phase III and IV clinical trials. It also spells out the criteria for moving candidate compounds from one stage of development to another. The program has undergone many changes and refinements over the years. Discussions will focus on the input side: (a) selection and acquisition of compounds, especially of synthetic origin; and (b) biological evaluation. Finally, the novel compounds that are in various stages of development will be described.

The flow of synthetic compounds occurs in three distinct stage: the acquisition phase, the preselection phase, and the anticancer evaluation phase. Several mechanisms are available for the input of novel compounds to the program, namely, voluntary submissions, active solicitations, contracts, and grants. The vast majority of compounds are acquired from industries, both domestic and foreign, on a voluntary basis under provisions of confidentiality. Continuous literature surveillance is also employed to select compounds on the basis of relevant chemical, biochemical, pharmacological, and biological criteria. These compounds encompass a large variety of structural types, prepared as synthetics or isolated from plants, fermentation broths, and marine organisms.

Anticancer Test Systems

The development of predictable animal tumor models for identifying clinical candidates continues to be a major challenge [4]. The biological systems that are used to evaluate new compounds for anticancer activity are summarized in Table 1. The mouse P388 leukemia model is used as a prescreen to select new compounds for secondary evaluation against a panel of tumors. Occasionally, the P388 prescreen is bypassed for compounds that have shown either (a) activities in antitumor screens not available at NCI or (b) other pertinent biochemical or biological activities. The tumor panel consisted of eight cancer models in mice—

231

Table 1. Biological systems used to evaluate new compounds for anticancer activity

Model	Code	Drug (rt./schedule)	Parameter	Active T/C% DN1(+)	Active T/C% DN2(+ +)
Prescreen					
IP P388 leukemia	3PS31	IP/Q1D × 5	Median survival time	≥ 120	≥ 175
Transplanted mouse tumors					
IP B16 melanoma	3B131	IP/Q1D × 9	Median survival time	≥ 125	≥ 150
SC B16 melanoma	3B132	IP/Q1D × 9	Median survival time	≥ 140	≥ 150
SC CD8F₁ mammary	3CDJ2	IP/Q1D × 1	Median tumor wt. change	≤ 20	≤ 0
	3CD72	IP/Q7D × 5	Median tumor wt. change	≤ 42	≤ 10
IP colon 26	3C631	IP/Q4D × 2	Median survival time	≥ 130	≥ 150
SC colon 38	3C872	IP/Q7D × 2	Median tumor wt. change	≤ 42	≤ 10
IC ependymoblastoma	3EM37	IP/Q1D × 5	Median survival time	≥ 125	≥ 150
IV Lewis lung	3LL39	IP/Q1D × 9	Median survival time	≥ 140	≥ 150
IP L1210 leukemia	3LE31	IP/Q1D × 9	Median survival time	≥ 125	≥ 150
	3LE21	IP/Q1D × 9	Mean survival time	≥ 125	≥ 150
SC M5 ovarian	3M572	IP/Q2D × 11	Median survival time	≥ 125	≥ 150
Human tumor xenografts					
SRC CX-1 colon	3C2G5	SC/Q4D × 4	Mean tumor wt. change	≤ 20	≤ 10
SC CX-1 colon	3C2H2	IP/Q4D × 3	Mean tumor wt. change	≤ 20	≤ 10
SRC LX-1 lung	3LKG5	SC/Q4D × 3	Mean tumor wt. change	≤ 20	≤ 10
SC LX-1 lung	3LKH2	IP/Q4D × 3	Mean tumor wt. change	≤ 20	≤ 10
SRC MX-1 mammary	3MBG5	SC/Q4D × 3	Mean tumor wt. change	≤ 20	≤ 10
SC MX-1 mammary	3MBH2	IP/Q4D × 3	Mean tumor wt. change	≤ 20	≤ 10

IP, intraperitoneal; SC, subcutaneous; IC, intracerebral; IV, intravenous; SRC, subrenal capsule; Q, query; D, day; Rt, route; T/C, Treatment/Control untreated; DN1, minimum activity level required for more detailed screening; DN2, minimum activity level required to consider for initial preclinical treatment.

five transplanted mouse tumors (L1210 leukemia, B16 melanoma, colon, breast, and lung) and three human xenografts (colon, breast, and lung) implanted under the kidney capsules of mice. As a result of retrospective analysis, the tumor panel has been modified recently: the current panel consists of three transplanted mouse tumors (L1210 leukemia, B16 melanoma, and M5076 sarcoma) and the mammary human tumor xenograft in athymic mice. Two different parameters are used for evaluating the activity of a compound, either the increase in life span of the treated versus the control mice or the reduction in tumor weight. In recent years, the human tumor colony-forming assay (HTCFA) has also been utilized to identify new compounds for clinical evaluation.

Preselection

A two-stage strategy has been developed to preselect compounds for screening, namely, (a) a computer model and (b) structure-activity analysis. The objective of preselection is to enhance the cost-effectiveness of the drug discovery process by decreasing the number of compounds acquired for screening in the tumor panel while improving the quality of the input.

A variety of criteria are used to select compounds for screening. The literature is extensively scanned to identify a rational basis for selection, e.g., antitumor activity reported in other screening programs or compounds reported to exhibit relevant biochemical and other biological activities and structural features suggestive of effects on enzymatic processes relevant to cancer chemotherapy. However, by and large, the majority of compounds come with only structural information. A computerized model has been developed that aids us in selecting compounds for screening on the basis of structural information alone [5].

Computer Model

The main features of the computer model are: (a) it evaluates a broad range of compounds; (b) it utilizes structural fragments (keys); (c) it utilizes the NCI screening experience with P388, L1210, and B16; and (d) it integrates the massive volume of structural data and screening experience to predict novelty and activity for each compound under consideration.

The structural features used are those routinely generated as keys for the substructure inquiry system. The system incorporates an open-ended feature set as opposed to a dictionary (roughly 8000 structural features). The main types of keys are: (a) augmented atom keys (AA), which consist of a central atom, its bonds, and the neighboring atoms attached to the bonds, all combinations of attachments being permitted; (b) ring keys; (c) two kinds of nucleus keys; and (d) individual element keys (Fig. 1). The method assigns weight to each feature

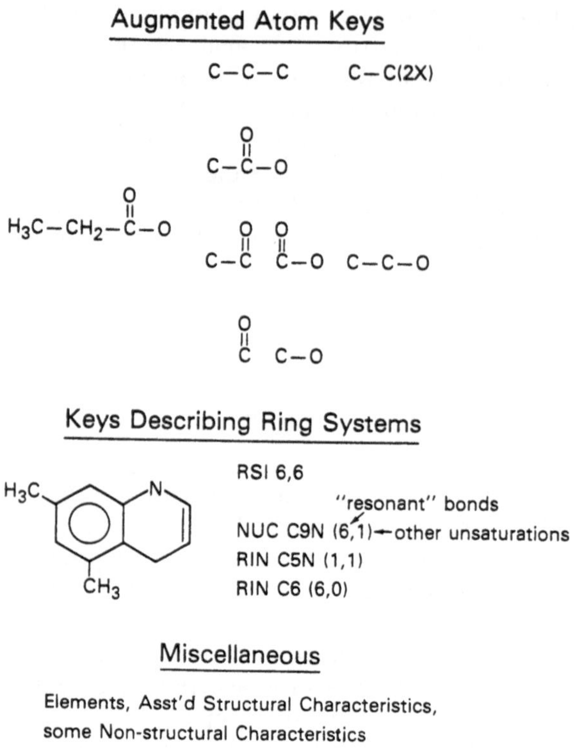

Augmented Atom Keys

C—C—C   C—C(2X)

$$C-\overset{\overset{\displaystyle O}{\|}}{C}-O$$

$$H_3C-CH_2-\overset{\overset{\displaystyle O}{\|}}{C}-O \qquad C-\overset{\overset{\displaystyle O}{\|}}{C} \ \ \overset{\overset{\displaystyle O}{\|}}{C}-O \ \ C-C-O$$

$$\overset{\overset{\displaystyle O}{\|}}{C} \ \ C-O$$

Keys Describing Ring Systems

RSI 6,6

"resonant" bonds

NUC C9N (6,1)←other unsaturations

RIN C5N (1,1)

RIN C6 (6,0)

Miscellaneous

Elements, Asst'd Structural Characteristics, some Non-structural Characteristics

Fig. 1. Structural fragments (keys) used in computer model for selection of compounds for screening

according to the statistical significance of its contribution to activity, using the P388, L1210, and B16 screening data. An unknown compound is scored by adding the weights of its dozen or so structural features. The score is not intended to estimate the strength of activity, but only to provide some measure of the likelihood of the compound having anticancer activity.

Regardless of activity, another useful measure supplied by the computer is an indication of novelty based on the large number of compounds tested against P388, L1210, and B16. Compounds are flagged as unique if they have a key which never occurred in all P388, L1210, and B16 testing. For each new compound, the feature that occurs least often is printed along with its frequency of occurrence. If the key occurring least often in the compound has appeared more than 100 times, the compound is considered adequately studied. Novelty scores are even more useful in selecting compounds for acquisition. It must be emphasized that although this method is computerized, it is not designed to automatically pass or reject compounds. It serves as a tool to aid the medicinal chemist in selecting compounds. In practice, the method is very useful for rejecting compounds. The acquisition/selection process is summarized in Fig. 2.

234

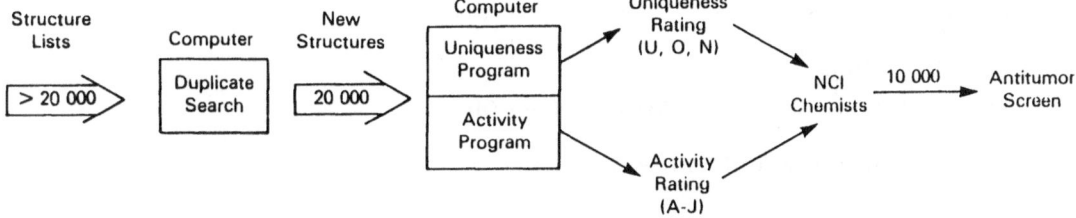

Fig. 2. Process of acquisition/selection of new compounds for screening

Structure-Activity Analysis

Detailed structure-activity analyses based on our large chemical-biological data base are an integral part of our acquisition and synthesis activities [6]. Large-scale analyses of NCI data files have become feasible because of the development of the chemistry-biology interlink and its active implementation during the past couple of years. Such activity analyses allow us to select compounds for screening maximizing structural uniqueness and anticancer potential. It also allows us to identify gap areas for further research.

New Anticancer Leads in Development

Figure 3 illustrates several examples of new anticancer leads that are currently under active development [7]. A brief description of these compounds is given below.

Mitoxantrone

The history of the development of dihydroxyanthracenedione (DHAQ, mitoxantrone) richly illustrates the value of screening in identifying new leads and the result of scientific collaboration and cooperation among a chemical company, a government agency, and a drug research team. The original compound, 1,4-bis(2-[(2-hydroxyethyl)amino]ethylamino)-9,10-anthracenedione, developed to be used as a ball-point ink, was shown to possess significant antineoplastic activity. Prior to the discovery of the above compound, antracenediones in general had shown very little, if any, anticancer activity. The high antineoplastic activity of the new lead compound made it an obvious candidate for analog studies, from which emerged DHAQ. DHAQ demonstrated outstanding anticancer activity against P388 and L1210 leukemias, B16 melanocarcinoma, and colon adenocarcinoma 26 in experimental animals. Tumor responses have been

235

MITOXANTRONE (DHAQ)

ANTHRAPYRAZOLE

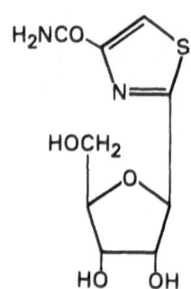

TIAZOFURIN

TETRAPLATIN

MERBARONE

TRIMETREXATE

ARA-AC

BIPHENQUINATE

$$H_3C - \overset{O}{\underset{\|}{C}} - NH \ (CH_2)_6 - NH - \overset{O}{\underset{\|}{C}} - CH_3$$

HEXAMETHYLBISACETAMIDE (HMBA)

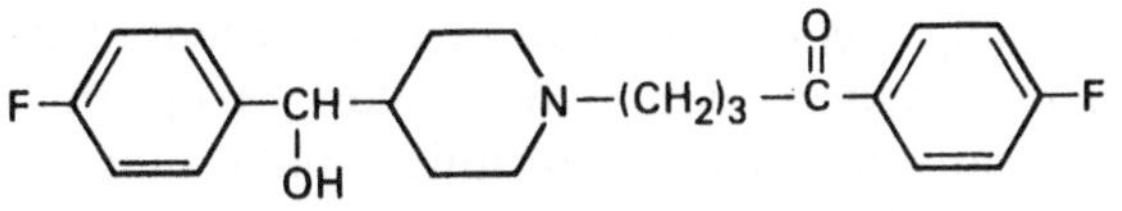

DIHYDROLENPERONE

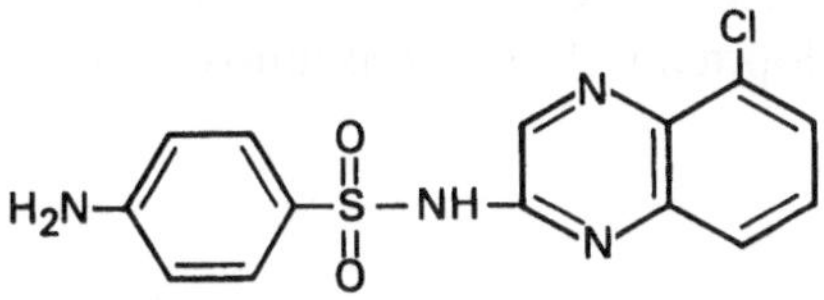

CHLOROQUINOXALINE SULFONAMIDE

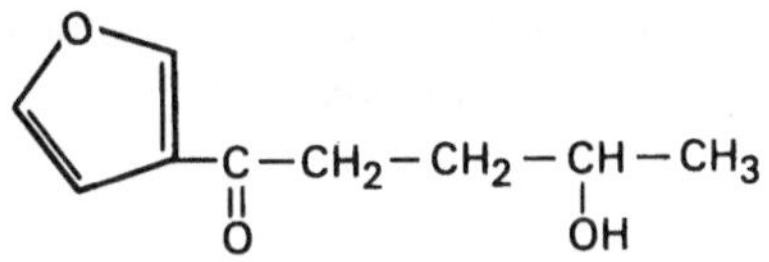

IPOMEANOL

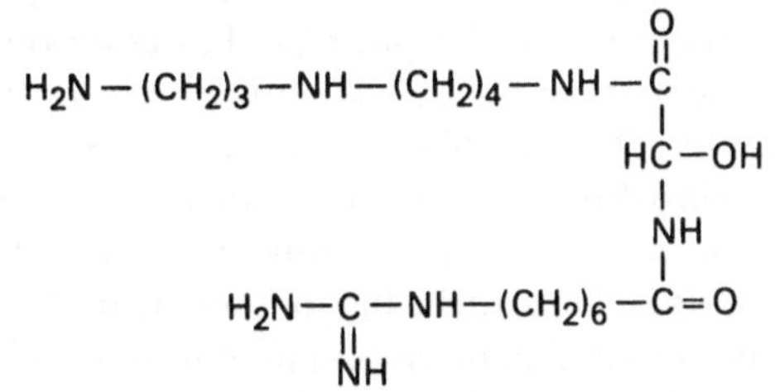

DEOXYSPERGUALIN

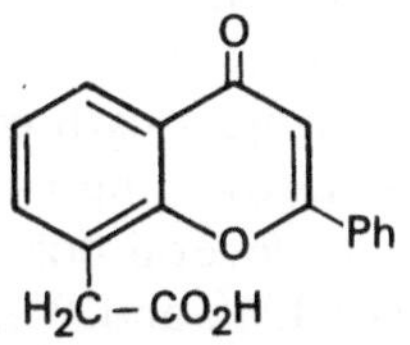

FLAVONE ACETIC ACID

Fig. 3. New anticancer leads currently under active development

achieved in phase I trials in a wide spectrum of tumors—leukemia, lymphoma, and solid tumors. Antitumor activity has been reported in phase II trials in metastatic breast cancer and adult and pediatric leukemia. This drug has been approved for use in several countries for treatment of carcinoma of the breast including locally advanced and metastatic diseases. In the USA it is approved for the treatment of acute nonlymphocytic leukemia.

Anthrapyrazoles

A series of 5-[(aminoalkyl)amino]–substituted anthra[1, 9-*cd*]pyrazol-6 (2*H*)-ones (anthrapyrazoles) were synthesized by the Warner-Lambert/Parke-Davis Co. in a congener program to modify the anthracenedione nucleus, in an effort to reduce the tendency to form semiquinone free radicals, which is believe to be the major cause of the cardiac toxicity of these compounds. Many of the compounds were highly active against a variety of preclinical tumor systems, e.g., L1210 leukemia, B16 melanoma, M5076 sarcoma, and MX-1 mammary xenograft. Several of the compounds studied were curative against every tumor of the above panel. Because of the high activity of the anthrapyrazoles as a class in the

237

NCI tumor panel, additional testing was necessary to identify potential clinical candidates, including mammary adenocarcinoma 16C, colon adenocarcinoma 11a, and Ridgway osteogenic sarcoma. These preclinical data suggest that anthrapyrazoles are similar to doxorubicin in both degree and spectrum of activity. On the basis of their high level of broad-spectrum activity, ease of formulation, possible lack of cross-resistance with doxorubicin, and potential lack of cardiotoxicity, three compounds in the series were selected for further preclinical evaluation and possible clinical development. Two compounds have entered phase I clinical trials.

Tiazofurin

Tiazofurin is another excellent example of discovery through screening. Compounds prepared as part of a targeted research effort to find new antiviral agents were selected by NCI for antitumor screening, on the premise that compounds known to exhibit certain types of biological activity may have an enhanced probability of exhibiting anticancer activity. From this effort emerged 2-β-D-ribofuranosylthiazole-4-carboxamide (Tiazofurin), which has shown remarkable activity against Lewis lung carcinoma in mice, producing ten out of ten long-term survivors at several dose levels. Also, Tiazofurin has demonstrated good activity against L1210 and P388 murine leukemias in vivo. The compound is of considerable biochemical interest since it has been shown to be a specific inhibitor of inosine monophosphate (IMP) dehydrogenase. The compound is metabolized to a nicotinamide adenine dinucleotide (NAD)-like structure, where the nicotinamide portion is replaced by thiazole-4-carboxamide. Tiazofurin is in phase II clinical trials.

Tetraplatin

Tetraplatin is a new platinum IV coordination complex with octahedral geometry in contrast to the square planar cisplatin. Unlike several other platinum complexes, the compound, is stable, water soluble, and can be obtained in good purity. The compound is about equal in potency to cisplatin, but it has slightly greater efficacy against intraperitoneally implanted L1210 leukemia. Interestingly, tetraplatin shows activity against a subline of L1210 leukemia which has acquired resistance to cisplatin, even to the point of producing long-term survivors. Renal biochemical toxicity studies are underway. The compound has been licensed to Upjohn company and is undergoing preclinical toxicology studies.

Merbarone

5-(N-phenylcarboxamide)-2-thiobarbituric acid (merbarone), in contrast to other barbiturates, has shown exceptional antitumor activity agaisnt the L1210 leukemia, as well as good activity against the B16 melanoma and M5076 sarcoma. Importantly, the compound shows curative activity against L1210 when the L1210 leukemia implant site is distant from the drug injection site (intraperitoneal administration for subcutaneous tumor). Merbarone is also active against resistant L1210 and P388 lines. However, the compound is only marginally active against intracerebrally implanted tumor. The lack of strong CNS effects, indicating that the compound does not penetrate the CNS, can be explained on chemical grounds. Even though the compound is a barbiturate, the absence of 5,5-disubstitution contributes to a pKa of 4.0 and renders it highly ionized at physiological pH. Studies of the mechanism of action of Merbarone indicate that it is neither an antimetabolite nor a DNA-binding agent. However, like a few other nonalkylating antitumor drugs, the compound has been shown to produce dose-related DNA single-strand breaks. Merbarone is undergoing phase I clinical trials.

Trimetrexate

Trimetrexate is an interesting 2,4-diaminoquinazoline derivative, which is being jointly developed by NCI and Warner-Lambert/Parke Davis. It is a prolonged inhibitor of dihydrofolate reductase; however, unlike MTX it is not polyglutaminated. Trimetrexate demonstrates activity equivalent to that of MTX against all MTX-sensitive cell lines and is also active against several MTX-resistant lines. In murine models, the anticancer effectiveness of trimetrexate is schedule dependent. In phase I clinical trials, partial responses have been observed in both colon and nonsmall-cell lung cancers. The compound is in phase II clinical trials.

Arabinosyl Azacytosine

Arabinosyl azacytosine is a rationally designed compound that combines the structural elements derived from both ara-C and 5-azacytidine. It shows good activity against P388 and L1210, intravenously implanted Lewis lung carcinoma, and the colon, lung, and mammary xenografts. Ara-AC is the only member of the group of related compounds to reproducibly inhibit the growth of all three xenografts by at least 90%. In addition, Arabinosyl azacytosine (ara-AC) was found to be very active against intracerebrally implanted L1210 leukemia. The compound has entered phase I clinical trials.

Biphenquinate

Substituted 4-quinoline carboxylic acids represent a new class of useful anticancer agents, which is being developed jointly by Dupont Co. and NCI. Biphenquinate was selected for further studies from over 200 related analogs because of

239

its broad spectrum of antitumor activity in several preclinical systems and its desirable pharmaceutical properties. The compound is active in the subrenal capsule assay against the human LX-1 lung, MX-1 mammary, and BL/STX-1 stomach tumors, and against the human HCT-15 colon tumor implanted subcutaneously in nude mice. Biphenquinate has entered phase I clinical trials.

Hexamethylbisacetamide

Evidence accumulated to date suggests that hexamethylbisacetamide (HMBA) is not effective in prolonging life or retarding tumor growth in animals bearing many of the transplantable tumors in common use in antitumor screening programs. Nevertheless, HMBA is highly efficacious in inducing differentiation of a number of cultured cell types, including human HL-60 promyelocytic leukemia. Preliminary data also suggest that HMBA may inhibit the process of tumor promotion. These results suggests a role for HMBA, either alone or in combination with other treatment modalities, in both chemoprevention and cancer therapy. HMBA is currently in phase II clinical trials.

Dihydrolenperone

Dihydrolenperone is a drug that was developed by Merrel Dow Co. as a CNS agent. The compound shows good activity in the HTCFA against lung tumors. The drug displays differential activity in vitro against human tumor cells versus mouse P388 cells. Dihydrolenperone is in phase I clinical trials.

Chloroquinoxaline Sulfonamide

Chloroquinoxaline sulfonamide shows activity in the HTCFA against melanomas and ovarian and lung tumors over a 3-log dosage range (0.1–100 mg/ml). Preclinical toxicology studies have been completed and the compound is expected to enter clinical trials shortly.

Deoxyspergualin

Deoxyspergualin is a novel antibiotic from the Microbial Chemistry Research Foundation in Japan, which shows excellent activity against both intraperitoneally and subcutaneously implanted L1210 leukemia, producing long-term cures. The mechanism of action of this polyamine derivative is not known; neither ornithine decarboxylase nor S-adenosylmethionine decarboxylase is inhibited. The compound undergoes metabolic oxidation by amine oxidases to produce the active agent. Deoxyspergualin is in phase I clinical trials.

240

Ipomeanol

Ipomeanol is a natural product isolated from moldy sweet potatoes. This furan derivative undergoes metabolic activation by the P450 system of the pulmonary Clara cells; it covalently binds to and acts as a specific toxin to these cells. Ipomeanol is being developed as a specific anticancer agent for tumors derived from the Clara cells, which are the stem cells for the bronchioalveolar tissue. The compound is about to enter clinical trials.

Flavone Acetic Acid

Flavone acetic acid is an exciting new lead, which is being developed rapidly. Flavone acetic acid given on days 2 and 9 at a dose of 267 mg/kg inhibited tumor growth completely in 60%–80% of mice with early-stage colon adenocarcinoma 38. The therapeutic efficacy of flavone against this tumor was retained when the sites of tumor implantation and drug administration were separated. Flavone acetic acid also caused regression of advanced (500-mg) colon 38 tumors. Unlike many other potential anticancer agents, only modest activity was observed for this compound against either P388 or L1210 leukemia. Based on the excellent activity observed against the highly refractory colon 38 model, flavone acetic acid is currently being evaluated phase I/phase II clinical trials. This trial is an important part of a prospective study to determine whether compounds identified by preclinical solid tumor models are more effective against human solid tumors than those agents identified by experimental leukemia models.

Future Directions

Recently, the United States NCI has undertaken a major restructuring of its anticancer drug-screening program. The restructuring represents a shift in emphasis from a compound-oriented strategy to a specific disease-oriented strategy focusing on major solid tumors for which there has been limited success in identifying active drugs. We will be replacing the mouse leukemia P388 prescreen with a new in vitro prescreen system consisting of panels of human tumor cell lines. The initial focus will be in vitro antitumor drug screening, utilizing a panel composed principally of human lung tumor cell lines. Compounds showing highly selective in vitro activity against a target tumor type would be earmarked for preclinical development and clinical trials in relevant target populations. Compounds showing a nonselective pattern of in vitro activity would be studied further in an in vivo tumor panel for antitumor activity.

In addition, biochemical prescreens—based, for example, on inhibition of oncogene expression, topoisomerases, protein kinases, and metastasis—would be utilized for the selection of materials for screening in the NCI disease-oriented anticancer drug discovery project. Thus, the future looks promising for the discovery of selective anticancer agents utilizing both screening and rational approaches based on principles emerging from new knowledge of tumor biology and modern medicinal chemistry.

References

1. Pinedo HM, Chabner BA (eds) (1984) Cancer chemotherapy, vol 6. Elsevier, New York
2. Jackson RC (1985) Mathematical modelling in drug design and utilization. Abstracts of the Eighth Annual Bristol-Myers Symposium on Cancer Research
3. Driscoll JS (1984) The preclinical new drug research program of the National Cancer Institute. Cancer Treat Rep 68: 63–76
4. Venditti JM, Wesley RA, Plowman J (1984) Current NCI preclinical antitumor screening in-vivo: Results of tumor panel screening, 1976–1982, and future directions. Adv Pharmacol Chemother 20: 1–20
5. Hodes L (1981) Computer-aided selection of compounds for antitumor screening: Validation of a statistical-heuristic method. J Chem Inf Comput Sci 21: 128–132
6. Nasr M, Paull KD, Narayanan VL (1984) Computer-assisted structure-activity correlations. Adv Pharmacol Chemother 20: 123–190
7. Lomax NR, Narayanan VL (1984) Chemical structures of interest to the Division of Cancer Treatment. NCI 4

12. New Drug Trials

G. Sarosy, L. Rubinstein, and B. Leyland-Jones

Introduction

Although most malignant tumors are either largely refractory to current chemotherapy (e.g., melanoma) or responsive but incurable (e.g., breast and small
cell lung cancer) some neoplasms such as choriocarcinoma, testicular cancer,
several childhood cancers and hemopoietic malignancies are curable by chemotherapy alone. The success in chemotherapy responsive tumors provides a
powerful incentive to continue to explore chemotherapeutic options in refractory cancers, and this, coupled to the continuing need to lessen toxicity without
compromising efficacy has resulted in major efforts to develop and evaluate new
cytoxic drugs, a process which requires the participation of numerous investigators at both preclinical and clinical levels.

Overview

The wide availability of an antineoplastic agent is the culmination of many years
of work. The agent must demonstrate activity in a preclinical screen, after which
its toxicities are established in several animal species. Based on this information,
the initial trials (phase I) in humans define the highest doses of the agent which
can be administered safely. Once the phase I trials are complete, phase II trials
are undertaken to determine whether the drug is active against individual tumor
types. Phase III trials then define the efficacy of the new agent in comparison
with standard therapy for the particular tumor type.

Preclinical Toxicology

Drugs undergo preclinical toxicology testing in order to establish a safe starting
dose for clinical trials, and help predict some of the toxicities that might be
expected in humans [1]. Initially, toxicology studies were conducted in rodents,

dogs, and monkeys [2]. In early phase I trials, the starting dose in humans was one-third of the toxic dose low (TDL) in the most sensitive large animal species. The TDL was defined as the lowest dose producing toxicity, assuming that doubling the dose did not cause lethality. Doses were established in milligrams per square meter (mg/m^2) because it was shown that body surface was more accurate than weight for interspecies conversion [3–5].

Recently, the manner in which the starting dose for phase I trials is established has been reevaluated. Freireich et al. [4] were the first to show that mice, rats, hamsters, dogs, and monkeys were equally predictive of the toxic doses in humans. This has been confirmed by several other investigators [3, 5, 6], and, based upon this work, the starting dose in phase I trials is now usually derived from murine data. A dose response curve for the new agent is developed in mice, and the lethal dose is defined for 10% (LD_{10}), 50%, and 100% of the mice treated.

The dose equivalent to the LD_{10} in mice in mg/m^2, the murine equivalent lethal dose in 10%, (or $MELD_{10}$) is then tested in another species, usually in dogs. If the $MELD_{10}$ produces no toxicity in dogs, then one-tenth of the $MELD_{10}$ is used as the entry level dose in the phase I trial. If the $MELD_{10}$ does cause toxicity in dogs, then the initial human dose is one-third of the lowest dose producing minimal toxicity in this species (TDL), or a fraction of one-tenth of the $MELD_{10}$ [1].

There are several problems inherent in defining the starting dose for a phase I trial. Firstly, the toxicity seen preclinically does not necessarily predict that which will be observed in humans. Whereas there is good correlation between the toxicity seen in rapidly dividing tissues such as bone marrow and gastrointestinal mucosa in mice, rats, dogs, and monkeys and that seen in similar tissues in humans, the correlation of toxicities of less rapidly dividing tissues is not as good [2]. In general, data from large animal species, such as dogs and monkeys, overpredict human renal and hepatic toxicity and underpredict cutaneous, cardiac, and peripheral nervous system toxicity in humans. Secondly, differences in life span cause another problem in translating preclinical data to humans [7]. The short life span of animals in which these agents are tested preclinically makes it difficult to predict the chronic and long term toxicities which may be observed in humans.

Schedule Selection

Once the human starting dose has been defined, a schedule of administration must be chosen. The number of separate schedules to be studied is determined by several factors: (a) evidence of schedule dependency in experimental in vivo systems, (b) pharmacokinetics, (c) existing clinical data for similar compounds suggesting superiority of a particular schedule, (d) patient convenience, and (e) other properties of the drug such as solubility.

Drugs which are highly schedule dependent in preclinical models undergo phase I evaluation in the schedule which appears optimal. However, preclinical schedule dependency has not been shown to predict the most active schedule in humans. In addition, no antitumor agent active against solid tumors has shown significant schedule dependency in humans. Prospective trials are ongoing to determine whether experimental models can predict the schedule dependency of efficacy and toxicity. Drugs which show no particular schedule dependency with respect to preclinical testing are initially tested in humans at two extremes of schedule, i.e., a single bolus dose per course and 5-day continuous infusion [8].

Phase I Trials

Objectives, and Patient Selection

Once the starting dose and schedules of administration have be established, phase I trials are undertaken. A phase I trial has two major goals: (a) to define the maximally tolerated dose (MTD) in humans and (b) to define and quantitate the human toxicities. Although phase I trials are conducted with therapeutic intent, antitumor activity is not a primary objective. Separate trials are performed in patients with acute leukemia and in those with solid tumors since a higher MTD is accepted for myelosuppressive drugs in patients with acute leukemia. In addition, separate phase I trials are undertaken in children since the MTD in a pediatric population is frequently higher, and the spectrum of toxicity may differ from that seen in adults. In general, pediatric phase I trials are not initiated until the adult phase I trials have been completed, and activity has been seen in adult phase I trials [9].

Because the primary goal of a phase I trial is to define the toxicity of new anticancer agents, the criteria for patient eligibility are strict. Only patients with microscopically confirmed malignancy in whom all conventional therapy has failed or for whom there is no effective therapy should be eligible. Patients must have normal organ function (adequate bone marrow reserve for patients with solid tumors, and normal hepatic, renal and cardiac function) so that toxicity of the new agent can be distinguished from disease. In patients with functional impairment of a major organ, drug administration may result in increased toxicity because of decreased clearance. Therefore, separate phase I trials are undertaken to define pharmacokinetics and safe doses for patients with abnormal organ function. These trials usually begin when the MTD has been defined in those with normal organ function. To conserve patient resources, these trials are frequently not initiated until the drug has shown evidence of activity in phase II trials.

Finally, before patients are enrolled on a phase I trial, they must give written informed consent, indicating that they are aware of the investigational nature of the agent they will receive, and aware that they may experience toxicity and no significant benefit. They must be aware that other treatment options, including no further therapy, would be equally satisfactory. In addition, a candidate for a phase I trial should ideally receive no concomitant medication which might influence the pharmacokinetic behavior of a new agent. Since this is unrealistic for most patients with advanced malignancies, concomitant medication should be minimized and carefully recorded.

In addition to possessing normal organ function, patients entering a phase I trial should have a sufficiently long life expectancy, i.e., 3 months, so that the toxicities of the new agent can be adequately assessed. In general, performance status is an indicator of life expectancy; therefore, patients should have a minimum Karnofsky performance status of 60%. Adequate time, e.g., 4 weeks, should have elapsed since prior therapy so that the patient has completely recovered from all toxicities associated with it. This should be extended to 6 weeks if the previous therapy included mitomycin C or a nitrosourea. Because a new drug may have unknown teratogenic effects, women of child-bearing potential should be specifically excluded.

Dose Escalation

Once the initial dose for a phase I trial has been selected, patients are treated in small cohorts at increasing dose levels. Most dose escalation schemes initially employ large dose increments which rapidly decrease when toxicity is observed, e.g., the modified Fibonacci scheme [10]. Another escalation scheme uses increments of 50% of the original dose, decreasing to 25% increments when toxicity is observed, but this has not been as widely tested as the modified Fibonacci scheme [11].

The aim of all dose escalation schemes is to define the MTD (the highest dose which can be given to man) in the smallest number of dose levels which can be safely administered. In such a fashion, the number of patients receiving sub-therapeutic doses is kept as low as possible.

At present, most phase I trials use a modified Fibonacci dose escalation scheme (Table 1). The dose increments may be made smaller if the drug has shown an unusually steep dose-toxicity curve during preclinical testing. Using this system, there is a great deal of variability in the number of dose increments required to achieve the MTD of various drugs. To minimize the number of dose levels required, yet maintain patient safety, alternative methods of dose escalation are being studied. Among the most promising is dose escalation based on preclinical pharmacology data, which will be discussed later in this chapter.

In any phase I trial, three patients previously untreated with the phase I agent are entered at each dose level because intrapatient escalation may confound interpretation of toxicity. For example, the toxicity experienced by a patient after the second course of an investigational agent given at the higher dose may represent the acute toxicity of one course of therapy at the higher dose, or the chronic toxicity of two courses of therapy. Because the administration of the agent at a new dose level may be associated with unknown toxicities, patients are

Table 1. Idealized modified Fibonacci dose escalation scheme

Dose level	Dose	Increase above previous dose level (%)
1	n	
2	$2n$	100
3	$3.3n$	67
4	$5n$	50
5	$7n$	40
6	$9n$	33
7	$12n$	33
8	$16n$	33

hospitalized and closely monitored for a minimum of 24 h following their first dose. In addition, escalation to a higher dose level should not occur until the safety of the current level has been established, in order to minimize the risk of toxicity occurring with increasing severity at two dose levels simultaneously. In general, this means that dose escalation should not take place until at least three patients have been observed for an entire treatment period (e.g., 3–5 weeks) at the previous dose level.

The precise dose escalation scheme varies among investigators, but a commonly used design proceeds as follows:

1. Three patients previously untreated with the phase I agent are placed on each succeeding dose level, until reversible moderate or severe (grade 3 or 4) toxicity is observed.
2. If one instance of grade 3 or 4 toxicity is observed among the initial three patients treated at a particular dose level, then up to three additional patients untreated with the phase I agent, are placed on that dose level. If no grade 3 or 4 toxicity is observed among the additional three patients, then dose escalation resumes in cohorts of three.
3. If two instance of grade 3 or 4 toxicity are observed while treating patients at a particular dose level, then the previous scheduled dose level is declared to be the MTD. (This design may be augmented at this point by testing at a new dose level between the one demonstrating two instances of grade 3 or 4 toxicity and the previous scheduled dose level.)

The rationale for the above design is as follows. It is felt that, in general, a rate of grade 3 or 4 toxicity not exceeding 20% is tolerable, while a rate exceeding 40% is excessive. The phase I design should have moderate power to discriminate between these two rates, while keeping at a minimum the number of patients treated at subtherapeutic dose levels. The above design yields a probability of 0.70 escalation at a given dosage level, if the underlying rate of grade 3 or 4 toxicity is 20%; it gives a probability of 0.31 of escalating at a given dosage level if the underlying rate of grade 3 or 4 toxicity is 40%.

End points

The endpoints of a phase I trial are very important since, as well as defining the toxicity of a new anticancer agent in humans, and the highest dose which can be safely administered, the results of a phase I trial permit determination of the dose recommended for further evaluation. The exact definition of the MTD varies among investigators; however, it is generally considered to be that dose which produces reversible moderate or severe (grade 3 or 4) toxicity in no more than one of six patients treated at the dose level. The recommended phase II starting dose is usually one level below. The MTD is frequently dependent upon the amount and type of prior therapy which a patient has had. Therefore, this should be carefully considered in analyzing the data from phase I trials and defining a phase II starting dose, which will be used to treat patients with minimal or no prior therapy. The concept of an MTD is based on the principle that for most cytoxic agents there is a monotonic relationship between the dose administered and the effect observed. However, for drugs which are used to modulate the effect of another, and for biologic response modifiers, increasing the concentration beyond a certain threshold may not increase the therapeutic effect. Therefore, the end point of a trial of a biochemical modulator should be the attainment of a level optimizing the desired effect in vivo, not necessarily the MTD based on toxicity.

In phase I trials, the number of patients treated at each dose level, including the dose recommended for phase II, is relatively small. Accordingly, it is important that continued careful monitoring takes place during phase II and III trials to identify less frequent acute toxicities, as well as cumulative and chronic toxicities [10].

Because the primary purpose of a phase I trial is to define the toxicities of a new agent, the absence of antitumor activity is not a reason to stop development of the drug. Many patients are treated at what are later found to be subtherapeutic levels and less than optimal schedules of drug administration. The patients entered onto phase I trials often have relatively drug-resistant tumors and frequently have received extensive prior therapy, which minimizes the chance of response. Hence, the only reason not to pursue phase II trials is unacceptable toxicity in phase I trials. Definition of the level of activity in each tumor type then takes place in phase II.

Preclinical Pharmacology as a Guide to Dose Escalation

The two objectives of a phase I trial—to establish an MTD as safely as possible and a recommended dose for phase II as quickly as possible—are contradictory. Rapid dose escalation prevents a large number of patients from receiving subtherapeutic doses of the new agent, and hastens the speed at which the drug enters phase II evaluation. However, if dose escalation occurs too rapidly, a new level may be lethal whereas the previous one was nontoxic.

The present method of establishing the phase I starting dose in humans, based on preclinical toxicology testing in rodents, has proved safe [1]. The same holds true for the modified Fibonacci scheme, which has permitted definition of an MTD without unacceptable toxicity [11]. Unfortunately, this system may permit patients to receive doses that are later recognized as being subtherapeutic. In a recent article, Collins et al. [12] have analyzed the results of a modified Fibonacci scheme for 17 drugs, when one-tenth of $MELD_{10}$ is the entry dose. For five of these drugs, ten or more dose escalations would be required to reach the MTD. An additional four to six escalation steps are required for those drugs (approximately half of all drugs that enter clinical trial) which begin phase I evaluation at one-third of one-tenth of $MELD_{10}$ [1]. Clearly, alternative methods of dose escalation are needed that protect patient safety but allow definition of dose limiting toxicities with markedly fewer dose escalations [12].

Collins et al. [12] have proposed a method of dose escalation based on murine pharmacokinetic data. By defining target plasma levels of drug in humans prospectively, one can attempt to attain these plasma levels in a more expeditious fashion.

Murine toxicology data have adequately predicted human toxicity overall, in view of the safety of the starting dose for human phase I trials based on the $MELD_{10}$ [6]. However, murine toxicology data have not been nearly as useful in predicting the behavior of individual drugs. If it were possible to identify the pharmacologic basis for this variation between species, murine pharmacologic data could be used to design a dose escalation scheme. Potential sources of difference include target cell sensitivity; duration of exposure to a critical drug concentration; and degree of protein binding, metabolism, or elimination. Differences in target cell sensitivity can be determined through in vitro testing. In a similar manner, schedule dependency testing can predict whether threshold effects will differ in mice and man. For those drugs for which preclinical testing suggests that there are no differences in threshold effects (i.e., a minimal concentration being required for pharmacologic effects) and target cell sensitivity, murine pharmacology data can be used to predict that level which is likely to cause toxicity in man. Underlying this assumption is the fact that the concentration-versus-time curve has been shown to correlate better with toxicity than peak plasma levels or absolute concentration [13]. In a retrospective analysis, Collins et al. [12] have shown that such an approach could reduce the number of escalation steps by about 20%–50% [12].

The Blood Level Working Group at the National Cancer Institute (NCI) has recently initiated this approach to dose escalation for those drugs for which it is appropriate. For example, merbarone, a conjugate of thiobarbituric acid, is undergoing phase I escalation. Because the severity of toxicity during preclinical evaluation appeared to increase with higher infusion rates, merbarone is being tested only in one schedule, a 120-h continuous intravenous infusion. In preclinical testing, murine and human target tissues did not differ in sensitivity to merbarone; furthermore, the two species did not differ in threshold effects. Hence, merbarone was an ideal drug for which to use murine data as an aid in defining a dose escalation scheme. The trial is ongoing, with dose escalations guided by murine pharmacology data, rather than by a modified Fibonacci scheme. A similar approach to dose escalation has been used with flavone acetic acid, deoxyspergualin, and oxanthrazole.

Phase II Trials

Objectives and Patient Selection

Once a drug has completed phase I evaluation, and if it is not associated with intolerable or unacceptably erratic toxicity, phase II trials are undertaken to screen for activity. Hence, only patients with objectively measurable disease are entered onto phase II trials. The principal goals of phase II trial are to define response rate and response duration and to record toxicities. Phase II trials should have the smallest possible number of patients permitting detection of a significant level of activity with reasonable confidence. Such a strategy permits rapid identification of active new agents while minimizing the chance of false-negative results.

Although a phase II trial defines the activity of a new agent, it does not assess efficacy. Definition of efficacy requires comparison with other agents used to treat the disease in question. Such a comparison requires a randomized phase III trial. However, since the screen for activity determines whether the drug will undergo further evaluation, the outcome of phase II trials is an important point in the drug's development [14].

In addition to defining the activity of a new anticancer agent, phase II trials provide further information concerning toxicity. Because a larger number of patients are treated than in phase I studies, previously unknown, rare acute toxicities may be observed. Chronic toxicities may be observed initially in patients with stable or responding disease who receive larger cumulative doses than are commonly administered in phase I [9].

During phase II testing, the agent is evaluated in a broad range of tumor types. However, during the past decade, there has been a trend away from broad phase II trials, into which large numbers of patients, heterogeneous with respect to tumor type and extent of prior therapy, were entered. Usually, the number of patients entered with each disease was so small that an estimate of activity against individual tumor types could not be reliably made. Phase II trials are now usually disease-specific, so that an estimate of activity can be made within diagnostic categories. Hence, a promising level of activity can be either established or excluded within reasonable confidence limits, thereby indicating whether the drug should be further investigated in that disease. An attempt is made to screen the drug in a large number of tumor types. At a minimum, this screen should include malignancies that are common, such as lung and breast cancer, and those that are generally considered either sensitive (e.g., lymphoma) or resistant (e.g., melanoma) to chemotherapy. An attempt is made to conduct two phase II trials for each tumor type to obtain a more reliable estimate of activity than can be made in a single trial.

Because the decision whether to pursue the evaluation of an agent rests on the outcome of phase II trials, it is essential that the drug is studied in the patient population most likely to respond. Recently, patient characteristics such as performance status and extent of prior therapy have been shown to be important determinants of response [14]. Hence, the patient population entered onto phase II trials must possess optimum performance status and the minimum amount of prior therapy consistent with good medical practice. If a patient has a malignancy for which potentially curative therapy exists, this should be administered prior to the investigational phase II agent. However, because for most common malignancies there is no treatment that is either curative or capable of providing long-term control, a phase II agent can often be given as initial or early therapy. For example, phase II trials in sensitive tumors—such as breast, ovary, and small-cell lung cancer, rhabdomyosarcoma, and non-Hodgkin's lymphoma—should ideally take place in those in whom no more than one prior regimen has failed. One can also justify initial treatment with a phase II agent in subgroups within these disease categories whose malignancies progress very slowly, and/or for whom therapy will not be curative. Such subgroups include some patients with metastatic breast cancer, stage IV ovary cancer, and indolent non-Hodgkin's lymphoma. If one chooses to treat these patients with a phase II agent initially, then one must administer standard therapy as soon as there is evidence of disease progression or nonresponse. Initial therapy with a phase II agent is unlikely to lessen the ability to respond to standard therapy. In addition, since therapy will not be curative, the delay in initiating palliative therapy is unlikely to affect survival. Similarly, in disease sites such as head and neck carcinoma in which chemotherapy yields a high response rate, but no improvement in survival, patient eligibility should be restricted to those with no prior therapy. In disease sites for which there is no effective therapy—such as malignancies of the colon, kidney, liver, and pancreas and melanoma—phase II trials should also be limited initially to patients with no prior therapy.

Requiring the demonstration of activity in an optimal patient population prior to more widespread administration prevents more heavily pretreated patients with poorer performance status from experiencing the toxicity of what may be an inactive drug. Also, screening for activity in patients with minimal prior therapy and maximal performance status—who are presumably at an earlier stage of the disease, when the tumor burden is less—facilitates the identification of active agents in the shortest period of time. Finally, in terms of patient numbers, it is unfortunate that in many phase II trials in the literature many more patients than were necessary to make an estimate of activity were entered; this is particularly unfortunate when the phase II agent is inactive [15, 16].

Statistical Design

We will describe briefly several statistical designs for phase II trials which are curently widely used. The oldest and most familiar is the two-stage design of Gehan [17]. The first stage for the trial is designed to allow the elimination of ineffective agents after treatment of the smallest number of patients. In particular, if one wishes to screen for a response rate of at least 20%, the first stage involves accrual of 14 patients. If no responses are observed among the initial 14 evaluable patients, then one can terminate accrual and rule out, with 0.95 confidence a 20% (or more) response rate for that agent (since a drug with a 20% response rate will yield at least one response among 14 patients with probability of 0.956). The second stage of the trial is designed to yield a certain maximum standard error for the response rate estimate. In particular, if at least one response is observed among the initial 14 evaluable patients, accrual of 11 additional patients will assure a standard error of no more than 0.1. Accrual of 40 evaluable patients, in total, will assure a standard error of no more than 0.08.

A more recent two-stage design is that of Fleming [18]. It assures adequate statistical power to discriminate between two prespecified response rates, the lower rate (P_0) being one for which further testing would be clearly unwarranted, and the upper rate (P_1) being one for which further testing would be clearly desirable. For diseases for which no active agents exist, such as colon cancer, P_0 and P_1 would typically be chosen to be 5% and 20%, respectively. On the other hand, for screening analogs in diseases for which there are active agents, P_0 and P_1 might be chosen to be 20% and 40%, respectively. The Fleming design also allows for early termination of the trial after a prespecified initial accrual stage, if the results are either extremely unpromising or extremely promising.

An example of a Fleming two-stage design, to discriminate between response rates of 5% and 20% is as follows. Thirty evaluable patients are accrued, and the agent is considered worthy of further testing if at least four responses (13% response rate) are observed. Accrual is terminated after the initial 15 patients if either no responses or at least four responses (27% response rate) are observed. The design gives a probability of 0.942 of a negative result if the true response rate is 5%, and gives a probability of 0.865 of a positive result if the true response rate is 20%. In general, if one wishes to limit to 5% the probability of a false-positive result (declaring the agent "active" when the true response rate is P_0) and to limit to 15%–20% the probability of a false-negative result (declaring the agent "inactive" when the true rate is P_1), the Fleming two-stage designs will require 25–45 patients, with provision for early termination about midway through the total potential accrual.

Randomized phase II trials, which adopt the small sample sizes and early stopping rules of the one-armed phase II designs, are gaining popularity for the reasons given by Simon, Wittes, and Ellenberg [19]. It is understood that these trials cannot be used for comparison of efficacy (which requires much larger phase III trials employing different end points). However, they can facilitate tentative comparisons of agents by reducing the differences in patient selection, and other factors, which make sequential phase II trials difficult to compare. Simon et al. give minimum sample sizes to assure that an agent with a response rate 15% greater than its randomized competitors will demonstrate a higher observed response rate with probability of at least 0.90. For trials involving two or three arms, this requires, in general, 30–55 patients per arm.

Phase III Trials

Objectives and Statistical Design

Based on the promising results in the phase II trials, phase III trials are undertaken to establish the efficacy of the new agent relative to standard therapy. These phase III comparsions can be designed with two different goals: randomized trials can define whether the new agent has activity equivalent to that of the standard therapy compound, but with less toxicity; alternatively, a phase III trial may establish whether the new agent has greater activity than standard therapy.

In general, trials which seek to demonstrate improved outcome provide more valuable information; for example, the lack of curative therapy for patients with metastatic breast cancer mandates a search for better therapy. If a new agent demonstrates superior activity, a potentially major advance in the treatment of the disease will have been made. If phase II trials suggest that the new agent and standard therapy have equivalent activity, phase III trials designed to demonstrate equivalence and differing toxicity may be reasonable. However, in such trials, it is imperative that there be adequate power to detect the minimal clinically significant decrease in efficacy which may result from use of the new agent. This difference may be smaller than the corresponding minimal difference one would have targeted in a positive outcome trial, since one may be more willing to err in the direction of preserving the established therapy; therefore, such equivalence studies will have larger sample sizes.

The most important end point of the activity comparison is survival. Survival percentages can be compared at a fixed time point, e.g., 1 year post randomization. However, a statistically more efficient technique is to compare the entire survival curves by means of the Mantel-Haenszel log-rank statistic [20]. The power of this test increases with the magnitude of the difference in median survival to be detected and with the expected number of deaths to be observed [21]. This means that trials in diseases with long median survivals require a far greater number of patients than do trials in diseases with short median survivals. For example, in a disease with a median survival of 6 months for the standard therapy, it may be felt sufficient to be able to detect an increase in median survival of 6 months for the experimental therapy. This twofold difference in median survival will be detected with 0.90 probability if 72 deaths are observed, and in such a rapidly lethal disease this may require the accrual of only slightly more than 100 patients. On the other hand, in a disease with a median survival of 3 years for the standard therapy, it may be felt that a 1.5-fold increase must be detectable for the experimental therapy. To detect a 1.5-fold difference in median survival with 0.90 probability requires 210 deaths, which could translate into a required accrual of 400–500 patients. Even scaling back one's requirement to detection of such a difference with 0.80 probability only reduces the required sample size by about 30%. Sometimes, this difficulty may be partially circumvented by using an earlier surrogate end point, such as disease-free survival.

In large trials such as those just described, it has become common to include rules for early termination in case one regimen should prove substantially less active. A commonly used design is that of Fleming, Harrington, and O'Brien [22], which allows for monitoring at several interim points prior to the scheduled termination of the trial. In general, this design is applied so that early termination occurs only for relatively extreme early differences in either direction, e.g., differences that are significant at the two-sided 0.005 level of probability. Thus, the final comparison generally preserves the statistical power it would have in the absence of early stopping rules.

A final consideration in new agent development is examination of the optimal drug dosages when the new agent is combined with other agents. One would like to compare alternative dosage ratios and determine the optimal combined dosage. This may be evaluated by means of the response surface designs of Carter, Wampler, and Stablein [23]. An example of such a design for a two drug regimen might involve the 16 different drug combinations created by varying each drug over four possible dosages, with sixteen patients randomized to each of the combinations. The results of the trial are then fitted to a parametric model of the effect of the drug dosages on survival (or response), and the fitted model is used to estimate the optimal dosage. Care must be taken to assure that the model may be adequately fitted to the data.

Analog Development

Because the identification of novel structures possessing significant anticancer activity is a rare event, there is a great deal of interest in developing analogs with greater potency, or less toxicity than the parent compound, or a different spectrum of clinical activity. For example, Selenazofurin, a selenium-substituted analog of Tiazofurin was studied because of greater potency in vitro [24]. On the other hand, 4'-deoxydoxorubicin has undergone clinical evaluation because of activity in a colon xenograft in which deoxorubicin was inactive [25]. Antifolate analogs such as piritrexim and trimetrexate have been designed in an attempt to overcome the biochemical basis for methotrexate (MTX) resistance, thereby increasing the degree and perhaps the spectrum of clinical activity [26]. Nevertheless, few analogs thus far have shown a different spectrum of activity, or increased potency clinically. As a result, decreased toxicity has become the major reason to develop most analogs.

Many of the anthracycline analogs, such as epirubicin, have undergone further evaluation based on the suggestion of decreased cardiotoxicity compared with doxorubicin [27, 28]. Platinum analogs, such as carboplatin, have been pursued clinically in an attempt to overcome the dose-limiting nephrotoxicity of the parent compound, cisplatin [29]. Regardless of the reason for which an analog is chosen for further development, one should seek to determine its efficacy relative to the parent compound in the smallest number of patients possible.

Development Strategy

We will use the development of antifolates as an example of drug class and trimetrexate as a specific example. Similar plans could be outlined for platinum and anthracycline analogs. This topic has been comprehensively reviewed in a recent article [30].

Because antifolate analogs have been developed to overcome the biochemical basis of MTX resistance, it would be most logical to test these analogs in resistant human tumors, and to determine whether the analog showed activity through the biochemical mechanism for which it was designed. Unfortunately, the measurement of such biochemical end points in a clinical trial is only beginning to be developed, and it presents great technical difficulties. Therefore, one must design a trial with clinical end points to establish the efficacy of the analog relative to MTX. One strategy to evaluate the efficacy of trimetrexate relative to MTX requires testing in three groups of diseases based on their sensitivity to MTX. Tailoring the testing of the analog to the activity of the parent compound permits rapid identification of any possible therapeutic advance. For example, one can divide the diseases in which one wishes to evaluate trimetrexate into three groups according to the role of MTX in standard therapy:

1. Tumors in which MTX is an important component of a standard regimen that has state-of-the-art effectiveness: lymphoma, osteosarcoma, breast, small-cell lung, (leukemia).
2. Tumors in which MTX has antitumor activity but no defined role in standard state-of-the-art regimens: head and neck, bladder, cervix.
3. Tumors in which MTX has insufficient activity to warrant its use alone or in combination: NSCLCA, colon, esophagus, stomach, brain, pancreas, prostate.

One can design a mehtod of evaluating trimetrexate in each of these three groups; such a strategy is also applicable to other analogs.

Group 1

The role of an analog is probably most difficult to determine in the first group of diseases. A precise way of evaluating the activity of trimetrexate relative to MTX would be a trial in which patients were randomized to a regimen containing MTX or to one identical except for the substitution of trimetrexate. However, such a trial requires large numbers of patients and a long follow-up period. In order to facilitate the establishment of the efficacy of the analog, an alternative plan was proposed for trimetrexate. Phase II trials in MTX-sensitive tumors were designed to indicate whether trimetrexate and MTX possessed equivalent activity. Phase II trials were also undertaken in patients in whom prior therapy with MTX had failed. The demonstration of activity in MTX-refractory disease would suggest that trimetrexate and MTX were at least partially noncross-resistant.

To illustrate how one might evaluate trimetrexate in diseases sensitive to MTX, one can examine a testing strategy in breast cancer. Phase II evaluation of trimetrexate in breast cancer could take place in three separate populations of patients with advanced disease: (a) previously untreated patients, (b) those in whom cyclophosphamide-doxorubicin-5-fluorouracil (CAF) therapy failed, and (c) those in whom cyclophosphamide-methotrexate-5-fluorouracil (CMF) therapy failed. The number of responses observed in previously untreated patients would provide the best estimation of the activity of trimetrexate. If the level of activity of trimetrexate appeared significantly higher than that of the parent compound, then a randomized phase III comparison would be an important priority. Activity in patients in whom CMF had failed would suggest that these two agents were at least partially noncross-resistant. If the results of phase II trials suggested that these two compounds had equivalent activity, and trimetrexate showed activity in patients previously treated with CMF, then development of salvage regimens containing the analog would become a priority.

Based on the results of these phase II trials, phase III trials are undertaken to establish more precisely the efficacy of trimetrexate relative to MTX. These phase III comparisons of a parent compound and analog can take the form of improved outcome or equivalence trials. Equivalence studies are more difficult to design, and the results are frequently difficult to interpret. The contribution of MTX to CMF has not been fully defined; as a result, a study demonstrating that CMF and cyclophosphamide-trimetrexate-5-fluorouracil (CTF) have equivalent activity but that CTF has less toxicity would not identify the role of trimetrexate in breast cancer.

Group 2

In the second group of diseases, phase II screening of the new agent does not provide useful information. In general, a study of the analog for 30 patients might merely indicate that the agent has activity similar to that to the parent compound within broad confidence limits.

An alternative approach is a randomized trial against the parent compound immediately after the dose limiting toxicities have been determined in phase I. Such a trial must have early stopping rules, so that the trial can be terminated if the analog appears less active. A particularly appropriate early stopping design in such a case is that of Ellenberg and Eisenberg [31], which would involve monitoring the trial at approximately the midpoint of accrual and terminating early if the analog failed to demonstrate greater activity. Such a rule can be applied in such a way that the power of the trial to detect a clinically significant improvement for the analog is not substantially decreased. However, this design is better applied to a trial with response rate, as opposed to survival, as the end point.

As an example of the above, a randomized trial of trimetrexate and MTX in head and neck cancer should quickly establish the relative efficacy and toxicity of trimetrexate. Since MTX has not been shown to improve survival in this group of patients, it is essential to establish quickly, and in the smallest number of patients possible, whether the analog provides a significant advantage.

Group 3

For this third group of diseases, evaluation is straightforward. Because MTX is inactive, demonstration of the relative activity and toxicity of the analog is unnecessary. Therefore, the analog is screened in a broad range of tumor types. Further testing is undertaken only if trimetrexate demonstrates significant activity.

Conclusions

The complexity of many modern chemotherapy regimens has increased the difficulty of defining both the degree of activity of new drugs as well as their precise role in the treatment of specific diseases. This necessitates a scrupulously scientific approach to the clinical evaluation of new drugs. Such an approach is the best way to ensure that the greatest number of patients receive the maximum benefit both from currently standard treatment approaches as well as from newly developed, active cytoxic drugs.

References

1. Greishaber CK, Marsoni S (1986) Relation of preclinical toxicology to findings in early clinical trials. Cancer Treat Rep 70: 65–72
2. DeVita VT (1985) Principles in chemotherapy. In: DeVitra V, Hellman S, Rosenberg SA (eds) Cancer principles and practice of oncology. J.B. Lippincott, Philadelphia, pp 257–285
3. Homan ER (1972) Quantitative relationships between toxic doses of antitumor chemotherapeutic agents in animals and man. Cancer Chemother Rep 3: 13–19
4. Freireich EJ, Gehan EA, Rall DP, Schmidt LH, Skipper HE (1966) Quantitative comparison of toxicity of anticancer agents in mouse, rat, hamster, dog, monkey, and man. Cancer Chemother Rep 50: 219–244
5. Penta JS, Rozencweig M, Guarino AM, Muggia FM (1979) Mouse and large animal toxicology studies of twelve antitumor agents: relevance to starting dose for Phase I clinical trials. Cancer Chemother Pharmacol 3: 97–101
6. Goldsmith MA, Slavik M, Carter SK (1975) Quantitative prediction of drug toxicity in humans from toxicology in small and large animals. Cancer Res 35: 1354–1364
7. Regulatory and Medicolegal Aspects of Investigational Cancer Chemotherapy (1980) In: Dorr RT, Fritz WL (eds) Cancer chemotherapy handbook. New York, Elsevier, pp 715–742
8. Investigator's Handbook (April 1987) Cancer Therapy Evaluation Program, DCT, NCI, NIH
9. Marsoni S, Wittes R (1984) Clinical development of anticancer agents—A National Cancer Institute perspective. Cancer Trest Rep 68: 77–85
10. Carter SK (1977) Clinical trials in cancer chemotherapy. Cancer 40(1): 544–557
11. Von Hoff DD, Kuhn J, Clark GM (1984) Design and conduct of phase I trials. In: Staquet M, Sylvester R, Buyse M. (eds) E.O.R.T.C. Oxford University Press, Oxford, pp 210–220
12. Collins JM, Zaharko DS, Dedrick RL, Chabner BA (1986) Potential roles for preclinical pharmacology in phase I clinical trials. Cancer Treat Rep 70: 73–80
13. Schlabel FM Jr, Griswold DP, Corbett TH, et al. (1983) Increasing therapeutic response rates to

anticancer drugs by applying the basic principles of pharmacology. Pharmacol Ther 20: 283–305

14. Wittes RE, Marsoni S, Simon R, Leyland-Jones B (1985) The phase II trial. Cancer Treat Rep 69: 1235–1239

15. Omura GA, Bartolucci AA, Lessner HE, et al. (1984) Phase II evaluation of amsacrine in colorectal, gastric, and pancreatic carcinomas: A Southeastern Cancer Study Group Trial. Cancer Treat Rep 68: 929–930

16. Kramer BS, Gams R, Birch R, et al. (1984) Phase II evaluation of mitoxantrone in patients with bronchogenic carcinoma: A Southeastern Cancer Study Group Trial. Cancer Treat Rep 68: 1295–1296

17. Gehan EA (1961) The determination of the number of patients required in a preliminary and follow-up trial of a new chemotherapeutic agent. J Chronic Dis 13: 346–353

18. Fleming TR (1982) One-sample multitude testing procedure for phase II clinical trials. Biometrics 38: 143–151

19. Simon R, Wittes RE, Ellenberg SS (1985) Randomized phase II clinical trials. Cancer Treat Rep 69: 1375–1381

20. Mantel N (1966) Evaluation of survival data and two new rank order statistics arising in its consideration. Cancer Chemother Rep 50: 163–170

21. Rubinstein LV, Gail MH, Santner TJ (1981) Planning the duration of a comparative clinical trial with loss to follow-up and a period of continued observation. J Chron Dis 34: 469–479

22. Fleming TR, Harrington DP, O'Brien PC (1984) Designs for group sequential tests. Controlled Clinical Trials 5: 348–361

23. Carter WH, Wampler GL, Stablein DM (1983) Regression analysis of survival data in cancer chemotherapy. Marcel Dekker, New York

24. Burchenal JH, Pancoast T, Carrol A, Elslager E, Robins RK (1984) Antileukemic antitumor and cross resistance studies of 2-B-D-ribofurananosyl-selenazole-4-carboxylamide (Selenazofurin) (abstract). Proc Am Assoc Cancer Res 25: 1375

25. Casazza AM, Savi G, Pratesi G, DiMarco A (1983) Antitumor activity in mice of 4'-deoxydoxorubicin in comparison with doxorubicin. Eur J Cancer Clin Oncol 19: 411–418

26. Jacksoin RC, Fry DW, Boritzki TJ, Besserer JA, Leopold WR, Sloan BJ, Elsgager EF (1984) Biochemical pharmacology of the lipophilic antifolate trimetrexate. Adv Enz Regul 22: 187–206

27. Casazza AM, Guiliani FC (1984) Preclinical properties of epirubicin. In: Bonnadonna G (ed) Advances in anthracycline chemotherapy: epirubicin. Maison, Milan, pp 31–40

28. Goldin A, Venditti JM, Geran R (1985) The effectiveness of the anthracycline analog 4'-epidoxorubicin in the treatment of experimental tumors: a review. Invest New Drugs 3: 3–21

29. Harrup KR (1985) Preclinical studies identifying carboplatin as a viable cisplatin alternative. Cancer Treat Rev 12 (Suppl A): 21–33

30. Leyland-Jones B, O'Dwyer PJ, Hoth DF, Wittes RE (1987) Clinical development of antifolate analogs. In: Symposium "Development of Folates and Folic Acid Antagonists in Cancer Therapy." NCI Monographs

31. Ellenberg SS, Eisenberg MH (1985) An efficient design for phase III studies of combination chemotherapies. Cancer Treat Rep 69: 1147–1154

13. Drug Delivery to Brain Tumors

N.H. Greig

Introduction

Primary malignant brain tumors occur at an annual rate of 4.5 cases per 100 000 members of the population, and metastatic brain tumors at a rate of 8.5 per 100 000 [42]. Several types of systemic malignancy (choriocarcinoma, testicular carcinoma, oat cell carcinoma of the lung, and breast cancer in women) can be successfully managed by chemotherapy even when disseminated to multiple sties; however, when the same responsive tumors are identified as metastatic foci in the brain, the effect of chemotherapy at the CNS sites has been minimal [11, 27]. The mainstays for the treatment of tumors within the brain remain surgery and radiation therapy. However, it is rare that patients are cured even after aggressive treatment. Malignant brain tumors are almost always fatal. The median survival time following surgery and radiation therapy for primary brain tumors is approx. 7.5–9.5 months. The prognosis for patients with metastatic brain tumors is even more pessimistic: median survival time is approx. 4–6 months after surgery and/or radiation therapy.

Chemotherapy failure is ultimately due to the overgrowth of resistant cells. For brain tumors, chemotherapy resistance is more likely to occur because the range of cytotoxic drugs which can be effectively delivered into the CNS is considerably narrower than that available for systemic treatment.

In this chapter, the difficulties associated with delivering anticancer drugs to brain tumors are reviewed, and techniques designed to optimize pharmacokinetics and circumvent the blood-brain barrier so that increased drug concentrations can be delivered to the brain are discussed. These techniques are by no means applicable to all chemotherapeutic agents since some anticancer agents are extremely neurotoxic [22], and brain uptake of these is to be avoided [26].

Factors Affecting Drug Delivery to the Brain

The concentration of a systemically administered drug which is achieved in the brain is determined by a number of factors, including the free, unbound, plasma concentration-time profile of the drug; the permeability of the blood-brain

259

barrier to the drug; and the rate of cerebral blood flow. The first two factors are a consequence of the compound's physicochemical characteristics [12].

Following systemic administration of a drug, its plasma concentration reaches a peak after an interval that varies according to the route of administration. The drug concentration then declines as the compound is redistributed, eliminated, and metabolized. The height and duration of the peak concentration are major determinants of the quantity of the compound that enters and remains in the brain. For some compounds, the brain is both an ideal and a major organ for drug uptake since it has a high rate of blood flow—approx. 20% of cardiac output. However, although highly perfused, the brain is different from other organs in that its blood vessels are comprised of endothelial cells that are joined by continuous belts of tight intercellular junctions [31]. Further, these endothelial cells contain few cytoplasmic vesicles, and there is good evidence that those present are not involved in transcapillary transport. This blood-brain barrier— which is also present in the circumventricular regions at the epithelial cell level, lying between the brain parenchyma and capillary endothelium—restricts the entry of most water-soluble and charged compounds into the brain. This includes most anticancer drugs [11], as well as neurotransmitters [12]. While specific and saturable transport systems exist at the level of the cerebrovascular endothelium to transport essential solutes into the brain (D-glucose, L-amino acids, and various ions), there has until recently been no evidence that drugs are similarly transported [8]. Consequently, only compounds that have an appreciable solubility in the lipid component of the endothelial cell membranes are able to cross the blood-brain barrier by diffusion and freely enter the brain [12].

Blood-Brain Barrier in Brain Tumors

The extent to which the blood-brain barrier is functional within brain tumors and the area directly surrounding them, which they invade, is controversial. There have been several reports of morphological alterations in brain endothelium at the microscopic level—including the presence of open tight junctions, fenestrations, and gap junctions—in both primary and secondary CNS tumors [11, 13, 15]. As a consequence, it has been suggested that the delivery of drugs to brain tumors is not a problem [43]. In apparent confirmation of this, iodinated radiocontrast agents are able to penetrate many metastatic brain tumors and high-grade gliomas, and partially delineate them during enhanced (i.e., by contrast agents) computerized tomographic (CT) scanning [13, 27]. Clinically, however, metastatic brain tumors often continue to grow despite regression of the primary tumor and systemic metastatic foci after chemotherapy. Further, small foci of metastatic brain tumors and low-grade gliomas appear to have relatively intact blood-brain barriers. Recent research indicates that the breakdown of the blood-brain barrier in brain tumors is not an all-or-nothing phenomenon [11, 13]. In large metastatic brain tumors and high-grade gliomas, breakdown is both regional and variable. Large areas of tumor often exist in which the barrier is either completely or partially intact. These areas are not enhanced by intravenous contrast agnets when imaged by CT scanning but can be detected by the measurement of local cerebral glucose utilization by positron emission tomography [4].

Even when the barrier within a CNS tumor is reduced or completely absent, drug distribution problems may still exist. There are several reasons for this:

1. Blood flow to brain tumors is often variable. The blood vessels are frequently ill formed, coiled, dead-ended, or sinuslike.
2. The intercapillary distance within the brain tumor is variable and generally increased [23]. When distances are great, the diffusion of oxygen and metabolic substrates, as well as drugs, into the tumor is compromised. As a consequence, cells often remain in G_0, resting state, in which they are insensitive to cell-cycle-dependent anticancer agents.
3. Tumor cells often infiltrate into the surrounding brain parenchyma and are fed by the vessels of the normal brain.
4. The permeability of the capillaries in the brain tissue directly surrounding the tumor may be reduced [23].
5. Both the normal brain surrounding the tumor and the CSF act as a diffusion sink for drugs, reducing their cytocidal concentration within the tumor.
6. Brain tumors have an efficient perivascular drainage.

Because these factors apply in tumors with disruption of the blood-brain barrier—and in addition, some tumors have only a partially disrupted or even completely intact barrier—it is important to choose nonneurotoxic anticancer agents that are able to penetrate normal brain, if tumors are to be effectively treated. For a drug to be effective against a tumor, not only must the malignant cells be sensitive to the drug, but the latter must reach its site of action in a cytotoxic concentration for an adequate time; this is the "concentration × time" (C × T) concept. In addition, if the anticancer agent is cell cycle phase specific, drug exposure must occur at the correct time. There are two major consequences of inadequate drug delivery: the first is a suboptimal cell kill, which results in a poor therapeutic response; the second is the induction of drug resistance in the surviving cells, caused by the emergence of drug-resistant clones.

Pharmacokinetic Parameters

Three major factors determine the delivery of a drug to the brain:

1. The time-dependent free plasma concentration profile of the drug, which is related to its route of administration.
2. The permeability of the blood-brain barrier to the compound. This is expressed formally as a lipid: water partition coefficient. Since only the unionized

and unbound fraction of a compound is free to penetrate a cell, this partition parameter (P) has been defined as the fractional concentration of the unionized and unbound fraction in the aqueous phase times the lipid solubility of the unionized agent, derived from its octanol:water partition coefficient [12, 32].

3. Local cerebral blood flow.

The cumulative effect of these three factors determines the actual concentration of drug that reaches the brain. The time-dependent distribution of a drug depends on its structure and on body mechanisms for its uptake, distribution, modification, and removal. After systemic administration, the plasma concentration of a drug reaches a peak and then declines as it is redistributed and metabolized. As mentioned, the amount of drug available to enter the brain is dependent on the peak plasma concentration achieved and its maintenance over time. A high steady-state concentration will optimize brain uptake, while a rapid clearance will minimize it, except in the case of intra-arterial drug administration. As demonstrated in Fig. 1, there is a linear relationship between the cerebrovascular permeability of a compound (i.e., its brain penetration) and its lipophilicity as determined by its octanol:water partition coefficient. Thus, in the case of a lipophilic drug with an octanol:water partition coefficient of greater

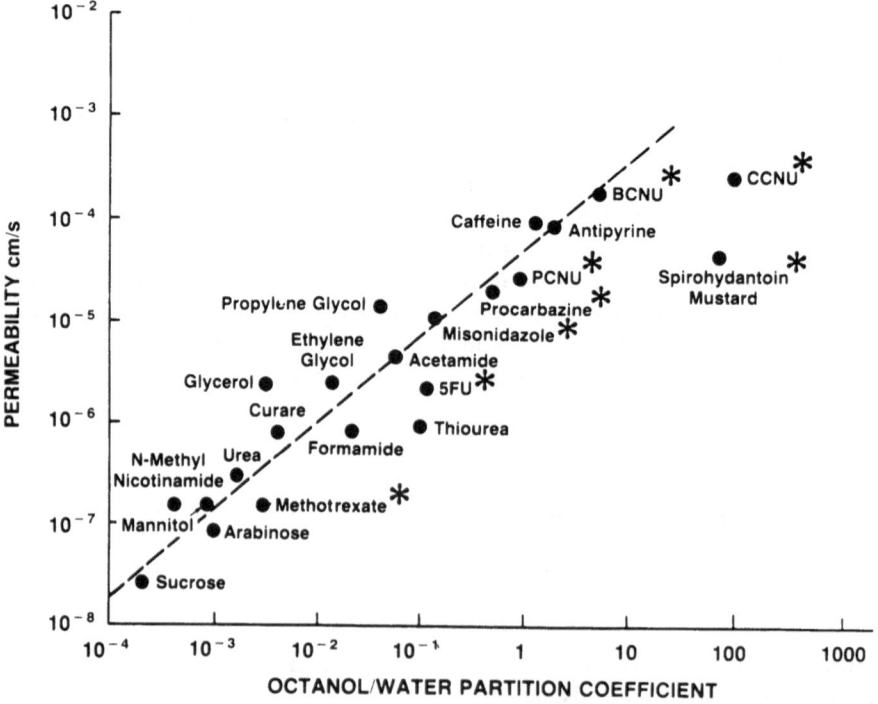

Fig. 1. Relationship between octanol:water partition coefficient and cerebrovascular permeability. *Asterisks* designate anticancer agents

than 1.0 (i.e., equal partition), its transfer across the blood-brain barrier is rapid, and its distribution from blood to brain is limited by the rate of local blood flow. The rate at which a lipid-insoluble polar compound whose octanol:water partition coefficient is lower than 0.1 enters the brain is limited by the permeability of the compound across the blood-brain barrier. For compounds whose octanol:water partition coefficients lie between these two limits, a combination of both blood flow and permeability limits their brain uptake. In each case, however, the final brain concentration of drug depends on the time-dependent profile of the free agent in plasma.

The pharmacokinetics and physicochemical characteristics of the commonly used anticancer agents have been extensively described by Chabner et al. [1], Dorr [5], and (for the brain) Greig [11]. This chapter will focus on experimental techniques relevant to the treatment of CNS tumors to optimize or manipulate the three described pharmacokinetic parameters—concentration-time profile, barrier permeability, and rate of local cerebral blood flow. The goal of such manipulations is to increase the brain uptake of specific anticancer agents in order to improve their efficacy against intracerebrally sequestered tumors.

Factors Governing the Concentration-Time Profile of a Drug

One problem with classical pharmacokinetic studies is that the most important aspect—the tumor tissue concentration of the active moiety of the drug over time—is a parameter which cannot easily be studied and may not necessarily be correlated with the classical plasma pharmacokinetic data that are routinely reported. While plasma drug concentrations give little knowledge of the absolute quantity of drug in the tumor, they do, together with the CSF levels, provide a valuable approximation. Should plasma drug concentrations either not reach or quickly fall below cytotoxic levels, it is unlikely that tumor cells in the brain would be reached by cytocidal drug concentrations.

Clinically, techniques to optimize the pharmacokinetics of drugs for brain entry are limited. They rely on altering the route of drug administration (i.e., systemic, intra-arterial, intrathecal, and intratumor) and the schedule. Anticancer agents are administered systemically for the treatment of most solid intraparenchymal brain tumors and some CSF-sequestered tumors. This route is less invasive, and the bioavailability of drug administered intravenously is superior to that after oral administration. Systemic administration results in drug delivery to multiple potential or actual metastatic sites and is necessary for the use of drugs such as cyclophosphamide, which must be activated in the liver. The major disadvantage of systemic drug administration is that drugs must penetrate the blood-brain barrier to reach all the tumor cells, and few drugs possess this ability [11, 12]. In addition, the availability of systemically administered drugs to the tumor will be reduced by drug binding to plasma constituents and other tissues, metabolism, and excretion. Systemic toxicity can also occur.

For most anticancer agents, the maintenance of steady-state plasma concentrations results in both a higher brain concentration and greater cytotoxicity. Techniques to achieve a steady state include repetitive dosing and continuous intravenous infusion. Interestingly, the maintenance of plasma drug concentrations versus the administration of a single high intravenous bolus can, depending on the agent and its mode of action, either reduce or increase systemic toxicity. For some agents (e.g., methotrexate and cytosine arabinoside), high-dose drug infusions, coupled with a rescue technique if necessary, can safely and significantly increase both brain and peripheral tissue drug delivery.

Following intravenous administration of methotrexate to humans, the compound minimally enters the brain, with a CSF:plasma concentration ratio of 0.0006 [35]. However, high-dose 24-h methotrexate infusions, in combination with leucovorin rescue 24–36 h later, have been shown to increase brain methotrexate levels to cytocidal concentrations and heighten the CSF:plasma ratio to 0.03 [1]. A combination of factors probably accounts for this increased brain uptake: (a) peak plasma concentrations are dramatically increased during high-dose therapy, (b) the saturation of binding sites leads to a reduction in plasma protein binding and a subsequent increase in free drug levels [40], and (c) infusion maintains plasma levels for sufficient time to allow the brain concentration to become uniformly high (no sink effect).

Since alkylating agents such as melphalan produce relatively little second-organ toxicity after their profound hematological toxicity, several investigators have similarly administered them in high-dose infusions, followed by autologous bone marrow rescue [3]. As yet, no data are available concerning the concentrations these agents attain in CSF. For reasons similar to those stated for methotrexate, one would expect increased brain levels.

Simple drug infusion alone will not necessarily increase the brain uptake of a drug to therapeutic levels, as demonstrated by 5-fluorouracil (5FU). Following its intravenous administration, the compound becomes rapidly deaminated to an inactive form. In studies which have not included methods to differentiate between these forms, it has been concluded that significant amounts of 5FU enter the brain. However, Hornbeck et al. [21] treated three patients with a 5FU infusion and found little or no 5FU in the CSF. Interestingly, Weinstein et al. [44] have reported high CSF: serum ratios (0.58) in patients administered cytosine arabinoside by continuous intravenous infusion. Cytosine arabinoside is similar to 5FU in that it is rapidly inactivated in vivo; however, unlike 5FU, the high cytosine arabinoside concentrations achieved during intravenous infusion probably saturate the inactivating enzyme system (the serum deaminases).

Intra-arterial administration of drugs to the brain is only of value for lipophilic compounds, particularly those that are rapidly metabolized in plasma, thereby reducing their systemic toxicity. The advantage of the arterial route is present only during the compound's initial passage through the brain, after which the drug enters the venous circulation, and its kinetics are identical to those pertaining after intravenous administration [12]. While the technique has proved of significant clinical value in the isolated limb perfusion of malignant melanoma and in the treatment of hepatic metastases, it is not commonly used for CNS tumors through lack of ideal compounds and technical expense. Of the anticancer agents available, carmustine (BCNU) is probably the most suitable.

Circumvention of the Blood-Brain Barrier

Few of the anticancer agents currently in clinical use possess the physicochemical properties required for adequate penetration of the brain. Consequently, appreciable brain concentrations are not achieved following systemic administration. This does not apply to the nitrosoureas, which have been the mainstay of brain tumor chemotherapy, but the effects of these agents on patient survival have been disappointing. There are a number of possible explanations for this, including tumor cell heterogeneity, initial insensitivity, acquired drug resistance, and inadequate drug delivery to avascular quiescent cells. Regardless of which paradigm is used to explain the failures of chemotherapy, it is not surprising that single-drug regimens at best only minimally increase patient survival. Both the cell kill [37] and the Goldie-Coldman [9] hypotheses predict that the best responses are likely to be achieved by combination therapies. However, the list of agents with appropriate physicochemical properties which could be used in combination with the nitrosoureas is meagre.

In addition to the design of novel lipophilic anticancer agents, a number of rational experimental approaches have recently been made to increase the brain uptake of the conventional anticancer agents, whose activities, pharmacokinetics, toxicities, and possible rescue techniques are already known. Since these agents are often effective against the systemic disease, they would appear to be potentially valuable against brain metastases, if delivery to the tumor site could be accomplished.

Intrathecal Chemotherapy

Intrathecal drug administration, by either the intralumbar or the intraventricular route, allows the immediate achievement of high CSF drug concentrations by bypassing the blood-brain barrier. In addition, since the volume of distribution of a drug delivered intrathecally is considerably smaller than that following systemic administration, a smaller initial drug dose will achieve a high CSF concentration without the associated systemic toxicity. Certain drugs, in particular methotrexate and cytosine arabinoside, have more favorable pharmacokinetics when administered intrathecally than when administered systemically for the treatment of some CNS diseases. The disappearance half-life of methotrexate in

265

CSF and plasma is biphasic, however, the initial phases being 4.5 h and 45 min, respectively. Likewise, the disappearance of cytosine arabinoside in CSF is far slower than in plasma.

In addition to metabolism, several other factors jointly determine the half-life of a drug in CSF. CSF is formed under pressure at the choroid plexuses. Thus, drugs injected into CSF are carried by bulk flow through the ventricular and cisternal systems of the brain and are excreted into the venous system at the sagittal sinus. As there is free exchange between brain extracellular fluid (ECF) and CSF, drugs are free to mix and distribute throughout the ECF of brain parenchyma during their passage, to enter cells and cross capillaries.

It is generally believed that the brain penetration of most anticancer agents administered into CSF is minimal since the extracellular space of the brain is extremely tortuous. Steady-state conditions would be required to achieve significant drug concentrations in all but marginal areas. The rate of a drug's brain penetration is determined by its aqueous diffusion constant. This is a physical characteristic of each compound and a function of its molecular weight [8]. Further, intrathecal drug administration, particularly by the lumbar route, is often contraindicated in the presence of solid intraparenchymal tumor due to the possibility of brain herniation.

The route of intrathecal drug administration is an additional factor that determines the distribution of a drug, both in CSF and (secondarily) in brain [12]. Although the intralumbar route does not require surgical placement of an Ommaya reservoir, which is essential for intraventricular drug administration [28], the lumbar approach has a variety of disadvantages [12].

Two adaptions of the Ommaya reservoir have been developed for intratumor drug administration and ventriculolumbar CSF perfusion. In the former, a catheter is inserted directly into an intraparenchymal tumor during its resection [28]. This is then attached to an Ommaya reservoir. The device may be of value in the treatment of well-localized single tumors. As yet, however, insufficient data exist to adequately assess its benefits. Recently, Poplack et al. [30] have developed an experimental CSF perfusion system in the monkey to attain artificially high CSF concentrations of drugs over a protracted period of time. Artificial CSF, containing drug, is infused intraventricularly via an Ommaya reservoir and removed via a lumbar cannula. Again, insufficient data exist to assess its potential clinical benefit adequately. Unless a significant advantage is demonstrated, its technical complexity and expense may prevent its widespread utilization.

Reversible Blood-Brain Barrier Modification

As described, the blood-brain barrier maintains the homeostatic environment of the brain. Consequently, the brain is not subjected to the large fluctuations in essential compounds which occur in the systemic circulation. Further, the barrier protects the brain from toxic systemic chemicals. While it is necessary for the normal functioning of the brain, its absolute and continuous integrity may not be essential. Two techniques that have proved consistently successful in innocuously and reversibly increasing the brain uptake of water-soluble anticancer agents are the osmotic opening and Metrazol opening techniques.

Osmotic Opening

Rapoport et al. [31, 32] have demonstrated that cerebral artery administration of a hyperosmotic water-soluble agent, either mannitol or arabinose, consistently and safely produces barrier opening throughout the entire cerebral capillary network supplied by the infused artery. To accomplish this, an osmotic threshold of 1.6 osmols was required over at least a 20 second infusion period, and the phenomenon was completely reversed within 4 h. Morphological studies utilizing the intravascular marker horseradish peroxidase demonstrated that the increased capillary permeability resulted from an osmotically induced shrinkage of the capillary endothelial cells, causing widening of the intercellular tight junctions [32]. The gradual rehydration of these cells after the osmotic load restores barrier integrity.

In extensive experiments in animal models, Rapoport et al. [32] demonstrated that the technique could increase the cerebral permeability of methotrexate by up to seven times. They also found that methotrexate levels could be additionally increased by a factor of 7 by administration of the drug into the cerebral artery infused with the hyperosmotic agent. Using this technique, Neuwelt et al. [27] were able to increase brain levels of methotrexate in dogs by up to 90 and 100 times, with hyperosmotic infusions of 25% mannitol followed by administration of methotrexate either into the carotid or vertebral arteries. In brain tumor models, Neuwelt et al. [27] and Hiesiger et al. [20] separately demonstrated that the osmotic opening technique could not only increase the distribution of methotrexate into normal brain but also into brain adjacent to tumor, which, as described, harbors invasive tumor cells. Most importantly, this technique also increased the delivery of methotrexate into the tumor itself [27]. In addition, Neuwelt et al. [27] reported that prior adrenal cortical steroid administration inhibited such increases. These experiments demonstrated several important points:

1. The osmotic technique could optimize drug delivery to intracerebral tumors and to the brain surrounding them.
2. Adrenal cortical steroids, generally given clinically for the management of cerebral edema associated with brain tumors, interfered with osmotic barrier modification in an undetermined manner.
3. Intracerebral tumors have a variable barrier, which while partially open can still be modified by the osmotic opening technique.

Neuwelt et al. [26, 27] have undertaken extensive neuropathological studies in the dog to determine which anticancer agents in conjunction with osmotic opening would be of clinical benefit. The neurotoxicity of several commonly used water-soluble anticancer agents was assessed, in doses from 5% to 100% of their normal systemic dose. Neurological observation and postmortem neuropathology was undertaken at intervals from minutes to months after their administration. Cis-platinum and doxorubicin hydrochloride (Adriamycin) proved to be extremely neurotoxic, causing brain tissue necrosis, hemorrhagic infarction, and cerebral edema. Cis-platinum was highly neurotoxic following its intracarotid infusion, even without barrier modification. It caused extravasation of the intravascular marker, Evans blue, and resulted in multiple areas of necrosis and hemorrhage. Following osmotic barrier modification, bleomycin and 5FU also proved to be neurotoxic, but to a lesser degree. Only methotrexate and cyclophosphamide (administered intravenously in order to achieve hepatic microsomal activation) were not associated with substantial neurotoxicity.

Neuwelt et al. [24, 26] have also carried out clinical studies. Since 1979, they have successfully undertaken more than 1000 barrier modifications on more than 100 patients. They have documented tumor regression, assessed by combined CT scan and neurological examination, in patients with glioblastoma, microglioma, medulloblastoma, CNS lymphoma, and CNS metastases from breast and lung and, additionally, have clearly demonstrated that the technique can significantly increase the duration of patient survival [27].

Metrazol Opening

The permeability of the blood-brain barrier can be reversibly increased by seizure activity. Greig and Hellmann [14] demonstrated that the CNS stimulant pentylenetetrazol (Metrazol) could increase the brain uptake of the intravascular markers horseradish peroxidase and radiolabelled albumin by a factor of 3. The effect was innocuous, temporary, and reversed within 4 h. They further demonstrated that pentylenetetrazol in combination with pentobarbital sodium (to reduce peripheral seizure activity) significantly enhanced the brain uptake of both razoxane and melphalan in the rat. This led to an increase in the therapeutic efficacy of razoxane against intracerebrally sequestered L1210 leukemia in mice [17].

Miscellaneous

A number of other chemical and physical insults have been reported to increase the permeability of the blood-brain barrier innocuously and reversibly. Many of these observations remain unsubstantiated, and several have since been refuted [11, 12, 18]. They have been extensively reviewed by Greig [11, 12].

Possibly of greatest interest is the question whether X-irradiation alters the permeability of the blood-brain barrier. Nair and Roth [24] demonstrated that a single dose of 100 Gy caused a slight barrier opening to both radiolabelled albumin and the anticonvulsant acetazolamide in rats; however, at clinical doses of X-rays (which are substantially lower), this acute effect was not observed. Thus, while there appears to be a synergism between radiotherapy and several anticancer agents—BCNU, which readily enters the brain, being particularly important in this regard—it is unlikely that the scheduling of chemotherapy directly after radiotherapy would increase the brain uptake of water-soluble anticancer agents.

Chronically, radiotherapy may indeed cause vascular alterations and permeability changes in the brain, as demonstrated by the occurrence of radiation necrosis. Such vascular alterations may be of relevance to neurotoxicity associated with combined modality treatment approaches. There is no doubt, for example, that the combination of radiotherapy and methotrexate, used in CNS prophylaxis, results in a higher incidence of neurotoxicity in patients with leukemia [22].

While the long-term sequelae of conventional X-radiation on both the brain and the cerebral vasculature remain largely unknown, it is probable that fast-neutron radiation detrimentally and irreversibly alters the cerebral vasculature chronically and possibly acutely [12].

Carrier-Mediated Transport at the Blood-Brain Barrier

As described, stereospecific, saturable, carrier-mediated transport systems exist at the level of the cerebral capillary endothelium to regulate and facilitate the brain uptake of essential water-soluble compounds (D-glucose, L-amino acids, neurotransmitter precursors, and ions). Greig et al. [16, 22] have recently demonstrated that for melphalan, a nitrogen mustard derivative of the large neutral amino acid L-phenylalanine, there is facilitated transport at the blood-brain barrier by the large neutral amino acid carrier system. Using an isolated brain perfusion technique, they were able to measure the cerebrovascular permeability of melphalan separately from the endogenous L-amino acids that compete for the carrier. Melphalan brain uptake demonstrated classical concentration-dependent transport, saturation, and inhibition by L-phenylalanine.

Melphalan's affinity for the carrier system was significantly less than that of the endogenous large neutral amino acids, and its facilitated transport was inhibited by these at physiological concentrations. Nevertheless, this is the first clear demonstration that an exogenous compound can make use of an existing facilitated transport system located at the blood-brain barrier to gain entry into the brain. It is possible that other amino acid drug analogs, such as the glutamine antimetabolite acivicin, are likewise transported. While melphalan is not a perfect substrate for the carrier system, research is continuing towards synthesizing further compounds that compete more readily for it.

Drug Design and Chemical Modification

The development of anticancer agents for the treatment of CNS-sequestered disease has recently progressed beyond the empirical approach, in which the random screening of drugs against a bank of proliferative tumor models is carried out. Currently, there is enough information in this field to embark upon "rational" drug design.

The design of anticancer agents specific for brain tumors can be divided into two categories: (a) novel lipophilic agents with anticancer activity and (b) classical anticancer agents with modified lipophilicity. In reality, the groups largely overlap, as the synthesis of a totally novel compound is rare.

Novel Lipophilic Agents

Two compounds that fit better into the category of novel lipophilic agents are spirohydantoin mustard (SHM) and aziridinylbenzoquinone (AZQ). SHM was developed by Peng et al. [29] to take advantage of the observation that the centrally acting anticonvulsive agent diphenylhydantoin, or phenytoin, readily enters the brain and distributes preferentially in primary brain tumors, reaching concentrations of up to four times that in normal brain. Diphenylhydantoin has an octanol:water partition coefficient of log 2.47. The addition of a nitrogen mustard group to the molecule significantly increased its partition coefficient to log 4.69, but the removal of an aromatic ring—giving the drug SHM—reduced the partition coefficient to approx. log 2.5. The optimal octanol:water partition coefficient for brain entry is considered to be in the range of log 1.5–2.5. SHM was found to penetrate the CSF of dogs in significant quantities following its intravenous administration and proved active against intracerebral ependymoblastoma in mice [11]. As yet, its activity in clinical trials has been hampered by dose-limiting CNS neurotoxicity, consisting of hallucinations and other symptoms resembling anticholinergic overdrive. Preliminary studies have indicated that physostigmine or haloperidol pretreatment might reduce these side effects [36]. Should the acute toxicity problem be overcome, allowing dose escalation, it will be interesting to assess whether the promising properties of SHM will translate into effectiveness against high-grade gliomas.

Driscoll et al. [6] and Chou et al. [2] have synthesized and tested a number of quinones against several brain and peripherally implanted tumor models. The quinone structure is a common chemical feature in doxorubicin, daunorubicin, mitomycin C, steptonigrin, and lapachol. A series of aziridinylbenzoquinones demonstrated significant anticancer activity, and AZQ was eventually chosen for pharmacokinetic studies and clinical trials. As AZQ is a small, unionized, and lipophilic compound, it was found to readily enter the brain [10]. Its clinical spectrum of activity has been reviewed by Greig [11]. AZQ has demonstrated some activity against primary brain tumors, but this was inferior to that of

BCNU. Analysis of the true value of AZQ awaits the completion of further clinical trials.

Modification of Lipophilicity

The second approach to the synthesis of CNS anticancer agents is to modify the lipophilicity of classical agents already in clinical use [12]. Chemical manipulations have led to the circumvention of resistance pathways (e.g., antimetabolite analogs) or alterations in drug distribution with resultant reduced toxicity (e.g., *cis*-platinum derivatives).

Nitrosoureas

The nitrosoureas, BCNU, lomustine (CCNU), and semustine (MeCCNU) (log octanol:water partition coefficient 1.53, 2.83, and 3.3, respectively) have formed the basis of chemotherapeutic treatment of brain tumors since they are among the few anticancer agents that readily enter the brain. Their brain uptake is limited by cerebral blood flow only. The brain pharmacokinetics and clinical activity of these compounds have been reviewed by Greig [11] and Edwards et al. [7], respectively. PCNU (log octanol:water partition coefficient 0.37), a newer nitrosourea, was originally brought into clinical trials to test a quantitative structure-activity relationship, based on extensive studies on intracerebral and other animal tumor models [19]. These investigations indicated that the activity of the nitrosoureas declined with increasing lipophilicity. Clinical studies have, in general, supported this paradigm and indicate that BCNU is more active than both CCNU and MeCCNU against brain tumors. PCNU demonstrated significant activity against intracerebral tumor models and appeared to readily enter the brain; however, its activity in clinical studies has proved disappointing. Its anticipated benefits were quickly reevaluated following greater than expected myelotoxicity. In phase II trials on both metastatic and primary brain tumors, its activity was not superior to that of BCNU or CCNU [11].

Methotrexate

Possibly the most extensive studies on the structural modification of a single agent have been undertaken by Rosowsky et al. [33, 34] on methotrexate. Methotrexate (log octanol:water partition coefficient 1.85) is restricted from entering the brain by the presence of two amine and carboxyl residues (Fig. 2), which become positively and negatively charged, respectively, at physiological pH. This indicates that the compound exists in the form of a dipolar ion. As a consequence, less than 0.1% of methotrexate exists in the unionized form under physiological conditions, which results in its low brain permeability. Rosowsky

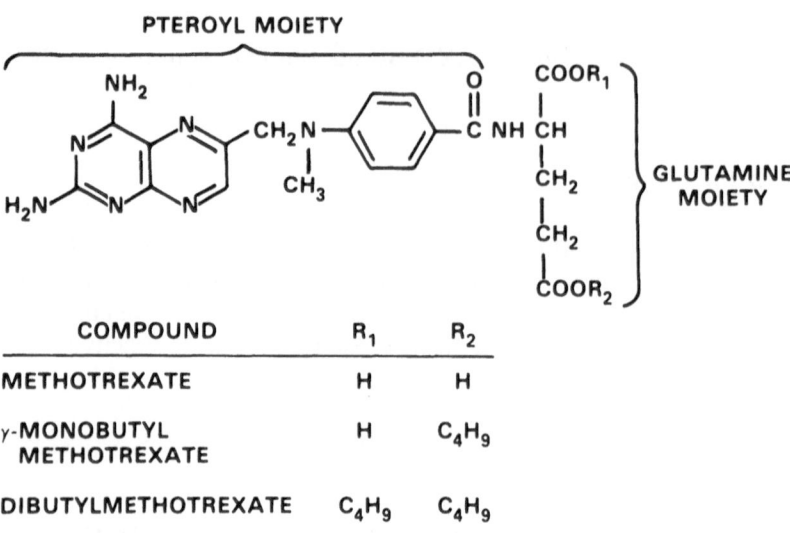

COMPOUND	R_1	R_2
METHOTREXATE	H	H
γ-MONOBUTYL METHOTREXATE	H	C_4H_9
DIBUTYLMETHOTREXATE	C_4H_9	C_4H_9

Fig. 2. Structure of methotrexate and γ-monobutyl and -dibutyl methotrexate derivatives

restricted his studies to alterations in the glutamine residue of methotrexate, and in particular to the two ionizable carboxyl groups. The replacement of these by hydrophobic esters offers an improved opportunity for drug uptake into the brain and also into tumor cells by passive diffusion. Methotrexate normally enters tumor cells by a carrier-mediated transport system. Alterations in this transport system lead to one form of methotrexate resistance. Chemical modification of the pteroyl moiety of methotrexate or the $C = O$ group in the amide bond separating the pteroyl and glutamine moieties considerably reduces the activity of the analog compared with methotrexate.

Rosowsky's manipulations of the glutamine moiety of methotrexate are too extensive to be adequately reviewed in this article, and consequently only a few will be discussed. The lipophilicity of methotrexate could be increased by esterification of the R_1 and R_2 carboxyl groups either singly or jointly to form α or γ monoesters or α or γ diesters, respectively (Fig. 2). The synthesis of a series of alkyl esters of C_4–C_{16} chain length demonstrated that increasing the alkyl chain length of the ester moiety decreased the ability of the analog to inhibit dihydrofolate reductase (DFR) in a cell free assay and increased its cytotoxicity against human leukemic lymphoblasts (CEM cells) in culture [34]. These results are not necessarily incompatible since greater amounts of the more lipophilic long-chain analogs would be expected to enter the tumor cells in vitro. The only detailed pharmacokinetic experiments undertaken with these analogs have involved the dibutyl and γ-monobutyl C_4 esters of methotrexate in the rhesus monkey [33]. Following intravenous administration, the dibutyl ester broke down principally to the monoester, methotrexate, but substantial quantities of unidentified products were also formed. Conversely, the γ-monobutyl ester formed methotrexate only. The γ-monobutyl ester bound heavily to plasma proteins ($> 99\%$), and the combined CSF level of both the parent compound and methotrexate was no greater than that following the equimolar intravenous adminstration of methotrexate. These experiments nevertheless demonstrate how chemical manipulation can substantially alter the cytotoxicity and distribution of a drug.

Chlorambucil

Extensive pharmacokinetic and activity experiments have been undertaken by Greig [12] on esters of chlorambucil to assess how the structural modifications of a single carboxyl group can alter the distribution of the compound. Unlike methotrexate, chlorambucil has only a single ionizable group. Since chlorambucil is an alkylating agent, chemical modification of the carboxyl group is unlikely to alter its activity, as unlike methotrexate it does not compete with endogenous substrates for a rate-limiting enzyme. As with methotrexate, increased brain concentrations of drug, brought about by reversible blood-brain barrier opening in rats (Greig, unpublished results), were not associated with neurotoxicity. Short-chain alkyl esters and simple aromatic esters of chlorambucil were rapidly metabolized in both rat and human plasma to release chlorambucil. Following the intravenous administration of these esters in rat, only chlorambucil and phenylacetic mustard (the active end product of chlorambucil β-oxidation) were detected in brain, and these concentrations were not significantly different from those following the equimolar administration of chlorambucil. In accord with this finding, the activity of these esters against intracerebral tumor implants was comparable with that of equimolar chlorambucil. The longer-chain (6 and 8 carbon length) alkyl chlorambucil esters were more stable in plasma, with half-lives of up to 10 min prior to ester hydrolysis to chlorambucil. Interestingly, neither the total brain alkylating concentration nor the brain activity of these compounds was signficantly different from equimolar chlorambucil. This is probably due to the fact that all are heavily bound to plasma proteins.

These experiments demonstrate anew several interesting points that have been shown with other compounds [12]:

1. Simple esters, with specific exceptions, are rapidly cleaved from drugs. While esterase activity is slower in humans than in rodents, it is often sufficiently rapid to ensure that minimal drug becomes localized to the brain.
2. Esterase hydrolysis declines with the increasing complexity of the ester or with steric hindrance.
3. Long-chain alkyl esters are often highly lipophilic, above the limit for optimal brain entry, and bind heavily to plasma proteins. They distribute to liver, bile, and fat depots and are difficult to administer.
4. Complex esters that bind heavily to plasma proteins can act as pro-drugs to maintain systemic drug concentrations of therapeutically useful agents over a protracted period of time after a single intravenous dose.

The approaches discussed are representative of those currently being undertaken with the objective of directing systemically administered anticancer agents to the brain. Similar approaches are being undertaken with other pharmacological agents [12]. It is to be hoped that advances made with these agents may establish general principles which will be of value in ensuring improved brain delivery of other (including new) therapeutic drugs.

Blood Flow

As described, the brain delivery of the unbound fraction of a lipophilic drug is limited solely by blood flow. Although the brain is small in mass, it is highly perfused. In addition, regional cerebral blood flow is heterogeneous and under most circumstances is closely linked to the local rate of energy utilization [39]. Since the rate of blood flow is a determinant of total drug delivery, it follows that systemically administered drugs, and in particular lipophilic ones, would be available for uptake in greater amounts in those regions with higher metabolic rates.

Elaborate studies by Soncrant et al. [40], utilizing the 2-deoxy-D-[^{14}C]-glucose technique to measure regional cerebral metabolism [38], have demonstrated that neurotransmitter agonists consistently increased and antagonists and anesthetic agents consistently decreased glucose utilization, and hence blood flow, in highly localized brain areas. The specific regions affected, the total number, and the degree depended on the drug and its mechanism of action, its initial concentration, and the time after its administration. These dose-response–time relations are complex; however, studies such as these are gradually elucidating the principles of how drugs affect local cerebral metabolism and how different brain regions interact, leading to a new and broader view than that inherent in the more classical drug-receptor binding studies. In addition, utilizing the 2-[^{18}F]fluoro-2-deoxy-D-glucose technique in humans [4], pharmacological agents are now being used as probes to assess how the brain responds to specific stimuli in health and disease.

Soncrant et al. [40] have posed an interesting question: can drugs, by their regionally specific actions on metabolism (and blood flow), alter either their own regional delivery or that of other drugs within the brain? This novel concept poses a series of further questions of relevance to the chemotherapy of brain tumors: as it is generally possible to localize the tumor in the brain of a patient by brain imaging, can prior administration of a specific drug that increases cerebral metabolism in the region surrounding the lesion enhance the delivery of anticancer drugs to it? Or conversely, can an agent that decreases cerebral metabolism in areas other than that surrounding the lesion protect distant brain from neurotoxicity? These questions highlight a few of the many possible manipulations, through drug synergism, that might enhance the delivery of therapeutically useful anticancer agents to brain tumors. At the present time, the practical utility of such approaches remains speculative.

Conclusions

It is finally being accepted that the blood-brain barrier, although of variable integrity, severely compromises the delivery of drugs to brain tumors. With this realization, progress is at last being made to increase the number of chemotherapeutic agents available to the neuro-oncologist. Osmotic blood-brain barrier modification has already been demonstrated to be both beneficial and safe in delivering hitherto CNS-restricted anticancer agents into the brain. In addition, drugs are now being rationally designed specifically for brain tumor treatment. Although the prognosis for patients with malignant brain tumors is presently bleak, there is hope that it will improve in the near future.

Acknowledgements. I wish to thank Drs. Deena Shapiro, Timothy Soncrant, and John Driscoll for their invaluable help during the preparation of this article.

References

1. Chabner B (1979) Antimetabolites. In: Pinedo H (ed) Cancer chemotherapy. Excerpta Medica, Amsterdam
2. Chou F, Khan H, Driscoll J (1976) Potential central nervous system anticancer agents: Aziridinylbenzoquinones-2. J Med Chem 19: 1302–1308
3. Cornbleet M, Leonard R, Smyth J (1984) High dose agent therapy: A review of clinical experiences. Cancer Drug Delivery 1: 227–238
4. DiChiro G, De LaPaz R, Brooks A et al. (1982) Glucose utilization of cerebral gliomas measured by (^{18}F)-fluorodeoxyglucose and positron emission tomography. Neurology 32: 1323–1329
5. Dorr R, Fritz W (1980) Cancer chemotherapy handbook. Elsevier, New York
6. Driscoll J, Dudeck L, Congleton G et al. Potential CNS antitumor agents VI: Aziridinylbenzoquinones III. J Pharm Sci 68: 185–188
7. Edwards M, Levin V, Wilson C (1980) Brain tumor chemotherapy: an evaluation of agents in current use for phase II and III trials. Cancer Treat Rep 64: 1179–1205
8. Fenstermacher J, Blasberg R (1981) Methods of quantifying the transport of drugs across brain barrier systems. Pharmacol Ther 14: 217–248
9. Goldie J, Coldman A (1979) A mathematical model for relating the drug sensitivity of tumors to their spontaneous mutation rate. Cancer Treat Rep 63: 172
10. Gormley P, Wood J, Poplack D (1981) Ability of a new anticancer agent AZQ to penetrate to cerebrospinal fluid. Pharmacology 22: 196–198
11. Greig N (1984) Chemotherapy of brain metastases: Current status. Cancer Treat Rev 11: 157–186
12. Greig N (1988) Drug delivery to the brain by blood-brain barrier circumvention and drug modification. In: Neuwelt E (ed) The clinical impact of the blood-brain barrier and its manipulation, vol I. Plenum Press, New York, pp 311–368
13. Greig N (1988) Brain tumors and the blood-tumor barrier. In: Neuwelt E (ed) The clinical impart of the blood-brain barrier and its manipulation, vol II. Plenum Press, New York

14. Greig N, Hellmann K (1983) Enhanced cerebrovascular permeability by Metrazol: Significance for brain metastases. Clin Exp Metast 1: 83–95
15. Greig N, Jones H, Cavanagh J (1983) Blood-brain barrier integrity and host responses in experimental metastatic brain tumors. Clin Exp Metast 1: 229–246
16. Greig N, Momma S, Smith Q et al. (1987) Facilitated transport of melphalan at the rat blood-brain barrier by the large neutral amino acid transport system. Cancer Res 47:1571–1576
17. Greig N, Newell D, Hellmann K (1984) Metrazol enhances brain penetration and therapeutic efficacy of some anticancer agents: Implications for brain metastases. Clin Exp Metast 2: 55–59
18. Greig N, Sweeney D, Rapoport S (1985) Inability of dimethylsulfoxide (DMSO) to increase the brain uptake of water-soluble compounds: Implications to chemotherapy of brain tumors. Cancer Treat Rep 69: 305–312
19. Hanasch C, Smith N, Engle R et al. (1972) Quantitative structure activity relationships of antineoplastic drugs: Nitrosoureas and triazenoimidazoles. Cancer Chemother Rep 56: 443–456
20. Hiesiger H, Voorhies R, Basler G et al. (1984) Comparison of ^{14}C-methotrexate delivery by intravenous vs intracarotid route with and without intracarotid mannitol in experimental rat brain tumors as measured by quantitative autoradiography. Proc Am Assoc Cancer Res 25: 363
21. Hornbeck C, Floyd R, Byfield J et al. (1982) Cerebrospinal fluid versus serum concentrations of 5FU, allopurinol, and oxypurinol, and radiation. Cancer Treat Rep 66: 571–573
22. Kaplan R, Wiernik P (1982) Neurotoxicity of antineoplastic drugs. Semin Oncol 9: 103–130
23. Levin V (1976) Pharmacological considerations in brain tumor chemotherapy. In: Fewer D, Wilson C, Levin V (eds) Brain tumor chemotherapy, Thomas, Springfield, Ill.
24. Nair V, Roth L (1964) Effect of x-irradiation and certain other treatments on blood-brain barrier permeability. Radiat Res 23: 249–264
25. Neuwelt E, Balaban P, Diehl J (1983) Successful treatment of primary central nervous lymphomas with chemotherapy after osmotic blood-brain barrier opening. Neurosurgery 12: 662–671
26. Neuwelt E, Glasberg M, Frenkel E et al. (1983) Neurotoxicity of chemotherapeutic agents after blood-brain barrier modification: Neuropathological studies. Ann Neurol 14: 316–324
27. Neuwelt E (1988) The blood-brain barrier: does it disruption have a role in the treatment of central nervous system neoplams? In: Neuwelt E (ed) The clinical impact of the blood-brain barrier and its manipulation. Plenum Press, New York
28. Ommaya A (1963) Subcutaneous reservoir and pump for sterile access to ventricular cerebrospinal fluid. Lancet 2: 983–984
29. Peng G, Marquez V, Driscoll J (1975) Potential central nervous system antitumor agents: spirohydantoin mustard. J Med Chem 18: 846–849
30. Poplack D, Bleyer W, Pizzo P (1979) Experimental approaches to the treatment of CNS leukemia. Am J Pediatr Hematol Oncol 1: 141–149
31. Rapoport S (1976) Blood-brain barrier in physiology and medicine. New York
32. Rapoport S (1980) Quantitative aspects of osmotic opening of the blood brain barrier. In: Weiss L, Gilbert H, Posner J (eds) Brain metastasis. Martinus Nijhoff, The Hague
33. Rosowsky A, Abelson H, Beardsley G et al. (1982) Pharmacological studies on the dibutyl and γ-monobutyl esters of methotrexate in the rhesus monkey. Cancer Chemother Pharmacol 10: 55–61
34. Rosowsky A, Forsch R, Yu C et al. (1984) Methotrexate analogues. 21. Divergent influence of alkyl chain length on the dihydrofolate reductase affinity and cytotoxicity of methotrexate monoesters. J Med Chem 27: 605–609
35. Shapiro W, Young D, Mehta B (1975) Methotrexate distribution in cerebrospinal fluid after intravenous, ventricular and lumbar injections. N Engl J Med 293: 161–166
36. Sigman L, Van Echo D, Egorin M et al. (1984) Phase I trial of spiromustine. Proc Am Soc Clin Oncol 3: 31
37. Skipper H, Schabel F, Wilcox W (1964) Experimental evaluation of anticancer agents VII: On the criteria and kinetics associated with "curability" of experimental leukemia. Cancer Chemother Rep 35: 1–111
38. Sokoloff L (1977) The (^{14}C)-deoxyglucose method for the measurement of local cerebral glucose utilization, procedure, and normal values in conscious and anesthetized albino rats. J Neurochem 28: 897–916

276

39. Sokoloff L (1977) Relationship between physiological function and energy metabolism in the central nervous system. J Neurochem 29: 13–26
40. Soncrant T, Pizzolato G, Battistin L (1986) The use of drugs as probes of cerebral function. In: Battistin L (ed) PET and NMR: New perspectives in neuroimaging and clinical neurochemistry. Alan R. Liss, New York, pp 131–149
41. Steele W, Lawrence J, Stuart J et al. (1979) The protein binding of methotrexate by the serum of normal subjects. Eur J Pharmacol 15: 363–366
42. Survey of Intracranial Neoplasms (1977) Office of Biometry and Epidemiology NINCDS. NIH, Bethesda, MD 20205, USA
43. Vick N, Bigner D (1977) Chemotherapy of brain tumors: The blood-brain barrier is not a factor. Arch Neurol 34: 523–526
44. Weinstein H, Griffin T, Feeney J et al. (1982) Pharmacokinetics of intravenous and subcutaneous infusion of cytosine arabinoside. Blood 59: 1351–1353

Biological Approaches to Therapy

14. The Evaluation of Biological Response Modifiers for Cancer Therapy

R.B. Herberman

Compass of Biological Response Modification

During the past several years, increasing attention has been devoted to the potential applications of biological response modifiers (BRMs) for treatment of patients with cancer. It has been suggested that BRMs might provide a novel approach to therapy and be an effective alternative and/or adjunct to therapy by conventional modalities, such as chemotherapy, radiotherapy, and surgery.

BRMs have been defined by the Subcommittee on BRMs to the Division of Cancer Treatment, National Cancer Institute (NCI) as "Those agents or approaches that modify the relationship between tumor and host by modifying the host's biological response to tumor cells with resultant therapeutic effects" [1]. BRMs include natural or synthetic agents (including genetically engineered molecules as well as chemicals) and can be divided into two main categories: (a) chemical and biological agents which can stimulate or otherwise affect the host resistance mechanisms that may be involved in the control of growth and/or metastases of tumor cells and (b) cellular products that can have direct antitumor effects.

Included within the first category are predominantly immunomodulators, which could mediate their effects by activating, increasing, and/or restoring reactivity of immunological effector mechanisms that are involved in resistance to tumor growth and metastasis. Immunomodulators might also act by inhibiting suppressor or other mechanisms which interfere with effective host resistance to tumors. This general category of BRMs includes chemical agents, tumor antigens, effector cells, antibodies, and cytokines (i.e., proteins produced by, and which affect various functions of, the immune system). Also included would be agents which increase the ability of the host to tolerate damage by chemotherapy or radiotherapy, e.g., by increasing or restoring hematopoiesis (various colony-stimulating factors or drugs).

Included within the second main category of BRMs would be effector cells, antibodies, or cytokines which have antitumor effects by (a) direct cytotoxicity against tumor cells, such as cytotoxic antibodies or cytokines, including lymphotoxin or tumor necrosis factor; (b) decreasing the state of transformation (i.e., the degree of "malignancy") or increasing the differentiation or maturation of tumor cells (optimally to a terminal, nonproliferative form), so that they manifest reduced potential for uncontrolled growth, invasion, and spread (retinoids and interferons, for example, have been shown to have such effects); and (c) increasing the sensitivity of tumor cells to control by host effector mechanisms, e.g., by inducing receptors for regulatory molecules.

It is apparent that many of the approaches and agents considered to be BRMs are immunologic, and therefore there is much overlap with immunotherapy. It is therefore worthwhile to review briefly the current status of immunotherapy, and to examine why the approaches to therapy with BRMs hold much promise despite the limitations of previous immunotherapeutic approaches.

Disappointments and Defects in Previous Immunotherapeutic Approaches

During the past few years, attitudes and expectations about immunotherapy of cancer have fluctuated dramatically. A high degree of optimism as to the ability of immunologic manipulations to cure residual disease and thereby provide a major supplement to surgery and other forms of conventional therapy has been largely replaced by widespread doubts as to the value or even the potential for immunotherapy.

It seems worthwhile to first reflect on some of the reasons for the initial hopes and expectations for major therapeutic advances as a result of immunotherapy:

1. In the 1960s and early 1970s, numerous studies were published which demonstrated tumor-associated transplantation antigens on a variety of experimental tumors, primarily in inbred strains of mice. With such tumors, it was possible to induce specific resistance to autologous or syngeneic tumor growth by removal of growing tumors or by immunization with tumor cells or tumor extracts. In some cases, this resistance was rather potent, such that the immunized animals were able to resist challenge by large numbers of tumor cells.

2. These in vivo demonstrations of effective and specific antitumor immunity were soon followed by reports which provided a considerable body of evidence for apparently specific cell-mediated immunity against tumor-associated antigens on such experimental tumors [2]. In addition, similar data was obtained with many human tumors, suggesting that human tumors might also have tumor-associated transplantation antigens that were immunogenic in the autologous host.

3. Further encouragement came from the successful results of immunotherapy with various agents in some experimental tumor systems. Particular attention was focused on treatment of certain transplantable tumors with the bacterial agents *Mycobacterium bovis* (BCG) and *Corynebacterium parvum*, but some successful results were also obtained by specific immunotherapy with tumor vaccines [3]. Most impressively, the immunotherapy often resulted in complete eradication of tumor and persistent immunity against subsequent tumor challenge.

4. From several preliminary studies, it appeared that similarly successful immunotherapy could be performed on cancer patients. Of particular note were reports of significant prolongation of disease-free intervals and/or survival in patients with acute lymphocytic or myelogenous leukemia after treatment with BCG plus allogeneic irradiated tumor cells [4], regressions of primary or metastatic skin tumors after elicitation of delayed hypersensitivity reactions by contact sensitizers or BCG applied to the tumor site [5], and increased survival of operable lung cancer patients given intrapleural BCG shortly after surgery [6]. Most recently, much attention has been given to antitumor effects of interferon in some cancer patients [7], with the likely possibility that these results were mediated by stimulation of host effector mechanisms.

Despite this apparently strong basis for immunotherapy, most oncologists and even many tumor immunologists are currently quite pessimistic about clinical immunotherapy. The most immediate cause for skepticism has come from larger-scale clinical immunotherapy trials, particularly several well-designed randomized controlled trials, in which it was not possible to verify the apparent clinical benefits that had been suggested by the initial studies [8]. Of particular concern has been the lack of convincing evidence for beneficial clinical results from immunotherapy with specific tumor vaccines. An additional fundamental concern has been the accumulating evidence against some of the basic assumptions providing the rationale for immunotherapy.

Much discussion has centered on the frequent failure to detect tumor-associated transplantation antigens on some types of tumors in experimental animals, particularly spontaneous tumors [9]. Most of the earlier positive results were obtained with tumors induced by oncogenic viruses or chemical carcinogens. Since almost all human tumors are, in the absence of a clearly defined etiology, considered to be spontaneous, the negative results with spontaneous rodent tumors have often been considered to be more clinically relevant [10]. There has also been considerable evidence against a central role for immune T cells in protection against a variety of tumors. For example, the incidence of spontaneous or chemical carcinogen-induced tumors has generally been the same in nude or neonatally thymectomized mice as in euthymic mice [11]. Since thymus-dependent immunity was frequently postulated to be of primary importance for immunosurveillance and for general host resistance against tumors, this has raised questions about the overall role of the immune system in antineoplastic defenses. Similarly, there has been increasing evidence that what had previously been thought to be specific cytolytic T cells reactive against human tumors were actually natural effector cells, especially natural killer (NK) cells [12]. Further discouragement has come from the failure to detect consistent and clear-cut alterations in immune parameters in patients receiving immunotherapy.

The above findings have been taken by many investigators and oncologists as sufficient reasons to abandon attempts at immunotherapy. However, although expectations for immunotherapy were initially inappropriately optimistic, there are a number of reasons to believe that immunotherapy may have a role in future approaches to cancer treatment, not the least being the recent major advances in the understanding of the tumor-host relationship, and the development of highly purified reagents, including monclonal antibodies and molecules obtained from bacteria containing appropriate genes inserted by recombinant DNA technology. A number of problems, however, need to be overcome. For example, despite the extensive data indicating therapeutic efficacy in some experimental animal tumor systems, there is a very wide gap between such systems and the clinical situations [13]. Almost all experimental immunotherapy studies have been done with transplantable tumor cell lines, particularly those which were initiated at least 15 years ago. Such tumors may have normal histocompatibility antigens that are different from those expressed in current inbred strains. Closer models for human tumors would seem to be primary tumors, with immunotherapy being performed on established, autochthonous tumors.

In addition, although two of the basic objectives of biological response modification are to restore deficiencies in immunologic functions or to augment reactivity about existing levels, almost all of the clinical trials so far conducted have employed empirically selected doses and schedules of administration of agents. Often, agents have been given at the maximal tolerable or available doses or at arbitrary doses and schedules.

Frequently, no clear hypothesis was formulated as to the expected immunologic effect to be achieved by the immunotherapy. When a rationale for a particular immunotherapy trial was stated, it was usually formulated in terms of attempts to augment T-cell-mediated immunity to tumor-associated transplantation antigens. Similarly, most efforts at immunologic monitoring of patients receiving immunotherapy were focused on alterations in the numbers and functions of T cells. Increasing evidence indicates that other types of effector cells and mechanisms may be important in resistance against tumor growth. Further, these may not even depend on the expression of tumor-associated transplantation antigens. Such alternative immune effector mechanisms include NK cells, macrophages, and possibly even granulocytes. These may all function as components of the natural cellular immune defense system, which can be rapidly activated and can react against a wide variety of tumor cells [14, 15]. In addition, there is a real possibility that some of the agents in current use for immunotherapy may also have biological response-modifying effects which are not manifested by way of the immune system, e.g., alterations in the production of various cellular growth factors [16]. For this reason, it is preferable to speak in terms of biological response modification rather than immunotherapy.

Performance of Future Trials Involving Biological Response Modifiers

The evaluation of BRMs as therapeutic agents requires of necessity a different approach from that employed for cytotoxic drugs. Even the screening of potentially useful agents is complicated by the fact that many BRMs are not effective in other species. This applies, for example, to most human interferons and, of course, monoclonal antibodies. With such agents, in vitro assessments and evaluation of effects on human xenografts in nude mice would comprise the preclinical phase of BRM testing. After appropriate in vitro and in vivo preclinical studies, potentially useful agents must then be subject to direct testing in patients. Prior to embarking upon large-scale clinical trials, it would seem essential to determine the dose and schedule for a particular agent that optimally augment for a sustained period one or more of the effector mechanisms considered important. This is of particular concern since a variety of agents may not only augment the activity of a particular immunologic function but under some conditions also cause depression via induction of activation of suppressor cells. It should be noted that there is little reason to expect that more of a particular agent will be better. The relevant principles for immunomodulation are likely to be quite different from those that have been developed for treatment with chemotherapeutic agents, where the highest possible dose is given.

One possible approach would be to determine the optimal immunomodulating dose for each of several effector functions and then set up and compare the therapeutic results of protocols based on such information. For example, one might compare the optimal schedule for augmenting macrophage cytolytic activity with that for augmenting NK or antibody-dependent cell-mediated cytotoxic activity. One aspect of this approach which should be taken into account is that many agents are pleiotropic in their effect on the immune system or other host functions, so that for a single compound it is advisable to assay several immunologic effects. The primary concern then in a phase I trial with a putative biological response-modifying agent would be to carefully monitor for the effects of the agent at various doses and schedules of administration. Although this would appear to be an obvious and straightforward approach, agents that have been brought to the clinical level so far have not been studied in this way.

It should also be noted that most previous and current phase I trials with BRMs have been performed in patients with advanced, widespread disease, in analogy with the approaches taken for initial evaluation of chemotherapeutic agents. Although studies in such patients can provide useful information about the possible toxic side effects of the agents, they are quite unlikely to provide any indications of antitumor efficacy. Although the susceptibility of many tumors to cure by chemotherapy varies inversely with tumor mass [17]—due to the increased likelihood of development of drug-resistant clones—drugs produce logarithmic, first-order kinetics of cytotoxicity against advanced, bulky tumors as well as against small, localized tumors. In contrast, immunologically mediated antitumor effects mainly seem to be subject to a threshold, with no discernible activity against tumors beyond a certain size or degree of tissue invasion. Most experience with animal tumor systems has indicated that effective immunotherapy or other forms of biological response modification are limited to small tumor burdens and micrometastatic disease. Even highly immunogenic tumors have usually been shown not to be susceptible to therapy when BRMs are first given at an advanced stage of disease [18]. Thus, development of clinical protocols to evaluate the effects of BRMs on micrometastatic disease, as an an adjunct to surgery and/or chemotherapy or radiation therapy, is more likely to provide positive results.

A major technical issue to be raised in regard to the monitoring of the effects of various agents on effector activity is the problem of substantial spontaneous fluctuation in reactivity in the assays over a period of time. Some of this may be attributed to technical variation from day to day in the assay itself, resulting, for example, in varying susceptibility of a target cell to lysis. In addition, there may be considerable biological fluctuation in reactivity [19]. Thus, there is a real need to carefully control the monitoring, to adequately discriminate between treatment-induced alterations and spontaneous fluctuations.

Once a decision is reached as to the main mechanism of action for a given BRM, the next major issue is the determination of the protocol that would induce optimal alterations of the relevant effector mechanism. This is the primary focus for the immunopharmacology of BRMs, and it goes beyond an assessment of the pharmacokinetics of the agent itself, with the main concern being the pharmacokinetics of the alteration of the biological response. It should be noted that whereas most mechanistic studies with a BRM are focused on the alterations in reactivity after a single dose, for development of effective therapeutic protocols one needs to determine the route and schedule of administration that would produce continued alterations in reactivity over a prolonged period. It is not as yet clear whether it would be necessary to have continuous and sustained alteration in reactivity or whether cyclic alterations would be sufficient. In any event, it seems critical to determine whether repeated administration of a BRM would lead to hyporeactivity or refractoriness to alterations upon repeated exposures. If such hyporeactivity were seen, it would be the important to understand the basis for the refractoriness and to develop protocols for avoiding or overcoming such effects.

Evaluation of Interferon as a Biological Response Modifier

One very instructive example of the potential and limitations of BRMs for therapy is interferon. Over the past several years, much attention has been focused on the potential therapeutic efficacy of various types of interferon. When clinical trials were initiated with interferon, the main rationale was the known ability of interferon to inhibit the proliferation of certain types of tumor cells. However, it soon became increasingly clear that interferon is a very pleiotropic agent, with the ability to act as a potent BRM, having effects on a variety of host responses—including activation of NK cells, macrophages, and T cells—as well as potential direct antitumor effects [20, 21]. The latter include an ability to modulate various cell surface structures, including major histocompatibility antigens and tumor-associated cell surface antigens.

Despite the increasing awareness of the possible importance of such indirect biological response-modifying effects of interferon, most clinical trials that have been performed to date have centered on the frequent administration, usually daily, of the maximum amounts of interferon that either were available or were tolerated by the patients. It is quite likely that such protocols are mainly optimal for direct cytostatic antitumor activity of interferon. These protocols have had early positive therapeutic effects on some types of cancer, with partial or complete regressions being seen in patients with extensive tumor burdens, who had become refractory to other forms of therapy. A substantial proportion of patients with non-Hodgkin's lymphoma—particularly nodular poorly differentiated lymphoma [22, 23] and cutaneous T-cell lymphoma [24]— and patients with hairy-cell leukemia [25] have been shown to respond to α-interferon. A similar range of antitumor effects has been observed so far in the phase I clinical trials of recombinant γ-interferon [26–30]. However, it has been quite disappointing that most patients with other types of cancer have shown little or no therapeutic benefits from interferon administration.

One of the possible explanations for the limited therapeutic efficacy that has been seen thus far is the use of protocols for administration of interferon that are not sufficiently effective for inducing sustained alterations of other important biological effects. This possibility is supported by the experience to date in regard to the effects of the interferon protocols on NK activity. Interferon has been demonstrated to be a major factor involved in the activation of NK cells and for augmentation of spontaneous reactivity [31]. This information, coupled with the increasing evidence for an important role of NK cells in resistance against tumors—particularly against metastases—has led to much interest in the effects of interferon administration on NK activity. Most clinical trials have now incorporated the monitoring of NK activity as a fundamental part of the study design. Unexpectedly, in view of the known ability of interferon administration to boost NK activity in mice, and the early reports of sustained augmentation of NK activity in patients with osteosarcoma receiving therapy with Cantell α-interferon [31], most clinical studies have revealed only transient augmentation of NK activity in patients receiving frequent, high doses of various forms of interferon. For example, in a clinical trial with highly purified recombinant leukocyte interferon clone A, augmentation of NK activity was seen in very few of the patients, and about 30% of the patients receiving interferon twice daily showed depressed NK activity below the spontaneous levels measured prior to initiation of therapy [19].

The explanation for the failure of interferon to cause sustained augmentation of NK activity in cancer patients is not yet clear, and the question is under active investigation. These results cannot be explained by a general refractoriness in the response of the cancer patients to interferon since in vitro treatment of the cells of most cancer patients resulted in substantial augmentation of NK activity. Further, it appears that administration of a single dose of interferon results in augmentation in most patients. Therefore, it appears that the repeated administration of interferon results in some form of hyporeactivity. Recent studies [32] have indicated that this is not due to a decrease in the number of circulating large granular lymphocytes (LGL), which mediate NK activity, or to a decrease in the proportion of LGL which can bind to NK-susceptible target cells. Rather, it appears that the LGL lose their ability to cause lysis of attached target cells and become refractory to augmentation of NK activity upon in vitro exposure to α-interferon.

A potentially useful animal model for exploring the mechanisms for this refractoriness has recently been developed. It has been found that a hybrid recombinant leukocyte interferon, A/D bgl, is able to boost NK activity of mouse cells as well as human cells [33]. Single doses of this hybrid recombinant interferon have caused substantial augmentation of NK activity in mice, whereas repeated daily doses of this preparation have led to progressively lower NK activity, particularly in the peripheral blood [34]. Further studies to elucidate the mechanism for this refractoriness to sustained boosting of NK activity and the likely development of strategies to overcome this hyporeactivity may be quite helpful in designing future clinical trials that might be efficacious. In addition, it is hoped that the extensive experience with interferon therapy will serve as a useful model for analogous attempts at therapy with other cytokines.

Evaluation of Interleukin 2 as a Biological Response Modifier

Another example of some current problems in the evaluation of BRMs has come from studies with another cytokine, interleukin 2 (IL-2). This is a product of T cells and LGL which can stimulate the growth and function of T cells and of NK cells, and by either one of these effects it might be quite useful therapeutically. The Biological Response Modifiers Program (BRMP) of the NCI decided in 1984 to become actively involved in clinical trials with IL-2, and as a first step, it seemed important to evaluate it in a series of preclinical tests. Preclinical evaluation of IL-2 has been easier than in the case of the interferons, since human IL-2 is active in mice and rats as well as in humans, so that it can be extensively tested both in vitro and in vivo in rodents as well as in humans. Detailed studies on how it might be effective in animal models are now being actively pursued. This should provide an extensive information base to help in the design of the clinical trials.

It has also been necessary to decide which IL-2 preparation to utilize for clinical studies. One question was whether to perform studies with natural IL-2, produced by lymphoid cells, or to proceed immediately to studies with the recombinant protein. On the one hand, recombinant IL-2 was attractive because of the potential availability of unlimited quantities of homogeneous factor, whereas natural IL-2 preparations are difficult to make in large amounts and to purify to homogeneity. However, one might expect that the lack of glycosylation of the recombinant protein and possible differences in its physical form might make it appreciably different from natural IL-2 in terms of biodistribution or functional activities. Upon surveying possible supplies of IL-2, the BRMP soon became aware of 12 different products, 6 natural and 6 recombinant. Since clearly it would not be practical to perform clinical trials with more than one or two of these preparations, a series of preclinical studies were performed to directly compare the potency of the different products in various functional assays and to examine them for possible contaminants or unexpected effects [35].

In order to adequately evaluated the relative potency of the various IL-2 preparations, they first had to be standardized in terms of their activity in assays of promotion or growth of T-cell lines. When the preparations were all compared with a BRMP standard preparation of IL-2, it was obvious that a unit of IL-2 from one company was considerably different from a unit of IL-2 from another company. Overall, there was more than 100-fold variation among the preparations in the relationship between the companies' stated units of activity and the BRMP reference units which were actually measured. In order to compare adequately the results of various trials with different IL-2 preparations, it will obviously be important to achieve standardization of the units of activity.

As well as standardizing the potency, it was also important to determine the possible presence of contaminants in the preparations. Although it is desirable to work only with homogeneous materials, there were no completely homogeneous natural IL-2 preparations available, and it was therefore necessary to screen for a number of other cytokine activities and other materials which might be contaminating the IL-2. Endotoxin was detected in some of the natural and recombinant preparations, which would clearly be undesirable for clinical use. Some of the natural products were found to have interferon activity, and if these were used in clinical trials, it would be difficult to determine whether any therapeutic effects were due to the IL-2 or to the interferon. In addition, after the IL-2 preparations were standardized to have the same potency in terms of their ability to grow T cells, they were still found to vary in regard to other biological activities. For example, there was much heterogeneity, more than 50-fold, in the ability of the preparations to augment NK cell activity, another important property of IL-2. Even among the recombinant IL-2 preparations, there was a 50-fold difference in NK-augmenting activity. Another unexpected result from this comparative study was the observation that most IL-2 preparations, including the recombinant materials, had macrophage- or monocyte-activating properties. This indicates an additional functional effect of IL-2 which might have therapeutic implications and will need to be monitored during clinical trials with IL-2.

Thus, even before entry into clinical trials, a number or potential pitfalls in the evaluation of IL-2 were apparent; many of these apply to other BRMs. A further problem which must be addressed in clinical studies is the in vivo ability of IL-2 (it has a serum half-life of only a few minutes) and the uneven distribution in the body.

The results of phase I trials with IL-2 have been reported [36–39], and, as might be expected for such preliminary dose-finding studies in patients with advanced cancer, little evidence for therapeutic efficacy in these trials was obtained.

Potential of Monoclonal Antibodies for Cancer Therapy

Monoclonal antibodies directed against tumor-associated antigens represent another promising approach to therapy. Although this technology has only been available for a few years, widespread and intensive efforts are being directed toward the development of therapeutically effective antibodies and protocols. Currently, the main challenge is to identify the parameters that are critical for in vivo antitumor efficacy.

The central issue with monoclonal antibodies is their specificity. Firstly, it is important for the antibodies to react well with tumor cells—preferably with high affinity—to recognize most or all neoplastic cells within a tumor, and to react with metastatic lesions as well as with primary tumors. Several of the currently available monoclonal antibodies to human tumor antigens have not been optimal in this regard because of considerable heterogeneity of expression of the relevant antigen on the tumor cells of a given patient [40]. Such heterogeneity would be expected to substantially limit the therapeutic efficacy, unless the heterogeneity correlates with some aspect of tumor cell behavior. For example, it is possible that some antigens might be well expressed on all clonogenic tumor cells and not on more differentiated progeny within the tumor. In such a case, the ability of antibodies to eliminate the stem cells might be a highly effective form of therapy.

The other key issue regarding specificity of monoclonal antibodies is the degree of reactivity with various normal cells, particularly with cell surface antigens. To maximize selective uptake by the tumor and to minimize toxicity, it would clearly be desirable to utilize antibodies with a high degree of specificity for tumor-associated antigens. It is of critical importance in screening potentially useful monoclonal antibodies to determine their specificity for tumor cells. In vitro screening of antibodies on tissue sections from tumors and normal tissues, utilizing an immunoperoxidase histochemical technique, can be very useful. However, this in vitro screening may not provide a sufficiently accurate indication of in vivo localization of the antibodies at the site of the tumor, and it may also fail to reveal potential problems with in vivo binding of the antibodies to certain normal tissues or circulating tumor antigen.

With regard to the degree of uptake of antibody by the tumor, very detailed information can be obtained with accessible lesions by performing biopsies at various times after antibody administration and examining the distribution of mouse immunoglobulins by immunoperoxidase staining. This procedure can provide direct indications of the degree of coating of tumor cells with the antibody and reveal whether some parts of the tumor are not detectably coated. Similarly, single-cell suspensions can be prepared from the biopsy material, and studies performed by fluorescence flow cytometry to determine the proportion of tumor cells which bind antibody. Such approaches provide considerably more information than can be obtained by radiolocalization of administered antibody coupled to a radioisotope. However, the radiolocalization technique has the particular advantage of also providing information about the proportion of the total antibody that actually reaches the tumor; i.e., it may be more sensitive than the in vitro procedures just described and can provide direct evidence of unwanted uptake in normal organs.

The potential toxicity of monoclonal antibodies still needs to be better understood. One would anticipate that toxic effects would be related to the proportion of antibody which did not reach the tumor, but rather bound to normal tissues; a major factor in this regard is the specificity of the antibody for tumor cells. However, even if few normal cells express the relevant antigen, circulating antigen may not only prevent access to tumor cells but also lead to the formation of immune complexes which will be taken up by liver and spleen. If monoclonal antibodies are coupled to drugs, toxins, or radionuclides, this could have serious consequences. In addition, monoclonal antibodies are currently produced predominantly in mice or rats, and problems resulting from this may be encountered. Antibodies that are produced in heterologous species may not discriminate tumor-associated specificities as effectively as human antibodies, and, as soon as the necessary technology is sufficiently developed, it is hoped that an array of human monoclonal antibodies to tumor-associated antigens can be developed. The dependence on rodents as the source of monoclonal antibodies also has the associated problem of inoculation of heterologous proteins into cancer patients. This might lead to the induction of anaphylactic reactions, serum sickness, or other immunologic manifestations of an immune response against the monoclonal antibody or contaminating proteins [41]. Further, the production, by the patient, of antibodies against mouse or rat immunoglobulins, with consequent inactivation, would appear to be a major limitation to the efficacy of repeated administration of such antibodies over a prolonged period.

Another major issue which must be addressed is the degree of modulation of antigens on tumor cells which is induced by monoclonal antibodies. Such modulation is not necessarily a disadvantage. On the one hand, decreased expression by the tumor cell of the antigens recognized by a monoclonal antibody would be expected to limit the efficacy of repeated doses of the antibody, a particular concern in trials involving administration of antibodies alone. On the other hand, however, antigenic modulation or endocytosis of the surface-bound antigen-antibody complexes could be a prerequisite for the toxic effects of most immunoconjugates since it is likely that the toxic moieties affect tumor cells only when introduced internally. Most instances of antigenic modulation that have been observed with monoclonal antibodies have been associated with leukemia and lymphoma cells. It is generally considered that solid tumors are not susceptible to antigenic modulation by monoclonal antibodies, and therefore the susceptibility of solid tumors to effective therapy with immunoconjugates has been questioned. However, there are recent indications that at least some monoclonal antibody conjugates directed toward specific solid tumors induce cytotoxicity. For example, marked antitumor effects have been observed in a guinea pig hepatocarcinoma treated with conjugates of a monoclonal antibody coupled to the A chain of either diphtheria toxin or abrin [42. 43]. Nevertheless, it seems necessary to screen for the particular antibody-tumor combination which shows antigenic modulation and, particularly, to demonstrate in vitro killing of tumor

291

cells by the immunoconjugate. Positive results in such studies would provide considerable encouragement for use in in vivo therapy. This issue of antigenic modulation would not seem so important for immunoconjugates of monoclonal antibodies with radioisotopes, where delivery of radiation in the region of the tumor cells might be sufficient to cause regression of radiosensitive tumors, although this would clearly depend upon the amount and energy of the radioactivity delivered.

In addition to the considerable potential for utilizing antibodies to deliver toxic agents to the site of tumor growth, there are several indications that administration of monoclonal antibodies alone may have antitumor effects. This might be mediated by direct cytostatic effects of the antibodies (e.g., if the target antigen is a growth factor receptor) or by complement-dependent cytolysis. Another likely basis for antitumor effects of monoclonal antibodies alone would be cooperation with effector cells to result in antibody-dependent cell-mediated cytotoxicity. From available evidence, it would appear that therapeutic effects of antibodies alone will be mainly observed when there is a low tumor burden [42, 43]. Lack of efficacy in more advanced disease might be related either to insufficient access of the antibody to bulky lesions or to depression of the needed effector cell mechanisms [44, 45].

A monoclonal antibody to a 250 000-dalton determinant associated with human malignant melanoma, 9.2.27, has been shown to have some therapeutic efficacy against human melanomas growing in nude mice [46]. These effects are presumed to be related to collaboration of the 9.2.27 antibody with either macrophages or NK/killer cells. The latter activity, particularly, is increased in nude mice treated with 9.2.27. A clinical trial is currently under way in the BRMP of the NCI with the 9.2.27 antibody, and administration of high doses of the antibody to patients has been found to result in substantial localization in tumor sites [47]. Thus far, however, as might be expected, no therapeutic efficacy has been observed in these patients, who all have advanced disease.

Another antibody which has been utilized in phase I clinical trials is T101 (CD5), directed against a 65 000-dalton protein that is relatively specific for normal T cells but is expressed on chronic lymphocytic leukemia of B-cell type as well as on T-cell leukemias and lymphomas. Based on preliminary reports of some antitumor effects in a few patients with chronic lymphocytic leukemia [48], a systematic clinical study has been initiated [49]. In contrast to the 9.2.27 antibody, the T101 antibody causes quite rapid modulation of the cell surface antigen. Administration of high doses over a prolonged infusion period led to a particularly dramatic loss of antigen expression on the leukemia cells. Some transient decreases in circulating leukemia cells were seen in patients receiving lower doses, administered rapidly. Among patients with cutaneous T-cell lymphomas, several showed transient improvement in skin lesions, but no major responses were observed. Although the clinical results obtained thus far with this antibody are not particularly encouraging, the ability of T101 to induce rapid modulation might provide the basis for a follow-up clinical trial with the antibody conjugated to a drug, toxin, or radioisotope.

292

Monoclonal antibodies have also been produced against idiotypic determinants on the surface immunoglobulins of some B-cell lymphomas. Administration of relatively small amounts of such antibody to a patient caused long-lasting regression [50]. Such antibodies provide a striking example of the potential for exquisite tumor specificity of some monoclonal antibodies, and in parallel with the early clinical studies, extensive studies are being performed with anti-idiotype monoclonal antibodies directed against mouse lymphomas. However, it has recently been reported that even the immunoglobulin idiotype of a tumor may be modified over time, so that this most promising of tumor-specific antigens may not be the ideal target for monoclonal antibody therapy. Further, the extreme specificity of the antibody is also a major limitation of this approach since production of a new antibody for each patient is required. Development of effective monoclonal antibodies against determinants shared by a wide variety of tumors, at least of the same histologic type, would seem to have greater potential for large-scale therapeutic applications.

In conclusion, the prospects for cancer therapy with biological response modification are quite good. However, it will probably be necessary to develop detailed understanding of the mechanisms of action of the various BRMs, and to better understand the immunoregulatory processes affected by these agents, if their potential is to be realized. Although the results to date in patients with advanced disease are unimpressive, a variety of BRMs have shown considerable antitumor effects in animal tumor model systems, particularly against micro-metastatic disease. The prevention of overt metastatic disease is a major clinical problem, and it is perhaps particularly in this area that further research into the role of BRMs may be expected to lead to significant advances in the treatment of patients with cancer.

References

1. Mihich E, Fefer A (eds) (1983) Biological response modifiers: Subcommittee report. NCI Monogr 63
2. Herberman RB (1974) Cell mediated immunity to tumor cells. Adv Cancer Res 19: 207–263
3. Baldwin RW (1982) Manipulation of host resistance in cancer therapy. Springer Semin Immunopathol 5: 113–125
4. Foon KA, Smalley RV, Riggs CW, Gale RP (1983) The role of immunotherapy in acute myelogenous leukemia. Arch Intern Med 143: 1726–1731
5. Klein E, Holtermann OA, Helm F, Rosner D, Milgrom H, Adler S, Stoll HL, Case RW, Prior RL, Murphy GP (1975) Immunologic approaches to the management of primary and secondary tumors involving the skin and soft tissues: review of a ten-year program. Transplant Proc 7: 297–315
6. McKneally MF, Maver CM, Kausel HW (1978) Regional immunotherapy of lung cancer using postoperative intrapleural BCG. In: Terry WD, Windhorst DB (eds) Immunotherapy of cancer: Present status of trials in man. Raven Press, New York, pp 180–188
7. Borden, E (1979) Interferons: Rationale for clinical trials in neoplastic disease. Ann Intern Med 91: 472–479

8. Terry WD, Rosenberg SA (eds) (1983) Immunotherapy of human cancer. Excerpta Medica, New York
9. Hewitt HB, Blake ER, Walder AS (1976) A critique of the evidence for active host defense against cancer, based on personal studies of 27 murine tumours of spontaneous origin. Br J Cancer 33: 241–259
10. Hewitt HB (1982) Animal tumor models and their relevance to human tumor immunology. J Biol Response Mod 1: 107–119
11. Stutman O (1979) Chemical carcinogenesis in nude mice: Comparison between nude mice from homozygous matings and heterozygous matings and effects of age and carcinogen dose. JNCI 62: 353–358
12. Herberman RB (ed) (1980) Natural cell-mediated immunity against tumors. Academic Press, New York
13. Herberman RB (1983) Counterpoint: Animal tumor models and their relevance to human tumor immunology. J Biol Response Mod 2: 39–46
14. Herberman RB Ortaldo JR (1981) NK cells and natural defenses against cancer and microbial diseases. Science 214: 24–30
15. Herberman RB (ed) (1982) NK cells and other natural effector cells. Academic Press, New York
16. Schlick E, Bartocci A, Chirigos MA (1982) Effect of azimexone on the bone marrow of normal and γ-irradiated mice. J Biol Response Mod 1: 179–186
17. Devita VT (1983) The relationship between tumor mass and resistance to chemotherapy. Implications for surgical adjuvant treatment of cancer. Cancer 51: 1209–1220
18. North RJ, Dye ES, Mills CD, Chandler JP (1982) Modulation of antitumor immunity—immunologic approaches. Springer Semin Immunopathol 5: 193–220
19. Maluish AE, Ortaldo JR, Conlon JC, Sherwin SA, Leavitt R, Strong DM, Weirnik P, Oldham RK, Herberman RB (1983) Depression of natural killer cytotoxicity following in vivo administration of recombinant leukocyte interferon. J Immunol 131: 503–507
20. Fogler WE, Fidler IJ (1983) Role of macrophages in host resistance against tumors. In: Herberman RB (ed) Basic and clinical tumor immunology. Martinus Nijhoff, The Hague, pp 83–106
21. Talmadge JE. Fidler IJ, Oldham RK (1985) Screening models for biological respoonse modifiers: methods and rationale. Martinus Nijhoff, Boston
22. Gutterman JB, Blumenschein G, Alexanian R, Yap H-Y, Buzdar AU, Casanillas F, Hortobagyi GN, Hersh EM, Rasmussen SL, Harmon M, Kramer M, Pestka S (1980) Leukocyte interferon-induced tumor regression in human metastatic breast cancer, multiple myeloma and malignant lymphoma. Ann Intern Med 93: 399–406
23. Foon KA, Sherwin SA, Abrams PG, Longo DL, Fer MF, Stevenson HC, Ochs JJ, Bottino GC, Schoenberger CS, Zeffren J, Jaffe ES, Oldham RK (1985) Treatment of advanced non-Hodgkin's lymphoma with recombinant leukocyte A interferon. N Engl J Med 311: 1148–1152
24. Bunn PA Jr, Foon KA, Ihde DC, Longo DL, Eddy J, Winkler CF, Veach SR, Zeffren J Sherwin S, Oldham R (1984) Recombinant leukocyte A interferon: An active agent in advanced cutaneous T-cell lymphomas. Ann Intern Med 101: 484–487
25. Foon KA, Maluish AE, Abrams PG, Wrightington S, Stevenson HC, Alarif A, Fer MF, Overton WR, Poole M, Schnipper EF, Jaffe ES, Herberman RB (1986) Recombinant leukocyte A interferon therapy for advanced hairy cell leukemia: therapeutic and immunologic results. Am J Med 80: 351–356
26. Kurzrock R, Rosenblum M, Sherwin S, Rios A, Talpaz M, Quesada J, Gutterman J (1985) Recombinant γ-interferon: Pharmacokinetics, single dose tolerance and biological activity in cancer patients. Proc Am Soc Clin Oncol 4: 222
27. Ogawa M, Yoshida Y, Shimoyama M, Yoshida S, Abe O, Kimura I, Sekiba K, Nishi M, Koyama Y (1985) A phase I trial of recombinant gamma interferon. Proc Am Soc Clin Oncol 4: 219
28. Trautman T, Kirkwood JM, Ernstoff MS, Davis C, Coval S, Reich S, Rudnick S, Fischer D (1985) Phase I-II trial of recombinant interferon gamma (IFNγ) by 2 or 24 hr infusion in 30 melanoma patients. Proc Am Soc Clin Oncol 4: 232
29. Vadhan-Raj S, Nathan C, Bhalla R, Pelus L, Al-Katiba A, Koziner B, Sherwin S, Oettgen H,

Krown S (1985) Phase I trial of recombinant interferon gamma (~ IFNγ) by 6 hour intravenous infusion. Proc Am Soc Clin Oncol 4: 228

30. Gockerman JP, Hood L, Bishop C, Huang AT, Triozzi P, Sedwick WD, Koren H, Borowitz H, Tso CY, Laszlo J (1985) Phase I studies of recombinant gamma interferon. Proc Am Soc Clin Oncol 4: 232

31. Einhorn S, Ahre A, Blomgren H, Johansson B, Mellstedt H, Strander H (1982) Enhanced NK activity in patients treated by interferon-α. Relation to clinical response. In: Herberman RB (ed) NK cells and other natural effector cells. Academic Press, New York, pp 1259–1263

32. Hizuta A, Maluish AE, Ortaldo JR, Herberman RB (1984) NK activity in patients receiving therapy with recombinant leukocyte A interferon. In: Hoshino T, Koren HS, Uchida A (eds) Natural killer activity and its regulation. Excerpta Medica, Tokyo, pp 453–458

33. Ortaldo JR, Mason A, Rehberg E, Kelder B, Harvey C, Osheroff P, Pestka S, Herberman RB (1983) Augmentation of NK activity with recombinant and hybrid recombinant human leukocyte interferons. In: De Maeyer E, Shellekens H (eds) The biology of the interferon system. Elsevier, Amsterdam, pp 353–358

34. Brunda MJ, Rosenbaum D (1984) Modulation of murine natural killer cell activity in vitro and in vivo by recombinant human interferons. Cancer Res 44: 597

35. Thurman GB, Maluish AE, Rossio JL, Schlick E, Onozaki K, Talmadge JE, Procopio ADG, Ortaldo JR, Ruscetti FW, Stevenson HC, Cannon GB, Iyer S, Herberman RB (1985) Comparative evaluation of multiple lymphoid and recombinant human IL-2 preparations. In: Sorg C, Schimpl A (eds) Cellular and molecular biology of lymphokines. Academic Press, New York, pp 767–777

36. Lotze MT, Robb RJ, Sharrow SO, Frana LW, Rosenberg SA (1984) Systemic administration of interleukin-2 in humans. J Biol Response Mod 3: 475–482

37. Lane HC, Siegel JP, Rook AH, Masur H, Gellmann EP, Quinnan GV, Fauci AS (1984) Use of interleukin-2 in patients with acquired immunodeficiency syndrome. J Biol Response Mod 3: 512–516

38. Mertelsmann R, Welte K, Sternberg C, O'Reilly R, Moore MAS, Clarkson BD, Oettgen HF (1984) Treatment of immunodeficiency with interleukin-2: initial exploration. J Biol Response Mod 3: 483–490

39. Kolitz JE, Holloway K, Welte K, Sykora KW, Miller G. Fiedler W, Bradley E, Konrad M, Engert A, Oettgen H, Clarkson BD, Mertelsmann R (1985) A multiple dose phase I trial of recombinant interleukin 2 in advanced malignancy. Proc Am Soc Clin Oncol 4: 228

40. Hand PH, Nuti M, Colcher D, Schlom J (1983) Definition of antigenic heterogeneity and modulation among human mammary carcinoma cell populations using monoclonal antibodies to tumor-associated antigens. Cancer Res 43: 728–735

41. Ritz J, Schlossman SF (1982) Utilization of monoclonal antibodies in the treatment of leukemia and lymphoma. Blood 59: 1–11

42. Bernhard MI, Foon KA, Oeltmann TN, Key ME, Hwang KM, Clarke GC, Christensen WL, Hoyer LC, Hanna MG Jr, Oldham RK (1983) Guinea pig 10 hepatocarcinoma model: characterization of monoclonal antibody and in vivo effect of unconjugated antibody and antibody conjugated to diphtheria toxin A chain. Cancer Res 43: 4420–4428

43. Hwang KM, Foon KA, Cheung PH, Pearson JW, Oldham RK (1984) Selective antitumor effect on L10 hepatocarcinoma cells of a potent immunoconjugate composed of the A chain of abrin and a monoclonal antibody to a hepatoma-associated antigen. Cancer Res 44: 4578–4586

44. Rosenberg SA, Terry WD (1977) Passive immunotherapy of cancer in animals and man. Adv Cancer Res 25: 323–388

45. Kirch ME, Hammerling U (1981) Immunotherapy of murine leukemias by monoclonal antibody. I. Effective passively administered antibody and growth of transplanted tumor cells. J Immunol 127: 805–810

46. Bumol TF, Wang OC, Reisfeld RA, Kaplan NO (1983) Monoclonal antibody and an antibody-toxin conjugate to a cell surface proteoglycan of melanoma cells suppress in vivo tumor growth. Proc Natl Acad Sci USA 80: 523–533

47. Oldham RK, Foon KA, Morgan AC, Woodhouse CS, Schroff RW, Abrams PG, Fer M,

295

Schoenberger CS, Farrell M, Kimball E, Sherwin SA (1984) Monoclonal antibody therapy of malignant melanoma: in vivo localization in cutaneous metastasis after intravenous administration. J Clin Oncol 2: 1235–1244

48. Dillman R O, Shawler DL, Sobol RE, Collins HA, Beauregard JC, Wormsley SB, Royston I (1982) Murine monoclonal antibody therapy in two patients with chronic lymphocytic leukemia. Blood 59: 1036–1045

49. Foon KA, Schroff RW, Mayer D, Sherwin SA, Oldham RK, Bunn PA, Hsu S-M (1983) Monoclonal antibody therapy of chronic lymphocytic leukemia and cutaneous T cell lymphoma: preliminary observations. In: Boss BD, Langman R, Trowbridge I, Dulbecco R (eds) Monoclonal antibodies and cancer. Academic Press, Orlando, pp 39–52

15. Biologic Response Modifiers in Cancer Therapy

J.W. Clark and D.L. Longo

Introduction

Biologic response modifiers (BRMs) encompass those agents or approaches that modify the biologic interaction between an individual and his malignancy with a resulting therapeutic effect. The host-tumor interaction can be modified by direct effects against the tumor, by modulating the host immunologic response against the tumor, or by modifying other aspects of the biology of the host-tumor interaction. Technologic advances over the past 15 years have led to the production of large amounts of highly purified specific biologic agents and to the rapid increase in the understanding of both the biology of the host-tumor interaction and how this interaction could be modified by various interventions. Hopefully, these approaches will provide effective new cancer treatments both alone and in combination with the established forms of cancer therapy—surgery, radiation therapy, and chemotherapy. In addition, these agents and approaches are providing, and should continue to provide, enhanced understanding of cancer cell biology, with resultant novel approaches to cancer therapy.

Historical Perspectives and Classical Immunotherapeutic Approaches

Prior to the development of the molecular biologic techniques that made gene cloning possible, with the resultant ability to produce large amounts of specific biologic agents, and the hybridoma technology that enabled highly specific monoclonal antibodies to be produced, the majority of trials with "BRMs" employed mixtures of ingredients aimed at modulating the host immune system in order to achieve an immunotherapeutic antitumor response. The ideas used in designing these clinical trials were often based on results generated from studies of immunotherapy of cancer in animals. In many of these animal studies, antitumor effects were measured soon after the inoculation of malignant cells into a healthy animal, models that have little correlation with the usual clinical situation of well-established tumors in cancer patients. Most studies in animals have suggested that immunotherapy against cancer is most successful when the tumor burden is small, so many of the attempts using immunotherapy have been in the adjuvant setting.

Clinical attempts at immunostimulation have primarily used one of two approaches: (a) specific stimulation of the host immune response against the tumor either *actively*—by injecting autologous or heterologous tumor cells that have been rendered nontumorigenic but remain viable, or by using cell surface antigens of malignant cells—or *passively*, by the administration of antibodies targeted against tumor antigens and (b) nonspecific stimulation of the immune response using viral, bacterial, or a variety of other antigenic materials. It has been difficult to identify, isolate, and purify specific tumor-associated antigens from human tumors, so that most early trials using tumor antigens as vaccines were with impure preparations of undetermined specificity. Tumor vaccines have been used either by themselves or more commonly in combination with other immune stimulants, such as inactivated viruses or bacille Calmette-Guérin (BCG), in an attempt to boost the immune response against tumor cells or tumor antigens [1]. Although occasional studies showing evidence of clinical benefit have been reported, these efforts have been largely unsuccessful due at least in part to the inability to stimulate a sufficiently strong host immune response against tumor antigens. However, the occasional positive clinical trials— such as one using treated autologous colon cancer cells in combination with BCG—raise [2] the hope that if vaccines with sufficient antigenicity can be developed, and vaccination conditions that maximize the host immune response defined, one might be able to induce a sufficient host antitumor response to be clinically beneficial; this might be especially true in the adjuvant setting. Animal studies showing synergy between chemotherapy and tumor cell vaccines, the ability to define tumor-associated antigens more readily using monoclonal antibodies, the availability of techniques to produce synthetic peptides based on the amino acid sequence of tumor antigens, and the availability of specific biologic agents [such as interleukin-2 (IL-2) or interferons] which can augment the immune response all provide future directions for developing therapeutic tumor vaccines.

Therapeutic attempts using passive, specific immunotherapy have included heteroantisera directed against specific tumor-associated antigens or, more recently, monoclonal antibody therapy directed against such antigens [3, 4]. The early studies using heteroantisera required large amounts of animal sera and had the problems of laborious and difficult purification of antibodies from these sera, variability in the amount of activity in the different purified lots, and the strong antigenicity of the infused antibodies. This approach was generally unsuccessful and has given way to monoclonal antibody therapy, which will be discussed later in this contribution.

A number of trials have investigated the use of nonspecific augmentation of the immune response in order to (hopefully) generate a concomitant host antitumor response. The most commonly used agent in these trials has been BCG or derivatives of BCG, although a variety of other agents have been used, including *Corynebacterium parvum*, bestatin (a low-molecular-weight dipeptide derived from fungus), levamisole, endotoxin, OK-432 (a streptococcal cell wall extract), viruses, and tuftsin (a natural four-amino acid peptide, which is primarily a macrophage activator) [1]. Several trials have indicated some clinical benefit with this approach, including trials using BCG in the adjuvant setting in acute myeloblastic leukemia (AML) and melanoma [1]. However, except for the use of BCG intravesically to treat superficial bladder cancer (especially post-fulguration)—which has been shown to be effective and has become one of the currently accepted treatments for this malignancy [5]—the overall clinical experience does not suggest strikingly beneficial results with any of these agents. Some of these agents—such as tuftsin, bestatin, and OK-432—have undergone only preliminary testing, and new agents, combinations, or methods of delivery may yet provide additional roles for nonspecific immunostimulation in anticancer therapy.

A variety of other approaches to immunotherapy have been attempted with only limited success: these include the inhibition of suppressor (T-) cell function by histamine-2 receptor antagonists (such as cimetidine) or chemotherapeutic agents (such as low-dose cyclophosphamide), the use of transfer factor in an attempt to transfer specific cellular immunity, and the use of subcellular RNA fractions (so-called immune RNA) in an attempt to transfer specific immunity. Attempts to develop better mehtods of inhibiting suppressor cell function and to combine this with immunostimulating agents are being pursued [6].

Just as the cumulative, largely negative results of traditional immunotherapeutic approaches were suggesting that new approaches were needed, technologic developments during the past 15 years led to a rebirth of interest in BRM approaches to cancer treatment. The two developments that have had the greatest impact are: (a) cloning and insertion of genes and the induction of expression of human gene products in bacterial, yeast, and other cells, which has made possible the production of large amounts of highly purified human proteins with high specific activity and (b) hybridoma technology that allows the production of large amounts of monoclonal antibodies with predefined specificity [7].

There has also been an immense increase in the understanding of biologic processes at the cellular and molecular levels over the past 15 years. This provides a more rational basis for determining which agents should be screened in preclinical studies, how these can best be used, and how they might be combined with other cancer treatment modalities to yield clinical benefit. One of the major fundamental concepts that this increased understanding has provided is that there are many approaches to biologic response modification in cancer patients other than strictly immunotherapeutic ones that it is critical to pursue (e.g., differentiating agents, attempts at inhibiting tumor metastasis, and biologic agents that have direct antitumor activity; Fig. 1). Continued basic research into the complex host-tumor interaction should provide a better understanding of how to manipulate this interaction in a clinically beneficial manner.

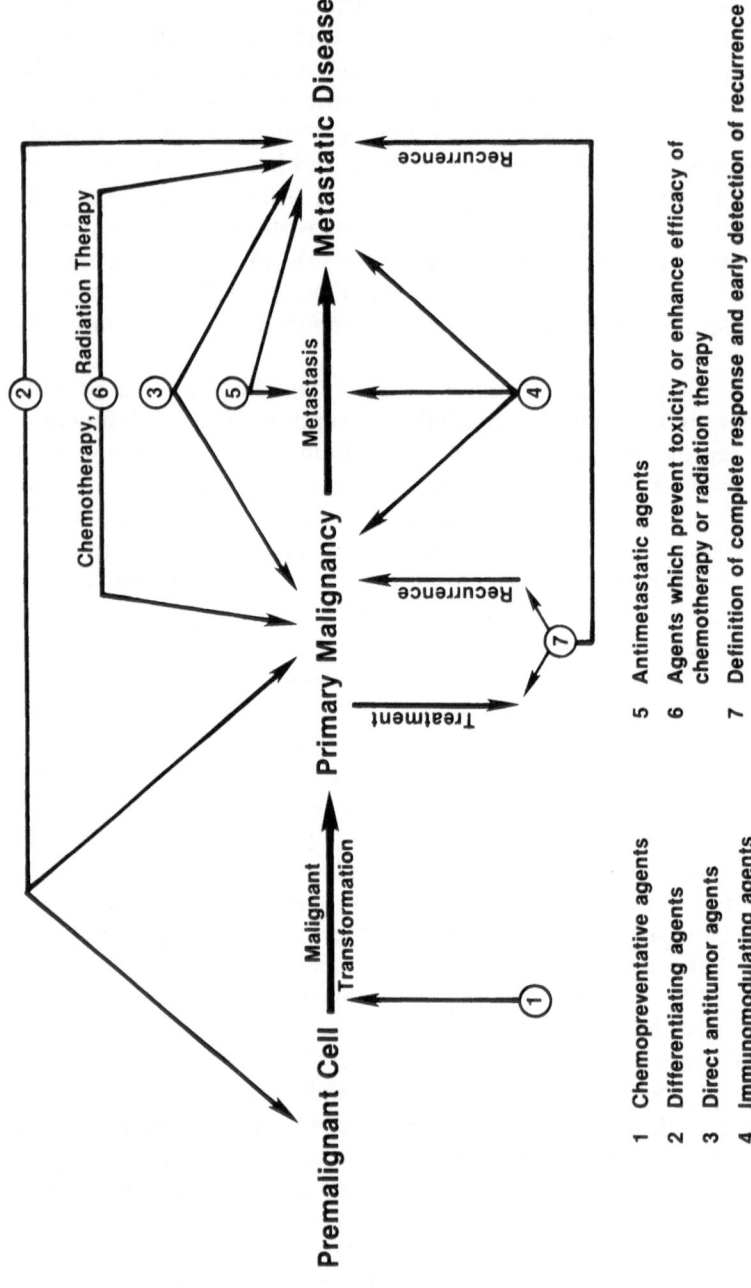

Fig. 1. Multiple areas where BRMs are involved in anticancer treatment

1 Chemopreventative agents
2 Differentiating agents
3 Direct antitumor agents
4 Immunomodulating agents

5 Antimetastatic agents
6 Agents which prevent toxicity or enhance efficacy of chemotherapy or radiation therapy
7 Definition of complete response and early detection of recurrence

Classification of Biologic Response Modifiers

BRMs can be divided into three major functional categories:

1. Agents that modulate, enhance, decrease the suppression of, or restore host immunologic mechanisms which might be involved in suppressing the growth or metastasis of malignant cells
2. Either cell products or cells that have direct antitumor effects [e.g., natural killer cells, lymphokine-activated killer cells, monoclonal antibodies, or tumor necrosis factor (TNF)]
3. Agents with various other biologic effects that modify host-tumor interactions by mechanisms other than immunologic or direct antitumor effects (agents that inhibit events such as oncogene expression which might be important in the initiation or maintenance of transformation, agents that interfere with the metastatic process or the establishment or growth of metastatases once they have occurred, differentiating agents, and agents that protect bone marrow cells or other normal tissues from cytotoxic effects of chemotherapy or radiation therapy).

Many agents have more than one biologic effect, and may act both directly and indirectly. They therefore have several mechanisms by which they might mediate an antitumor response. Good examples of this are the interferons, which have a number of biologic effects, including direct antiproliferative effects against cancer cells, various immunomodulating effects, differentiating effects on certain cells, inhibition of expression of certain oncogenes, and potentially indirect effects through interaction with other cells (e.g., the stimulation of TNF receptors on cell surfaces by γ-interferon) [8]. Therefore, it is often extremely difficult to determine by which mechanism or mechanisms these agents are mediating their antitumor effects. The precise mechanism may differ with dose and schedule of administration of the agent. If one can define the mechanisms important in the antitumor response mediated by the different agents and against different tumors, then this should lead to more rational approaches using these agents in treating cancer. Table 1 lists some of the BRMs and the mechanisms by which they are felt to be mediating their antitumor effects.

Current Therapy with Biologic Response Modifiers

The following is a discussion of selected BRMs—especially those which are highly purified, such as recombinant interferons, recombinant IL-2, and monoclonal antibodies—that have undergone clinical testing. Clearly, there are many other BRMs, and each BRM has some unique properties that must be considered in performing and evaluating clinical trials. However, the general principles that have evolved in bringing the agents discussed here from the

Table 1. Biologic response modifiers

Agents with primarily immunomodulating activity
    Nonspecific immune modulators (BCG, *C. parvum*, OK-432, tuftsin, etc.)
    Cytokines/lymphokines [thymic factors, interleukins (IL-1, IL-2), etc.]
    Suppression of inhibitors of immune function [agents which inhibit suppressor cell function (low-
        dose Cytoxan, H-2 receptor blockers), removal of immune complexes, etc.]
    Specific transfer of immunity (transfer factor, immune RNA)
    Active specific immunization (tumor cells or tumor cell surface antigens with or without additional
        adjuvant immunotherapy)
Agents with primarily direct antitumor effects
    Tumor necrosis factor
    Monoclonal antibodies
    Adoptive immunotherapy (IL-2 + LAK, γ-interferon + monocytes, etc.)
Agents with other biologic effects
    Differentiating agents (retinoids, vitamin D derivates, 5-azacytidine, etc.)
    Agents which affect expression of certain genes (inhibitors of oncogenes, growth factors, etc.)
    Agents which decrease toxicity (especially bone marrow cell protectors) or enhance efficacy of
        antitumor agents (GM-CSF, G-CSF, L-histidinol, etc.)
Agents with combination of effects
    Interferons (have all of above effects)

---

laboratory to patient treatment can be used as a framework in which to view the clinical approach to other BRMs.

Preclinical Screening

The large number of BRM agents and the need to take only those agents with promise of activity into clinical trials means that extensive preclinical evaluation of the agent is required. The particular preclinical studies that need to be done depend on the nature of the agent being used. For immunomodulating agents, these include in vitro studies of the effects on various immune functions and studies in animals evaluating both immunomodulating effects and direct anti-tumor activity. For agents that have direct antitumor effects, both in vitro studies (including clonogenic assays) and evaluation of in vivo antitumor effects are needed. For agents with other biologic effects, the relevant effect (e.g., dif-ferentiation or inhibition of oncogene expression) needs to be studied in vitro and in vivo, and one also has to evaluate for antitumor efficacy. Since, as men-tioned previously, many BRMs have a variety of potential modes by which they might mediate their antitumor effects, a variety of studies are usually needed to fully evaluate the mechanisms of action and therapeutic potential of the agent. One also has to evaluate the toxicity of these agents in animals to determine a safe starting dose for human clinical trials. Although it is always difficult to extrapolate from in vitro and animal studies to the human situation—and this is compounded in the evaluation of biologic agents, which often have highly species-specific activities and toxicities—these studies are essential in evaluating activity, the immunomodulating properties which should be monitored, and the toxicities which might be expected in human trials.

Clinical Trials

As is true of all agents being tested in clinical trials, BRMs undergo phase I/II/III trials [1]. In addition to evaluating toxicity, maximal tolerated dose, pharmacokinetics, and whether there is any suggestion of clinical activity in the phase I trials, one has to evaluated BRMs with immunomodulating properties for that dose which most effectively modulates the immune system [9]. This optimal immunomodulating dose might differ from the maximal tolerated dose; it might be the dose that has maximal therapeutic benefit and therefore be a dose for testing in phase II studies. As mentioned, these agents often affect more than one immune function, and the dose which optimally stimulates one of these functions may suppress others. Moreover, interpersonal as well as intrapersonal differences occur over time in immunomodulatory responses to any given agent. It has therefore proved very difficult to define the optimal immunostimulatory dose for any given compound. Furthermore, a patient's overall immune function is difficult to assess by examining only the function of cells or the levels of particular molecules in the peripheral blood. Techniques for evaluating and quantitating immune function in the target organs are not available. In addition, evaluations of immune function in clinical trials are difficult and expensive. Therefore, one must carefully use the preclinical studies to determine which measures of immune function should be performed and at what time points these should be determined. Better understanding of how each of these agents mediates its effects on various immune functions and more accurate, as well as more reproducible, evaluations of immune function may make the determination of the most effective immunomodulatory dose more feasible in the future.

Therapy with Specific Biologic Response Modifiers

Interferons

Interferons (α, β, γ) are a family of glycoproteins produced by mammalian cells in response to viral infections and a variety of other inducers [8]. They can be viewed as the prototypic BRM agents because of their multitude of biologic effects, which include antiproliferative, direct antitumor, differentiating, and various immunomodulatory effects (some of these diverse actions possibly being mediated through the inhibition of oncogene expression). In addition, they have antiviral properties, which could also conceivably play a therapeutic antitumor role in those malignancies where viruses are felt to play an etiologic role. With these multiple possible modes of antitumor activity, it has been difficult to determine which ones are important for mediating interferon's antitumor effects against a particular malignancy, and clearly, different effects or a combination of effects may be involved for different malignancies and different sites of disease. Most of the data from clinical studies to date suggest that for most malignancies responsive to α-interferon, the antitumor effect is a direct one; however, the evidence for this is largely indirect.

All classes of interferons (α, β, and γ) have undergone preclinical and clinical testing. On the preclinical level, the various α-interferons and β-interferon have similar properties and activities for the most part. In addition to the properties it shares with α- and β-interferons, γ-interferon appears to be a more potent immunomodulating agent, especially with respect to its ability to stimulate class II major histocompatibility complex surface expression and to activate monocytes.

Clinically, the initial interferon trials were with natural interferons. Although these were purified and consisted largely of one class of interferon, they still contained a variety of interferons, in addition to other proteins. This made it difficult to be certain that both the antitumor effect and all of the toxicities seen were being mediated by a single subclass of interferon. Trials with these natural interferons suggested sufficient antitumor activity to encourage the rapid cloning and production of recombinant interferons once the techniques were available. The recombinant α-interferons, and especially the α_2 subclass, have been the most extensively studied. Early phase trials have also been completed for recombinant β- and γ-interferons. Overall, pharmacokinetics of different interferons are roughly similar, with rapid clearance from the blood after IV administration and more prolonged serum levels after IM administration, at least for α- and γ-interferon. Although biologic effects are seen after IM administration of recombinant β-interferon, serum levels are usually low or nondetectable. Subcutaneously administered α-interferons have kinetics similar to those after IM administration, while the bioavailability of subcutaneously administered β- and γ-interferon is still being determined.

Side effects, although varying somewhat qualitatively and quantitatively between the interferons, are also largely similar, with fever, fatigue, chills, and/or myalgias occurring in the majority of patients. Except for fatigue, the frequency and severity of these symptoms usually lessen with continued therapy, and they are also controllable by pretreatment plus frequent treatment with acetaminophen. Fatigue generally does not lessen and, especially at high doses, is one of the major dose-limiting side effects. Other toxicities occur less frequently; of these, anorexia, weight loss, and (much less commonly) central nervous system side effects (confusion, etc.) are the most common side effects that lead to discontinuation of therapy. Although some differences exist, similar side effects are seen with most of the biologic agents that have been used. Table 2 gives the side effects of interferon therapy.

Therapeutic Response to α-Interferon

Table 3 lists those diseases with reasonable response rates to α-interferon therapy. Of these, the most gratifying results so far have been seen in hairy-cell leukemia (HCL), where α-interferon has taken its place as one of the important treatment modalities and clearly prolongs survival [10]. High clinical response rates have also been seen in patients in the chronic phase of chronic myelogenous leukemia (CML), malignant pancreatic endocrine tumors, and carcinoid tumors [8]. However, it is not yet known whether these high response rates will translate into meaningful improvements in survival. The other two

Table 2. Side effects of interferon therapy

Acute
  Fever[a]/chills[a]/myalgias[a]
  Nausea/vomiting/diarrhea
  Hypotension/hypertension/arrhythmias/myocardial infarction[b]
  Headaches/dizziness/seizures[b]
  Local inflammation/urticaria
  Reactivation of oral herpes/stomatitis
Subacute to chronic
  Anorexia[a]/weight loss[a, c]
  Lethargy[a, c]/decreased concentrating ability[a]
  Altered taste
  Mood alterations/peripheral neuropathy
  Mild alopecia

[a] Frequent.
[b] Uncommon.
[c] Often dose limiting.

Table 3. Response rates of diseases to interferon

High (> 50%)
  Hairy-cell leukemia
  Chronic myelogenous leukemia (chronic phase)
  Carcinoid tumors
  Malignant endocrine pancreatic tumors
Medium (> 20% < 50%)
  Low-grade non-Hodgkin lymphoma
  Cutaneous T-cell lymphoma
  Kaposi's sarcoma
  Glioma
  Ovarian cancer (interferon given IP)
Low (> 10% < 20%)
  Melanoma
  Renal cell carcinoma
Minimal (< 10%)
  Breast cancer
  Colon cancer
  Lung cancer

diseases where therapeutic results may be most relevant clinically at the present time, although they have low overall response rates (15%–25%) to interferon, are metastatic melanoma and renal cell carcinoma since these are malignancies that have been refractory to most forms of therapy [8].

There are several interesting features concerning the responses of malignancies to α-interferon that may provide insights into how α-interferon might be mediating its antitumor effects. The most responsive tumors (HCL, CML, and malignant endocrine pancreatic tumors) respond to relatively low doses (3–6 million units/m^2 daily), raising the possibility that effects other than or in addition to direct antitumor ones may be important in the responsiveness of these tumors [8]. However, careful dose escalation trials have not been done in these malignancies to determine whether higher doses might produce more frequent or more prolonged responses that might suggest a direct antitumor effect. The mechanism or mechanisms involved in α-interferon's antitumor effects against these or any other malignancies still remain unknown. For several of the other malignancies [especially renal cell carcinoma, non-Hodgkin lymphoma (NHL), and Kaposi's sarcoma], there is a suggestion of a dose-response effect which is consistent with the possibility that for these malignancies the major mechanism of response may be a direct antitumor one. Most responses to α-interferon are partial ones, with a lower percentage of complete responses; this is even true of the most responsive malignancies. There may be disease stabilization in some patients, so that some beneficial effect may occur even in individuals who do not have measurable responses. Another interesting feature is that responses can occasionally take several months to occur, again raising the possibility that mechanisms other than or in addition to direct antitumor ones may be involved in some of the responses. Median duration of response varies by disease, with the more responsive diseases having longer response durations. For example, as long as patients continue receiving α-interferon therapy, the median response duration has not yet been reached in HCL. For most solid tumors, the median duration of response is 4–12 months despite continued interferon treatment, although occasional patients have prolonged responses lasting several years.

A potential problem with interferon (or any BRM) therapy is the development of antibodies against the agent, which might then limit its effectiveness. Studies have shown that antibodies develop in a proportion of patients receiving α-interferon therapy, and less commonly, neutralizing antibodies develop which can inhibit interferon activity [11]. Most patients who develop antibodies do not appear to have loss of interferon activity, but there are patients in whom the development of neutralizing antibodies has correlated with a loss of interferon activity. What is not known is the overall frequency of antibody development (although it appears to be low) and whether it might vary by subclass of α-interferon. Antibodies have also been detected in patients receiving β-interferon, but the overall frequency with which this occurs has not been established [12]. Preliminary studies suggest that patients receiving γ-interferon have a very low rate of antibody formation [13].

In summary, α-interferon has sufficient activity against HCL for it to have become one of the major treatment modalities for this disease. High (> 50%) response rates are also seen against the chronic phase of CML, malignant endocrine pancreatic tumors, and carcinoid tumors, although it is not yet known whether these will translate into survival benefits. Response rates in the 30%–50% range are seen for low-grade NHL, cutaneous T-cell lymphoma (CTCL), and AIDS-associated Kaposi's sarcoma, all diseases which are also responsive to chemotherapy and radiation therapy, so that the exact role of interferons in the overall treatment of these diseases still needs to be established. Lower response rates are seen in a variety of malignancies, including metastatic melanoma and renal cell carcinoma, where even these low response rates are somewhat encouraging since these diseases are largely refractory to all current forms of therapy. Very low response rates are seen in patients with lung, colon, and breast cancer.

306

β- and γ-Interferon

Results from preliminary studies using β and γ-interferon indicate some anticancer activity for each of these agents—primarily against malignancies which are responsive to α-interferon [8]. One exception may be HCL, in which preliminary studies suggest that β-, but not γ-interferon, produces responses. Whether these interferons might have unique antitumor activity not seen with α-interferon has not yet been determined.

Future Directions with Interferons

Studies evaluating (a) whether one interferon might be more effective than another for a given malignancy; (b) the mechanism or mechanisms of interferon's antitumor effects for each malignancy; (c) whether combinations of interferons with each other, with other BRMs, or with chemotherapy (all of which have been shown to be synergistic in various combinations) might have synergistic antitumor activity; and (d) whether the use of interferons (especially γ-interferon, with its more potent immunomodulating properties) in the adjuvant setting might be beneficial are all ongoing or planned. Despite several years of study, the best way to integrate interferon therapy into anticancer treatment still needs to be defined.

Interferon Inducers

A variety of interferon inducers, most notably polyinosinic polycytidylic acid in poly-L-lysine solubilized in carbonylmethylcellulose) (poly IC:LC) and poly-adenylic poly-uridilic acid (poly AU), have also been used to treat cancer patients [1]. Detectable interferon levels have not been reproducibly induced by any of these agents, and response rates have been low. However, it is not yet clear whether the interferon inducers have been optimally administered, in the fashion that would maximize the chances of detecting significant antitumor effects.

Interleukin-2 and Interleukin-2 plus Lymphokine-Activated Killer Cell Therapy

An ever-increasing number of products secreted by monocytes and lymphocytes have been discovered which have been named interleukins because they mediate interactions between hematopoietic and lymphoid cells. Interleukin-2 (IL-2) is a lymphokine produced by T cells with multiple effects on the immune system, including activation of other T cells, natural killer (NK) cells, and lympokine-activated killer (LAK) cells. [14] LAK activity is mediated by human blood leukocytes which are lytic for fresh autologous, syngeneic, and allogeneic primary tumors when tested in vitro. The LAK cell precursors do not have T- or B-lymphocyte markers, and LAK activity appears to be generated by several lymphocyte subsets. After activation with IL-2, the majority of LAK activity appears to be mediated by cells bearing NK surface markers, but a minor contribution also comes from cells bearing some T-cell surface markers. Both of these subsets express the Leu 19+ surface marker. IL-2 is also an essential factor for the growth of T cells and augmentation of various T-cell functions, it supports the proliferation and augments the function of NK cells, and as IL-2 receptors are found on other cells including monocytes, IL-2 clearly affects many cells of the immune system both directly and indirectly.

Animal studies have shown that IL-2 can restore immunologic responsiveness in certain immune-deficient states, and at high doses it has antitumor effects. A variety of human studies have used IL-2 alone in a number of doses and schedules to treat cancer patients [14, 15]. At low doses (up to 1 million units/m^2 daily), there has been minimal therapeutic activity. Higher doses of IL-2 (from 3 million units/m^2 daily to 0.1 million units/kg every eight hours) have produced responses in cancer patients. Overall, melanoma appears to be the disease most responsive to IL-2 used alone. The variability in doses and schedules used and the small numbers of individuals treated in each study make it impossible to define a response rate for melanoma for any dose and schedule of IL-2. Occasional patients with renal cell carcinoma have also responded, but most patients with renal cell cancer and malignancies other than melanoma who have been treated with IL-2 alone have not responded [14, 15]. There is some evidence that 1 million units/m^2 administered on a weekly basis can result in significant long-term augmentation of immune function, but it is not yet clear whether this will result in antitumor effects. There are a number of ongoing studies attempting to define the best dose, route, and schedule of IL-2 therapy for maximal antitumor response, and whether combination with other agents (such as cyclophosphamide, various interferons, or monoclonal antibodies) will yield higher response rates.

In an attempt to enhance the efficacy of immunotherapy in the treatment of cancer, one can directly activate immune cells ex vivo, which can then be infused into the patient to mediate an antitumor response either directly or indirectly—so-called adoptive immunotherapy. In the past, a variety of approaches have been used to do this on a limited scale without much success. The availability of highly purified BRMs with potent ability to activate cells (such as γ-interferon, which primarily activates monocytes and NK cells, and IL-2, which primarily activates T cells, NK, and LAK cells) has renewed interest in this approach.

An adoptive immunotherapy approach piloted by Steven Rosenberg at the National Cancer Institute (NCI) utilizes LAK cells in combination with IL-2 [14]. Studies in animals had shown that this combined approach decreased the number of metastases and prolonged survival to a greater extent than either LAK cells or IL-2 alone. Several human malignancies have been treated with this therapy. It appears to have greatest activity against renal cell cancer; melanoma; perhaps indolent, non-Hodgkin lymphoma; and to a lesser extent colon cancer [14]. Overall response rates for both renal cell carcinoma and melanoma are in the 15%–33% range, whereas colon cancer response rates are in the 10%–20% range. Three of four evaluable patients with nodular lymphomas who have been treated have responded, whereas one with diffuse histiocytic lymphoma did not. This therapy has been tried in a limited number of patients with other malignancies, with partial responses being reported in patients with Hodgkin's disease and lung, parotid, and ovarian cancer [16]. However, too few patients with any of these diseases have been treated to know what the overall response rates or durations will be.

The toxicities associated with this treatment are significant. The mechanisms of all of the toxicities seen have not been clearly elucidated. However, one major mechanism appears to be related to increased capillary permeability induced by IL-2 or a lymphokine product of IL-2-stimulated cells. Related to this, the majority of patients develop hypotension requiring vasopressors, over one-third of patients gain over 10% of their body weight in retained fluid, and a significant percentage have decreased urine output requiring fluid and dopamine treatment. Other toxicities include abnormal liver function (both transaminases and bilirubin elevations) in over 50% of patients, diffuse pruritic desquamating skin rash in most patients, anemia requiring red blood cell transfusions in 60%, thrombocytopenia in 28%, and alterations in mental function ranging from confusion to psychosis in approximately one-third of patients. Cardiac arrhythmias have been seen in about 13%, and angina or myocardial infarctions in 6%. All of these toxicities except for the myocardial infarctions are promptly reversible upon discontinuation of the IL-2.

In an attempt to deliver high concentrations of IL-2 plus activated cells locally while minimizing systemic toxicity, the Biological Response Modifiers Program of the NCI has begun studying the intraperitoneal administration of LAK cells plus IL-2 in patients with peritoneal carcinomatosis from ovarian and colon cancer [17]. Five patients with ovarian cancer are evaluable at this time, and two have demonstrated partial responses. Partial responses have also been seen in two of five patients with colon cancer with intraperitoneal carcinomatosis. Although these studies are preliminary, this approach would appear to hold some promise, with qualitatively similar but quantitatively less toxicity than is seen with systemic IL-2 plus LAK therapy.

There are many questions that still need to be answered concerning IL-2 plus LAK therapy. What role are LAK cells (or other adoptively transferred cells) playing in the antitumor response? Can improvements be made in dose, schedule, or route of administration of the IL-2 which might decrease toxicity or enhance activity? Can the cells be activated to a greater degree or more efficiently? Might IL-2 or IL-2 plus LAK be particularly effective in the adjuvant setting when the host tumor burden is low? What will the overall response rate be in NHL, and are there other tumor types that might be responsive? Will maintenance therapy or repeated treatment cycles yield more durable responses? Combinations with other treatment modalities—including chemotherapeutic agents such as cyclophosphamide or doxorubicin, or other BRMs such as interferons, which have shown synergistic activity in vitro in combination with IL-2—are ongoing or planned.

Another approach using adoptively transferred cells is the isolation and expansion of tumor-infiltrating lymphocytes (TILs), which have been shown to have 50–100 times greater activity than LAK cells do against the specific tumor from which they were derived [18]. Hopefully, these can be given with lower doses of IL-2, thus reducing toxicity, while still retaining high antitumor activity. Only future clinical trials will reveal how effective this approach might be.

In summary, preliminary studies have shown some activity for IL-2 alone or in combination with LAK cell therapy in the treatment of various malignancies, but especially melanoma, renal cell carcinoma, and possibly low-grade NHLs. This is encouraging since metastatic melanoma and renal cell carcinoma are malignancies which have low response rates to all therapies attempted to date. The adoptive transfer of LAK cells and IL-2 is a new form of immunotherapy about which much still needs to be learned in order to maximize its efficacy. Very preliminary results have shown an overall response rate of approximately 20%. The regimen as currently given has moderate to severe toxicity. Attempts are ongoing in the laboratory and through a variety of clinical trials to improve the efficacy of this therapy, to decrease toxicity, and possibly to combine this therapy with other treatment modalities to help establish what role IL-2 alone or in combination with LAK cells might have in the overall treatment of cancer.

Other Cytokines/Lymphokines

A large number of cytokines/lymphokines have been described, but the evaluation of most of these is still at the laboratory level [19]. A few have undergone clinical study. Thymosins are hormonelike peptides derived from the thymus, which have multiple in vitro and in vivo effects on the immune system but especially that of enhancing T-cell-mediated immune effects. Clinical studies to date, although limited, have not shown substantial antitumor activity [1, 19]. Tumor necrosis factor (TNF) is a glycoprotein produced by macrophages in response to sequential stimulation with any of a variety of priming agents (such as BCG) and then endotoxin, and it appears to be one member of a family of proteins— similar to the situation with interferons [6]. It has preferential cytotoxicity against transformed cells as opposed to normal cells and can produce hemorrhagic necrosis of murine and human tumor grafts in mice. TNF receptors have been demonstrated on tumor cells, and TNF has been shown to have direct antitumor activity against human tumors in clonogenic assays. It has also been shown to have significant antiviral activity. TNF has been cloned, and phase I trials have been performed with TNF, showing that it can be given at tolerable doses. Antitumor activity so far has been limited, but further studies are needed to define the overall antitumor activity of TNF alone. In addition, TNF and γ-interferon have marked synergistic antitumor activity in vitro and in vivo, and combination therapy using these two agents in patients are planned in the near future. Other cytokines/lymphokines include (a) interleukin-1 (IL-1), a protein produced by macrophages (among other cells) with both a variety of immuno-modulating properties (such as activation of various lymphoid cells) and a large number of other biologic effects (such as fibroblast proliferation or bone resorption) and (b) colony-stimulating factors [granulocyte/macrophage (GM-CSF) and granulocyte (G-CSF)] which have a variety of biologic effects, including the terminal differentiation of leukemic cells, macrophage activation, and—probably most importantly from an immediate clinical standpoint—augmentation of marrow generation of granulocytes and macrophages [19]. These cytokines/lymphokines have been cloned and are undergoing preclinical testing to determine whether they might play a role in cancer treatment. As more are discovered, purified, and characterized, they should provide an ever-expanding pool of agents, which can be used to modify the host-tumor interaction in a large variety of ways.

Monoclonal Antibodies

Monoclonal antibody cancer therapy is extensively discussed elsewhere in this volume, so it will be discussed only briefly here. The concept behind monclonal antibody therapy is an attractive one, with the theoretical ability to deliver treatment specifically targeted for a given tumor. One attempts to develop an antibody targeted against a surface antigen present either only on malignant cells or at least in much higher concentrations on malignant cells than on normal ones so that there is relatively specific targeting of these cells. Hopefully, the binding of the antibody to these cells will lead to immune-mediated killing of the cells; alternatively, the monoclonal antibody can be used to deliver cytotoxic agents (radioisotopes, toxins, chemotherapeutic agents, hormonal or antihormonal agents, or other biologic agents) specifically to these cells.

However, despite multiple clinical studies, the attempts to make this therapy clinically effective have been largely unsuccessful. It has been difficult to define tumor-associated antigens which are both sufficiently specific and present in sufficient concentrations on malignant cells to allow significant antibody binding. Even when these can be defined, and monoclonal antibodies developed against them, a number of remaining problems can be listed. Rapid modulation of cell surface antigens off the malignant cells frequently occurs, effectively removing the target for the monoclonal antibody (especially in leukemias and lymphomas). Most antibodies used so far have been murine antibodies that poorly activate human immune effector cells which might be important in the antitumor response. Insufficient numbers of host effector cells may be present locally when the tumor is large. There may be sufficient circulating tumor antigen in the serum to bind most of the monoclonal antibody before it can bind to the malignant cells. Clearance of the antibodies by the reticuloendothelial system (especially liver and spleen) may occur before they can bind to malignant cells.

Antimouse-immunoglobulin antibodies may develop. Finally, there may be im-
munoselection for the outgrowth of malignant cells which either do not express
the particular antigen targeted by the monoclonal antibody or express it at very
low levels. All of these factors could allow the tumor to escape attack by monoclonal antibodies. Therefore, it is not surprising that although a few patients have
had a good therapeutic response to unconjugated monoclonal antibody therapy,
most responses have been partial and transient. Even for B-cell lymphomas—
where one has a highly specific antigen, the immunoglobulin idiotype (antigen
recognition site), against which specific antibodies can be developed, and where
one patient did obtain a prolonged complete response when treated with anti-
idiotype antibody, the ability to achieve clinically significant responses has been
limited by problems with modulation of the antigen and selection for outgrowth
of cells with minor differences in the antigen recognition region of the surface
immunoglobulin molecule [3].

The major attempt at improving monoclonal antibody therapy has been to
conjugate them to various compounds (toxins, radioisotopes, or chemothrapeu-
tic agents) in an attempt to specifically deliver these agents to malignant cells
while limiting their delivery to normal tissues [4]. These conjugates potentially
take advantage of internal modulation of surface antigens by malignant cells,
leading to accumulation of these compounds within cells or concentration of
radioisotopes in the proximity of tumor cells. There still remain significant technical problems that have limited monoclonal-conjugate therapy (e.g., designing
highly stable antibody-conjugate bonding to prevent dissociation of the complex
in vivo and nonspecific uptake of the monoclonal antibody by the reticuloendothelial system in organs such as liver and lung, with accumulation of large
amounts of the toxin, drug, or radioisotope in these organs). Despite these
difficulties, several studies have used monclonal antibodies conjugated with
radioisotopes or toxins with limited success so far. One study using antiferritin
antibodies linked to ^{131}I did show some promise in the treatment of hepatocellular cancer [20], but as antibody-conjugates would be expected to accumulate
nonspecifically in the liver, it is not clear what the specific monoclonal antibody
contributed to the response.

Although monoclonal antibodies have not yet been dramatically effective
when used therapeutically, they have achieved a useful role in a variety of diagnostic applications in cancer therapy. These include their use in the immunohistologic determination of the tissue of origin of certain tumors; radioimaging
of metastases in malignancies which express known tumor antigens on their cell
surface (e.g., CA125 in ovarian cancer); and radioimmunoassays to detect the
presence of various tumor markers, which have been especially useful in detecting relapses in certain malignancies post-treatment [4]. Therapeutically, they
have been used either through complement fixation or conjugated to toxins to
eliminate cells from bone marrow (either malignant cells in autologous transplants or normal T cells to prevent graft-versus-host disease in allogeneic ones)
prior to bone marrow transplantation.

A variety of approaches are being used to try to improve the efficacy of
monoclonal antibody therapy in cancer therapy. These include antibody frag-

312

ments, which are specific but have decreased antigenicity; chimeric antibodies (mouse variable regions combined with human constant ones), which retain the antigen specificity of the mouse variable region while having the benefits of decreased antigenicity and improved activation of human immune effector functions; better methods of in vitro priming of human lymphoid cells, which to date have generally produced IgM antibodies of low affinity; heteroconjugates combining an antitumor antibody with an antibody directed against an effector cell (such as a cytotoxic T cell), leading to enhanced antigen-specific lysis of the tumor by the T cell; antibodies against growth factor receptors; combinations of antibodies against several antigens to prevent escape of the tumor by modulation of one antigen or the selection for outgrowth of cells which do not express that specific antigen; and combination therapy, using antibodies combined with chemotherapy or other biologic agents, such as interferon, IL-2, and/or effector cells. These approaches and those yet to be developed should lead to an enhanced role for monoclonal antibody therapy in the treatment of cancer in the future.

Differentiating Agents

A fair amount of information has been acquired from in vitro studies on the effects of various agents on cell differentiation and maturation [21]. A large number of compounds or combinations of compounds have been shown to induce differentiation in various cell systems. These agents include growth factors (such as nerve growth factor), interferons, prostaglandins, hormones, chemotherapeutic agents, retinoids, vitamin D analogues, endotoxin, and polar solvents like dimethylformamide. However, clinical trials using these agents have been limited. Most commonly studied have been retinoid derivatives, which have not shown a high degree of clinical activity against established malignancies, possibly because these compounds might have their greatest efficacy in the precancerous or early cancerous state. Studies of retinoids as chemopreventative agents are ongoing. Also, it is not clear what relevance the ability of differentiate a particular cell in vitro has to attempts to differentiate other types of malignant cells in patients. Work is in progress attempting to define and develop more potent cell-specific differentiating agents for use in cancer therapy.

Antimetastatic Therapy

The metastatic capacity is unique to malignant cells, and metastases are responsible for most cancer therapeutic failures. Several approaches are being studied to either prevent metastases from occurring or inhibit the ability of metastases to grow once they have occurred. The metastatic process is complex, with several steps which can be potentially attacked. The approaches include inhibition of platelet/coagulation factors involved in the binding of metastatic lesions to endothelial cell surfaces; inhibition of tumor angiogenesis to prevent metastatic foci from becoming established; inhibition of the action of autocrine motility factor, which allows the tumor cell to move through the basement membrane; and the use of laminin (a basement membrane component) fragments or antibodies against laminin receptors to block these receptors on malignant cells and inhibit their attachment to the basement membrane [22]. Animal studies have shown laminin receptors to be important in the metastatic process of at least certain malignancies, and blocking them with laminin fragments decreases the number of metastases in these animal systems [22]. Laminin receptors have been demonstrated on human breast cancer cells, so the animal models would appear to have relevance to the human situation.

Protection or Regeneration of Bone Marrow Cells from Toxic Effects of Chemotherapy/Radiation Therapy

Although a variety of compounds have been shown in animals to protect or increase the rate of recovery of bone marrow cells from the effects of chemotherapy or radiation therapy, the cloning of the CSFs (G-CSF and GM-CSF, as mentioned previously) has again raised the hope that bone marrow cells in humans might be either protected or induced to regenerate more rapidly from the toxic effects of chemotherapy or radiation therapy [19]. This would allow the delivery of higher and/or more frequent doses of these treatments, with greater dose intensity and hopefully improved antitumor efficacy. There are a number of agents in addition to the CSFs which might also have a role in bone marrow protection, and this is an area which is being actively studied.

Summary

Despite various attempts over the years to use immunotherapy in treating patients with cancer, and despite the demonstration of clinical benefit in some patients with a variety of approaches aimed at modifying the host-tumor interaction, the only BRMs well-established in cancer treatment are α-interferon used in the treatment of patients with hairy-cell leukemia and BCG used intravesically for the treatment of superficial bladder cancer. The rapid and large increase over the past 15 years in the understanding of biologic factors important in the host-tumor interaction and the production of large amounts of purified biologic agents with a wide variety of functions has led to a renewal of interest and reevaluation of the role of biologic response modification in the treatment of cancer. Prior to this time, the major therapeutic approach in this area was the attempt to induce or augment either specific or nonspecific immune responses which would hopefully lead to an immunotherapeutic response against the malignancy. This approach had been largely unsuccessful. Although improving immunotherapeutic methods remains a critical component of the application of BRM therapy to cancer, there are also multiple other possible approaches, including agents which have direct antitumor effects and agents which affect various other aspects of the host-tumor interaction (e.g., differentiating tumor cells). In vitro and animal models suggest that novel applications using all of these approaches should have value in the treatment of cancer patients. The accumulating demonstrations of anticancer activity of various BRM approaches (interferons, IL-2, IL-2 plus LAK, and monoclonal antibodies), although limited in number (so far), argue that as improvements in these approaches are made, as new agents and ideas are developed, and as these treatments are combined with each other and with other forms of cancer therapy, they will provide new effective cancer treatments.

References

1. Mihich E, Fefer A (eds) (1983) Biological response modifiers: Subcommittee report. NCI Monogr 63
2. Hoover Jr HC, Surdyke MG, Gengel RB, Peters LC, Hanna Jr MG (1985) Prospectively randomized trial of adjuvant active specific immunotherapy for human colorectal cancer. Cancer 55: 1236
3. Levy R (1985) Biologicals for cancer treatment: monoclonal antibodies. Hosp Pract 20: 67
4. Longo DL (1987) Immunomodulators in clinical medicine: monoclonal antibodies. Ann Intern Med 106: 421–433
5. Pinsky CM, Camacho FJ, Kerr D, Geller NL, Klein FA, Herr HA, Whitmore WF, Oettgen HF (1985) Intravesical administration of Bacillus Calmette-Guerin in patients with recurrent superficial carcinoma of the urinary bladder: report of a prospective randomized trial. Cancer Treat Rep 69: 47
6. Mihich E (1986) Future perspectives for biological response modifiers: viewpoint. Semin Oncol 13: 234
7. Oldham RK (1985) Biologicals and biologic response modifiers: new approaches to cancer treatment. Cancer Invest 3: 53
8. Goldstein D, Laszlo J (1986) Interferon therapy in cancer: from imaginon to interferon. Cancer Res 46: 4315
9. Urba WJ, Maluish AE, Longo DL (1987) Strategies for immunological monitoring. Cancer Chemother Biol Response Modif Annu 9: 484
10. Quesada JR, Reuben JR, Manning JT, et al. (1984) Alpha interferon for the induction of remissions in hairy-cell leukemia. N Engl J Med 310: 15
11. Quesada JR, Rios A, Swanson D et al. (1985) Antitumor activity of recombinant-derived interferon alpha in metastatic renal cell carcinoma. J Clin Oncol 3: 1522
12. Vallbracht A, Treuner J, Flehring B et al. (1981) Interferon neutralizing antibodies in a patient treated with human fibroblast interferon. Nature 289: 496

13. Vadhan-Ray S, Al-Katib A, Bhalla R et al. (1986) Phase I trial of recombinant interferon gamma in cancer patients. J Clin Oncol 4: 137
14. Rosenberg SA, Lotze MT, Muul LM et al. (1987) A progress report on the treatment of 157 patients with advanced cancer using lymphokine-activated killer cells and interleukin-2 or high-dose interleukin-2 alone. N Engl J Med 316: 889
15. Sondel PM, Hank JA, Kohler PC (1987) Status and potential of interleukin-2 for the treatment of neoplastic disease. Oncol 1(6): 41
16. West WH, Tauer KW, Yannelli Jr et al. (1987) Constant-infusion recombinant interleukin-2 in adoptive immunotherapy of advanced cancer. N Engl J Med 316(15): 898
17. Steis, R, Bookman M, Clark J et al. (1987) Intraperitoneal lymphokine activated killer cell and interleukin-2 therapy for peritoneal carcinomatosis: toxicity, efficacy, and laboratory results. Proc ASCO 6: 250 (Abs)
18. Rosenberg SA, Speiss P, Lafreniere P (1986) A new approach to adoptive immunotherapy of cancer with tumor-infiltrating lymphocytes. Science 233: 1818
19. Gillis S, Conlon PJ, Cosman D, Hopp TP, Dower SK, Price V, Mochizuki DY, Urdal DL (1986) Lymphokines: from conjecture to the clinic. Semin Oncol 13: 218
20. Order SE, Klein JL, Leichner PK (1987) Hepatoma: model for radiolabeled antibody in cancer treatment (International Symposium on Labeled and Unlabeled Antibody in Cancer Diagnosis and Therapy.) Natl Cancer Inst Monogr 3: 37
21. Sachs L (1986) Growth, differentiation and the reversal of malignancy. Sci Am 254: 40
22. Liotta L (1984) Tumor invasion and metastasis: role of the basement membrane. Am J Pathol 117: 339

16. The Potential Value of Radiolabelled Monoclonal Antibodies in Cancer Therapy

A.M. Keenan and S. M. Larson

Introduction

The use of radionuclides for therapy in human subjects depends on sufficient accumulation of atoms with effective radiation characteristics at a precise anatomical location. This has traditionally been achieved by direct introduction of radioisotopes to the site of disease, such as intracavitary administration of radiocolloids, or by the exploitation of existing metabolic pathways, such as iodine concentration in thyroid tissue. In recent years, particularly since the development of monoclonal antibodies, the possibility of targeting of radionuclides by immunologic means has become a real one. Not only are monoclonal antibodies highly specific, but they can be produced on a commercial scale by mass culture techniques using the hybridoma cells from which they are derived, and they can be readily purified.

Basic Principles

The ideal tumor-specific antigen for radioimmunotherapy is one which is present exclusively on tumor cells and is exposed in large numbers to the intravascular space (Table 1). For practical purposes, an antigen that is expressed on tumor cell surface in more than 100-fold concentration compared with normal tissues, is not found on circulating blood cells, and is present in quantities of at least 100 000 molecules per cell is considered adequate [1].

Radiolabeled antibodies must bind to tumor antigens in sufficient quantities for target-specific therapy to occur. The radioactivity remains at the antigenic site as a function of the binding kinetics of the antibody and antigen, the stability of the radiolabel, and the metabolic fate of the antigen-antibody complex. Circulating antigens may compete with tumor-bound antigens, and, if present in sufficient quantities in serum, they may provide a barrier that is difficult for the antibody to penetrate. Undoubtedly, this particular problem will vary from patient to patient, and its actual clinical impact is unclear.

In addition, poor vascular delivery and several other factors can also interfere with tumor-specific localization of antibodies:

Table 1. Some tumor-associated antigens under consideration for antibody targeting

Antigen	Expressed in
Prostatic acid phosphatase	Prostate cancer
Human chorionic gonadotropin	Choriocarcinoma
α-Fetoprotein	Hepatoma
Carcinoembryonic antigen	Colon and pancreatic carcinoma
p97, others	Melanoma
CD5	T-cell lymphoma and chronic lymphocytic leukemia

Antigen expression
Antigen accessibility
Tumor vascularity
Plasma antibody concentration
Cross-reactivity with nontarget tissue
Circulating antigens
Nonspecific antibody binding
Labeled irrelevant proteins
Unincorporated isotope
Antigen-antibody binding kinetics
Antigen-antibody complex stability
Persistence of radiolabel

Cross-reactivity with normal tissues, nonspecific binding and host derived antibodies directed against the infused monoclonal antibody can all reduce tumor uptake. Therefore, careful screening of antibodies against normal human tissues, animal studies of in vivo pharmacokinetics, and human studies with tracer doses are necessary in the evaluation of an antibody for therapeutic applications.

Another problem which can give rise to significant nonspecific binding is the presence of Fc receptors on a broad range of tissue types. This can theoretically be overcome by cleaving the Fc portion from the antibody molecule, yielding immunoreactive Fab or F(ab')$_2$ fragments [2, 3]. These fragments retain the antigen-specific sites and function as monovalent or divalent agents, respectively. Although nonspecific binding can be diminished in this manner, more rapid blood clearance occurs, which, in some situations, leads to higher target-to-background ratios [4]. However, rapid blood clearance also reduces the exposure time of tumor antigens to the circulating antibodies, and monovalent antibody fragments may bind more weakly to tumor antigens. Both whole immunoglobulin [5] and Fab fragments [6] have been employed in therapy, and each type of murine protein has its own properties.

Clinical Experience

Most clinical studies have utilized ^{131}I-labeled anticarcinoembryonic antigen (CEA) or antiferritin derived from the serum of immunized goats, horses, or rabbits. Order et al. have conducted several studies in patients with primary hepatic malignancies [5, 7, 8]. They have been able to document tumor regression by serial computerized axial tomography (CAT) in the majority of their patients, but none have achieved long-lasting remission. The majority of these studies were conducted as combined multimodality therapeutic trials and included external irradiation and chemotherapy to shrink the tumor prior to antibody infusion. This presumably increases the tumor concentration of immunoglobulin by reducing the tumor mass relative to the limited quantity of labeled antibody that can be administered at one time [7]. Their data suggest that maximum tumor uptake is reached between 48 and 72 h after injection, and that the effective half-life ranges from 5 to 8 days, resulting in a tumor dose of 20–30 Gy [8]. This produces a relatively low dose rate of approximately 0.05–0.07 Gy/h, compared with 0.4 Gy/h from iridium or radium implants.

Clinical toxicity from therapeutic doses of radiolabeled antibodies appears to be dose related. Ettinger et al. [9] reviewed data from 14 patients receiving up to 157 mCi ^{131}I-labeled antiserum to CEA or ferritin and found that the degree of leukopenia and thrombocytopenia was dependent on the dose of radioactivity administered. Hematologic toxicity, particularly thrombocytopenia, was the most significant side effect and appeared to result from circulating radioactivity rather than bone marrow localization of labeled antibodies. Whole-body radiation doses ranged from 1.1 to 2.2 Gy, primarily due to circulating radioactivity with an effective serum half-life of approximately 3 days [5, 9]. Mild hepatotoxicity was inferred from transient elevations in liver enzymes in 72% of the patients and probably resulted from radiation doses to the liver calculated to be in the range of 4–10 Gy per infusion. Allergic reactions and immune complexes were not clinically evident in this group of patients.

It is important to realize that the side effects experienced by patients treated with radiolabeled polyclonal antisera may differ from those encountered with radiolabeled monoclonal antibodies, particularly with regard to the therapeutic index. Polyclonal antibody preparations are heterogeneous in antibody content and at best are 70% immunospecific even after affinity chromatography purification [10]. Tumor radiation doses of 20–30 Gy at low dose rates from 100 to 150 mCi labeled antibody have proven inadequate for cure, and doses above 150 mCi have been associated with potentially life-threatening hematologic consequences, presumably due to circulating labeled antibodies lacking immunoreactivity [9].

Polyclonal antibodies can only be produced in limited quantities, requiring an animal colony to maintain a continuous supply. Monoclonal antibodies, on the other hand, can be generated in unlimited quantities at the bench top or in small animals and can be readily purified to homogeneity. Immunospecificity is inherently greater, usually 90% or more, even after radiolabeling, and a much

319

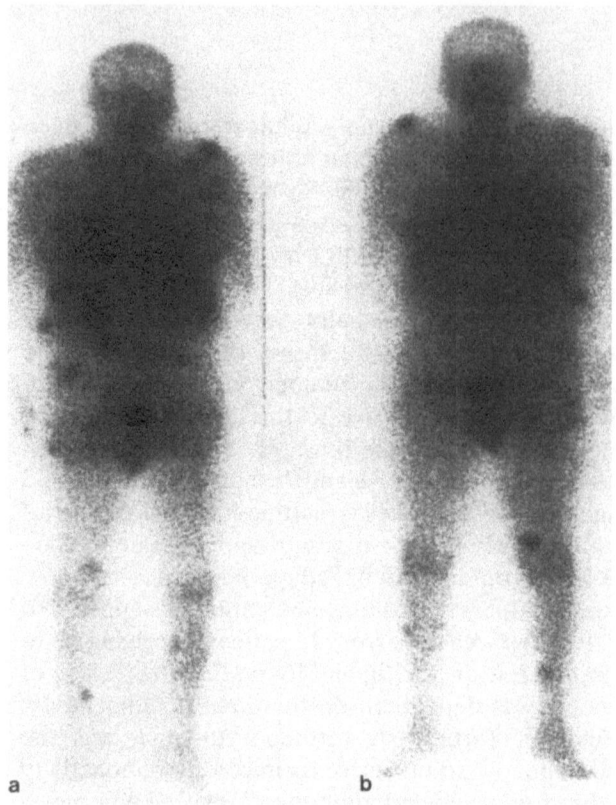

Fig. 1a, b. Whole-body posterior (**a**) and anterior (**b**) images of a patient showing multiple sub-cutaneous melanoma metastases were obtained 48 h after intravenous injection of a therapeutic dose of ^{131}I-labeled Fab fragments (100 mCi labeled to 50 mg) directed against the p97 melanoma antigen. The visualized lesions varied from 2 to 4 cm in diameter. Diffuse body background of radioactivity is seen throughout the extracellular space and liver, and free iodide is concentrated in thyroid, stomach, and bladder. This pattern of uptake was reproducible, being seen on three other occasions—once after a diagnostic dose prior to therapy and again following two other therapeutic doses. (From [12])

larger percentage of the radioactivity is bound to reactive antibody due to the lack of irrelevant proteins.

Larson et al. have successfully used ^{131}I-labeled monoclonal IgG and Fab fragments directed against the p97 antigen of melanoma for imaging and treatment of metastatic disease [2, 6] (Fig. 1). These investigators have safely infused up to 340 mCi ^{131}I at a time, with cumulative doses of more than 800 mCi. High specific activities, ranging from 10 to 20 mCi ^{131}I per milligram of antibody, have been achieved. Experience with labeled fragments indicates that the more rapid plasma clearance of Fab fragments results in less hematologic toxicity, allowing administration of larger therapeutic doses [2]. Whole-body clearance occurred with a biologic half-life of approximately 33 h, whereas tumor clearance was determined to be 46 h, suggesting that weekly therapeutic doses might be optimal.

Practical Considerations

When considering therapy with radiolabeled antibodies, additional evaluation of the patient is required beyond the usual diagnostic and staging studies. Whenever possible, immunohistologic staining of biopsy material or immunologic studies of fresh tumor cells is desirable to measure the reactivity of the antibody to be used with the tumor tissue.

Imaging studies with diagnostic doses of the radiolabeled antibodies may be the best means of predicting the efficacy of the planned therapy in each patient. Relative distribution throughout the body and biologic clearance from tumor, blood, and critical organs are required for dosimetric calculations, and this data can be obtained from computer analysis of serial gamma camera images. The optimal milligram dosage of antibody has not been established and may vary significantly for different antibodies, antigens, or other tumor properties. Recent studies have employed doses in the range of 5–10 mg protein [2]. In general, antibodies should be labeled to the highest possible specific activity with a radionuclide to ensure adequate tumor radiation doses.

Large-scale labeling procedures require facilities that provide adequate shielding and a remote-controlled labeling apparatus [11]. Highly trained personnel must devote large amounts of time for consistency of product quality. The specific activity of the final product will depend on the optimal milligram quantity of antibody, which is limited by the total radioactivity that can be administered at one time and tempered by the sensitivity of the antibody to radiolabeling. Different antibodies lose immunoreactivity at different specific activities [11]; thus, each antibody requires individual evaluation.

The process of developing a radiolabeled monoclonal antibody for clinical use is a long, complicated, and expensive endeavor. Tumor-specific antigens are difficult to isolate and purify, and the development of a viable hybridoma clone generating the desired antibody can require painstaking work. Optimal labeling procedures must be determined individually for each new antibody, and studies in an appropriate animal model are necessary to characterize in vivo pharmacokinetics. Extensive screening is required to rule out cross-reactivity with normal human tissues.

Important Considerations for Future Studies

Several issues remain to be resolved before radiolabeled monoclonal antibodies come into clinical practice [12]. Selection of the most appropriate target antigen

321

and antibody in any given disease is perhaps the most critical of these. Selection of the best radionuclide to couple to the antibody is also very important, as is the determination of the optimal schedule of administration. Other issues, such as the use of antibody fragments, need to be considered as well.

New antigens are continually being identified and characterized. Those with the most abundant expression on tumor cells and with a narrow range of expression on normal cells with result in the highest target-to-background ratio. Antigens that modulate internally, carrying the radiolabeled antibody with them, offer the greatest potential for cell destruction. To avoid the problem of an antigen not being expressed on all tumor cells, the use of mixtures of monoclonal antibodies directed towards several antigens expressed by a tumor needs to be considered. This approach has been demonstrably more effective in purging tumor cells from bone marrow in vitro [13].

Antibodies generated to a particular antigen can have distinct properties according to their isotype, subclass, and binding characteristics. Antibodies with a high affinity and avidity are generally preferable, and these properties can be measured in vitro using well-established techniques. Although current antibodies have yielded tumor-to-tissue ratios of approximately 10:1, calculations of the maximum achievable uptake for high-affinity antibodies indicates that ratios between 100:1 and 1000:1 are theoretically obtainable [1].

Antibody fragments will continue to play a larger role in future studies, but several issues remain to be settled. Fab fragments clear more rapidly from the circulation, reducing background activity from the blood pool [2], but shorter circulation times may also reduce the time of exposure of antigen to the antibodies, and the avidity of binding may be less than with divalent antibodies. Smaller molecules provide fewer labeling sites, which may reduce the potential for high specific activities. On the other hand, removal of the Fc portion of the antibody molecule reduces the potential for nonspecific binding. For these reasons, it has been suggested that $F(ab')_2$ fragments may represent the best compromise between whole antibodies and small, monovalent Fab fragments [3]. Murine monoclonal antibodies have so far been the only antibodies available for human use, but present work with human-human hybridomas may soon provide human monoclonal antibodies which may have a longer half-life and less potential for allergic responses [14]. Batteries of monoclonal antibodies may become available for "crossmatching" of patient tumor samples, and it is possible to envisage the individualization of antibody mixtures for individual tumors; however, it seems more practical at present to develop antibody "cocktails" as appropriate for each histologic entity.

Labeling methods with radioiodine are well established, and both ^{131}I and ^{125}I have therapeutic potential. The beta radiation from ^{131}I can act within a radius of several cell diameters, and this can enhance the overall tumoricidal effect in tumors with heterogeneous expression of antigen. A single cell with ^{131}I concentrated on its surface can irradiate surrounding cells that lack antibody accumulation. The short-range Auger electrons of ^{125}I could provide effective therapy if delivered in close proximity to the nucleus of each and every tumor cell, and they may reduce irradiation to adjacent nontumor tissue [15].

Techniques for conjugating bifunctional chelates such as diethylenetria-minepentaacetic acid (DTPA) to antibody molecules have allowed chelation of a number of metallic radionuclides [16], and many beta- and alpha-emitters have come into consideration for radioimmunotherapy. In addition to its beta radiation, ^{47}Sc has abundant 160-keV photons for imaging. ^{212}Bi is both an alpha- and beta-emitter that is available as a generator product of ^{212}Pb. ^{109}Pd has shown great promise for therapy in preliminary animal studies due to its predominant beta radiation, 13-h half-life, and ready availability in large quantities. ^{67}Cu and ^{90}Y have also been proposed as possible candidates for therapeutic applications, but ^{67}Cu has the advantage of gamma radiation, which can be imaged to monitor biodistribution. The search for novel radionuclides for medical applications will no doubt continue. The suitability of the radiation characteristics of an individual radionuclide will depend to a large extent upon the pharmacokinetics of the antibody or antibody fragment to be used.

The delivery of an antibody to a tumor antigen after intravenous administration is dependent on the vascularity of the tumor, the percentage of the cardiac output recieved by the tumor, and the plasma concentration of antibody. Clearance of antibodies from the circulation reduces the time during which the delivery process can occur. Preferential distribution can be achieved through the use of intra-arterial or intracavitary catheters and through intralymphatic infusion or subcutaneous injection, thus directing the delivery of antibodies to tumor, organs, body spaces, or lymph nodes. These methods have several advantages over intravenous administration: (a) smaller administered dose, (b) less systemic toxicity, (c) less competition by circulating antigens, (d) less cross-reactivity with antigens expressed on normal cells, and (e) faster localization [17].

Clearly, much work remains to be done to bring radioimmunotherapy into routine clinical use, but ongoing efforts in tumor immunology, hybridoma technology, and radiolabeling techniques provide hope that effective primary or ancillary therapy with immune-targeted radionuclides will become a reality.

References

1. Larson SM, Carrasquillo JA, Reynolds JC (1984) Radioimmunodetection and radioimmunotherapy. Cancer Invest 2: 363–381
2. Larson SM, Carrasquillo JA, Krohn KA et al. (1983) Localization of I-131-labeled p97-specific Fab fragments in human melanoma as a basis for radiotherapy. J Clin Invest 72: 2101–2114
3. Moldofsky PJ, Powe J, Mulhern CB et al. (1983) Metastatic colon carcinoma detected with radiolabeled F(ab')$_2$ monoclonal antibody fragments. Radiology 149: 549–555
4. Larson SM, Brown JP, Wright PW et al. (1983) Imaging of melanoma with I-131-labeled monoclonal antibodies. J Nucl Med 24: 123–129
5. Order SE, Klein JL, Ettinger D et al. (1980) Use of isotopic immunoglobulin in therapy. Cancer Res 40: 3001–3007
6. Larson SM, Carrasquillo JA, Krohn KA (1982) Radiotherapy with "anti-p97" iodinated monoclonal antibodies in melanoma. In: Raynau (ed) Proceedings of the Third World Congress in Nuclear Medicine and Biology, vol 4. Pergamon Press, New York, pp 3666–3669

7. Order SE, Klein JL, Ettinger D et al. (1980) Phase I–II study of radiolabeled antibody integrated in the treatment of primary hepatic malignancies. Int J Radiat Oncol Biol Phys 6: 703–710

8. Order SE, Klein JL, Leichner PK (1981) Anti-ferritin IgG antibody for isotopic cancer therapy. Oncology 38: 154–160

9. Ettinger DS, Order SE, Wharam MD et al. (1982) Phase I-II study of isotopic immunoglobulin therapy for primary liver cancer. Cancer Treat Rep 66: 289–297

10. Order SE (1982) Monoclonal antibodies: potential role in radiation therapy and oncology. Int J Radiat Oncol Biol Phys 8: 1193–1201

11. Ferens JM, Krohn KA, Beaumier PL et al. (1984) High-level iodination of monoclonal antibody fragments for radiotherapy. J Nucl Med 25: 367–370

12. Larson SM (1985) Radiolabeled monoclonal anti-tumor antibodies in diagnosis and therapy. J Nucl Med 26: 538–545

13. Reynolds CP, Black AT, Saur JW et al. (1985) An immunomagnetic flow system for selective depletion of cell populations from marrow. Transplant Proc 17: 434–436

14. Olsson L, Kaplan HS (1980) Human-human hybridomas producing monoclonal antibodies of predefined antigenic specificity. Proc Natl Acad Sci USA 77: 5429–5431

15. Saenger EL, Kereiakes JG, Sodd VJ et al. (1979) Radiotherapeutic agents: properties, dosimetry, and radiobiologic considerations. Semin Nucl Med 9: 72–84

16. Krejcarek GE, Tucker KL (1977) Covalent attachment of chelating groups to macromolecules. Biochem Biophys Res Commun 77: 581–585

17. Weinstein JN, Steller MA, Covell DG et al. (1984) Monoclonal antibodies in the lymphatics. Cancer Treat Rep 68: 257–264

17. Monoclonal Antibody Conjugates with Cytotoxic Agents for Cancer Therapy

V.S. Byers and R.W. Baldwin

Introduction

The difference in the cytotoxicity of chemotherapeutic agents between tumor cells and normal cells is generally not sufficient to permit curative doses of drug to be administered without producing unacceptable toxicity. Methods are being sought, therefore, for selective delivery of antineoplastic agents in order to improve their therapeutic potential. This approach also opens up the possibility of using agents such as naturally occurring plant and bacterial toxins, which hitherto would not have been acceptable in view of their very significant toxicity.

Antibody-targeted therapy, in which drug-tissue interactions are restricted to tumor sites by linking cytotoxic agents to antibodies reacting with tumor cells, was proposed many years ago. In the past, this approach had limited, if any, practical significance in view of the difficulties in producing antibody preparations of sufficient purity and in the amounts needed for drug conjugation. The technique of immortalizing individual clones of antibody-secreting cells by fusing them with cultured myeloma cells to form hybridomas which continuously secrete antibody [49] has for the first time made possible the reproducible production of antibodies. Firstly, these hybridomas can be maintained continuously in culture or as ascites in mice, allowing the production of monoclonal antibodies on an appropriate multigram scale. Secondly, since the hybridomas are produced by fusion of a single antibody-producing lymphocyte, the "monoclonal" antibody is directed against a single epitope on the antigen molecule; therefore, the problem of separating antibodies of different specificities is obviated. This means that an antibody produced against a cancer cell-associated antigen will be specific for that antigen, and cross-reactivity with normal tissues will only occur if the epitope to which it binds is also expressed in these tissues.

Monoclonal Antibodies to Human Tumor-Associated Antigens

Monoclonal antibodies have been produced which react with a wide range of human cancers [7, 8]. Typically, these are murine antibodies produced by hybridomas formed following fusion of spleen cells from immunized mice with mouse myeloma cell lines. Donor mice have been immunized with whole human tumor cells, subcellular fractions, or secretory products such as carcinoembryonic antigen (CEA). Antibodies have been produced which react with many types of solid tumor, including carcinomas of colon, rectum, breast, ovary, lung, pancreas, and bladder, as well as malignant melanoma and bone and soft tissue sarcomas. Antibodies reacting with leukemia cells have also been generated. It is important to recognize that antibodies generated by immunizing mice with human tumor cells or subcellular fractions do not necessarily recognize tumor-specific antigens. Rather, they may react with normal or modified tissue antigens which are either preferentially or inappropriately expressed upon malignant cells. In most instances, the nature and function of the tumor-associated antigens recognized by monoclonal antibodies is unknown.

One class of "neoantigen", the so-called oncofetal antigens, are tumor cell products expressed on fetal and malignant cells but either absent from or expressed at low levels in normal adult tissues [36]. These are typified by CEA, a complex molecule expressing both protein and carbohydrate determinants [65], which is widely associated with colorectal cancer. Another oncofetal antigen used to generate monoclonal antibodies is α-fetoprotein, found in the serum of patients with hepatocellular carcinoma and teratoblastomas of testis and ovary [71].

Other tumor-associated antigens against which monoclonal antibodies have been generated include glycoproteins and glycolipids associated with colorectal cancer [37] and high-molecular-weight mucins associated with breast and ovarian cancer [15, 59].

Monoclonal antibodies produced against these antigens are not tumor specific, and they may react to a certain degree with a number of normal tissues. Monoclonal antibodies produced against human milk fat globule membrane (HMFG) react with breast and ovarian cancer cells but also with normal tissues. For example, HMFG1, recognized by a monoclonal antibody generated against human milk fat globule membrane, is present upon breast carcinoma cells and also in a number of normal secretory epithelial cells, including lactating breast epithelium [15].

It is important to recognize that many of the murine monoclonal antibodies being developed for drug targeting do have some normal tissue reactivity since this has to be taken into account when evaluating immunoconjugates for therapy. Furthermore, as described later, immunoconjugate evaluation by reaction with cultured tumor cells and by treatment of human tumor xenografts in athymic mice does not provide any assessment of potential toxicity for normal human tissues. This can only be derived from phase I clinical trials, together with knowledge of normal tissue reactivity derived primarily from immunohistological studies.

It has been proposed that human monoclonal antibodies may be more appropriate for drug targeting, and methods for generating hybridomas secreting human monoclonal antibodies are now available [18]. This involves fusion of sensitized B-lymphocytes from the human donor (e.g., peripheral blood lymphocytes or lymphocytes derived from lymph nodes draining a tumor) with human

326

myeloma cell lines to produce a human-human hybridoma, or with mouse myeloma cell lines to produce a heterohybridoma, both of which secrete human antibody. There are numerous obstacles in this approach, including hybridoma stability (a particular problem with heterohybridomas) and the generation of hybridomas which produce acceptable levels of antibody.

A more fundamental problem is whether human tumors do express neo-antigens which are recognized by the tumor-bearing patient [6]. Opinions on this issue remain divided, but there is still little, if any, evidence that human tumors evoke tumor-specific T-cell responses or specific antibodies in patients. Moreover, hybridomas have not been produced which secrete antibody specific for cell surface antigens on human cancer cells. Most of the antibodies described show cross-reactivity with normal cells and seem to recognize cytoplasmic antigens. For example, more than 4350 human immunoglobulin (Ig)-secreting hybrids have been produced in one study [25], and of the 305 reacting with tumors, only 5 antibodies reacted with the cell surface.

Tumor Localization of Monoclonal Antibodies: Immunoscintigraphy

Monoclonal antibody targeting of drugs to tumor requires that the antibody localizes in the tumor following systemic administration. The most convincing evidence for this comes from trials in which patients are injected with radio-labelled monoclonal antibodies. Images obtained with a gamma camera have clearly show tumor localization of radioisotope [6, 11, 35, 55, 60].

For most tumor-imaging studies, patients have received 0.1–10 mg monoclo-nal antibody labelled with 2–6 mCi ^{131}I, ^{123}I, ^{111}In, or ^{99}Tc^m. Imaging is then carried out 2–3 days later, using either a gamma camera or rectilinear scanner to produce planar images, or tomographic cameras which allow construction of image slices similar to those generated by X-ray or computerized tomographic (CT) scanning [55].

A representative sample of radiolabelled monoclonal antibodies which have been used in imaging studies is given in Table 1. The primary objective of these studies is to evaluate immunoscintigraphy as a diagnostic procedure, but they also provide a means of establishing the tumor-localizing capacity of selected monoclonal antibodies. Numerous studies have demonstrated that anti-CEA monoclonal antibodies localize in colorectal cancer [11, 28]. The localization of a monoclonal antibody (791T/36) which recognizes a tumor glycoprotein (gp72) has also been demonstrated in extensive trials with ^{131}I- and ^{111}In-labelled anti-body [1–3]. Other monoclonal antibodies shown to localize in colorectal cancer include antiglycolipid antibodies 19-9 and 17-1A [21–23].

Imaging of ovarian cancer has been reported in several trials using monoclo-nal antibody HMFG-2 produced against human milk fat globule membrane [53] and anti-placental alkaline phosphatase antibody [27, 34]. Monoclonal antibody

Table 1. Clinical imaging with radiolabelled monoclonal antibodies

Tumor type	Antibody designation[a]	Antibody subclass	Radiolabel[b]	Lesions examined (n)	Positive rate (%)	Reference
Colorectal carcinoma	YPC-121 (CEA)	IgG$_{2a}$	^{131}I with ^{99}Tc^m (blood pool subtraction)	28	60	[72]
	MAB-35 (CEA)	F(ab')$_2$ Fab	^{123}I	44	86	[28]
	17-1A (glycolipid)	IgG/ F(ab')$_2$	^{131}I with ^{99}Tc^m (blood pool subtraction)	46	59	[21–23]
	19-9	IgG1/ F(ab')$_2$	^{131}I with ^{99}Tc^m (blood pool subtraction)	29	66	[21–23]
Ovarian carcinoma	HMFG-2 (milk fat globule membrane)	IgG	^{123}I	18	90	[53]
	NDOG (placental alkaline phosphatase)	IgG	^{123}I	15	73	[27]
	791T/36 (gp 72 glycoprotein)	IgG2b	^{111}In or ^{131}I with ^{99m}Tc^m (blood pool subtraction)	123	75–87	[58]
Breast carcinoma	3E1.2	IgM	^{131}I	9	100	[76]
	M8 (Milk fat globule membrane)	IgG1	^{111}In/^{123}I	Multiple sites	100	[61]
Malignant melanoma	8.2 (p97 membrane)	IgG1 Fab	^{131}I with ^{99}Tc^m (blood pool subtraction)	25	88	[50, 51]
Osteogenic sarcoma	225-28S	F(ab')$_2$	^{111}In	412	92	
	971T/36 (gp72)	IgG2b	^{111}In	5	100	[4]

791T/36 has also been used extensively in imaging primary and recurrent ovarian cancers [58, 75], while anti-HMFG antibodies have also been used to image breast cancer [33, 61]. Several antibodies have been used to image malignant melanoma [14, 50, 51], and monoclonal antibody 791T/36 has been used for imaging bone and soft tissue sarcomas [4].

A more direct assessment of tumor localization of monoclonal antibody in humans has been feasible in instances where patients with primary tumors have undergone imaging with radioisotope-labelled monoclonal antibodies prior to surgical resection of a tumor [1–3, 35]. In this case, it is possible to directly determine the levels of radioactivity in tumor, compare them with normal tissue, and so construct a tumor-to-normal tissue ratio of radioactivity (antibody) levels. This is illustrated by trials in patients with colorectal cancer, where the tumor-to-normal colon ratios of radioactivity were found to range up to 10:1 following injection of ^{131}I-labelled monoclonal antibody 791T/36 [1–3].

Immunotoxins

Ribosome-inactivating protein toxins of plant and bacterial origin represent a class of highly cytotoxic agents which can be used for linking to monoclonal antibodies to form immunotoxins [39, 40, 79, 81]. One type of toxin, typified by ricin (from castor beans), consists of two polypeptides (A and B chains) linked through a disulfide bond. In the natural course of events, the toxin binds through a site on the B chain to receptors which are expressed upon essentially all cells in a susceptible host. The A chain is then internalized, probably through the endosome, and produces cell kill by inactivation of protein synthesis. This process is highly efficient at terminating the metabolic activity of a cell, so that one molecule of toxin entering the cytoplasm is sufficient to produce a lethal response [79, 81].

Immunotoxins constructed by linking the whole toxin (holotoxin) to antibody are highly toxic, and their activity may even exceed that of the native toxin. However, since these immunotoxins contain the B chain, which binds to most mammalian cells, they lack the specificity of the antibody component. One approach to this problem is to "block" the interaction of the B chains with cell receptors. For example, ricin B chain "recognizes" galactose-terminating glycoproteins or glycolipids, and this interaction can be blocked by the presence of high levels of free galactose or lactose [78, 80]. This can readily be achieved when immunotoxins are used in vitro for purging T-lymphocytes or malignant cells from bone marrow [16], but it is less practicable for in vivo immunotoxin therapy. An alternative approach, therefore, is to separate the A- and B-chain polypeptides following enzymatic cleavage of the whole toxin. The A-chain component is then linked to antibody to form an A-chain immunotoxin [79, 81]. The coupling is generally effected by introducing an activated disulfide reside (e.g., dithiopyridine) into the antibody, which is then reacted with free sulfydryl

329

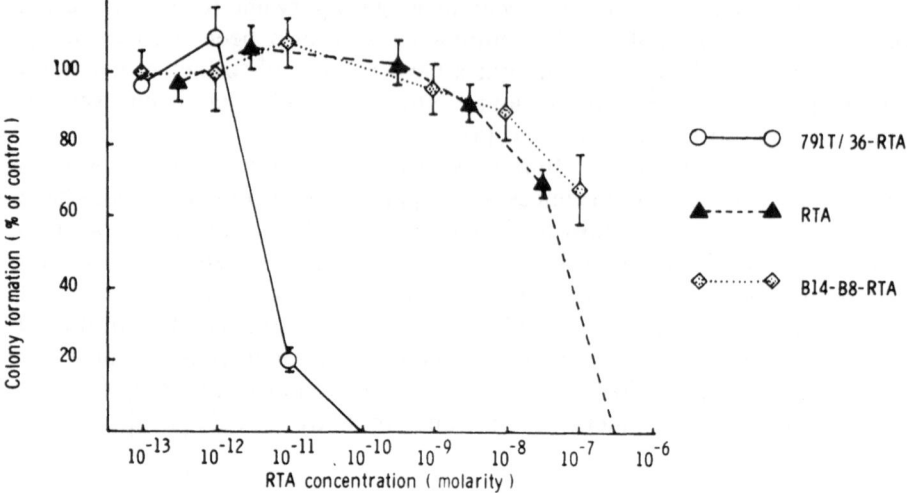

Fig. 1. Cytotoxicity of an immunotoxin constructed by linking monoclonal antibody 791T/36 to ricin A chain (*RTA*) [32]. Osteogenic sarcoma 791T cells were incubated with immunotoxin (*791T/36-RTA* or *B14-B8-RTA*) or free ricin A chain for 5 days. Colony formation by treated tumor cells was then determined

groups of the toxin A chain. This forms a conjugate in which the A-chain toxin is linked to antibody through a disulfide bond.

Immunotoxins containing ricin A chain (RTA) linked to monoclonal antibody have been produced which are cytotoxic for many types of solid human tumor, including carcinoma of colon, breast, lung, and ovary; malignant melanoma; and osteogenic sarcoma [32, 39, 40, 44]. Immunotoxins cytotoxic for leukemic cells have also been synthesized [20, 47, 62, 63, 74]. When tested in vitro, these immunotoxins are exquisitely specific for target tumor cells which express the antigen reacting with the antibody component. This is illustrated in Fig. 1, showing that an immunotoxin constructed by linking RTA to monoclonal antibody 791T/36 is highly cytotoxic for tumor cells (e.g., osteosarcoma 791T) which express the gp72 antigen recognized by this antibody [32]. The dose of immunotoxin producing 50% inhibition of tumor cell growth (colony formation) was 4.5×10^{-12} M, compared with 6.3×10^{-8} M with free RTA.

There are multiple steps in immunotoxin-directed cell cytotoxicity, the first being immunotoxin binding to target cell antigen. For cytotoxicity to occur, it is then necessary for the bound immunotoxin to be internalized by the target cell in order for the A-chain component to be released and inactivate the 60S subunit of ribosomes [78, 79]. With whole ricin, the B chain plays an important but as yet ill-defined role in the internalization of the toxin, so that A-chain immunotoxins may lack the high cytotoxicity of intact toxin. The cytotoxicity of A-chain immunotoxins can, however, be potentiated by synergistically acting B-chain conjugates [80]. Other agents may potentiate cytotoxicity, and this phenomenon can be utilized most effectively in in vitro systems [19, 20, 41]. This is illustrated by the use of potentiating agents in conjunction with an immunotoxin containing

RTA linked to monoclonal antibody T101 (CD5) for eliminating leukemic cells from bone marrow. The in vitro cytotoxicity of the immunotoxin for leukemic cells was potentiated some 6700 times by inclusion of ammonium chloride in the incubation medium. Even more pronounced potentiation is achieved with carboxylic ionophores, so that monensin produced a 50 000-fold increase in cytotoxic potency [19]. These potentiating agents probably function by modifying the fate of immunotoxins following their entry into cells through the endosome.

RTA and to a lesser extent diphtheria A chain have been used quite extensively for designing immunotoxins [44, 82]. This has led to a search for other ribosome-inactivating proteins (RIPs). RIPs which occur naturally as single polypeptide chains (A chains) have a pragmatic advantage since this obviates the necessity to purify A chain from contaminating B chain, which may produce toxic side effects in vivo. Naturally occurring A-chain RIPs include gelonin from *Gelonium multiforum* seeds and saporin from *Saponaria officinalis* (soapwort) seeds [73]. There are, in addition, other plant RIPs which, like ricin, occur naturally as two polypeptide chains. These include abrin from *Abrus precatorius* (jequirity bean) seeds and modeccin from *Adenia digitata* roots.

In addition to plant RIPs, considerable effort is being devoted to extending the range of immunotoxins containing bacterial toxins. This work stems predominantly from original studies with diphtheria toxin [44], and some success has been achieved, as exemplified by an immunotoxin containing pseudomonas exotoxin linked to antitransferrin receptor antibody, which is cytotoxic to cultured ovarian carcinoma cells [57].

Immunotoxins have also been constructed by linking the antibiotic neocarzinostatin to an antimelanoma antibody [52]. Neocarzinostatin (M_r 10 000) consists of a protein and nonprotein chromophore, the latter being the biologically active component which interacts with DNA. The neocarzinostatin-antibody conjugates are highly cytotoxic in vitro for melanoma cells, 50% inhibition of tumor cell survival being obtained with 5–6 ng/ml, compared with 480 ng/ml with free neocarzinostatin.

In Vivo Efficacy

The in vivo efficacy of immunotoxins administered systemically is being evaluated against human tumor xenografts in T-cell-deficient (athymic) mice. Only a limited number of immunotoxins have reached this stage of evaluation and been shown to be therapeutically effective. This is illustrated by trials with an immunotoxin containing monoclonal antibody 791T/36, which recognizes a tumor membrane glycoprotein (gp72), linked to RTA [32]. Treatment of sarcoma 791T xenografts by daily intraperitoneal injections of immunotoxin produced a significant inhibition of tumor growth (Fig. 2). In contrast, unconjugated RTA or an immunotoxin containing an antimelanoma antibody not reacting with the target cells did not inhibit 791T tumor growth [17]. The antimelanoma immunotoxin did suppress growth of human melanoma xenografts.

The gp72 antigen reacting with monoclonal antibody 791T/36 is expressed

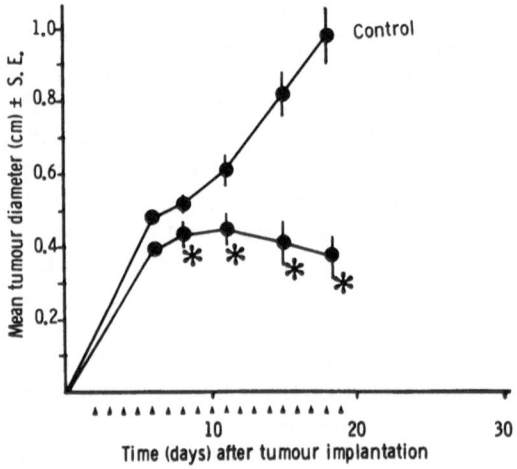

Fig. 2. Suppression of osteogenic sarcoma xenografts in athymic mice treated with immunotoxin [17]. Mice in which 791T xenografts were implanted were treated daily with 5 mg/kg 791T/36-RTA i.p. (▲), and tumor growth was measured at termination of the experiments. Tumors were measured in control and treated groups, and the influence of immunotoxin was determined from the T/C ratio, i.e., the weights of tumors in treated and control groups, respectively. At termination, T/C was 0.30 (*P* < 0.001). *P < 0.05

upon a wide range of human tumors, including colorectal and ovarian carcinomas [29]. This antibody has also been shown in extensive immunoscintigraphy trials to permit the imaging of colorectal [1, 3] and ovarian [58, 75] cancer. The potential value of the RTA-791T/36 immunotoxin in the treatment of these tumors is demonstrated by its ability to suppress the growth of colorectal carcinoma xenografts [9].

Therapeutic efficacy has also been observed after the systemic administration of immunotoxins reacting with malignant melanoma and breast carcinoma [39, 40]. In addition, immunotoxins administered intraperitoneally have suppressed peritoneal growth of human ovarian tumor cells in immunodeficient mice. These include an immunotoxin containing antitransferrin receptor monoclonal antibody linked to pseudomonas exotoxin [38] and RTA linked to monoclonal antibody 791T/36 (Byers and Baldwin, unpublished work).

Monoclonal Antibody-Drug Conjugates

Chemical conjugation of cytotoxic drugs to monoclonal antibodies requires that the compound has a reactive functional group such as an amino, hydroxyl, or carboxyl group available for protein conjugation. Also, these reactive groups should not be required for drug action or, if so, they should become available following intracellular release of the drug from the antibody conjugate. Cytotoxic drugs are much less active than the plant toxins used to construct immunotoxins. It is therefore necessary to couple the maximum number of drug residues to the antibody molecule whilst retaining as much as possible of the antibody binding activity. Since some of the functional groups in the antibody which can be linked to drug are likely to contribute to the functioning of the immunoglobulin

332

—either as a component of the forces retaining its three-dimensional structure or as part of the binding site of the antibody—the optimal molar substitution ratio (moles of drug bound per mole of immunoglobulin) represents a compromise between the desire to maximize toxicity and to minimize reduction in antibody specificity. Substitution ratios of up to 32 have been reported for immunoglobulins with retention of a proportion of antibody reactivity. Generally, however, substitution of more than ten drug residues per antibody molecule will produce an unacceptable degree of antibody damage [5, 10, 31, 67].

Several classes of cytotoxic drugs have been investigated for drug-antibody conjugate design, including alkylating agents, such as chlorambucil [5]; cis-platinum [45]; anthracyclines [42]; and antimetabolites, e.g., methotrexate (MTX) [43, 48], cytosine arabinoside [5], and the vinca alkaloid analog vindesine (desacetyl vinblastine amide) [67, 68]. These drugs have either been directly linked to antibody or linked via an intermediate carrier between drug and antibody, which has been used to increase the amount of drug which can be coupled to immunoglobulin. A variety of carriers have been used for this purpose, including dextran, human serum albumin (HSA), and poly-L-lysine [5, 10, 67].

MTX has been directly coupled to antibodies using mixed anhydride, water-soluble carbodiimide, and active ester methods [43]. Of these, the active ester method appears to be most favorable since it is sufficiently mild for drug not to be degraded and for antibody polymerization to be avoided. This procedure has been used to conjugate MTX to a range of monoclonal antibodies, including 250–306 and 791T/36—which react with human colorectal carcinoma cells—and an antitransferrin receptor antibody [43, 48].

MTX-carrier conjugates have been prepared by initially linking drug to HSA using water-soluble ethyl carbodiimide. Since the HSA does not have any essential biological activity, it is possible to produce highly substituted conjugates containing up to 40 mol MTX per mole HSA. The MTX-HSA conjugate is then coupled to monoclonal antibody to yield MTX-HSA-antibody conjugates. This synthesis has been utilized with monoclonal antibody 791T/36 to produce MTX-HSA-791T/36 conjugate containing up to 35–40 mol MTX per mole antibody [43].

These MTX conjugates with monoclonal antibody 791T/36 are cytotoxic in vitro for tumor cells expressing the target (gp72) antigen, including osteosarcoma and colon carcinoma cells. Clinical trials with MTX linked directly or using HSA carrier with antibody 791T/36 are in progress, and initial studies have shown localization of the directly linked conjugate in colorectal tumors [54]. In 15 colorectal cancer patients injected with ^{131}I-labelled MTX-791T/36 conjugate, immunoscintigraphy examination and radiochemical analysis of resected tumor specimens demonstrated tumor uptake, with tumor-to-normal tissue ratios of radioactivity ranging up to 7.9 : 1. These findings, together with studies on conjugates prepared with monoclonal antibodies reacting with experimental tumors, demonstrate the therapeutic potential of MTX conjugates [5, 10].

Vinca alkaloid conjugates with monoclonal antibodies have been prepared using either azide or active ester conjugation [13, 30, 67, 68]. Initially, desacetyl vinblastine hydrazide was converted to the azide and reacted with monoclonal antibody. Alternatively, an active ester method was used, in which 4-succinyl-vindesine was reacted with antibody. This active ester method produces conjugates with a greater substitution ratio for the same efficiency of reaction and with comparable retention of antibody-binding reactivity. These procedures have been used to construct vindesine conjugates with several monoclonal antibodies, including an anti-CEA antibody (11.285.14) and 791T/36—which react with colorectal cancer—and antimelanoma antibody 96.5 [67, 68]. Lung monoclonal antibody KS1/4 has also been conjugated to 4-succinoyl-vinblastine [13]. These conjugates retain antibody-binding reactivity and inhibit in vitro growth of tumor cells. Trials with vindesine linked to anti-CEA antibody (11.285.14), antimelanoma antibody 96.5, and 791T/36 have shown that these conjugates suppress growth of colorectal carcinoma, melanoma, and osteogenic sarcoma xenografts, respectively [68].

The anthracyclines doxorubicin (Adriamycin) and daunomycin have been conjugated to antibodies by a number of different methods [5, 10, 42]. In one approach, the sugar ring of daunomycin is cleaved by periodate oxidation to leave aldehyde functional groups in the drug, which can then be coupled to antibody [5]. In another approach, glutaraldehyde has been used to cross-link the anthracycline sugar amino group to antibody. In both of these methods, the resulting bonds were stabilized by reduction with sodium borohydride [5]. An alternative approach involves conjugation through the 14-carbon position, and in studies with monoclonal antibody 791T/36, four different procedures were compared [42]. 14-Bromo-daunomycin was linked to antibody amino groups directly by nucleophilic substitution, or dithiopyridyl residues are introduced into the monoclonal antibody using N-succinimidyl-3 (2-pyridyldithio) propionate. Free sulfydryl groups were then generated by mild reaction with dithiothreitol and reacted with 14-bromodaunomycin to produce thioether bonding through the drug side chain. Conjugation was also effected through the sugar amino group of daunomycin. For this purpose, daunomycin was reacted with cis-aconitic acid or succinic anhydride, and the carboxyl groups of these derivatives were linked to the amino groups of the lysine side chains of antibody using carbodiimide to produce peptide bonding.

Daunomycin and doxorubicin conjugates have also been synthesized using dextran and HSA as drug carriers [5]. The dextran carrier (dextran T10, M_r 10 000) was oxidized by sodium periodate and reacted first with daunomycin and then with antibody. This conjugation, viewed as involving Schiff base formation between aldehyde groups in protein and the sugar residue of daunomycin, was stabilized by partial reduction with sodium borohydride. Conjugates involving HSA as carrier were prepared by linking HSA to daunomycin through several intermediates, including 14-bromo-daunomycin, cis-aconityl, and succinyl ester (Baldwin and Ogunmuyiwa, unpublished work).

Conjugates containing daunomycin or doxorubicin linked directly to antibody or through a polymeric carrier are cytotoxic in vitro for tumor cells and show a degree of inhibitory activity when tested in vivo against experimental tumors or human tumor xenografts [5, 10, 42, 56]. In general, however, the studies suggest that direct linkage of anthracycline to antibody does not permit sufficient drug

334

targeting to effect a significant therapeutic response. The carrier systems show that sufficient drug can be attached to antibody to effect tumor cell kill. However, these conjugates do not have optimal properties with respect to in vivo biodistribution. Improvements in design are therefore being investigated with respect to both the carrier system and the anthracycline analog, the goal being to improve therapeutic effectiveness.

Cis-platinum has been complexed to antibodies to yield conjugates cytotoxic for tumor cells [45]. The conjugation procedure is not satisfactory, however, and, as shown in Table 2, conjugates produced with monoclonal antibody 791T/36 do not show high levels of reactivity. Carboxymethyl-dextran has also been investigated as a carrier for *cis*-platinum [69, 70]. Carboxymethyl-dextran complexes were formed by reacting *cis*-diaminedichloro platinum II (*cis*-DPP) and *cis*-diaminediaquo platinum nitrate (*cis*-aq) with two dextran carriers, dextran T10 (M_r 10 000) and dextran T40 (M_r 40 000). The dextran was substituted with carboxymethyl groups, and complexes were formed by interaction with *cis*-DPP or *cis*-aq. These complexes containing platinum compounds bound in a reversible manner were cytotoxic for tumor cells and, in view of earlier work on anthracycline-dextran antibody conjugates [5], may provide carrier systems for antibody targeting of *cis*-platinum complexes.

Conclusions and Discussion

Direct conjugation of cytotoxic drug to monoclonal antibodies generally results in a substantial reduction of drug activity when compared with that of free drug. This is illustrated in Table 2, which compares the concentrations of a range of

Table 2. Cytotoxicity of monoclonal Antibody 791T/36-drug conjugates

Conjugate[a]	Molar substitution ratio	Cytotoxicity[b] IC_{50}(ng/ml)	
		Free drug	Conjugate[c]
Methotrexate–791T/36	3:1	5	180
Vindesine–791T/36	6:1	10	10 000
Doxorubicin–791T/36	4:1	10	15 000
Daunomycin–791T/36	4:1	30	3 000
Cis-platinum–791T/36	1.5:1	100	2 000
Ricin toxin A chain–791T/36	1.5:1	5000	5

IC_{50}: concentration inhibiting [75Se] selenomethionine incorporation by 50%
[a] Drugs directly linked to antibody.
[b] Determined using an in vitro assay. Tumor cell survival determined by [75Se] selenomethionine incorporation [31, 32].
[c] Expressed in terms of nanograms of drug content per millilter.

drugs in free form or conjugated to monoclonal antibody 791T/36 producing a 50% inhibition (IC_{50}) of cytotoxicity for tumor 791T cells. For example, the IC_{50} of MTX is increased from 5 to 180 ng/ml following antibody conjugation. With other drugs such as vindesine and the anthracyclines, the influence of antibody conjugation is even more marked. In this respect, it should be noted that the situation is completely reversed with the plant toxin RTA, where antibody conjugation produces a 1000-fold increase in cytotoxicity [32]. This is because the toxin A chain is not readily internalized in the absence of the B chain. In contrast, antibody conjugation of cytotoxic drugs essentially abrogates their normal pathways for entry into a cell, which is probably more efficient than antibody-mediated endocytosis. The aim of antibody targeting of drugs, however, is to deliver drugs specifically to tumor cells, and it is envisaged that the introduction of this specificity will compensate for loss of drug activity.

Unfortunately, it is often the case that insufficient amounts of the drug can be directly linked to antibody to effect a significant cytotoxic response in the target cell. The dose is based upon calculations of the amount of drug which can be attached to antibody without damaging immunoreactivity, the number of antibody-binding sites on a tumor cell, and the amount of drug required to effect a cytotoxic response. For example, with MTX-mediated cytotoxicity for tumor 791T cells, it has been calculated that approximately a million molecules of drug are required to delivered to the intracellular compartment to effect a cytotoxic response (Durrant, personal communication). There are approximately 2×10^5–10^6 antibody 791T/36-binding sites on the target cell [64], and since maximum MTX substitution ratios of 4:1 can be achieved, it is not considered feasible to deliver cytotoxic doses of drug using drug directly linked to antibody.

Two avenues of approach are being explored which aim to improve drug delivery by monoclonal antibodies. Firstly, drug carrier systems are being developed, this being exemplified by the use of HSA with MTX, and dextran with a range of cytotoxic drugs [5, 10]. This provides the means for conjugating greater levels of drug to antibody, but in so doing it increases the size of the conjugate. This in turn alters the pharmacokinetics of the conjugates and may reduce their capacity to extravasate and localize in tumor. For example, the half-life in the circulation of conjugates containing MTX directly linked to monoclonal antibody 791T/36 in colorectal cancer patients is not markedly different from that of the antibody [54]. In contrast, conjugates prepared with MTX linked to HSA as a carrier are rapidly eliminated from blood, with liver uptake being the major route of metabolism. This effect is thought to be influenced by changes in the net charge of conjugates. Based upon these observations, modifications in conjugate design are being investigated, the aim being to produce conjugates which preferentially localize in tumors. This is one of the problems being addressed in the design of other immunotoxins which are preferentially taken up into liver.

The alternative approach for improving the therapeutic efficacy of drug-antibody conjugates is to use drugs with much greater cytotoxicity. Second-generation drug conjugates are being designed, taking advantage of the large range of synthetic agents which have been synthesized but not brought to clinical trial simply because they were too toxic. In this way, it should be practicable to

336

synthesize conjugates of a single antibody or antibody combinations with a range of cytotoxic drugs operating through different metabolic pathways.

Significant progress has been made in the use of immunotoxins. RTA conjugates with antimelanoma antibody and 791T/36 [9, 17] have proven efficacy against tumor xenografts and are now in phase I/II clinical trials in melanoma and colorectal cancer patients [9]. Also, RTA linked to an anti-T-lymphocyte monoclonal antibody directed against the CD5 antigen has been shown to be effective in vivo for the treatment of acute graft versus host disease (GVHD) in allogeneic bone marrow transplantation [16]. A phase I clinical trial is in progress in which bone marrow transplant recipients with grade II–IV steroid-resistant GVHD are treated with immunotoxin (Byers et al., to be published). The treatment was well tolerated and was accompanied by a drop in circulating T cells throughout the course of infusion (14 days). Target tissue clearing was seen, with skin, gut, and liver lesions responding to treatment.

Refinements in immunotoxin design may be expected to further improve their efficacy. Pharmacokinetic studies of a range of RTA-containing immunotoxins have shown that they rapidly localize in liver [12, 77]. This is because the RTA component has a mannose-contained oligosaccharide structure, which is recognized by mannose receptors on hepatic Kupffer's cells [77]. It follows from these findings that RTA in which the mannose receptor is blocked or eliminated may have an improved blood survival and result in increased therapeutic efficacy.

The efficiency of immunotoxin internalization into target cells is clearly an important factor, and with some antibodies, potentiators are required to produce high cytotoxic activity. This has proved to be a requirement with some of the immunotoxins acting against leukemic cells and T-lymphocytes in bone marrow purging [16, 47]. In contrast, potentiators have not proved of any benefit with some immunotoxins, e.g., RTA-791T/36 active against solid tumors.

It is appropriate that a range of immunotoxins containing other plant and bacterial products are being evaluated. These include pseudomonas exotoxin [38, 57] and plant toxins such as gelonin and saporin [73]. One anticipates that further toxins will be introduced for antibody conjugation, and from what is already known with RTA-containing immunotoxins, it is hoped that they will have cytotoxicities at least comparable to, if not better than, that of ricin.

The potential of monoclonal antibodies for targeting cytotoxic agents in cancer treatment has been substantiated with immunotoxins and drug conjugates. Further research will be directed towards developing new antibody conjugates and refining existing products. In addition, it is conceivable that cocktails of immunotoxins and drug conjugates will be used to resolve problems related to antigenic heterogeneity of tumors [29]. RTA conjugates have been prepared with monoclonal antibodies reacting with CEA and the anti-gp72 antigen expressed on colon carcinoma cells. Already, therefore, it is possible to use these immunotoxins together for the treatment of colorectal cancer [9].

Finally, one of the outstanding problems in the use of monoclonal antibody conjugates for repeated treatment is the generation of antimouse antibody response. Even low doses of radiolabelled murine antibody administered for patient imaging have resulted in the generation of antimouse antibody responses, especially anti-idiotype antibodies [26, 55, 66]. The importance of this is illustrated by tests on the treatment of renal allograft patients with the murine anti-T-lymphocyte antibody OKT3 (CD3), where the generation of anti-OKT3 (anti-idiotype) antibodies abrogated its therapeutic activity [24, 46]. Chemical immunosuppression, such as treatment with corticosteroids and azathioprine in the case of OKT3 antibody trials [46], is one approach. Immunotoxin trials are being devised in conjunction with immunosuppressive drugs, so allowing patient retreatment to be carried out. In addition, trials are in progress aimed at devising protocols for inducing unresponsiveness to murine antibodies and other foreign proteins such as RTA.

Design of antibody conjugates with cytotoxic drugs and toxins has advanced rapidly over the past 5 years. It is evident that numerous problems remain to be solved, but nevertheless immunoconjugates have been designed for clinical trial in the treatment of cancer. RTA-containing immunotoxins are in phase I/II clinical trials in the treatment of colorectal cancer and malignant melanoma and for ablating GVHD in patients receiving allogeneic bone marrow transplantation. Drug-antibody conjugates are also in trials in colorectal and lung carcinoma patients. These trials now in progress justify all the efforts in the basic research designing and evaluating immunoconjugates. It is anticipated that the clinical trials, together with studies on the biodistribution of immunoconjugates, will lead to the design of even more effective conjugates for cancer treatment.

References

1. Armitage NC, Perkins AC, Pimm MV, Farrands PA, Baldwin RW, Hardcastle JD (1984) The localisation of an anti-tumour monoclonal antibody (791T/36) in gastrointestinal tumours. Br J Surg 71: 407
2. Armitage NC, Parkins AC, Hardcastle JD, Pimm MV, Baldwin RW (1985) Monoclonal antibody imaging in malignant and benign gastro-intestinal diseases. In: Baldwin RW, Byers VS (eds) Monoclonal antibodies for cancer detection and therapy. Academic Press, London, p 129
3. Armitage NC, Perkins AC, Pimm MV, Wastie ML, Baldwin RW, Hardcastle JD (1985) Imaging of primary and metastatic colorectal cancer using an ^{111}In-labelled antitumour monoclonal antibody (791T/36). Nucl Med Comm 6: 623
4. Armitage NC, Perkins AC, Pimm MV, Wastie M, Hopkins JS, Dowling F, Baldwin RW, Hardcastle JD (1986) Imaging of bone tumours using a monoclonal antibody raised against human osteosarcoma. Cancer 58: 37
5. Arnon R, Hurwitz E (1985) Monoclonal antibodies as carriers for immunotargeting of drugs. In: Baldwin RW, Byers VS (eds) Monoclonal antibodies for cancer detection and therapy. Academic Press, London, pp 367–382
6. Baldwin RW (1985) Immunotherapy of cancer. Cancer Chemother Annu 7: 192
7. Baldwin RW, Byers VS (eds) (1985) Monoclonal antibodies for cancer detection and therapy. Academic Press, London
8. Baldwin RW, Byers VS (1986) Monoclonal antibodies in cancer treatment. Lancet 1: 603
9. Baldwin RW, Byers VS (1987) Monoclonal antibodies in the diagnosis and therapy of colorectal cancer. In: Levin B (ed) Current approaches for the diagnosis and treatment of gastrointestinal cancer. Unis Texas Press, Houston

10. Baldwin RW, Embleton MJ, Gallego J, Garnett M, Pimm MV, Price MR (1986) Monoclonal antibody drug conjugates for cancer therapy. In: Roth J (ed) Monoclonal antibodies in cancer; advances in diagnosis and treatment. Futura, New York, p 215
11. Begent RHJ (1985) Recent advances in tumour imaging: use of radiolabelled antitumour antibodies. Biochim Biphys Acta 780: 151
12. Bourrie JP, Casellas P, Blythman HE, Jansen FK (1986) Study of the plasma clearance of antibody-ricin-A-chain immunotoxins. Eur J Biochem 155: 1–10
13. Bumol TF, Apelgren LD, Boder GB, Varkki N, Walker LE, Reisfeld RA, Cullinan GJ (1984) Development and characterization of a vinblastine monoclonal antibody conjugate directed at human lung adenocarcinoma. Proc Am Cancer Res 25: 356
14. Buraggi GL, Callegaro L, Turrin A, Cascinelli N, Attili A, Emanuelli H, Gasparini M, Deleide G, Plassio G, Dovis M, Mariani G, Natali PG, Scassellati GA, Rosa U, Ferrone S (1984) Immunoscintigraphy with ^{123}I, ^{99m}Tc and ^{111}In-labelled F(ab')2 fragments of monoclonal antibodies to a human high molecular weight-associated antigen. J Nucl Med Allied Sci 28: 283
15. Burchell JM, Taylor-Papadimitriou J (1985) Monoclonal antibodies to breast cancer and their application. In: Baldwin RW, Byers BS (eds) Monoclonal antibodies for cancer detection and therapy. Academic Press, London, chap 1
16. Byers VS (1987) Bone marrow transplantation. In: Byers VS, Baldwin RW (eds) Immunology of malignant disease. MTP Press, Lancaster, p 55
17. Byers VS, Pimm MV, Scannon PJ, Pawluczyk IZA, Baldwin RW (1987) Inhibition of growth of human tumor xenografts in athymic mice treated with ricin toxin A chain-monoclonal antibody 791T/36 conjugates. Cancer Res 47: 5042–5046
18. Carson DA, Freimark BD (1986) Human lymphocyte hybridomas and monoclonal antibodies. Adv Immunol 38: 275
19. Casellas P, Bourrie BJP, Cros P, Jansen K (1984) Kinetics of cytotoxicity induced by immunotoxins. J Biol Chem 259: 9359–9384
20. Casellas P, Canat X, Fauser AA, Gros O, Laurent G, Poncelet P, Jansen FK (1985) Optimal elimination of leukemic T cells from human bone marrow with T101-ricin A-chain immunotoxin. Blood 65: 289
21. Chatal J-F, Saccavini J-C, Fumoleau P, Douillard J-Y, Curtet C, Kremer M, Le Mevel B, Koprowski H (1984) Immunoscintigraphy of colon carcinoma. J Nucl Med 25: 307
22. Chatal JF, Douillard JY, Saccavini JC, Kremer M, Curter C, Aubrey J, Le Mevel B (1985) Clinical prospective study with radio-iodinated monoclonal antibodies directed against colorectal cancer. In: Baldwin RW, Byers VS (eds) Monoclonal antibodies for tumour detection and drug targeting. Academic Press, London, p 159
23. Chatal JF, Thedrez P, Blottiere H, Kremer M, Bianco-Arco A, Douillard JY, Curtet C, Maurel C, Le Mevel B (1986) Comparative characteristics of 17-1A and GA-733 monoclonal antibodies for immunoscintigraphic application. Hybridoma [Suppl 1] 5: S87
24. Chatenoud L, Baudrihaye MF, Chkoff N, Kreis H, Goldstein G, Bach J-F (1986) Restriction of the human in vivo immune response against the mouse monoclonal antibody OKT3. J Immunol 137: 820
25. Cote RJ, Morrissey DM, Houghton AN, Thomson TM, Daly ME, Oettgen HF, Old LJ (1986) Specificity analysis of human monoclonal antibodies reactive with cell surface and intracellular antigens. Proc Natl Acad Sci USA 83: 2959
26. Courtenay-Luck NS, Epenetos AA, Moore R, Larche M, Pectasides D, Dhokia B, Ritter MA (1986) Development of primary and secondary immune responses to mouse monoclonal antibodies used in the diagnosis and therapy of malignant neoplasms. Cancer Res 46: 6489
27. Davies JD, Davies ER, Howe K, Jackson PC, Pitcher EM, Sadowski CS, Stirrat GM, Sunderland CA (1985) Radionuclide imaging of ovarian tumours with ^{123}I-labelled monoclonal antibody (NCOG$_2$) directed against placental alkaline phosphatase. Br J Obstet Gynaecol 92: 277
28. Delaloye B, Bischof-Delaloye A, Buchegger F, von Fliender V, Grob J-P, Volant J-C, Pettavel J, Mach J-P (1986) Detection of colorectal carcinoma by emission-computerized tomography after injection of ^{123}I-labelled Fab or F(ab')$_2$ fragments from monoclonal anti-carcinoembryonic antigen antibodies. J Clin Invest 77: 301
29. Durrant LG, Robins RA, Armitage NC, Brown A, Baldwin RW, Hardcastle JD (1986) Association of antigen expression and DNA ploidy in human colorectal tumors. Cancer Res 46: 3543

30. Embleton MJ, Rowland GF, Simmonds RG, Jacobs E, Marsden CH, Baldwin RW (1983) Selective cytotoxicity against human tumor cells by a vindesine-monoclonal antibody conjugate. Br J Cancer 47: 43–49

31. Embleton MJ, Garnett MC (1985) Antibody targeting of anti-cancer agents. In: Baldwin RW, Byers VS (eds) Monoclonal antibodies for cancer detection and therapy. Academic Press, London, p 317

32. Embleton MJ, Byers VS, Les HM, Scannon P, Blackhall NW, Baldwin RW (1986) Sensitivity and selectivity of ricin toxin A chain-monoclonal antibody 791T/36 conjugates against human tumor cell lines. Cancer Res 46: 5524

33. Epenetos AA, Mather S, Granowska M, Nimmon CC, Hawkins LR, Britton KE, Shepherd J, Taylor-Papadimitriou J, Durbin H, Malpas JS, Bodmer WF (1982) Targeting of iodine-123-labelled tumour-associated monoclonal antibodies to ovarian, breast and gastrointestinal tumours. Lancet 2: 999

34. Epenetos AA, Carr D, Johnson PM, Bodmer WF, Lavender JP (1986) Antibody-guided radiolocalisation of tumours in patients with testicular or ovarian cancer using two radioiodinated monoclonal antibodies to placental alkaline phosphatase. Br J Radiol 59: 117

35. Epenetos AA, Snook D, Durbin H, Johnson PM, Taylor-Papadimitriou J (1986) Limitations of radiolabeled monoclonal antibodies for localization of human neoplasms. Cancer Res 46: 3183

36. Evered D, Whelan J (eds) (1983) Fetal antigens and cancer. Ciba Found Symp 96

37. Feizi T (1985) Demonstration by monoclonal antibodies that carbohydrate structures of glycoproteins and glycolipids are onco-developmental antigens. Nature 314: 53

38. Fitzgerald DJ, Willingham MC, Pastan I (1986) Antitumor effects of an immunotoxin made with Pseudomonas exotoxin in a nude mouse model of human ovarian cancer. Proc Natl Acad Sci USA 83: 6627

39. Frankel AE (1985) Antibody-toxin hybrids: a clinical review of their use. J Biol Response Mod 4: 437

40. Frankel AE, Houston LL (1987) Immunotoxin therapy of cancer. In: Carlo D (ed) Immunoconjugates and cancer. Academic Press, Orlando

41. Fulton RJ, Uhr JW, Vitetta ES (1986) The effect of antibody valency and lysosomotropic amines on the synergy between ricin A chain- and ricin B chain-containing immunotoxins. J Immunol 136: 3103

42. Gallego J, Price MR, Baldwin RW (1984) Preparation of four daunomycin monoclonal antibody 791T/36 conjugates with anti-tumour activity. Int J Cancer 33: 737

43. Garnett MC, Baldwin RW (1986) An improved synthesis of a methotrexate-albumin-791T/36 monoclonal antibody conjugate cytotoxic to osteogenic sarcoma cell lines. Cancer Res 46: 2407

44. Gilliland DG, Steplewski Z, Collier RJ, Mitchell KF, Chang TH, Koprowski H (1980) Antibody-directed cytotoxic agents: use of monoclonal antibody to direct the action of toxin A-chains to colorectal carcinoma cells. Proc Natl Acad Sci USA 77: 4539

45. Hurwitz E, Kashi R, Wilcheck M (1982) Platinum-complexed antitumor immunoglobulins that specifically inhibit DNA synthesis of mouse tumor cells. JNCI 69: 47

46. Jaffers GJ, Fuller TC, Cosimi AB, Russell PS, Winn HJ, Colvin RB (1986) Anti-idiotypic and non-anti-idiotypic antibodies to OKT3 arising despite intense immunosuppression. Transplantation 41: 572

47. Jansen FK, Laurent G, Liance MC, Blythman HE, Berthe J, Canat X, Carayon P, Carriere D, Casellas P, Derocq JM, Dussossoy D, Fauser AA, Gorin NC, Gros O, Gros P, Laurent JC, Poncelet P, Remandet B, Richer G, Vidal H (1985) Efficiency and tolerance of the treatment with immuno-A-chain toxins in human bone marrow transplantations. In: Baldwin RW, Byers VS (eds) Monoclonal antibodies for cancer detection and therapy. Academic Press, London, p 224

48. Kanellos J, Pietersz GA, McKenzie IFC (1985) Studies of methotrexate-monoclonal antibody conjugates for immunotherapy. JNCI 75: 319

49. Kohler G, Milstein C (1975) Continuous cultures of fused cells secreting antibodies of predefined specificity. Nature 256: 494

50. Larson SM, Brown JP, Wright PW, Carrasquillo JA, Hellstrom I, Hellstrom KE (1983) Imaging of melanoma with I-131-labeled monoclonal antibodies. J Nucl Med 24: 123

51. Larson SM, Carrasquillo JA, Krohn KA, Brown JP, McGuffin RW, Ferens JM, Graham MM, Hill LD, Beaumier PL, Hellstrom KE, Hellstrom I (1983) Localization of ^{131}I-labelled p97-specific Fab fragments in human melanoma as a basis for radiotherapy. J Clin Invest 72: 2101

52. Luders G, Kohnlein W, Sorg C Bruggen J (1985) Selective toxicity of neocarzinostatin-monoclonal antibody conjugates to the antigen-bearing human melanoma cell line in vitro. Cancer Immunol Immunother 20: 85

53. Pateisky N, Philipp K, Skodler WD, Czerwenka K, Hamilton G, Burchell J (1985) Radioimmunodetection in patients with suspected ovarian cancer. J Nucl Med 26: 1369

54. Perkins AC, Pimm MV, Ballantyne KC, Garnett MC, Clegg JA, Hardcastle JD, Baldwin RW (1987) In vivo imaging of a monoclonal antibody drug conjugate (791T/36-methotrexate): Experimental and clinical studies. In: Greten H, Klapder R (eds) Proceedings of the 4th Hamburg symposium on cancer markers. Thieme, Stuttgart

55. Pimm MV (1987) Immunoscintigraphy: tumour detection with radiolabelled anti-tumour monoclonal antibodies. In: Byers VS, Baldwin RW (eds) Immunology of malignant diseases. MTP Press, Lancester, p 21

56. Pimm MV, Jones JA, Price MR, Middle JG, Embleton MJ, Baldwin RW (1982) Tumour localization of monoclonal antibody against a rat mammary carcinoma and suppression of tumour growth with adriamycin-antibody conjugates. Cancer Immunol Immunother 12: 125

57. Pirker R, Fitzgerald DJP, Hamilton TC, Ozols RF, Willingham MC, Pastan I (1985) Anti-transferrin receptor antibody linked to pseudomonas exotoxin as a model immunotoxin in human ovarian carcinoma cell lines. Cancer Res 45: 751

58. Powell MC, Perkins AC, Pimm MV, Jetaily A, Wastie ML, Durrant L, Baldwin RW, Symonds EM (1987) Diagnostic imaging of gynaecological tumours using the monoclonal antibody 791T/36. Am J Obstet Gynecol 157: 78–84

59. Price MR (1987) Breast cancer associated antigens defined by monoclonal antibodies. Subcell Biochem 12

60. Primus FJ, Deland FH, Goldenberg DM (1984) Monoclonal antibodies for radiommunodetection of cancer. In: Wright GL Jr (ed) Monoclonal antibodies and cancer. Dekker, New York, p 305

61. Rainsbury RM, Ott RJ, Westwood JH, Kalirai TS, Coombes RC, McCready VR, Neville AM, Gazet J-C (1983) Localisation of metastatic breast carcinoma by a monoclonal antibody chelate labelled with indium-111. Lancet 2: 8356

62. Raso V, Lawrence J (1984) Carboxylic ionophores enhance the cytotoxic potency of ligand- and antibody-delivered ricin A chain. J Exp Med 160: 1234

63. Raso V, Ritz J, Basala M, Schlossman SF (1982) Monoclonal antibody ricin A chain conjugate selectively cytotoxic for cells bearing the common acute lymphoblastic leukemia antigen. Cancer Res 42: 457

64. Roe R, Robins RA, Laxton RR, Baldwin RW (1985) Kinetics of divalent monoclonal antibody binding to tumour cell surface antigens using flow cytometry: standardization and mathematical analysis. Mol Immunol 22: 11

65. Rogers GT (1983) Carcinoembryonic antigen and related proteins: molecular aspects and specificity. Biochim Biophys Acta 695: 227

66. Rowe RE, Pimm MV, Baldwin RW (1985) Anti-idiotype antibody responses in cancer patients receiving a murine monoclonal antibody. IRCS 13: 936

67. Rowland GF, Simmonds RG (1985) Effects of monoclonal antibody-drug conjugates on human tumour cell cultures and xenografts. In: Baldwin RW, Byers VS (eds) Monoclonal antibodies for cancer detection and therapy. Academic Press, London, p 345

68. Rowland GF, Simmonds RG, Gore VA, Marsden CH, Smith W (1986) Drug localization and growth inhibition studies of vindesine-monoclonal anti-CEA conjugates in a human tumour xenograft. Cancer Immunol Immunother 21: 183

69. Schechter B, Pauzner R, Arnon R, Wilcheck M (1986) Cis-platinum (II) complexes of carboxymethyl-dextran as potential antitumor agents. I. Preparation and characterization. Cancer Biochem Biophys 8: 277

70. Schechter B, Pauzner R, Wilchek M, Arnon R (1986) Cis-platinum (II) complexes of

carboxymethyl-dextran as potential antitumor agents. II. In vitro and in vivo activity. Cancer Biochem Biophys 8: 289

71. Sell S (1980) Alphafetoprotein. In: Sell S (ed) Cancer markers: diagnostic and developmental significance. Humana Press, New Jersey, p 249

72. Smedley HM, Finan P, Lennox EJ, Ritson A, Takei F, Wraight P, Sikora K (1986) Localization of metastatic carcinoma by a radiolabelled monoclonal antibody. Br J Cancer 47: 253

73. Stirpe F, Barbieri L (1986) Ribosome-inactivating proteins up to date. FEBS Lett 195 (1/2): 1

74. Strong RC, Youle RJ, Vallera DA (1984) Elimination of clonogenic T-leukemic cells from human bone marrow using anti-M_r 65,000 protein immunotoxins. Cancer Res 44: 3000

75. Symonds EM, Perkins AC, Pimm MV, Baldwin RW, Hardy JD, Williams DA (1985) Clinical implications for immunoscintigraphy in patients with ovarian malignancy: a preliminary study using monoclonal antibody 791T/36. Br J Obstet Gynaec 92: 270

76. Thompson CH, Lichtenstein M, Stacker SA, Leyden MJ, Saleri N, Andrews JT, McKenzie IFC (1984) Immunoscintigraphy for detection of lymph node metastases from breast cancer. Lancet 2: 1245

77. Thorpe PE, Detre SI, Foxwell BMJ, Brown ANF, Skilleter DN, Wilson G, Forrester IA, Stirpe F (1985) Modification of the carbohydrate in ricin with metaperiodate-cyanoborohydride mixtures. Eur J Biochem 147: 197

78. Uhr JW (1984) Immunotoxins: harnessing nature's poisons. J Immunol 133: 1

79. Vitetta ES, Uhr JW (1985) Immunotoxins. Annu Rev Immunol 3: 197

80. Vitetta ES, Cushley W, Uhr JW (1983) Synergy of ricin A chain-containing immunotoxins and ricin B chain-containing immunotoxins in in vitro killing of neoplastic human B cells. Proc Natl Acad Sci USA 80: 6332

81. Vitetta ES, Krolick KA, Miyama-Inaba WC, Cushley W, Uhr JW (1983) Immunotoxins: a new approach to cancer therapy. Science 219: 644

82. Youle RJ, Uckun FM, Vallera DA, Colombatti M (1986) Immunotoxins show rapid entry of diphtheria toxin but not ricin via the T3 antigen. J Immunol 136: 93

18. Bone Marrow Purging

M.C. Favrot and T. Philip

Introduction

In the management of leukemia and malignant solid tumors [if one excepts the graft-versus-leukemia (GVL) effect of an allograft], bone marrow transplantation (BMT) is not therapeutic per se, but is simply a method designed to overcome myelotoxicity after high-dose chemotherapy. The main limitations of this method are graft-versus-host disease (GVHD) in allogenic BMT and the contamination of the graft by residual malignant cells in autologous BMT. A common approach, so-called purging, has been proposed to eliminate unwanted cells from the BM before its reinjection—either allogenic normal T cells responsible for GVHD or autologous malignant cells.

This ex vivo manipulation only represents one step of a complete process that includes high-dose chemotherapy and BMT. The indications and future of the purging procedures, especially for autografting, are thus closely linked to those of high-dose chemotherapy, an approach which continues to be controversial with regard to its place in the treatment of leukemia or solid tumors. It remains to be proved, for example, whether the results of high-dose chemotherapy and BMT would be better than those of conventional therapy in high-risk patients early in the clinical course of the disease (i.e., in first complete remission) and whether the toxicity could be reduced to acceptably low levels. At present, methods of sufficient sensitivity are not available to determine whether, in such clinical conditions, the autologous BMT is free of disease, i.e., whether purging is indicated, especially in leukemia. If, on the other hand, autologous BMT, especially in solid tumors, were restricted to high-risk patients in partial remission, relapse, or with progressive disease, purging would presumably be necessary in most cases. However, the clinical relevance and efficacy of such a procedure could not be demonstrated unless high-dose chemotherapy were sufficiently effective to eliminate residual disease outside the BM.

A third approach to the use of autologous BMT is to harvest the BM early in the course of the disease, but to reserve BMT for relapsing patients. Even if theoretically ideal, and feasible in some patients, this approach is unlikely to be applicable on a large scale in solid tumors because of considerations of cost and availability of resources. It is worthy of consideration, however, in leukemia.

In this brief review, we will first describe the purging techniques and then consider the experimental and clinical aspects of the major methods used either

343

for T-cell depletion in allogeneic BMT or for removing malignant cells from autologous BM grafts.

Purging Techniques

In considering bone marrow purging, it is usual to distinguish between physical, chemical, and immunological methods, as follows:

1. *Physical separation.* Techniques such as percoll or bovine serum albumin (BSA) gradients were the first methods described, and more recently, techniques such as counterflow centrifugation have been published [1]. The selection of hematopoietic precursors for reinfusion is based on their density, and these methods can be used as a preliminary step in purging. Sheep red blood rosetting or soybean lectin separation have more restricted applications in T-cell depletion [2], although soybean lectin separation has been shown to allow a poor elimination of neuroblastoma cells or T and B acute lymphoblastic leukemia (ALL) cells [3].

2. *Chemical methods.* Chemotherapeutic agents may destroy malignant cells with at least a partial preservation of normal hematopoietic progenitors [4]. Although this last point is still very unclear [5], active derivates of cyclophosphamide, either 4-hydroperoxycyclophosphamide (4-HC) or mafosfamide (ASTA Z 7557), are now extensively used in clinical trials for autografting in ALL or acute myeloid leukemia (AML), as well as for non-Hodgkin malignant lymphoma (NHL) or neuroblastoma [6–10]. Other chemotherapeutic agents, such as etoposide, which have been tested experimentally have not yet been used systematically in clinical trials [11]. Some nonchemotherapeutic agents are of potential interest, among them merocyanine 540, a DNA dye with lytic activity after photoactivation [12] and 6-hydroxydopamine (13).

3. *Immunological methods.* Unwanted cells are specifically targeted by monoclonal antibodies (MoAbs) directed against cell surface antigens. These cells are then eliminated by various mechanisms.

a) Complement-dependent lysis. MoAbs (IgM or IgG2a isotypes) lyse targeted cells in the presence of rabbit complement [14–17]. Some of these MoAbs—such as rat antibodies campath-1 or AL_2 and mouse MoAbs $RFAL_3$, RFB_7, BA_1, BA_2, BA_3, and BG_6—are claimed to be lytic in the presence of human complement [15, 18–20].

b) Immunomagnetic depletion. Magnetic particles (either macroparticles or colloids) covered with antimouse immunoglobulins bind malignant cells through a linkage between the antimouse immunoglobulins and the MoAbs. The magnetic particles, coated with cells, are removed by a magnetic field [21–25]. A few other methods derive from the same principle: for example, malignant cells can be absorbed in a column via MoAbs attached to a solid phase through avidin-biotin linkages [26].

c) Immunotoxins. MoAbs are conjugated to various plant toxins. Ricin, from the castor bean *Ricinus communis*, is the one most commonly studied and used

344

in clinical trials [27]. This consists of two chains: the toxic A chain acts inside the cell by inhibiting protein synthesis on the 60S subunit of ribosomes; the B chain permits cell entry since it binds to galactose and N-galactosamine residues on the cell surface, like a monovalent lectin. The lytic activity of the ricin A chain is long (1 or 2 days) and is influenced by the presence or absence of the B chain, the affinity of the MoAbs, and the temperature and pH of incubation [28–31]. In spite of these disadvantages, immunotoxins are probably the most efficient agents. Other toxins coupled to MoAbs or activators with potential clinical interest have been more recently described [32–35].

Purging Procedures in Allogenic Bone Marrow Transplantation

The aim of T-cell-purging procedures is not necessarily to achieve an absolute depletion of T cells since experience has shown that a depletion which results in less than 10^{-6} T cells per kilogram being injected into the recipient is associated with a low level of GVHD (Table 1). It remains to be determined whether the GVL effect is separable from the broader GVHD, and whether heavy preconditioning regimens can decrease the risks both of graft rejection and of relapse in recipients of T-cell-depleted marrow [36]. Although safe engraftment can be achieved and GVHD also prevented, the therapeutic possibilities remain very limited; despite enthusiastic preliminary reports, several groups have given up attempts to prevent GVHD by such BM manipulations in matched transplantations. In mismatched haploidentical BMT, T-cell depletion does not entirely solve the problem since GVHD is not fully prevented, and the rate of nonengraftment is very high. A transient suppression of the immune reaction at the time of BMT by in vivo therapy with a MoAb directed against the alpha subunit of the human leukocyte functional antigen (LFA-1) permits the engraftment of T-cell-depleted haploidentical BM in patients suffering from severe immunodeficiency [37]. This approach has not yet been tested for leukemia and aplastic anemia. Autologous BMT, where the availability of matched donors is not limiting, is an alternative strategy for patients with malignant diseases, especially with solid tumors.

Bone Marrow Purging Procedures for Autologous Bone Marrow Transplantation

In the standardization of purging methods for autologous BMT, two different aspects have to be considered: the technique itself and a model for testing its efficiency. A clear distinction must be made between experimental models and clinical assessment: it should be emphasized that the efficiency of purging differs when the method is used on cell lines as opposed to fresh tumor samples. The

Table 1. Purging methods for allogenic grafting

Methods	Experimental assays		Clinical assays			
	Method of quantification	Elimination	Patients(n)	Acute GVHD (grade 3)(n)	Graft rejection(n)	Ref.
Physical						
Soybean agglutination + agglutination with sheep red blood cells	E rosette formation, alloreactivity (CML)	>99% [3]	3 (HLA-identical)	0	1	[2]
			129 (86 HLA-identical) (43 HLA-haploidentical)	0 1	8 13	[56]
Agglutination with sheep red blood cells	Immunofluorescence	>97%	8 (HLA-haploidentical)	0	1[a]	[37]
Counterflow centrifugation	Rosette formation	95%	26 (HLA-identical)	2	0	[1]
Immunological						
Rabbit complement						
CD6, CD8, 8 anti-T-cell antibodies	Immunofluorescence	95%–99%	56 (HLA-identical)	1	4	[36, 57]
	PHA (phytohemagglutinin) culture (7 days) + immunofluorescence	2–3 log	20 (HLA-identical)	3	7	[58]
CD2 + CD3 CD5 + CD2 + CD7	Immunofluorescence	94% ± 4%	32 (HLA-identical)	1	0	[59] [60]
Human complement						
Campath I	E rosette formation, immunofluorescence	95%–99%	11 (HLA-identical)	0	2	[18]
Immunotoxins						
Ricin chain A + B and TA1, UCTH, T101	Generation of CTL	> 2 log	2 (HLA-identical) 17 (HLA-identical)	0 0	0 10%–30%	[27, 61]

CML, chronic myelocytic leukemia; CTL, cytotoxic thymus-dependent lymphocytes
[a] One patient presented with a B-cell lymphoproliferative syndrome.

potentially optimal method may vary from one disease to another, depending upon the features of the malignant cells studied (Table 2).

The development of rigorous methods to detect and eliminate malignant cells is necessary if an extensive or even randomized multicentric study is being considered. Indeed, in only a few clinical situations where autografting has been used have malignant cells been detected in the graft, warranting the efforts made to remove such cells. Thus, the logical criteria for using a purging method are that the efficiency and the lack of toxicity for hematopoietic precursors have been proven experimentally, and that the method is reproducible in clinical practice in the presence of excess normal BM cells.

Experimental Models

Initial experiments on animal models suggested that purging methods can eliminate leukemic cells from an autograft and predicted the feasibility of autologous BMT [38, 39]. However, none of the animal models studied to date provides a precise analogue for autologous BMT in humans, and syngeneic tumor transplants have been studied rather than primary autochthonous tumors. The capacity of various methods to kill a malignant population has been evaluated using the ^{51}Cr-release assay or the measurement of thymidine incorporation or ^{125}I-labelled UDR uptake.

More recently, efforts have been made to demonstrate the efficiency of the purging methods in models closer to the clinical situation, i.e., bone marrow samples contaminated with 1%–10% malignant cells from various malignant cell lines. Either semisolid or liquid culture assays allow the quantification of up to a 6 log elimination, using limited dilutions and pre-B, T, and null or common ALL cell lines or Burkitt's lymphoma (BL) cell lines [14, 16, 33]. However, the use of carefully selected cell lines known to have a high clonogenic efficiency does not permit measurement of variations due to the heterogeneity of the tumor samples. When the clonogenic efficiency is very low (i.e., cell lines established from solid tumors), staining of the malignant cells with the vital dye Hoechst 342 before their admixture with the BM is an alternative method which permits their objective and rapid detection. In this artificial model, Reynolds et al. [40] described the detection of as few as 10^{-6} residual malignant cells stained with Hoechst 342 by a computerized analysis. Visual analysis permits detection of 10^{-4} residual cells within the normal BM [17]. However, this method is useful only for the measurement of the immediate elimination of malignant cells (i.e., by complement lysis or immunomagnetic depletion) and is inappropriate for testing the efficiency of purging with drugs.

Clinical or Preclinical Assessment of Purging Methods

Some methods of detection are applicable to the evaluation of the efficacy of purging methods both on BM artificially contaminated with cultured malignant

Table 2. Purging methods for autologous bone marrow transplantation: experimental and clinical assays

Methods	Model	Experimental assays			Clinical assays			Reference
		Method of quantification[a]	(limit of detection)	Elimination	Patients(n)[b]	Toxicity[c]		
						Neutrophils	Platelets	
Complement-dependent lysis								
MoAbs								
J_5 (CD_{10})	C-ALL	^{51}Cr (BM + 1% tumor cells or 1% Nalm1)	(2 log)	99%	24	44(16–78)	50(16–103)	[65]
BA_1 (CD_{24}) BA_2 (CD_9) BA_3 (CD_{10})	C-ALL Pre-B-ALL	Clon. assay (BM + 5% KM_3, HPB-null, Nalm6)	(>4 log)	2–4 log	23	22(16–64)	34(7–78)	[14, 66]
J_5 (CD_{10}) J_2 (CD_9) B_1 (CD_{20})	BL	Clon. assay (BM + 1% Namalwa)	(>5 log)	1–3.5 log	8 (NHL)	30(14–57)	28(18–60)	[16, 67]
B_1 (CD_{20}) Y29/55 AL_2 (CD_{10})	BL	Liquid culture assay (BM + 1% daudi, Raji, Ly_{67}, IARC BL_{17}, BL_{63}, BL_{93} or tumor cells)	(4–5 log)	1–4 log	12	17(5–22)	33(13–56)	[17, 41, 68]
Y29/55	B-CLL	IF (tumor cells)	(2.5 log)	2.5 log	7 (BL)	14(10–36)	27(8–117)	[69]
$RFAL_3$ or CD_7 (+ second Ab when required)	C-ALL T-ALL	TdT assay (tumor cells)	(>4 log)	>4 log	18	24(15–66)	36(24–140)	[15, 14]

Immunomagnetic depletion

MoAbs

Method/MoAbs	Disease	Assay		Depletion				Ref.
UJ13A, UJ223.8 UJ127.11, UJ181.4, Thy-1, H11	Neuroblastoma	IF Clon. assay (BM + 1% CHP100)	(?)	99.9%	17 4 (grafted after relapse)	22(14–36) 46	33(14–43) 81.5	[21, 62]
UJ13A, UJ223.8 UJ127.11, UJ181.4, Thy-1, H11	Neuroblastoma	Physical parameters defined on BL model (see text)	(5 log)	4–5 log on BL model	44	24	39	[48] [23, 24]
Ab390, Ab459, HSAN 1.2, BA_1, RFB_{21-7} ($\pm BA_2$, Leu 7)	Neuroblastoma	Hoechst 342 (BM + 20% LAN-1, SHS-KCNR, SH-S KANR, LA-N-5)	(4 log)	3–4 log	14	?	?	[24, 63]

Chemical methods

Method/MoAbs	Disease	Assay		Depletion				Ref.
4-HC or mafosfamid	AML	Rat model (LCFU-S)		5–6 log	25	29(16–63)	57(23–191)	[6]
	AML	Clon. assay (100% tumor cells)	(?)	?	14 16	34(19–47) 27(14–50)	150(55–330) 45(13–90)	[7, 64] [8]
	AML	Clon. assay (BM + 5% tumor cells)	(?)	Lack of specific reactivity for malignant cells				[4]
	ALL	Clon. assay (BM + cell lines)	(8 log)	6 log	21	25(13–60)	33(14–33)	[34]
	ALL				5	(15–28)	(25–35)	[9]
	ALL				8	19(11–30)	50(23–90)	[8] [7]

a Experiments were performed either on 100% cells or on a mixture of irradiated marrow and malignant cells; "tumor" refers to noncultured malignant cells; cell lines are entered under reference name. ^{51}Cr, measure of ^{51}Cr-release; Clon. assay, clonogenic assay with limited dilutions; IF, immunofluorescence

b When the experimental model and the clinical model are different, the disease is defined in parentheses.

c Median number of days necessary to obtain 0.5×10^9 neutrophils/liter or 50×10^9 platelets/liter, except for experiments marked, for which the median number of days necessary to reach 1×10^9 neutrophils/liter and 25×10^9 platelets/liter is given. Ranges are given in parentheses.

cells and on marrow samples freshly obtained from patients. The interest of these assays is that they each allow a relatively quick and reproducible evaluation of the potential efficacy of any purging procedure for individual patients. We recently developed a liquid cell culture assay, restricted to the BL model, which enabled us to detect one residual malignant cell in a million normal BM cells in short-term culture (10 days), and to detect a single residual BL cell in the BM sample in long-term culture (21 days). The BM can be contaminated with Epstein-Barr virus (EBV)(−) or EBV(+) cell lines recently established from our patients who are candidates for an autograft, or even with the patient's own noncultured tumor cells from the primary tumor [41]. Such an assay allows the quantification, in experimental or in clinical assays, of the elimination of up to 5 logs of malignant cells from BM contaminated with 1% BL cells. Other published assays usually quantify the purging efficiency on populations of 100% tumor cells. In such culture assays, the clonogenicity of malignant cells is usually very low, ranging from 1%–3%, and for this reason other groups developed methods based on immunostaining [42, 43]. Campana and Janossy [44] showed that double staining with TdT (terminal deoxynucleotidyl transferase) and a specific membrane marker allows the quantification of the elimination of more than 4 logs of leukemic cells. BuDR (bromodeoxyuridime) incorporation by malignant cells permits one to verify that these cells are really proliferating. Similarly, and as described by others [45], we showed that 10^{-4} to 10^{-5} residual neuroblastoma cells can be detected in the BM by immunocytochemical staining or double immunofluorescence staining.

Even more important with regard to the whole concept of reinjection of a purged autograft, immunostaining methods or culture assays (if the clonogenic efficiency is sufficient, as in our BL model) make it possible to determine whether or not the BM contains residual malignant cells (as few as 10^{-4}–10^{-5}) when harvested, and to demonstrate their elimination by purging.

If one wants to evaluate the efficacy of any purging method for autografting, it is fundamental to distinguish clearly in published reports between patients treated in relapse or partial remission (PR) with BM involvement but receiving an autograft taken in first complete remission (CR) and those rarely reported patients treated with BM harvested and grafted in PR or relapse, presumably with residual malignant cells in the BM before the purging procedure. For example, in none of our stage IV BL cases does the BM contain BL cells detectable by the liquid cell culture assay when the patients achieve first CR; consequently, if harvested at such a time, the BM would probably not need purging. On the other hand, in 40% of patients examined at the time of relapse, the cytologically normal BM does contain growing BL cells; consequently, in 2 of our 30 patients where BM was harvested and grafted either in PR or in second CR, the harvested BM contained BL cells detected only by the liquid cell culture assay before the purging procedure and eliminated after purging [46, 47]. Similarly, in two ALL patients receiving transplants in relapse, Janossy et al. demonstrated a contamination of the BM by TdT positive blast cells before the purging procedure and their reduction, after purging, to a level undetectable by immunostaining [15, 44].

In our group of 50 unselected patients with stage IV neuroblastoma entered in the autograft program, 16 had pathological BM when it was harvested. In 8 of them, malignant cells were detectable only in the trephine biopsy samples, whereas in 8 others, clumps of neuroblasts were also detectable by immunocytology in the harvested mononuclear BM cells before purging [48]. The clinical course of those patients who had pathological BM at the time of harvesting and grafting and who further achieved a BM CR following high-dose chemotherapy supports the rationale of using a purging procedure. Indeed, the patients would have received at least 10^4 malignant cells per kilogram in the absence of purging. Even if the percentage of malignant cells able to find an appropriate microenvironment for regenerating the malignant clone once they were reinjected into the patient is unknown, it seems unlikely that none of the tumor cells would have been clonogenic after reinjection.

Comparison of Purging Methods and their Combinations

In the BL model as in B-cell ALL (B-ALL), the combination of an immunological purging procedure with MoAbs and complement or an immunotoxin and a chemical procedure with mafosfamide improved the malignant cell elimination [33, 49, 50]. However, in these systems, the activity of mafosfamide might be overestimated, as the target cells that were used are rapidly dividing cell lines, different from some resting cells within the leukemic population.

We recently compared the efficiency of two different immunological procedures, complement lysis and immunomagnetic depletion (IMD), in the BL model (Table 3). When complement lysis was assayed with the two cocktails $RFB_7 + SB_4$ or $B_1 + Al_2 + Y29/55$, the cytoreduction was better with $RFB_7 + SB_4$, which resulted in a complete elimination of BL cells in almost all experiments, as demonstrated by inhibition of their growth. Using IMD, B_1 as a single MoAb allowed a 4- to 5-log reduction when a mononuclear BM cell fraction, rather than buffy coat, and a double-depletion procedure were used [22, 23]. The BL_{99} and BL_2 cell lines were very sensitive to complement lysis, and in contrast, the BL_{93} cell line was partially resistant to it, irrespective of the cocktail of MoAbs selected. In the case of BL_{93}, an optimal BL cell elimination was achieved with the immunomagnetic method. It appears, therefore, that the two immunological procedures are complementary [51]. The different classes of MoAbs required (i.e., IgM for complement lysis and IgG for magnetic beads) may explain the results. Whereas some MoAbs, such as SB_4, are highly cytotoxic with rabbit complement, even when the antigen they react with is weakly expressed, the immunomagnetic procedure requires MoAbs of high affinity and antigens of high density on the cell surface. Preliminary experiments even suggest that the use of MoAb cocktails does not necessarily improve the efficiency of immunomagnetic depletion and may even decrease its depleting power [23].

Various groups have suggested combining these complementary methods; we, however, do not advocate this. Indeed, the fact that some of the purging methods described above are capable, when combined, of removing large quantities of malignant cells is only of theoretical interest. BM contamination reflects a resistance of malignant cells to chemotherapy, and, similarly, the residual dis-

Table 3. Comparison of cytoreduction achieved in two immunological purging procedures (expressed in decimal logarithms)

Cell line	Complement-dependent lysis procedure		Immunomagnetic depletion
	$RFB_7 + SB_4$	$B_1 + AL_2 + Y29/55$	
BL_{99} ($n = 8$) EBV(+) Caucasian	>5	5	4
BL_{93} ($n = 5$) EBV(−) Caucasian	3	2.5	5
BL_2 ($n = 5$) EBV(−) Caucasian	>5	5	4

The efficiency of the procedure was evaluated by the liquid cell culture assay in short- and long-term culture, and results are expressed in decimal logarithms (means of 5–8 experiments). (When BL cell growth was fully inhibited and all BL cells then eliminated fom the sample, cytoreduction was recorded as >5 log.) Experiments with complement lysis and IMD where performed on the same samples and on the same day. Irradiated normal BM samples were contaminated with 1% BL cells from 3 different cell lines recently established from our patients. See refs 8, 14, 22

ease outside the BM is likely to be resistant to high-dose chemotherapy. The most successful clinical application of purging is therefore likely to be on BM harvested from patients when the involvement is minimal (i.e., BM containing 1% or less malignant cells). The only value in combining procedures will thus be to overcome, for a few patients, the possible resistance of malignant cells to one procedure or the other. However, such an approach will give rise to practical difficulties if applied to all patients and is likely to increase damage to the harvested BM simply by doubling the duration of the BM manipulation and the number of successive incubations and washings. An alternative approach might be to select the most effective MoAbs, or even the most suitable procedure, to be used on malignant tumor samples from each individual patient with relatively quick and reproducible assays such as those described above. The determination of the efficiency of the purging procedure for these patients will permit more accurate and meaningful analysis of the clinical outcome.

Conclusion

Results recently published by Yeager et al. [6] on the use of autologous BMT in AML patients in relapse or in second CR provide evidence that the

4-HC purging procedure, shown to be efficient experimentally, may have beneficial effects in this disease. However, in most clinical models, it is difficult to
demonstrate that purging has been useful on the basis of the clinical results
obtained. When relapse does occur, it is impossible to ascertain whether it is due
to residual disease resistant to chemotherapy or to tumor cells reinjected with
the BM. Until recently, in most clinical trials, there was no proof that the BM
was infiltrated by tumor and thus needed to be purged and also no method for
demonstrating total freedom from tumor. Partial answers will be obtained in
clinical models only if rigorously controlled purging procedures are used and if
the presence or absence of residual malignant cells in the BM is assayed with
very sensitive methods before and after purging. Such a rigorous analysis of the
clinical value of purging methods is fundamental both to the future prospects for
this approach and to a meaningful assessment of the role of high-dose chemotherapy and autologous BMT in the management of malignant proliferations.

Selective in vitro maintenance of normal hematopoietic progenitors [52] or
the positive selection of such progenitors with relevant MoAbs [53] could be an
alternative to the reinjection of the whole BM mononuclear cell fraction after a
purging procedure. Transplantation with peripheral blood hematopoietic stem
cells could be another alternative, as long as there are no demonstrable circulating malignant cells [54]. Some experimental therapeutic approaches, such as in
vitro immunostimulation of the patient's effector cells, involve ex vivo manipulation of either peripheral or BM mononuclear cells [55]; thus, the autografting
techniques developed in the last decade appear to be a preliminary but essential
step which may permit the introdution of new immunological approaches to
therapy.

References

1. DeWitte T, Hoogenhout J, De Pauw B, Holdrinet R, Jansen J, Wessels J, Van Daal W, Hustinx
   K, Haanen C (1986) Depletion of donor lymphocytes by counterflow centrifugation successfully
   prevents acute graft-versus-host disease in matched allogeneic marrow transplantation. Blood
   67: 1302
2. Reisner Y, Kapoor D, Kirkpatrick D, Pollack MS, Cunningham-Rundles S, Dupont B, Hodes
   MZ, Good RA, O'Reilly RJ (1983) Transplantation for severe combined immunodeficiency
   with HLA-A, B, D, DR incompatible parental marrow cells fractionated by soybean agglutinin
   and sheep red blood cells. Blood 61: 341
3. Reisner Y (1983) Differential agglutination by soybean agglutinin of human leukemia and
   neuroblastoma cell lines: potential application to autologous bone marrow transplantation. Proc
   Natl Acad Sci USA 80: 6657
4. Korbling M, Hess AD, Tutschka PJ, Kaiser H, Colvin MO, Santos GW (1987) 4-
   hydroperoxycyclophosphamide: a model for eliminating residual human tumour cells and T-
   lymphocytes from the bone marrow graft. Br J Haematol 52: 89
5. Kluin-Nelemans HC, Martens ACM, Lowenberg B, Hagenbeek A (1984) No preferential sensitivity of clonogenic AML cells to Asta Z 7557. Leuk Res 8: 723
6. Yeager AM, Kaizer J, Santos GW, Saral R, Colvin OM, Stuart RK, Braine HG, Burke PJ,
   Ambinder RF, Burns WH (1986) Autologous bone marrow transplantation in patient with acute

non-lymphocytic leukemia, using ex vivo marrow treatment with 4-hydroperoxycyclophosphamide. N Engl J Med 315: 141

7. Gorin NC, Douay L, Laporte JP, Lopez M, Mary JY, Najman A, Salmon C, Aagerter P, Stachowiak J, David R, Pene F, Kantor G, Deloux J, Duhamel E, Van den Akker J, Gerota J, Parlier Y, Duhamel G (1986) Autologous bone marrow transplantation using marrow incubated with Asta Z 7557 in adult acute leukemia. Blood 67: 1367

8. Hervé P, Cahn JV, Plouvier E, Flesch M, Tamayo E, Leconte des Floris R, Peters A (1984) Autologous bone marrow transplantation for acute leukemia using transplant chemopurified with metabolite of oxazaphosphorines (ASTA Z 7557, INN mafosfamide). First clinical results. New Drugs 2: 245

9. Kaizer H, Stuart RK, Brookmeyer R, Beschorner WE, Braine HG, Burns WH, Fuller DJ, Korbling M, Mangan KF, Saral R, Sensenbrenner L, Shadduck RK, Shende AC, Tutschka PJ, Yeager AM, Zinkham WH, Colvin OM, Santos GW (1985) Autologous bone marrow transplantation in acute leukemia: a phase I study of in vitro treatment of marrow with 4-hydroperoxycyclophosphamide to purge tumor cells. Blood 65: 1504

10. Hartmann O, Kalifa C, Beaujean F, Bayle C, Benhamou E, Lemerle J (1985) Treatment of advanced neuroblastoma with two consecutive high-dose chemotherapy regimens and ABMT. In: Evans AE, D'Angio O, Seeger RC (eds) Advances in neuroblastoma research. Alan R, iss, New York, pp 565–568

11. Chang TT, Gulati SC, Chou TC, Vega R, Gandola L, Ezzat Ibrahim SM, Yopp J, Colvin M, Clarkson BD (1985) Synergistic effect of 4-hydroperoxycyclophosphamide and etoposide on a human promyelocytic leukemia cell line (HL-60) demonstrated by computer analysis. Cancer Res 45: 2434

12. Sieber F, Spivak JL, Sutcliffe AM (1984) Selective killing of leukemic cells by merocyanine 540-mediated photosensitization. Proc Natl Acad Sci USA 81: 7584

13. Reynolds CP, Reynolds DA, Frenkel EP, Graham Smith R (1982) Selective toxicity of 6-hydroxydopamine and ascorbate for human neuroblastoma in vitro: a model for clearing marrow prior to autologous transplant. Cancer Res 42: 1331

14. Lebien TW, Stepan DE, Bartholomew RM, Stong RC, Anderson JM (1985) Utilization of a colony assay to assess the variables influencing elimination of leukemic cells from human bone marrow with monoclonal antibodies and complement. Blood 65: 945

15. Janossy G, Campana D, Galton J, Burnett A, Hann I, Grob JP, Prentice HG, Totterman T (1987) Applications of monoclonal antibodies in bone marrow transplantation (BMT). 3rd Workshop on Leucocyte Differentiation Antigens, Oxford, Sept 1986 (in press).

16. Bast RC, De Fabriities P, Lipton J, Gelber R, Maver C, Nadler L, Sallan S, Ritz J (1985) Elimination of malignant clonogenic cells from human bone marrow using multiple monoclonal antibodies and complement. Cancer Res 45: 499

17. Favrot MC, Philip I, Philip T, Pinkerton R, Lebacq AM, Forster K, Adeline P, Doré JF (1986) Bone marrow purging procedure in Burkitt lymphoma with monoclonal antibodies and complement. Quantification by a liquid cell culture monitoring system. Br J Cancer 64: 161

18. Waldman H, Hale G, Cividalli G, Weshler Z, Manor D, Rachmilewitz EA, Polliak A, Or R, Weiss L, Samul S, Brautbar C, Slavin S (1984) Elimination of graft-versus-host disease by in vitro depletion of alloreactive lymphocytes with a monoclonal rat anti-human lymphocyte antibody (Campath-1). Lancet 2: 483

19. Stepan DE, Bartholomew RM, Lebien TW (1984) In vitro cytodestruction of human leukemic cells using murine monoclonal antibodies and human complement. Blood 63: 1120

20. Saarinenu M, Coccia PF, Gerson SL, Pelley R, Cheung NKV (1985) Eradication of neuroblastoma cells in vitro by monoclonal antibody and human complement: method for purging autologous bone marrow. Cancer Res 45: 5969

21. Treleaven JG, Gibson FM, Ugelstad J, Rembaum A, Philip T, Caine GD, Kemshead JT (1984) Removal of neuroblastoma cells from bone marrow with monoclonal antibodies conjugated to magnetic microspheres. Lancet 14: 70

22. Favrot MC, Philip I, Combaret V, Maritaz O, Philip T (1987) Experimental evaluation of an immunomagnetic bone marrow purging procedure using the Burkitt lymphoma model. Bone Marrow Transplantation 2: 56–59

354

23. Combaret V, Favrot MC, Kremens B, Laurent JC, Philip I, Philip T (1987) Elimination of Burkitt cells from excess bone marrow with an immunomagnetic purging procedure. Selection of monoclonal antibodies is a critical step. In: Proceedings of the Third International Symposium on ABMT, Houston, pp 443–448

24. Reynolds PC, Seeger RC, Vo DD, Black AT, Wells J, Ugelstad J (1986) Model system for removing neuroblastoma cells from bone marrow using monoclonal antibodies and magnetic immunobeads. Cancer Res 46: 5882

25. Poynton CH, Dicke KA, Culbert S, Frankel LS, Jagannath S, Reading CL (1983) Immumomagnetic removal of CALLA positive cells from human bone marrow. Lancet 1: 524

26. Berenson RJ, Bensinger WI, Kalamasz D, Martin P (1986) Elimination of Daudi lymphoblasts from human bone marrow using avidin-biotin immunoadsorption. Blood 67: 509

27. Filipovich AH, Vallera DA, Youle RJ, Quinones RR, Neville DM, Kersey JH (1984) Ex-vivo treatment of donor bone marrow with anti-T cell immunotoxins for prevention of graft-versus-host disease. Lancet 1: 469

28. Casellas P, Canat X, Fauser AA, Gros O, Laurent G, Poncelet P, Jansen FK (1985) Optimal elimination of leukemic T cells from human bone marrow with T101-ricin A chain immunotoxin. Blood 65: 289

29. Stong RC, Youle RJ, Vallera DA (1984) Elimination of clonogenic T-leukemic cells from human bone marrow using anti-Mr 65,000 protein immunotoxins. Cancer Res 44: 3000

30. Myers CD, Thorpe PE, Ross WCJ, Cumber AJ, Katz FE, Tax W, Greaves MF (1984) An immunotoxin with therapeutic potential in T cell leukemia: WT1-Ricin A. Blood 63: 1178

31. Muirhead M, Martin PJ, Torok-Storb B, Uhr JW, Vitetta ES (1983) Use of an antibody-ricin A-chain conjugate to delete neoplastic B cells from human bone marrow. Blood 62: 327

32. Coombes RC, Buckman R, Forster JA, Shepherd V, O'Hare MJ, Vincent M, Powles TJ, Neville AM (1986) In vitro and in vivo effects of a monoclonal antibody-toxin conjugate for use in autologous bone marrow transplantation for patients with breast cancer. Cancer Res 46: 4217

33. Uckun FM, Ramakrishnan S, Houston LL (1985) Increased efficiency in selective elimination of leukemia cells by a combination of stable derivative of cyclophosphamide and a human B-cell-specific immunotoxin containing pokeweed antiviral protein. Cancer Res 45: 69

34. Ramakrishnan S, Houston LL (1984) Inhibition of human acute lymphoblastic leukemia cells by immunotoxins: potentiation by chloroquine. Science 223: 58

35. Bjorn MJ, Groetsema G, Scalapino L (1986) Antibody-pseudomonas exotoxin A conjugates cytotoxic to human breast cancer cells in vitro. Cancer Res 46: 3262

36. Janossy G, Prentice HG, Grob JP, Ivory K, Tidman N, Grundy J, Favrot M, Brenner MK, Campana D, Blacklock HA, Gilmore MJML, Patterson J, Griffiths PD, Hoffbrand AV (1986) T lymphocyte regeneration after transplantation of T cell depleted allogeneic bone marrow. Clin Exp Immunol 63: 577

37. Fischer A, Griscelli C, Blanche S, Le Deist F, Veber F, Lopez M, Delaage M, Olive D, Mawas C, Janossy G (1986) Prevention of graft failure by an anti-HLFA-1 monoclonal antibody in HLA-mismatched bonemarrow transplantation. Lancet 2: 1058

38. Thierfelder S, Rodt H, Netzel B (1977) Transplantation of syngeneic bone marrow incubated with leucocyte antibodies. Transplantation 23: 459

39. Hagenbeek A, Van Bekkum DW (eds) (1977) Proceedings of an International Workshop on comparative evaluation of the L5222 and the BNML rat leukemia models and their relevance for human acute leukemia. Leuk Res 1: 75–78

40. Reynolds CP, Black AT, Woody JN (1986) Sensitive method for detecting viable cells seeded into bone marrow. Cancer Res 46: 5878

41. Philip I, Favrot MC, Philip T (1987) Use of a liquid cell culture assay to quantify the elimination of Burkitt lymphoma cells from the bone marrow. J Immunol Methods 97: 11

42. Ajani JA, Spitzer G, Tomasovic B, Drewinko B, Hug VM, Dicke K (1986) In vitro cytotoxicity patterns of standard and investigational agents on human bone marrow granulocyte-macrophage progenitor cells. Br J Cancer 54: 607

43. Uckun FM, Gajil-Peczalska KJ, Kersey JH, Houston LL, Vallera DA (1986) Use of a novel colony assay to evaluate the cytotoxicity of an immunotoxin containing pokeweed antiviral pro-

tein against blast progenitor cells freshly obtained from patients with common B-lineage acute lymphoblastic leukemia. J Exp Med 163: 347

44. Campana D, Janossy G (1986) Leukemia diagnosis and testing of complement fixing antibodies for bone marrow purging in acute lymphoid leukemia. Blood 68: 1264–1271

45. Moss TJ, Seeger RC, Kindler-Rohrborn A, Marangos PJ, Rajevsky MF, Reynolds CP (1985) Immunohistologic detection and phenotyping of neuroblastoma cells in bone marrow using cytoplasmic neuron specific enolase and cell surface antigens. In: Evans AE, d'Angio O, Seeger RC (eds) Advances in neuroblastoma research. Alan R Liss, New York, p 367

46. Philip I, Philip T, Favrot MC, Vuillaume M, Fontanière B, Chamard D, Lenoir GM (1984) Establisment of lymphomatous cell lines from bone marrow samples from patients with Burkitt's lymphoma. JNCl 73: 835

47. Philip I, Favrot MC, Combaret V, Laurent JC, Kremens B, Philip T (1986) Use of a liquid cell culture assay to measure the in vitro elimination of Burkitt's cells from the BM in preclinical and clinical procedures. In: Proceedings of the Third International Symposium on ABMT, Houston, pp 351–358

48. Philip T, Bernard JL, Zucker JM, Pinkerton R, Lutz P, Bordigoni P, Plouvier E, Robert A, Carton R, Philippe N, Philip I, Favrot MC (1987) High dose chemotherapy with bone marrow transplantation as consolidation treatment in neuroblastoma: an unselected group of stage IV patients over one year of age. J Clin Oncol 5: 266

49. De Fabriitis P, Bregni M, Lipton J, Greenberger J, Nadler L, Rothstein L, Korbling M, Ritz J, Bast RC (1985) Elimination of clonogenic Burkitt's lymphoma cells from human bone marrow using 4-hydroperoxycyclophosphamide in combination with monoclonal antibodies and complement. Blood 5: 1064

50. Lebien TW, Anderson JM, Vallera DA, Uckun FM (1986) Increased efficacy in selection elimination of leukemic cell line clonogenic cells by a combination of monoclonal antibodies BA-1, BA-2, BA-3 plus complement and mafosfamid (ASTA Z 7557). Leuk Res 10: 139

51. Favrot MC, Philip I, Poncelet P, Combaret V, Kremens B, Janossy G, Philip T (1987) Comparative efficiency of an immunomagnetic procedure and a rabbit complement lysis for eliminating BL cells from the bone marrow. In: Proceedings of the Third International symposium on ABMT, Houston, pp 359–364

52. Chang J, Coutinho L, Morgenstein G, Scarffe JH, Deakin D, Harrison C, Testa NG, Dexter TM (1986) Reconstitution of haemopoietic system with autologous marrow taken during relapse of acute myeloblastic leukaemia and grown in long-term culture. Lancet 1: 294

53. Berenoson RJ, Andrews RG, Bensinger WI, Kalamasz D, Knitter G, Bernstein ID (1986) In vivo reconstitution of hematopoiesis in baboons using 12.8 positive marrow cells isolated by avidin-biotin immunoadsorption (Abstr 1025). Blood 68: 287

54. To LB, Haylock DN, Kimber RJ, Juttner CA (1984) High levels of circulating haematopoiesis stem cells in very early remission from acute non-lymphoblastic leukaemia and their collection and cryopreservation. Br J Haematol 58: 399

55. Rosenberg SA, Lotze MT, Muul LM, Leitman S, Chang AE, Ettinghausen SE, Matory YL, Skibber JM, Shiloni E, Vetto JT, Seipp GA, Simpson C, Reichert CM (1985) Observations on the systemic administration of autologous lymphokine-activated killer cells and recombinant interleukin-2 to patients with metastatic cancer. N Engl J Med 313: 1485

56. O'Reilly RJ, Kernan N, Collins N, Brochstein J, Cunningham I, Castro-Malaspina H, Laver J, Emanuel D, Gulati S, Flomenberg N, Keever C (1986) Abrogation of both acute and chronic GVHD following transplants of lectin agglutinated, E-rosette depleted (SBA-E-) marrow for leukemia (Abstr 1041). Blood 68: 291

57. Prentice HG, Janossy G, Price-Jones L, Tregdosiewicz LK, Panjwani DI, Graphokos S, Ivory K, Blacklock HA, Gilmore MJ, Tidman N, Skeggs DBL, Ball S, Patterson J, Hoffbrand AV (1984) Depletion of T-lymphocytes in donor marrow prevents significant graft versus host disease in matched allogeneic leukaemic marrow transplant recipients. Lancet 1: 472

58. Martin PJ, Hansen JA, Buckner CD, Sanders JE, Deeg HJ, Stewart P, Appelbaum FR, Clift R, Fefer A, Witherspoon RP, Kennedy MS, Sullivan KM, Flournoy N, Storb R, Thomas ED (1985) Effects of in vitro depletion of T cells in HLA-identical allogeneic marrow grafts. Blood 66: 664

356

59. Hervé P, Cahn JY, Flesch M, Plouvier E, Racadot E, Noir A, Couteret Y, Goldstein G, Bernard A, Lenys R, Bresson JL, Leconte des Floris R, Peters (1987) Successful GVHD prevention without graft failure in 32 HLA-identical allogeneic bone marrow transplantations with marrow depleted of T-cells by monoclonal antibodies and complement. Blood 69: 388–393

60. Racadot E, Hervé P, Beaujean F, Vernant JP, Flesch M, Plouvier E, Andreu G, Rio B, Philippe N, Souillet G, Pico J, Bordigoni J, Ifrah N, Paitre ML, Lutz P, Morizet J, Bernard A (1986) Prevention of graft versus host disease in HLA matched bone marrow transplantation for malignant diseases. A multicentric study of 62 patients using 3 pan-T monoclonal antibodies and rabbit complement. J Clin Oncol 5: 426–435

61. Quinones RR, Youle RJ, Kersey JH, Zanjani ED, Azemove SM, Soderling CCB, Lebien TW, Beverley PCL, Neville DM, Vallera DA (1984) Anti-T cell monoclonal antibodies conjugated to ricin as potential reagents for human GVHD prophylaxis: effect on the generation of cytotoxic T cells in both peritoneal blood and bone marrow. J Immunol 132: 1322

62. Kemshead JT, Heath L, Gibson FM, Katz F, Richmond F, Treleaven J, Ugelstad J (1986) Magnetic microspheres and monoclonal antibodies for the depletion of neuroblastoma cells from bone marrow: experiences, improvements and observations. Br J Cancer 54: 771

63. Seeger RC, Wells J, Lenarsky C, Feig SA, Selch M, Moss TJ, Ugelstad J, Reynolds CP (1986) Bone marrow transplantation for poor prognosis neuroblastoma (Abstr 20). J Cell Biochem 10D: 215

64. Douay L, Gorin NC, Laporte JP, Lopez M, Najman A, Duhamel G (1984) ASTA Z 7557 (INN mafosfamide) for the in vitro treatment of human leukemic bone marrows. Invest New Drugs 2: 187

65. Bast RC Jr, Sallan SE, Reynolds C, Lipton J, Ritz J (1985) Autologous bone marrow transplantation for CALLA-positive acute lymphoblastic leukemia: an update. In: Dicke KA, Spitzer G, Zander AR (eds) Autologous bone marrow transplantation. ND Anderson Hospital, Houston, pp 3–6

66. Ramsay N, Lebien TW, Nesbit M, McGlave P, Weisdorf D, Kenyon P, Hurd D, Goldman A, Kim T, Kersey (1985) Autologous bone marrow transplantation for patients with acute lymphoblastic leukemia in second or subsequent remission. Results of bone marrow treated with monoclonal antibodies BA-1, BA-2 and BA-3 plus complement. Blood 66: 508

67. Nadler LM, Takvorian T, Botnick L, Bast RC, Finberg R, Hellman S, Canellos GP, Schlossman SF (1984) Anti-B_1 monoclonal antibody and complement treatment in autologous bone marrow transplantation for relapsed B-cell non-Hodgkin's lymphoma. Lancet 2: 427

68. Philip T, Biron P, Philip I, Favrot M, Souillet G, Frazppaz D, Jaubert J, Bordigoni P, Bernard JL, Laporte JP, Le Mevel A, Plouvier E, Marguerite G, Pinkerton R, Brizard CP, Freycon F, Forster HK, Philippe N, Brunat-Mentigny M (1986) Massive therapy and autologous bone marrow transplantation in pediatric and young adults Burkitt's lymphoma (30 courses in 28 patients: a 5-year experience). Eur J Cancer Clin Oncol 22: 1015

69. Baumgartner C, Brun del Re G, Forster HK, Bucher U, Delaveu B, Hirt A, Imbach P, Luthy A, Stern AC, Wagner HP (1985) Autologous bone marrow transplantation for pediatric non-Hodgkin's lymphoma: in vitro purging of the graft with anti-Y29/55 monoclonal antibody and complement. In: Dicke KA, Spitzer G, Zander AR (eds) Autologous bone marrow transplantation. ND Anderson Hospital, Houston, pp 377–381

19. Future Prospects for the Treatment of Hormone-Responsive Tumors

G. Wilding and M.E. Lippman

Introduction

Hormone-responsive epithelial tumors account for more than 230 000 new cases each year and approximately 60 000 deaths yearly [60] (Table 1). Other tumors, such as the lymphomas and leukemias, also show varying degrees of hormone (glucocorticoid) responsiveness but are treated primarily with cytotoxic agents. The most common forms of hormone-responsive cancers—adenocarcinomas of the breast, endometrium, and prostate—affect a patient population covering the entire adult age range, although the median age for the development of breast cancer is 59 years, and for prostate cancer 70. The fact that some human neoplasms are responsive to endocrine manipulation was recognized in the nineteenth century, but the exact role of the hormones in the genesis and growth of cancer remains incompletely understood. Hormonal control of cancer cell growth has been well documented, and, more recently, it has attracted added attention, with experimental findings suggesting that growth stimulation occurs via autocrine or self-stimulating polypeptide growth factors [27].

Attempts to alter progression of hormone-dependent tumors have concentrated on (a) altering the hormonal milieu by inhibiting hormone production, (b) competitive inhibition of hormone-receptor interactions, and (c) additive hormonal therapy. Using these approaches, current hormone therapy achieves clinical responses in one-third of all metastatic breast cancer patients and two-thirds of patients with metastatic prostate cancer [60]. Unfortunately, a substantial number of patients do not respond to hormonal therapy. Even in those in whom a tumor regression is achieved, the responses are not durable, lasting, in general, only 1 year before hormone-independent clones emerge.

This chapter will focus on several aspects of the role hormones play in cancer. First, we will briefly review the clinical and epidemiologic evidence implicating hormones in carcinogenesis and promotion of carcinomas of the breast, endometrium, and prostate. Second, we will describe the cellular response to hormone stimulation as it has been explored in experimental human breast and prostate cancer model systems, emphasizing the hypothesis that polypeptide growth factors may be common mediators of growth control for both hormone-responsive and hormone-independent tumors. Finally, the clinical experience of the past and the experimental foundation of the present will be used to formulate future therapeutic approaches to hormone-responsive cancers and their hormone-independent counterparts.

Table 1. Hormone-responsive cancer [5]

Tumor	Incidence (X10³ cases per year)	Mortality (X10³ cases per year)	Prevalence (cases per 10^5 members of population)
Breast	120	38	847[a]
Endometrium	38	3	273[a]
Prostate	75	24	372[b]
Leukemias	24	17	140
Lymphomas[c]	31	15	—

[a] Female population.
[b] Male population.
[c] All lymphomas included.

The treatment approaches discussed are the result of an intensive effort to understand the basic mechanisms by which hormones stimulate growth, and to understand how cells, initially dependent on hormones, achieve hormone independence and proliferate without hormonal limitation. Because these basic studies have identified a series of events resulting in sustained cell proliferation, we can now devise strategies to disrupt the growth cycle at multiple points, thereby increasing our chances of achieveing tumor regression and avoiding the development of resistance. In addition, by combining these treatment approaches with existing therapies, noncross-resistant regimens can be established. The current status of hormonal therapy in breast cancer and cancer of the prostate is summarized elsewhere in this volume.

Hormones and Cancer Etiology

Breast Cancer

Breast cancer is one of the leading causes of cancer death in women. In 1987, there will be 120 000 new cases of breast cancer in the United States, and approximately one-third of these cases will eventually be fatal. The role hormones play in carcinogenesis is uncertain; however, three aspects of hormone action may be important in the eventual development of a malignant tumor [60]. First, estrogens may serve as true carcinogens by covalently binding to DNA and resulting in mutations and a heritable malignant phenotype. Second, hormones can function as promoters of the carcinogenic action of other primary carcinogens. Third, hormones may have a permissive action in allowing carcinogenic events to occur. For example, breast cancer occurs in women who have never had functional ovaries with only 1% of the frequency seen in women with functioning ovaries. Thus, estrogens are stimulatory, at least initially, in nearly all breast cancer. However, the permissive and promotional roles of estrogens often cannot be distinguished in clinical settings. Experimental breast cancer induced by dimethylbenzanthracene in rats provides substantial insight into this process. These animals develop breast cancer when fed the carcinogen shortly after they become sexually mature. The carcinogen is ineffective if given before puberty or to males. It is also ineffective if the animals are castrated shortly after the administration of the carcinogen.

Epidemiologic studies have provided information concerning genetic, chemical, viral, and hormonal factors which affect the risk of breast cancer [49, 63]. The risk factors in which endocrine influences may be significant include geographical variation, reproductive history, familial clustering, and hormonal milieu. Unfortunately, no single factor or combination of factors can accurately predict which women would benefit from prophylactic intervention. In fact, the absence of all risk factors does not rule out the possibility of breast cancer.

Endometrial Cancer

Endometrial cancer is responsible for 3000 deaths a year in the United States, with 38 000 new cases diagnosed annually. As a hormone-dependent tissue, the uterine endometrium responds to estradiol and progesterone with cyclical changes in its growth and morphology. As with breast cancer, estrogens are implicated as carcinogenic, permissive, and promotional agents [60]. Prolonged or unopposed estrogenic stimulation from either endogenous or exogenous sources increases the risk of developing endometrial cancer. Epidemiologically, this is evident by the association of endometrial cancer with late menopause and with the continuous use of estrogens after menopause. Depending on the length of estrogen supplementation, the relative risk of developing endometrial cancer increases four- to ninefold in postmenopausal women. In addition to the length of estrogen exposure, the continuity of the estrogenic stimulation is important. The appearance of endometrial cancer in women with gonadal dysgenesis treated with estrogens alone is further evidence for this concept. The usual interruption of estrogen stimulation by progesterone-induced sloughing of the endometrium may play a protective role. For example, the resumption of cyclic ovarian function in response to ovarian wedge resection in the polycystic ovary syndrome results in regression of endometrial hyperplasia; progesterone can also reverse estrogen-induced endometrial hyperplasia.

After menopause, the predominant blood estrogen is estrone, which is largely derived from androstenedione secreted by the adrenal cortex. The percentage of androstenedione converted to estrone by peripheral tissues increases with age and weight. Since adipose tissue has the enzymatic capacity to convert androstenedione to estrone, obesity is a risk factor for endometrial cancer.

Prostate Cancer

The influence of hormones in the etiology of prostate cancer has long been debated. Evidence supporting the importance of hormone factors is provided by

360

several observations: (a) prostate cancer does not develop in eunuchs; (b) the incidence of latent prostatic cancer is lower than expected in male cirrhotics, who have elevated blood levels of endogenous estrogens [26]; and (c) many cases of metastatic cancer of the prostate are hormone dependent [72]. However, epidemiologic evidence suggests that environmental factors may also play a role in the etiology of clinical prostate cancer [72]. For example, the mortality for American blacks from prostate cancer is significantly higher than that for American whites, and the incidence of prostate cancer in American blacks is six times higher than that in Nigerian blacks. In contrast, the incidence of latent prostatic cancer is the same in all these populations. This environmental influence is further supported by the finding that Japanese living in Hawaii have a higher incidence of clinical cancer of the prostate than their counterparts living in Japan despite a similar incidence of latent carcinoma of the prostate.

The central role of steroid hormones in the etiology, maintenance, and treatment of a variety of tumor types afflicting thousands of patients each year is evident from the above discussion. To develop strategies for preventing and treating these tumors in the future, an extensive effort to understand the mechanisms of the cellular hormonal response is warranted. The remainder of this contribution will be devoted to a review of the cellular response to steroid hormones as we understand it today, and a discussion as to how this knowledge may be utilized in the development of future therapeutic strategies.

Cellular Responses to Steroid Hormones

Despite the high incidence of hormone-responsive cancers and the formulation of effective hormonal therapies, the exact nature of the cellular response to steroid hormones has not been completely defined. At the cellular level, steroid hormones modulate a wide variety of physiological functions—such as metabolism, differentiation, and proliferation—by regulating the expression of specific genes. By understanding the pathways by which steroids exert their effects, the role of hormones in carcinogenesis can be better understood, and more efficacious means of preventing and treating hormone-responsive tumors developed.

Hormone Receptors

Steroids exert their influence via an intracellular protein receptor. Following association with receptor, an "activation" step permits the steroid-receptor complex to interact with DNA and chromatin proteins and alters the expression of specific genes. Early studies of the estrogen receptor proposed that the unoccupied receptor was located in the cytoplasm, and that, following ligand occupation, the receptor's affinity for chromatin increased and tanslocation to the nucleus occured [80]. This concept may require revision since recent immunolocalization studies using monoclonal antiestrogen receptor antibodies [53] have shown the apparent presence of unoccupied receptors in the nucleus of MCF-7 breast cancer cells [34]. Both forms of the estrogen receptor, occupied and unoccupied, are now thought to reside in the nucleus. In either case, activation by altering the affinity of the receptor for nuclear components permits interaction with the genome.

Recently, cDNAs of the estrogen, glucocorticoid, and progesterone receptors have been cloned [13, 28, 31, 43, 85]. The human estrogen receptor mRNA is 6322 nucleotides in length and contains an open reading frame of 1785 nucleotides, which codes for a 595-amino acid protein of 66 182 daltons. Of interest, the mRNA also contains a long, 4305-nucleotide, 3'-untranslated region of unknown significance [29]. Other steroid receptors, such as the glucocorticoid and progesterone receptors, have similar structures [31, 43]. Comparison of chicken and human estrogen receptor sequences shows 80% amino acid homology, with the putative hormone- and DNA-binding regions showing 94% and 100% homology, respectively [55]. When the sequences of these two regions of the estrogen receptor were examined, one region (region E) contained all of the sequences necessary to bind estradiol with high affinity. Another region (region C) was rich in cysteine and basic amino acids, and it contained structural characteristics thought to be important for DNA binding in other eucaryotic transcriptional regulatory proteins [56].

Amino acid sequence comparison of the estrogen receptor, glucocorticoid receptor, progesterone receptor, and the *v-erb A* oncogene product of the avian erythroblastosis virus has shown that there are extensive regions of homology between the four genes [55]. The most striking region of homology is region C of the estrogen receptor, thought to be the DNA-binding region. This region was shown to be 61% homologous to the corresponding region of the glucocorticoid receptor and 53% homologous to *v-erb A* [25, 55, 56]. This suggests that *c-erb A*, the cellular counterpart of *v-erb A*, belongs to a multigene family of transcriptional regulatory proteins and is derived from a common primordial ancestral regulatory gene. Isolation of the steroid receptor genes will open many new avenues of investigation into the process of steroid-induced cellular changes. Understanding such control mechanisms will allow us to develop new strategies for the treatment of hormone-responsive cancers.

Hormone Effects on Macromolecules

Using cloned human breast cancer cell lines, the effects of estrogen on cell growth, gene activation, and enzyme activity have been explored. Cell lines such as MCF-7 respond to physiologic concentrations of estradiol by increasing their rate of proliferation [2, 62]. These results can be duplicated in defined medium devoid of serum constituents [4]. Potent antiestrogens are capable of inhibiting estrogenic stimulation of cells containing estrogen receptors. This effect can be prevented by the simultaneous administration of estrogen and reversed by subsequent estrogen administration [61]. A similar mitogenic response has been demonstrated in human prostate cancer cells containing androgen receptors and treated with testosterone or dihydrotestosterone in vitro [33]. In contrast, lymphoid cells are commonly inhibited by glucocorticoids.

The mitogenic response of breast cancer cells to estrogen is maintained by an increase in the activity of a variety of enzymes involved in both scavenger and de novo DNA synthetic pathways. They include DNA polymerase, thymidine and uridine kinases, thymidylate synthetase, aspartate transcarbamylase, carbamyl phosphate synthetase, dihydrooratase, and dihydrofolate reductase [2]. Additional proteins whose activities are altered by estrogens are progesterone receptor; plasminogen activator; and several secreted proteins 7000, 24 000, 52 000 and 160 000 daltons in size [35, 42, 87]. Though progesterone receptor is not directly growth modulatory, its presence appears to be coupled to growth regulation by estrogen, and the progesterone receptor content of breast tumors is used clinically as a marker for hormone therapy responsiveness. Plasminogen activator, a serine protease, is thought to contribute to tumor progression and growth by allowing the tumor to digest and traverse basement membranes [58]. In purified form, the 52 000-dalton secreted glycoprotein has been shown to be mitogenic for beast cancer cells in vitro [87]. The function of the other induced proteins is unknown, though the activity of most can be shown to be unnecessary for cell proliferation through the use of clonal variants in tissue culture [15]. Like breast cancer, secreted proteins are induced by androgen therapy of human prostate cells in culture [9]. One of these, the prostate-specific antigen, is also a serine protease [86].

Several enzymes are regulated at the transcriptional level; these include thymidine kinase and dihydrofolate reductase. Using cDNA probes, estrogens can be shown to increase the mRNA levels of these enzymes [47, 57]. For thymidine kinase, message levels increase as a result of increased transcription rather than stabilization of the message. Estrogens also exert transcriptional control over a 600-base pair message, pS2, as demonstrated by Jakowlew et al. [42]; the function of the protein product of pS2 is unknown. Of recent interest has been the demonstration that the laminin receptor protein is increased by estrogen treatment of MCF-7 cells [3]. The laminin receptor is thought to mediate attachment of cells to basement membranes, a function important to the metastatic process. Finally, several investigators have isolated a collection of cDNA clones representing mRNA species which are induced within 6 h of estrogen stimulation of human breast cancer cells [14, 67]. In prostate cancer, Montpetit et al. [69] have produced data suggesting that androgens increase the mRNA levels of a variety of genes in rat prostate tissue. Viola et al. [84] have demonstrated a correlation between histological grade and the level of the oncogene product of *ras*, p21, in human prostate cancers.

Autocrine-Stimulated Growth

Several pieces of evidence support the hypothesis that hormones may stimulate a growth response via intermediate factors which serve as effectors of hormone

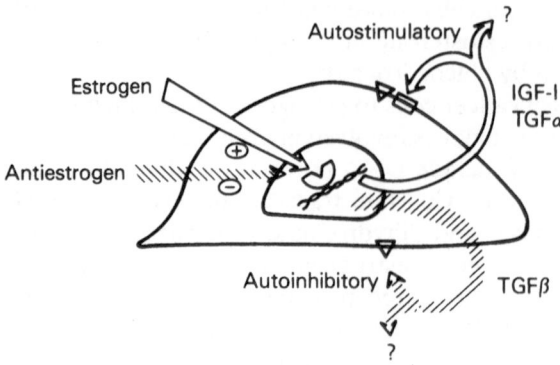

Fig. 1. Possible autocrine growth control loops in breast cancer. (From [17a])

treatment (Fig. 1). First, the rate of proliferation of MCF-7 breast cancer cells is increased by plating at higher densities [41], suggesting conditioning of the media by the cells with factors which support growth. Second, using anchorage-independent growth to assay for activities capable of inducing a malignant transformed phenotype, a number of growth factor activities have been isolated. These can be grouped into the following different activities: platelet-derived growth factor (PDGF), epidermal growth factor and transforming growth factor α (TGF α), insulinlike growth factors, transforming growth factor β (TGF β), and the fibroblast growth factor (FGF) family [27]. Third, some of these peptide growth factors alter the phenotype of human breast cancer cells in vitro and, in many instances, are produced by the breast cancer cells stimulated with estrogen [18].

Though studied much less extensively, prostate cancer cells in vitro transcribe TGF α, and Bulbul et al. [11] and Maehama et al. [64] have isolated additional prostate-derived growth factors. Kaighn et al. [45] demonstrated that two human hormone-unresponsive prostate cancer cell lines respond to a variety of peptides, including luteinizing hormone-releasing hormone (LHRH) and FGF, but do not require the presence of any of these factors to grow. The characteristics and effects of each of these activities are described below.

Human breast cancer cells produce PDGF. When conditioned media from human breast cancer cells are applied to quiescent fibroblasts, DNA synthesis is initiated. In addition, the human breast cancer cell lines express RNA complementary to *c-sis*, and specific antiserum against PDGF will precipitate a protein with the same molecular weight, heat, and reducing agent stability as authentic PDGF. Production of this activity may be under estrogen control [27]. The potential influence of *c-sis* in human malignancies has been demonstrated by Gazit et al. [24], who showed that human *c-sis* is able to induce cellular transformation. When a similar human *c-sis* clone under the control of a retroviral long terminal repeat (LTR) was transfected into NIH 3T3 cells, high titers of transforming activity were observed, and the transformants expressed human *c-sis* translational products.

The insulinlike growth factor (IGF I and II) are found in the blood and mediate the anabolic effects of human growth hormone. They are polypeptides with molecular weights of 7600 and 7500 daltons, respectively, which have considerable homology to proinsulin and appear to interact with specific cell surface receptors. Authentic serum-derived IGF I stimulates the proliferation of four human breast cancer cell lines—MCF-7, MDA-MB-231, ZR-75-1, and Hs578T. In addition, each of these lines produces and secretes IGF I. The two highly tumorigenic, estrogen-independent cell lines, MDA-MB-231 and Hs578T, produced two- to tenfold more IGF I activity than the estrogen-responsive and less tumorigenic cell linese, MCF-7 and ZR-75-1 [18]. Estradiol increases IGF I secretion in hormone-dependent human breast cancer cell lines, and secretion is inhibited by antiestrogens. Thus, IGF I is hormonally regulated and may function as an autocrine growth factor [36].

Epidermal growth factor (EGF), with a molecular weight of 6045 daltons, has been shown to stimulate a wide variety of cells to proliferate, differentiate, or both [79]. It shares 40%–45% homology with another factor, termed TGF α, which is itself produced by transformed cells. Both interact with a common receptor located on the cell surface. The EGF receptor is an integral membrane protein, which serves to transmit signals via an intrinsic EGF-stimulated tyrosine kinase. Receptor clustering may also be involved in signal transduction. Autoregulation of the receptor may occur by phosphorylation of specific regulatory sites, by receptor degradation, or by sequestration of the receptor. The EGF receptor appears to be the proto-oncogene to the v-erb B oncogene of the avian erythroblastosis virus.

The role of EGF and its receptor in carcinogenesis is complex. Clearly, the addition of EGF to many cell types elicits responses associated with neoplastic transformation, such as proliferation, partial loss of density-dependent inhibition of growth and decreased dependency on serum for growth, loss of fibronectin, and enhanced secretion of plasminogen activator [79]. For these reasons, EGF and TGF α serve as prime candidates for autocrine control factors.

Secretion of TGF α by a large variety of tumor cells suggests involvement of TGF α in cell transformation and provides evidence supporting an autocrine-stimulatory model. More direct evidence was provided by Rosenthal et al. [71], who transfected Fischer rat fibroblasts with a human TGF α cDNA construct. Synthesis and secretion of TGF α by these cells resulted in the loss of anchorage-dependent growth and induced tumor formation in nude mice. In addition, anti-human TGF α antibodies prevented the expressing cells producing TGF α from forming colonies in soft agar.

Human breast cancer cell lines show a proliferative response to EGF and TGF α [19]; in fact, they also secrete material of the EGF/TGF α class [73]. As shown by Bates et al. [8], hormone-dependent and -independent breast cancer cells produce a major species of approximately 30 000 daltons as well as a smaller species of TGF α. Estrogen induces this activity in estrogen-responsive cell lines, whereas it is secreted constitutively by hormone-independent breast cancer cell lines.

Two androgen-independent prostate cancer cell lines, PC3 and DU145, do not respond to exogenously added EGF or TGF α with increased growth. However, both express TGF α mRNA and contain EGF receptors. A hormone-responsive prostate cancer cell line, LNCAP, does, however, respond to EGF and TGF α with a proliferative response [88]. It is not known if these cells also produce TGF α. Thus, ample evidence exists that this growth factor family may serve as an autocrine or paracrine growth stimulator in hormone-responsive tumors. Strategies for future therapeutic manipulations based on these data will be discussed in a later section.

Additional stimulatory activities have been isolated from mammary and prostatic tumor systems. For example, using an SW13 human adrenal carcinoma soft agar cloning assay, Swain et al. [82] isolated a factor with an apparent molecular weight of 60 000 daltons, which is secreted in large quantities by the hormone-independent breast cancer cell line MDA-MB-231. This factor is distinct from mammary-derived growth factor [7], endothelial cell growth factor (ECGF) [75], and FGF. It is not hormonally regulated in hormone-responsive cell lines.

Using Balb/c 3T3 fibroblasts to assay for mitogenic activity, Tackett et al. [83] initially noted activity in tissue extracted from normal and malignant prostatic tissue. Subsequent characterization has revealed an affinity for heparin similar to basic FGF and ECGF [11]. Unlike the breast cancer factor of Swain [82], which was secreted most by poorly differentiated cells, this prostate-derived growth factor was present at higher activity in well-differentiated prostate tumors than in poorly differentiated tumors. Studies on the hormone-responsive human prostate cell line, LNCAP, have shown that the heparin-binding growth factors, basic FGF and ECGF, stimulate thymidine incorporation, though to a much lower extent than dihydrotestosterone (88).

In addition to autocrine-stimulated growth, estrogens may stimulate the production of growth factors in other estrogen-responsive tissues, which could then directly stimulate the proliferation of mammary tissue, as well as hormone-responsive breast cancer cells. A series of peptides, estromedins, which are mitogenic in vitro for MCF-7 cells have been purified from uteri and pituitaries [17, 39]. Estrogen-potentiating factor has been characterized as a pituitary growth factor for estrogen-responsive breast cancer cells and is secreted by normal pituitary cells as well as pituitary tumors. Unrelated to known pituitary hormones, this factor potentiates growth of estrogen-responsive breast cancer cells in the presence of estrogen in vivo and in vitro [17]. Therre is no direct evidence that these peptides function in vivo as estromedins.

TGF β is a multifunctional peptide that controls proliferation, differentiation, and other functions in many cell types. Many cells synthesize TGF β, and essentially all of them have specific receptors for this peptide. TGF β regulates the actions of many other peptide growth factors and determines the positive or negative direction of their action [77]. Human breast cancer cells secrete TGF β. However, antiestrogens and glucocorticoids, both inhibitory to MCF-7 cells, may inhibit cell growth by increasing TGF β levels and by lowering TGF α and IGF I levels. Furthermore, several MCF-7 clones, as well as estrogen-independent breast cancer cell lines, are inhibited by the exogenous addition of TGF β [54]. A mutant MCF-7 clone, Ly2 [10], which is antiestrogen resistant,

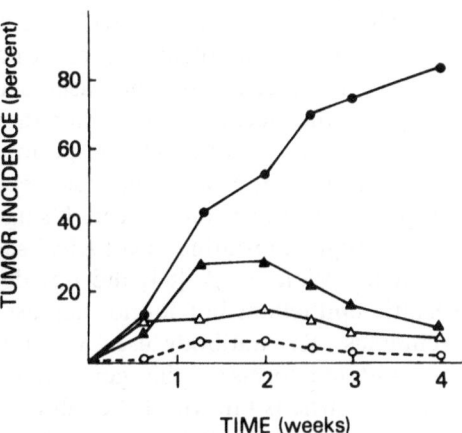

Fig. 2. Time dependence of estradiol-treated conditioned medium (CME2) activity. CME2 (▲) or untreated conditioned medium (△) was placed in Alzet minipumps and implanted along with MCF-7 cells in nude mice. Other groups of animals were treated with unconditioned negative control medium (0) or with a 0.5-mg estradiol pellet (●) to stimulate MCF-7 tumor formation. After 14 days, fresh pumps and estradiol pellets were reimplanted. Tumor incidence was observed over a 4-week period. Twenty or more animals were included in each group. (From [20])

fails to show induction of TGF β when treated with antiestrogens. These experiments suggest that TGF β is an important autocrine growth inhibitor. Resistance to its activity may occur through the loss of production of TGF β or the loss of its receptor. In addition to TGF β, Gaffney et al. [23] have found a 68 000-dalton growth inhibitor for MCF-7 cells in bovine serum.

The MCF-7 human breast cancer cell line requires the presence of estrogen to form tumors in the nude mouse model. As reviewed above, these cells, in vitro, produce a variety of peptide growth factors in response to treatment with estrogen. This raises the question as to whether these growth factors, produced and secreted into the media after estrogen stimulation in vitro, can replace the requirement for estrogen and support tumor formation in vivo. When the biological activity of serum-free, estrogen-free, conditioned medium from estrogen-treated MCF-7 cells was tested using Alzet mini-infusion pumps in nude mice, it contained sufficient growth activity to stimulate tumor growth, thus partially replacing estradiol [20] (Fig. 2). However, while early tumor growth was indistinguishable from estrogen-induced growth, the incidence of conditioned media-induced tumors was lower, they were smaller, and they tended to regress after 2 weeks despite reimplantation of infusion pumps every 7 days. When the conditioned medium was replaced with purified IGF I or EGF, tumor incidence rose above controls in the absence of estradiol, again suggesting that growth factors may act as estrogen-induced "second messengers" in estrogen-induced growth in human breast cancer.

Oncogene Expression

Further evidence supporting the role of growth factors as mediators of hormone stimulation of cancer has been provided by experiments in which the *v-H-ras* gene was transfected into MCF-7 cells [46]. The resultant cells express *v-H-*

367

ras mRNA and viral p21 and will give rise to tumors in nude mice without the need for estrogen supplementation. In addition, although they retain estrogen receptors, these cells have increased secretion of growth factor activities, suggesting that the mechanism by which they have become hormone independent is that of increased growth factor secretion.

A clinically important role has been suggested for the expression of *ras* oncogene p21 in prostate cancer. Using an immunohistochemical assay for the *ras* p21 antigen in routine histological sections of benign and malignant prostate specimens, Viola et al. [84] did not detect *ras* p21 in normal or hyperplastic prostatic epithelium but found increased levels of p21 in high-grade prostatic carcinomas. The antibody used was not able to distinguish wild-type *ras* p21 from mutated forms of this gene, known to be associated with transforming activities. Little is known of the effects of *ras* expression on growth factor production in human prostate cancer cells, and it has not been established whether *c-ras* or mutated *ras* play a critical role in prostate cancer.

In view of the hormone-independent tumorigenicity of *v-H-ras*-transfected MCF-7 cells, it is intriguing that Liotta et al. [59] have demonstrated the secretion of a cell motility factor (AMF) in NIH 3T3 cells transfected with *ras*. This autocrine motility factor is 55 000 daltons in size, its activity is neither replaced nor blocked by known growth factors, and it is also made by human A2058 melanoma cells. Its role in human breast and prostate cancers, however, remains unknown.

The role of the nuclear proto-oncogenes has not been defined in hormone-responsive cancer. The expression of such proto-oncogenes, coding for nuclear-associated proteins, has been implicated in the control of cell proliferation and differentiation in thyroid cells treated with thyroid-stimulating hormone [12], promyelocytic leukemia cells treated with dexamethasone [70], and others. The critical role nuclear oncogene products play in proliferation has been confirmed by two recent, independent sets of experiments. First, growth of NIH 3T3 mouse fibroblasts is inhibited by the induction of transfected antisense *fos* RNA [32]. Second, Studzinski et al. [81] have shown that replicative DNA synthesis is effectively inhibited in isolated nuclei in the presence of antibodies directed specifically against the *c-myc* protein. Understanding the relationship between hormone-induced growth factor production and growth factor-induced *c-fos* or *c-myc* induction may allow us to further elucidate the mechanisms of hormone-induced cell proliferation.

Recently, a member of the tyrosine kinase oncogene family, designated *neu*, was found to be amplified in the human mammary carcinoma MAC 117 [52]. The *neu* oncogene, identified initially in the ethylnitrosourea-induced rat neuroglioblastomas, has homology to the *erb-B* gene coding for the EGF receptor, but *neu* is distinct from the *erb-B* gene and is located on chromosome 17 [74]. In addition, this gene was shown to be amplified in a human salivary gland adenocarcinoma [76]. The 185 000-dalton protein product contains cell surface domains accessible to antibodies. The relationship of the *neu* gene amplification to the etiology of breast cancer has not been determined.

368

Table 2. Hormone therapy [22]

Therapy	Tumor type		
	Breast	Prostate	Endometrium
Ablative	Oophorectomy, adrenalectomy, hypophysectomy	Orchidectomy	—
Additive	Estrogens, progestogens, glucocorticoids, androgens	Estrogens, progestogens	Progestogens
Antihormonal	Antiestrogens	Antiandrogens	—
Steroidogenesis inhibitors	Aminoglutethimide	Aminoglutethimide, ketoconazole	—
Releasing hormones	LHRH agonists	LHRH agonists	—

LHRH, luteinizing hormone-releasing hormone.

Future Prospects for Therapy

Current efforts to control hormone-responsive tumors, which are centered on the inhibition of steroidogenesis or interference with hormone-receptor binding, fail universally when hormone-independent clones emerge (Table 2). As evident from in vitro studies, one mechanism by which tumors may become hormone unresponsive is by constitutively activating autocrine growth pathways normally under hormonal control. The elucidation of autocrine growth pathways has created a wide array of new therapeutic approaches aimed at disrupting the hormonal cellular response. This section will focus on new therapies designed to disrupt the hormonal response and autocrine pathways by utilizing the products of hormone stimulation as specific targets for antibodies, including growth factors, their receptors, or gene products whose expression is induced by the binding of growth factors to their receptors. For the most part, the therapeutic strategies discussed are still being evaluated in the laboratory and in animal studies. However, a number of monoclonal antibody trials have been initiated to investigate nonhormonally controlled tumor systems.

Antibody Therapy

Several distinct approaches to the use of antibodies designed to achieve antitumor activity have been explored. Initially, antibodies against tumor-associated antigens were employed. These antibodies were targeted against specific molecules on the cell surface. Cytotoxicity can be markedly enhanced by attaching to the antibody a nonspecific toxin, such as ricin A chain or pseudomonas endo-

369

toxin; radioisotopes; or chemotherapeutic agents, such as methotrexate or doxo-rubicin (Adriamycin). Thus, via the specificity of the antibody, the nonspecific toxin is directed to the tumor cells. A second approach is to use an IgG_{2a} isotype to achieve cytotoxicity immunologically by activating host macrophages and complement. This approach has been applied to human tumors by Koprows-ki [1, 78] and will be discussed in this section as it pertains to anti-EGF receptor antibody activity in animals. A third approach is to aim specifically at interfering with growth factor-stimulated growth. This includes the effective removal of growth factor by forming antibody-growth factor complexes and by blocking growth factor receptors with antibodies.

Antibody-Toxin Conjugates

The hormone-dependent tumors offer a unique opportunity to employ anti-bodies conjugated to drugs, radioisotopes, or toxins, in that they express a num-ber of cellular proteins in response to hormone stimulation which may serve as antigens. For example, human prostatic acid phosphatase is produced in large quantities by hormone-responsive prostate tumors and is measurable in the blood of many patients. Using the LNCAP human prostatic cancer cell line in a nude mouse mode, Deguchi et al. [16] conjugated methotexate to an IgG1 monoclonal antibody specific for human prostatic acid phosphatase (PAP) while retaining both the PAP-binding activity of the antibody and the dihydrofolate reductase-inhibitory activity of methotrexate. In vitro, this conjugate was taken up by the LNCAP cells with resultant inhibition of DNA synthesis, although to a lesser degree than free methotrexate. When injected into nude mice bearing xenografted LNCAP tumors, the methotrexate-antibody conjugate preferential-ly accumulated in the tumor. Preliminary results showed retardation of tumor growth in the treated animals. Other proteins, such as the prostate-specific anti-gen [86] and the numerous secreted proteins found in hormone-dependent breast cancer cells, are also candidates for this therapeutic approach.

A number of problems must be overcome for this approach to be successful. Since many of the available antigens are secreted proteins, administered anti-bodies which bind to extracellular protein are effectively neutralized. Large quantities of the antibody must be administered to overcome this. Second, anti-bodies that bind surface proteins which are not internalized may fail to exert a toxic effect, although this does not apply to radionuclides. Likewise, antibodies directed against intracellular proteins may not have access to their targets. Final-ly, most hormone-dependent tumors progress towards hormone independence as a consequence of the emergence of hormone-unresponsive clones as the pre-dominant cell type. This may be associated with the loss of some tissue-specific, hormone-induced proteins.

Anti-growth Factor Antibodies

Since the proliferation of many tumor cells is controlled by growth factors which bind to specific surface receptors, autocrine growth loops provide antigenic targets which are required by the cell for growth and which, therefore, are less

370

likely to be modulated during the development of hormone-independent clones. Autocrine pathways can be disrupted by directing antibodies towards the ligand or its receptor. With the availability of antibodies directed against EGF, TGF α, and other growth factors, the kinetics of growth factor-antibody interactions can be further evaluated. For example, the use of antibodies against EGF is unlikely to lower EGF levels because of the very fast turnover rate of EGF in vivo (half-life, 1.5 min) [30]; therefore, it would be preferable to use antibodies against the EGF receptor.

Insight into the potential utility of this approach was provided by Johnson et al. [44], who treated human fibroblasts transformed with simian sarcoma virus (SSV) with antibodies against PDGF. In these experiments, cells transfected with SSV—which contains the coding region for p28^{sis}, the product of the *sis* oncogene—showed transformation characteristics such as increased proliferation and focus formation. Treatment of the transformed cells with anti-PDGF IgG resulted in decreased thymidine incorporation and proliferation, as well as diminished focus formation. For unknown reasons, however, anti-PDGF only suppressed focus formation if the cells were treated within 12 days of infection.

Anti-receptor Antibodies

Because a specific receptor located at the cell surface is required for a growth factor to interact with a cell, antibodies directed against receptors which block ligand binding or which interfere with signal transmission after ligand binding occurs offer a new approach to deprive cells of proliferative signals. The feasibility of this approach has been demonstrated by the studies of Masui et al. [65, 66] concerning the antitumor effects of anti-EGF receptor monoclonal antibodies (anti-EGF-R Ab) on human A431 xenograft tumors in nude mice. Treatment with anti-EGF-R Ab prevented tumor formation in athymic nude mice by A431 cells implanted subcutaneously if the antibody therapy was started on the day of tumor cell inoculation. If antibody administration was initiated when the tumors had grown to 1 cm^3, then tumor growth was arrested, but only as long as the antibody therapy continued.

This differential response with regard to the timing of the antibody therapy raises several questions as to the mechanisms of antitumor activity. Does the antibody prevent the tumor from becoming established when therapy is initiated at the time of tumor cell inoculation, or is the antibody cytotoxic to tumor cells? In addition, once the tumor has been established, is the tumor growth prevented by cytostatic or cytotoxic means? Using the A431 cell system, the above investigators have addressed these questions. First, in vitro, anti-EGF-R Ab are cytostatic, not cytotoxic, to A431 cells. Second, antibodies of the IgG2a isotype may activate macrophages or complement, which, in turn, could contribute to the antitumor activity of the antibody. In vitro, while both IgG2a and IgG1 antibodies inhibit the proliferation of A431 cells, complement enhanced the effect of the IgG2a, but not the IgG1, antibody by inducing cytotoxicity. Of interest, cytotoxicity was not observed when the A431 cells were allowed to become confluent before the addition of IgG2a antibody and complement [68].

In the presence of IgG2a antibody, macrophages showed a high degree of cytotoxicity, >80% at a macrophage-to-A431 ratio of 40:1. In contrast, in the presence of IgG1 antibody, macrophages showed very little cytotoxicity. Macrophages required activation for IgG2a-mediated toxicity to occur. These results would favor the use of an IgG2a antibody.

Though A431 cells are epidermoid in origin, their inhibition by anti-EGF receptor antibodies is relevant to adenocarcinomas, such as breast cancer, which possess EGF receptors and whose growth appears regulated by autocrine pathways involving TGF α. It is not clear which parameters determine whether a tumor will respond to this form of therapy. For example, while a number of EGF receptor-bearing human epidermoid tumor xenografts are inhibited by antibody therapy, others are not inhibited [68].

Because of their proven ability to transform cells, oncogenes coding for cell surface receptors provide important targets for monoclonal antibodies. Several examples of inhibition or reversion of the transformed phenotype in vitro are available. Using *neu* oncogene-transformed NIH 3T3 cells, Drebin et al. [21] demonstrated the rapid but reversible loss of both cell surface and total cellular p185 *neu* protein product when cells were treated with monoclonal antibodies against p185. More important was the reversion of the *neu*-transformed cells to a nontransformed phenotype, as determined by the loss of anchorage-independent growth.

Antibody therapy holds great potential as a treatment against hormone-responsive tumors, whose growth is dependent on autocrine growth mechanisms. In addition, it offers a point of attack in the cascade of events leading to a hormonally initiated proliferative response, a point of considerable importance in tumors which have achieved hormone independence but still maintain active autocrine growth loops.

Receptor Antagonists

An alternative strategy to blocking the binding of growth factors to their receptors is the use of growth factor antagonists, i.e., molecules which bind to the receptor with high affinity, do not activate the signalling process, and prevent other ligands from binding to the receptor (e.g., a small peptide containing the binding domain of the native growth factor and modified to inhibit degradation and increase the serum half-life). Obviously , this sort of pharmacological approach would involve the synthesis and screening of numerous compounds to distinguish the antagonists from the partial agonists and agonists.

Additive Growth Factor Therapy

Additive growth factor therapy with TGF β represents another novel approach to growth factor therapy. Found in platelets in large quantities, TGF β is thought to play an important role in wound healing, especially in view of its mitogenic effect on fibroblasts. Growth of breast cancer cells in culture, however, is inhibited by exogenously added TGF β, and these cells produce additional TGF β when treated with antiestrogens or dexamethasone, both of which are inhibitory. Either the administration of TGF β synthesized in large amounts by recombinant DNA technology or modifications to the parent molecule so that its high receptor-binding affinity is retained but the serum half-life is lengthened would be worthy of experimental exploration.

Prevention of Attachment and Invasion

A number of cell surface receptors have been shown to be important for cell attachment and invasion through basement membranes. Two proteins, laminin and fibronectin, are components of basement membranes and subendothelial cell matrices and serve as attachment points for cells with the appropriate receptors. The binding of a cell's laminin receptor to laminin, for example, may facilitate the exit of that tumor cell from its tissue of origin and aid it in its penetration through other basement membranes, resulting in a metastatic lesion. In addition, the secretion of proteases, such as plasminogen activator and prostate-associated antigen, by tumor cells may enable them to digest surrounding fibrin and penetrate barriers more easily.

Hormone-responsive tumors produce a number of these molecules, and hormones can alter the levels of some of them, theraby affecting the metastatic phenotype of the tumor cells. For example, MCF-7 human breast cancer cells produce more plasminogen activator activity and laminin receptor in response to estrogen treatment. A treatment strategy aimed at flooding attachment receptors such as laminin receptor with laminin fragments and inhibiting the formation of metastases would have far-reaching potential. The feasibility of this approach was demonstrated by Humphries et al. [38] when they diminished metastatic tumor formation in mice injected with melanoma tumor cells by treating the animals with intravenous injections of fibronectin fragments. A pentapeptide sequence appears to be critical for cell interaction with fibronectin and inhibits the formation of lung colonies in mice injected with B16-F10 murine melanoma cells. Inhibition by this peptide was dose dependent, noncytotoxic, and specific to an exact pentapeptide sequence since closely related pentapeptides displayed little activity.

Differentiation

The cloning of the hormone receptor genes creates a variety of exciting, new investigative approaches to hormone therapy. For example, compounds such as the retinoids and 5-azacytidine have long been recognized for their ability to induce differentiation in a variety of cell types. The hormone receptor cDNA clones could be used to probe for renewed expression of a hormone receptor gene following treatment with differentiating agents. If this proved feasible, a hormone-responsive phenotype would be maintained, or reinstituted. In addition, since the hormone receptor complex may induce growth factor gene expression by binding to growth factor gene control regions, the cloned hormone receptor genes should permit the mechanisms of hormone-induced growth factor expression to be elucidated. In the future, such knowledge might be used to block hormone-induced gene expression and cell proliferation.

Antisense Gene Therapy

RNA molecules containing sequences complementary to a portion of or all of the RNA transcribed from a specific gene have been used successfully to decrease the concentration of the target gene's product. Antisense RNAs, introduced by DNA transfection techniques, have been shown to inhibit expression of cellular genes for *c-src*, *c-fos*, thymidine kinase, and actin [6, 32, 40, 51]. Though the inhibition of translation probably results from the formation of RNA-RNA duplexes, mRNA transport from the nucleus and processing within the nucleus may also be affected. This form of technology offers exciting new possibilities for the control of cell growth through inhibition of the translation of autocrine growth factors. Studies investigating such therapy are ongoing in in vitro experiments.

Supraphysiologic Hormone Therapy

Some patients with breast cancer respond to very high doses of estrogen or androgen; in fact, remission rates of 30%–37% have been reported when estrogen has been used as initial therapy [50]. Remission rates of 10% have been seen with androgen therapy. The duration of response to estrogen is generally greater than that seen with androgens, and the estrogen responsiveness increases with years after menopause and with increasing length of the preceding disease-free interval. The chances of response to addition hormonal therapy after relapse from other therapy are less than 10%. In addition, responses following withdrawal of estrogen or androgen therapy have been recorded [48]. The growth-stimulatory and/or -inhibitory effects of pharmacologic doses of steroids have been demonstrated in vitro in breast cancer cells with and without hormone receptors [37]. Unfortunately, the mystery of how these receptor-independent hormone effects are mediated remains unsolved. Understanding such clinical phenomena would provide clues to future therapeutic approaches towards the hormone-responsive tumors.

References

1. Adams DO, Hall T, Steplewski Z, Koprowski H (1984) Tumors undergoing rejection induced by monoclonal antibodies of the IgG2$_A$ isotype contain increased numbers of macrophages activated for a distinctive form of antibody-dependent cytolysis. Proc Natl Acad Sci USA 81: 3506

2. Aitken SC, Lippman ME (1982) Hormonal regulation of net DNA synthesis in MCF-7 human breast cancer cells in tissue culture. Cancer Res 42: 1727

3. Albini A, Graf JO, Kitten T, Kleinman HK, Martin GR, Veillette A, Lippman ME (1986) Estrogen and v-ras^H transfection regulate the interactions of MCF-7 breast carcinoma cells with basement membrane. Proc Natl Acad Sci USA 83: 8182

4. Allegra JC, Lippman ME (1978) Growth of a human breast cancer cell line in serum free medium and response to cytotoxic chemotherapy in patients with metastatic breast cancer. Cancer Res 38: 3823

5. American Cancer Society (1983) Facts and figures. American Cancer Society

6. Amini S, DeSeau V, Reddy S, Shalloway D, Bolen JB (1986) Regulation of pp60^{c-src} synthesis by inducible RNA complementary to c-src mRNA in polyomavirus-transformed rat cells. Mol Cell Biol 6: 2305

7. Bano, M, Salomon DS, Kidwell WR (1985) Purification of a mammary derived growth factor from human milk and human mammary tumors. J Biol Chem 260: 5745

8. Bates SE, McManaway ME, Lippman ME, Dickson RB (1986) Characterization of estrogen responsive transforming activity in human breast cancer cell lines. Cancer Res 46: 1707

9. Berns EMJJ, de Boer W, Molder E (1986) Androgen-dependent growth regulation of and release of specific protein(s) by the androgen receptor containing human prostate tumor cell line LNCaP. Prostate 9: 247

10. Bronzert DA, Greene GL, Lippman ME (1985) Selection and characterization of breast cancer cell line resistant to the antiestrogen LY 117018. Endocrinology 17: 1409

11. Bulbul M, Heston W, Mirenda C, Fair W (1986) A prostate derived growth factor partially purified by heparin affinity and anion exchange chromatography. Am Assoc Cancer Res 27: 852

12. Colletta G, Cirafici AM, Vecchio G (1986) Induction of the c-fos oncogene by thyrotropic hormone in rat thyroid cells in culture. Science 233: 458

13. Conneely OM, Sullivan WP, Tuft DO, Birnbaumer M, Cook RG, Maxwell BL, Zarucki-Schulz T, Greene GL, Shrader WT, O'Malley BW (1986) Molecular cloning of the chicken progesterone receptor. Science 233: 767

14. Davidson NE, Wilding G, Lippman ME, Gelman EP (1985) Isolation of estrogen regulated cDNA clones from human breast cancer cells. Proc Am Soc Clin Invest Clin Res 33: 577

15. Davidson NE, Bronzert DA, Chambon P, Gelman EP, Lippman ME (1986) Use of two MCF-7 cell variants to evaluate the growth regulatory potential of estrogen-induced products. Cancer Res 46: 1904

16. Deguchi T, Chu TM, Leong SS, Horoszewicz JS, Lee C (1986) Effect of methotrexate-monoclonal anti-prostatic acid phosphatase antibody conjugate on human prostate tumor. Cancer Res 46: 3751

17. Dembinski TC, Leung CKH, Shiu RPC (1985) Evidence for a novel pituitary factor that potentiates the mitogenic effect of estrogen in human breast cancer cells. Cancer Res 45: 3083

17a. Dickson RB, Lippman ME (1986) Role of estrogens in the malignant progression of breast cancer: new perspectives. Trends Pharmacol Sci 7(8): 294

18. Dickson RB, Lippman ME (1987) Estrogenic regulation of growth and polypeptide growth factor secretion in human breast carcinoma. Endocr Rev (in press)

19. Dickson RB, Huff KK, Spencer EM, Lippman ME (1986) Induction of epidermal growth factor-related polypeptides by 17$_B$ estradiol in MCF-7 human breast cancer cells. Endocrinology 118: 138

20. Dickson RB, McManaway M, Lippman ME (1986) Estrogen induced growth factors of breast cancer cells partially replace estrogen to promote tumor growth. Science 232: 1540

21. Drebin JA, Link VC, Stern DF, Weinberg RA, Greene MI (1985) Down modulation of an oncogene protein product and reversion of the transformed phenotype by monoclonal antibodies. Cell 41: 695

22. Feldman AR, Kessler L, Myers MH, Naughton MD (1986) The prevalence of cancer. Estimates based on the Connecticut Tumor Registry. N Engl J Med 315: 1394

23. Gaffney EV, Grimwald MA, Pigott DA, Dell'Aguila M (1980) Inhibition of growth of human breast cancer cell line MCF-7 by serum derived calcium chloride clotted plasma. JNCI 65: 1215

24. Gazit A, Igarashi H, Chiu I, Srinivasan A, Yaniv A, Tronick SR, Robbins KC, Aaronson SA (1984) Expression of the normal human sis/PDGF-2 coding sequence induces cellular transformation. Cell 39: 89

25. Giguere V, Hollenberg SM, Rosenfield MG, Evans RM (1986) Functional domains of the human glucocorticoid receptor. Cell 46: 645

26. Glantz GM (1964) Cirrhosis and carcinoma of the prostate gland. J Urol 91: 291

27. Goustin AS, Leof EB, Shipley GD, Moses HL (1986) Growth factors and cancer. Cancer Res 46: 1015

28. Greene GL, Gilna P, Waterfield M, Baker A, Hort Y, Shine J (1986) Sequence and expression of human estrogen receptor complementary DNA. Science 231: 1150

29. Greene S, Walter P, Kumar V, Krust A, Bornert JM, Argos P, Chambon P (1986) Human oestrogen receptor cDNA: sequence, expression and homology to v-erb-A. Nature 320: 134

30. Gregory H, Walsh S, Hopkiss CR (1979) The identification of urogastrone in serum, saliva and gastric juice. Gastroenterology 77: 313

31. Hollenberg SM, Weinberger C, Ong ES, Cerelli G, Orol A Lebo R, Thompson ED, Rosenfield MG, Evans RM (1985) Primary structure and expression of a functional human glucocorticoid receptor cDNA. Nature 318: 635

32. Holt JJ, Venkat GT, Moulton AD, Nienhaus AW (1986) Inducible production of *c-fos* antisense RNA inhibits 3T3 cell proliferation. Proc Natl Acad Sci USA 83: 4794

33. Horoszewicz JS, Leong SS, Kawinski E, Karr JP, Rosenthal H, Chu TM, Mirand EA, Murphy GP (1983) LNC$_a$P model of human prostatic carcinoma. Cancer Res 43: 1809

34. Horwitz KB, McGuire WL (1978) Estrogen control of progesterone receptor in human breast cancer. J Biol Chem 253: 2223

35. Huff KK, Lippman ME (1984) Hormonal control of plasminogen activator secretion in ZR-75-1 human breast cancer cell in culture. Endocrinology 114: 1665

36. Huff KK, Kaufman D, Gabbay KH, Spencer EM, Lippman ME, Dickson RB (1986) Human breast cancer cells secrete an insulin like growth factor I related polypeptide. Cancer Res 46: 4613

37. Hug V, Drewinko B, Hortobaggi GN, Blumenschein G (1985) Regulation of breast tumor growth by high dose estrogen is independent of the presence of estrogen receptors. Breast Cancer Res Treat 6: 237

38. Humphries MJ, Olden K, Yamada KM (1986) A synthetic peptide from fibronectin inhibits experimental metastasis of murine melanoma cells. Science 233: 467

39. Ikeda T, Liu QF, Danielpour D, Officer JB, Ho M, Leland FE, Sirbasku DA (1982) Identification of estrogen inducible growth factors (estromedins) for rat and human mammary tumor cells in culture. In Vitro 18: 961

40. Izant JG, Weintraub H (1985) Constitutive and conditional suppression of exogenous and endogenous genes by anti-sense RNA. Science 229: 345

41. Jakesz R, Smith CA, Aitken S, Huff KK, Schuette W, Shackney S, Lippman ME (1984) Influence of cell proliferation and all cycle phases on expression of estrogen receptor in MCF-7 breast cancer cells. Cancer Res 44: 619

42. Jakowlew SB, Breathnack R, Jeltsch J, Masiakowski P, Chambon P (1984) Sequence of the pS2 mRNA induced by estrogen in the human breast cancer cell line MCF-7. Nucleic Acid Res 12: 2861

43. Jeltsch JM, Krozowski Z, Quirin-Stricker C, Gronemeyer H, Simpson RJ, Garnier JM, Krust A, Jacob F, Chambon P (1986) Cloning of the chicken progesterone receptor. Proc Natl Acad Sci USA 83: 5424

44. Johnson A, Betsholtz C, Heldin CH, Westermark B (1985) Antibodies against platelet-derived growth factor inhibit acute transformation by simian sarcoma virus. Nature 317: 438

45. Kaighn ME, Kirk D, Szalay M, Lechner JF (1981) Growth control of prostate carcinoma cells in serum-free media: Interrelationship of hormone response, cell density and nutrient media. Proc Natl Acad Sci USA 78: 5673

46. Kasid A, Lippman ME, Papageorge AG, Lowy DR, Gelman EP (1985) Transfection of v-ras^H DNA into MCF-7 cells bypasses their dependence on estrogen for tumorigenicity. Science 228: 725

47. Kasid A, Davidson N, Gelman E, Lippman M (1986) Transcriptional control of thymidine kinase gene expression by estrogen and antiestrogen in MCF-7 human breast cancer cells. J Biol Chem 261: 5562

48. Kaufman RJ, Escher GC (1961) Rebound regression in advanced mammary carcinoma. Surg Gynecol Obstet 113: 635

49. Kelseg JL (1979) A review of the epidemiology of human breast cancer. Epidemiol Rev 1: 74

50. Kennedy BJ (1965) Diethylstilbesterol versus testosterone proprionate therapy in advanced breast cancer. Surg Gynecol Obstet 120: 1246

51. Kim SK, Wold BJ (1985) Stable reduction of thymidine kinase activity in cells expressing high levels of anti-sense RNA. Cell 42: 129

52. King CR, Kraus MH, Aaronson SA (1985) Amplification of a novel *v-erb B* related gene in a human mammary carcinoma. Science 229: 974

53. King WJ, Greene GL (1984) Monoclonal antibodies localize estrogen receptor in nuclei of target cells. Nature 307: 745

54. Knabbe C, Wakefield L, flanders K, Kasid A, Derynck R, Lippman M, Dickson RB (1987) Evidence that TGF$_\beta$ is a hormonally regulated negative growth factor in human breast cancer. Cell 48: 417–428

55. Krust A, Green S, Argos P, Kumar V, Walter P, Bornert JM, Chambon P (1986) The chicken oestrogen receptor sequence: Homology with v-erb A and the human oestrogen and glucocorticoid receptors. EMBO J 5: 891

56. Kumar V, Green S, Staub A, Chambon P (1986) Localization of the oestradiol-binding and putative DNA-binding domains of the human oestrogen receptor. EMBO J 5: 2231

57. Levine RM, Rubalcaba E, Lippman ME, Cowan KH (1985) Effects of estrogen and tamoxifen on the regulation of dihydrofolate gene expression in a human breast cancer cell line. Cancer Res 45: 1

58. Liotta LA (1985) Tumor invasion and metastases: role of the extracellular matrix. Proc Am Assoc Cancer Res 26: 385

59. Liotta LA, Mandler R, Murano G, Katz DA, Gordon RK, Chiang PK, Schiffmann E (1986) Tumor cell autocrine motility factor. Proc Natl Acad Sci USA 83: 3302

60. Lippman ME (1985) Endocrine responsive cancers of man. In: Williams RH (ed) Textbook of endocrinology. Saunders, Philadelphia, 1309

61. Lippman ME, Bolan G, Huff K (1972) Interactions of antiestrogens with human breast cancer in long term tissue culture. Cancer Treat Rep 60: 1421

62. Lippman ME, Bolan G, Huff K (1976) The effects of estrogens and antiestrogens on hormone responsive human breast cancer in long-term tissue culture. Cancer Res 36: 4595

63. MacMahon B, Cole P. Brown J (1973) Etiology of human breast cancer: a review. JNCI 50: 21

64. Maehama S, Li D, Nanri H, Leykam JF, Deuel TF (1986) Purification and characterization of prostate derived growth factor. Proc Natl Acad Sci USA 83: 8162

65. Masui H, Kawamoto T, Sato JD, Wolf B, Sato G, Mendelsohn J (1984) Growth inhibition of human tumor cells in athymic mice by anti-epidermal growth factor receptor monoclonal antibodies. Cancer Res 44: 1002

66. Masui H, Morogama T, Mendelsohn J (1986) Mechanism of antitumor activity in mice for anti-epidermal growth factor receptor monoclonal antibodies with different isotypes. Cancer Res 46: 5592

67. May FEB, Westley BR (1986) Cloning of estrogen-regulated messenger RNA sequences from human breast cancer cells. Cancer Res 46: 6034

68. Mendelsohn J, Masui H, MacLeod C (1985) Anti-EGF receptor monoclonal antibody 528 inhibits proliferation of a subset of human tumor cells in xenografts. Proc Am Assoc Cancer Res 26: 287

69. Montpetit ML, Lawless KR, Tennisweed M (1986) Androgen-repressed messages in the rat ventral prostate. Prostate 8: 25

70. Muller R, Curran T, Muller D, Guilbert L (1985) Induction of *c-fos* during myelomoncytic differentiation and macrophage proliferation. Nature 314: 546

71. Rosenthal A, Lindquist PB, Bringman TS, Goeddel DV, Derynck R (1988) Expression in rat

377

fibroblasts of a human transforming growth factor-α cDNA results in transformation. Cell 46: 301

72. Rotkin ID (1977) Studies in the epidemiology of prostatic cancer: expanded sampling. Cancer Treat Rep 61: 173

73. Salomon DS, Zwiebel JA, Bano M, Losonczy I. Felnel P, Kidwell WR (1984) Presence of transforming growth factors in human breast cancer cells. Cancer Res 44: 4069

74. Schechter AL, Hung M, Vaidymnathan L et al. (1985) The *neu* gene: an *erb B* homologous gene distinct from and unlinked to the gene encoding the EGF receptor. Science 229: 976

75. Schreiber AB, Kenney J, Kowalski J, Thomas KA, Gimenez-Gallego G, Rios-Candelore M, DiSalvo J, Bamitault D, Courty J, Courtois Y, Moemer M, Loret C, Burgess WH, Mehlamn T, Friesel R, Johnson W, Macirg T (1985) A unique family of endothelial cell polypeptide mitogens: the antigenic and receptor cross-reactivity of bovine endothelial growth factor and eye-derived growth factor II. J Cell Biol 101: 1623

76. Semba K, Kamata N, Toyoshima K, Yamamoto T (1985) A *v-erb B* related proto-oncogene is amplified in a human salivary gland adenocarcinoma. Proc Natl Acad Sci USA 82: 6497

77. Sporn MB, Roberts AB, Wakefield LM, Assoian RK (1986) Transforming growth factor B: biologic function and chemical structure. Science 233: 532

78. Steplewski Z, Lubeck MD, Korprowski H (1983) Human macrophages armed with murine immunoglobulin G_{2A} antibodies to tumors destroy human cancer cells. Science 221: 865

79. Stoscheck CM, King LE Jr (1986) Role of epidermal growth factor in carcinogenesis. Cancer Res 46: 1030

80. Strobl JS, Thompson EB (1985) Mechansim of steroid hormone action. In: Auricchio F (ed) Sex steroid receptors. Field Educational Halia Acta Medica, Rome, pp 9–36

81. Studzinski GP, Brelvi ZS, Feldman SC, ,Watt RA (1986) Participation of *c-myc* protein in DNA synthesis of human cells. Science 234: 467

82. Swain S, Dickson R, Lippman M (1986) Anchorage independent epithelial colony stimualting activity in human breast cancer cell line. Proc Am Assoc Cancer Res 27: 844

83. Tackett RE, Heston WDW, Parrish RF, Pletscher LS, Fair WR (1985) Mitogenic factors in prostatic tissue and expressed prostatic secretion. J Urol 133: 45

84. Viola MV, Fromowitz F, Oravez S, Deb S, Finkel G. Lundy J, Hand P, Thor A, Schlom J (1986) Expression of *ras* oncogene p21 in prostate cancer. N Engl J Med 314: 133

85. Walter P, Green S, Greene G, Krust A, Bornert JM, Jeltsch JM, Straub A, Jensen E, Scrace G, Waterfield M, Chambon P (1985) Cloning of the human estrogen cDNA. Proc Natl Acad Sci USA 82: 889

86. Watt KWK, Lee PJ, Timkulu T, Chan WP, Loor R (1986) Human prostate specific antigen: structural and functional similarity with serine proteases. Proc Natl Acad Sci USA 83: 3166

87. Westley B, Rochefort H (1980) A secreted glycoprotein induced by estrogen in human breast cancer cell lines. Cell 20: 353

88. Wilding G, Knabbe C, Freter C, Zugmaier G, Chen M, Gelmann EP (1987) Stimulation of human prostate cancer cells in vitro by transforming growth factor alpha. The Endocrine Society, Indianapolis

Potential Approaches

20. Tumor Invasion and Metastases: Biochemical Mechanisms

L.A. Liotta, M.L. Stracke, E. Kohn, S. Aznavoorian, and U.M. Wewer

Multistep Cascade of Metastases

A metastatic colony is the end result of a complicated series of tumor-host interactions (Fig. 1). Primary tumor initiation and progression is followed by the transition from in situ to locally invasive cancer and angiogenesis [1–6]. Newly formed tumor vessels are often defective and easily invaded by tumor cells within the primary mass. At the invasion front, tumor cells also invade preestablished host blood vessels. Tumor cells are discharged into the venous drainage in single-cell form and in clumps. From rapidly growing tumors 1 cm in size, millions of tumor cells can be shed into the circulation every day. Fortunately for the patient, only a very small percentage (<0.01%) of circulating tumor cells initiate metastatic colonies. Tumors generally lack a well-formed lymphatic network; therefore, communication of tumor cells with lymphatic channels occurs only at the tumor periphery and not within the tumor mass. Tumor cells entering the lymphatic drainage are carried to regional lymph nodes, where they arrest in the large lymphatics of the subcapsular sinus. Within 10–60 min after initial arrest in the lymph node, a significant fraction of the tumor cells detach and enter the efferent lymphatics. These tumor cells eventually end up in the regional or systemic venous drainage due to the existence of numerous lymphatic-hematogenous communications. Thus, the regional lymph node does not function as a true mechanical barrier to tumor dissemination. Lymphatic and hematogenous dissemination occur in parallel.

Circulating tumor cells utilize a variety of means to arrest in the vessels of the target organ where they will initiate metastatic colonies (Table 1). Approximately 80% of the circulating tumor cells are in single-cell form and attach directly to the intact endothelial surface or to preexisting regions of exposed subendothelial basement membrane. Clumps of circulating tumor cells or tumor cells aggregated with host leukocytes, fibrin, or platelets can directly embolize in the precapillary venules by mechanical impaction. Tumor cells in single-cell or clump form adhere to the endothelial luminal surface of arterioles. The fate and time course of the arrested tumor cells differs, depending on the mechanism and location of lodgement. Tumor cells adherent to the surface of venule or capillary endothelium rapidly (in 1–4 h) induce the active retraction of the endothelial cells. The tumor cells then attach avidly to the exposed basement membrane. Once the tumor cells have attached, the adjacent endothelial cells extend over

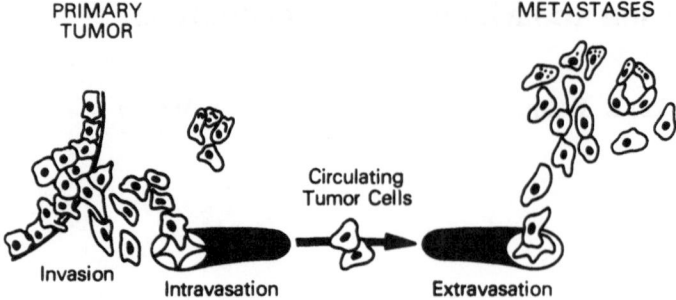

PRIMARY TUMOR

METASTASES

Circulating Tumor Cells

Invasion   Intravasation   Extravasation

Fig. 1. Multistep metastatic cascade. Following transition from in situ to invasive carcinoma, tumor cells gain access to host blood vessels and lymphatics. Tumor cells enter the bloodstream directly (or indirectly via lymphatic-hematogenous communications) and are carried to the distant organ site. Here, they arrest in the vascular bed, extravasate, and initiate a metastatic colony. Continued growth of the metastases requires angiogenesis and escape from host defenses

the tumor cells and separate them from the bloodstream. Tumor cells located between the endothelium and the basement membrane are held up in this location for 8–24 h. Local dissolution of the basement membrane is then observed, in association with tumor cell pseudopodia traversing the basement membrane. This step is soon followed by complete extravasation of the tumor cell and, quite often, reestablishment of blood flow in the breached vessel. Tumor cells arrested in the arterial tree can remain in this location for 2–3 weeks. Endothelial retraction does not occur following arterial arrest. Intraarterial tumor cells can actually proliferate and expand as colonies. As the tumor colonies enlarge, they become covered by a host endothelial surface which lacks a basement membrane. Once the tumor colony fills the arteriole, mechanical damage to the endothelium occurs, and this exposes the basement membrane. Tumor cells at the periphery of the intraarterial colony then invade through the basement membrane and the elastic lamina of the arteriole wall to gain an extravascular position.

At all stages of the metastatic cascade, tumor cells must overcome host defenses [3–5]. Although tumor-specific antigens have been identified in animal models, it still remains unclear whether similar antigens play a role in human tumors, and whether the recognition of these antigens can be boosted by adjuvant immunotherapy. Limited effectiveness of adjuvant immunotherapy for metastases may be due to tumor antigen heterogeneity, tumor antigen shedding, or absence of tumor cell immunogenicity. "Nonspecific" host defenses such as macrophages and natural killer cells may be more effective against heterogeneous tumor cell populations. In animal models, these effector cells play an important role in the elimination of circulating tumor cells and the destruction of micrometastases.

Extravasated tumor cells proliferate as colonies but require a new vascular supply to grow larger than 0.5 mm. Thus, angiogenesis is necessary at the beginning and the end of the metastatic cascade. Metastases can themselves metastasize, further amplifying the level of disease progression. Numerous clinical

Table 1. Potential mechanisms of the metastatic cascade of events

Metastatic cascade event	Potential mechanisms
Tumor initiation	Carcinogenic insult, oncogene activation or derepression, chromosome rearrangement
Promotion and progression	Karyotypic, genetic, and epigenetic instability, gene amplification; promotion-associated genes and hormones
Uncontrolled proliferation	Autocrine growth factors or their receptors, receptors for host hormones such as estrogen
Angiogenesis	Multiple angiogenesis factors, including known growth factors
Invasion of local tissues, blood and lymphatic vessels	Serum chemoattractants, autocrine motility factors, attachment receptors, degradative enzymes
Circulating tumor cell arrest and extravasation	Tumor cell homotypic or heterotypic aggregation
Adherence to endothelium	Tumor cell interaction with fibrin, platelets, and clotting factors, adhesion to RGD-type receptors
Retraction of endothelium	Platelet factors, tumor cell factors
Adhesion to basement membrane	Laminin receptor, thrombospondin receptor
Dissolution of basement membrane	Degradative proteases, type IV collagenase, heparanase, cathepsins
Locomotion	Autocrine motility factors, chemotaxis factors
Colony formation at secondary site	Receptors for local tissue growth factors, angiogenesis factors
Evasion of host defenses and resistance to therapy	Resistance to killing by host macrophages, natural killer cells, and activated T cells; failure to express, or blocking of, tumor-specific antigens; amplification of drug resistance genes

reports provide circumstantial evidence for the existence of dormant metastases [1]. Up to one-third of the mortality from breast cancer, for instance, occurs more than 5 years after removal of the primary tumor. Three potential mechanisms of tumor dormancy have been distinguished in animal models: (a) immunologic restraint, such that the tumor population death rate equals its growth rate; (b) constitutive dependency of tumor cells on host growth factors; and (c) avascularity causing the metastasis to be limited in size due to deficiency in nutrient diffusion.

Organ Tropism for Metastases

The distribution of metastases varies widely, depending on the histologic type and anatomic location of the primary tumor (Table 2). The most frequent organ location of distant metastases in many types of cancer appears to be the first capillary bed encountered by the circulating cells. Major pathways of metastasis determined directly by anatomic considerations are as follows:

Table 2. Frequency of metastases at autopsy

Organ of metastases	Primary tumor (%)			
	Lung	Colon	Breast	Melanoma
Liver	30–50	50–60	40–60	58–70
Lung	20–40	25–40	60–80	66–80
Bone	30–45	5–10	50–90	30–48
Brain	15–43	0–1	15–30	40–55
Adrenal	17–38	14	38–54	40–47
Pituitary	0–2	0–1	20	18
Ovary	0–2	14	15–30	10–15
Kidney	16–23	8	13	31–35
Spleen	9	5	17	31

1. Sarcomas arising in the extremities metastasize primarily to the lungs. Sarcoma cells entering the tumor venous drainage are carried into the inferior vena cava, enter the right ventricle, and are carried via the pulmonary artery to the lungs (Fig. 2).
2. Lung cancer disseminates widely to multiple organs, including brain. Lung cancer is the only tumor that has direct access to the general arterial circulation via the pulmonary vein through the left ventricle [3] (Fig. 2).
3. Colorectal carcinomas tend to metastasize to the liver. Colorectal carcinoma cells enter the mesenteric lymphatics and portal venous system and are carried to the liver [1, 3] (Fig. 2).
4. Tumors of the testicle metastasize via the lymphatics to lymph nodes of the periaortic area and then enter the subclavian veins by lymphatic-hematogenous communications. Tumor cells entering the subclavian veins go to the right ventricle and then to the lungs [1–3].
5. Prostate cancer metastasizes primarily (90%) to vertebral bone. The anatomic route is via Batson's plexus of paravertebral veins [2]. Tumor cells entering the prostatic plexus of veins are carried to the veins about the sacrum, ilium, and lumbar spine.
6. Patterns of head and neck cancer metastases correspond primarily to the regions of local lymphatic drainage [1].
7. Ovarian cancer remains confined for long periods in the abdominal cavity. Local spread occurs to the peritoneal surfaces, the posterior gutters, and the diaphragm. These tumors invade the liver in only a small percentage of cases at a very late stage. The liver is usually invaded directly from omental disease or by mesenteric venous emboli derived from omental implants [1].
8. Breast cancer metastases are frequently found in vertebral bone. Based on dye injection studies, it has been demonstrated that the mammary venous drainage can communicate with Batson's plexus of paravertebral veins [2]. When dye was injected into a small mammary vein, the dye was found in the clavicles, intercostal veins, head of humerus, cervical vertebrae, and transverse cranial sinuses.

Fig. 2. Organ pattern of metastases is in part determined by blood flow patterns. Sarcomas arising in the extremity disseminate tumor cells into the venous drainage which are carried through the right heart to the lungs. Carcinomas arriving in the bowel discharge tumor cells into the portal vein and the thoracic duct. Lung carcinomas disseminate systemically to other organs including the brain.

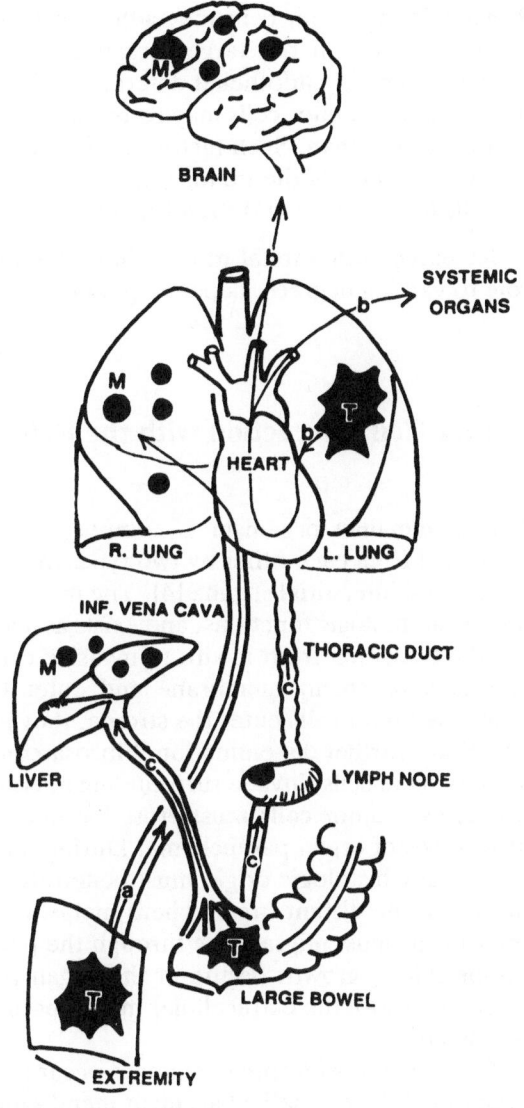

However, there are many metastatic sites which cannot be predicted on the basis of anatomic considerations alone, and which can be considered to be examples of organ tropism. For example, clear-cell carcinoma of the kidney often metastasizes to bone and thyroid, and ocular melanoma frequently metastasizes to the liver. Theoretical mechanisms for organ tropism include the following [3, 5]:

1. Tumor cells disseminate equally in all organs, but grow preferentially only in specific organs. Preferential growth may be induced by local growth factors or hormones present in the target organ for metastases.

2. Circulating tumor cells may adhere preferentially to the endothelial luminal surface only in the target organ for metastases. This hypothesis predicts organ-specific endothelial determinants.
3. Circulating tumor cells may respond to soluble factors diffusing locally out of the target organ. Such factors could act in a chemotactic fashion to promote extravasation of the tumor cells. They could also cause the circulating tumor cells to aggregate and therefore embolize in the target organ.

Research with animal models indicates that all of these mechanisms play a role to varying degrees, depending on the tumor model system [3, 5].

Tumor Cell Interaction with the Extracellular Matrix

The mammalian organism is composed of a series of tissue compartments separated from each other by two types of extracellular matrix: basement membranes and interstitial stroma [4]. The matrix determines tissue architecture, has important biologic functions, and exists as a mechanical barrier to invasion. During the transition from in situ to invasive carcinoma, tumor cells penetrate the epithelial basement membrane and enter the underlying interstitial stroma. Once the tumor cells enter the stroma, they gain access to lymphatics and blood vessels for further dissemination. Fibrosarcomas and angiosarcomas, developing from stromal cells, invade surrounding muscle basement membrane and destroy myocytes. Tumor cells must cross basement membranes to invade nerve and most types of organ parenchyma. During intravasation or extravasation, tumor cells of any histologic origin must penetrate the subendothelial basement membrane. In the distant organ where metastic colonies are initiated, extravasated tumor cells must migrate the through the perivascular interstitial stroma before tumor colony growth occurs in the organ parenchyma. Therefore, tumor cell interaction with the extracellular matrix occurs at multiple stages in the metastatic cascade.

General and widespread changes occur in the organization, distribution, and quantity of the epithelial basement membrane during the transition from benign to invasive carcinoma. The human breast is a particular example: benign proliferative disorders of the breast—such as fibrocystic disease, sclerosing adenosis, intraductal hyperplasia, fibroadenoma, and intraductal papilloma—are all characterized by disorganization of the normal epithelial stromal architecture. Extreme forms can mimic the appearance of invasive carcinoma. However, no matter how extensive the architectural disorganization is, these benign disorders are always characterized by a continuous basement membrane separating the epithelium from the stroma. In contrast, invasive ductal carcinoma, invasive lobular carcinoma, and tubular carcinoma consistently possess a defective extracellular basement membrane, with zones of basement membrane loss around the invading tumor cells in the stroma. The basement membrane is also markedly defective adjacent to tumor cells in lymph node and organ metastases. In some focal regions of well-differentiated carcinoma, partial basement membrane formation by differentiated structures can be identified. These findings are of direct application to diagnostic problems in surgical pathology, such as the differentiation of tangential sections of in situ lesions from true invasion, or that of severe adenosis from invasive carcinoma. Loss of basement membranes in human carcinomas significantly correlates with increased incidence of metastases and poor 5-year survival.

Three-Step Theory of Invasion

A three-step hypothesis has been proposed to describe the sequence of biochemical events during tumor cell invasion of extracellular matrix. The first step is tumor cell attachment to the matrix. Attachment may be mediated by specific glycoproteins such as laminin and fibronectin which interact with tumor cell plasma membrane receptors. Following attachment, the tumor cell secretes hydrolytic enzymes (or induces host cells to secrete enzymes) which can locally degrade the matrix (including degradation of the attachment glycoproteins). Matrix lysis most likely takes place in a highly localized region close to the tumor cell surface where the amount of active enzyme outbalances the natural protease inhibitors present in the serum and in the matrix itself. In contrast to the invasive tumor cell, the normal cell or benign tumor cell, once attached to the matrix, may respond by shifting into a resting or differentiated state. The third step is tumor cell locomotion into the region of the matrix modified by proteolysis. The direction of the locomotion may be influenced by chemotactic factors and autocrine motility factors (AMF). The latter are a newly described class of proteins (see "Autocrine Motility Factors" below), which bind to a cell surface receptor and profoundly stimulate motility [4]. They are distinct from known growth factors, and their mechanism of action involves a membrane guanine nucleotide (G) protein pathway which can be inhibited by pertussis toxin. The chemotactic factors derived from serum, organ parenchyma, or the matrix itself [3, 6] may influence the organ specificity of metastases. Continued invasion of the matrix may take place by cyclic repetition of these three steps.

Autocrine Motility Factors

Cell motility is necessary for tumor cells to be able to traverse many stages in the complex cascade of invasion. Such stages could include the detachment and subsequent infiltration of cells from the primary tumor into adjacent tissue, the migration of the cells through the vascular wall into the circulation (intravasation), and the extravasation of the cells to a secondary site. The movement of cells through biologic barriers such as the endothelial basement membranes of the vasculature may well occur by means of chemotactic mechanisms. Indeed, studies on in vitro chemotaxis of some tumor cells report that a variety of compounds such as complement-derived materials, collagen peptides, formyl peptides, and certain connective tissue components can act as chemoattractants [7, 8]. While these agents may well contribute to the directional aspects of a motile response, they are not sufficient to initiate the intrinsic locomotion of tumor cells. The availability of soluble attractants to the tumor cell is greatly dependent upon the host, even in those cases in which the production of attractants is the result of tumor cell-host tissue interaction. At best, it seems that the cell would have access to such motility stimuli at sporadic and irregular intervals, conditions unfavorable to a sustained migration of highly invasive cells.

With these considerations in mind—and stimulated by the studies of Anzano et al. [9] in which they demonstrated autocrine growth factors for transformed cells—we investigated the possibility that such cells could elaborate AMF. The action of these substances might, in part, explain both the markedly invasive character and the metastatic property of malignant cells. Thus, under the influence of such an autocrine material, a tumor cell might move out into the surrounding host tissue and also exert a "recruiting" effect on adjacent tumor cells in the presence of a gradient of attractant. Conceivably, such factors might also attract fibroblastic cells of the host, resulting in the phenomenon of desmoplasia, characteristic of invasive tumors.

We have found that in culture, the human melanoma cell line A2058 and human breast carcinoma cells produce a material that markedly stimulates their own motility [10]. These cells respond in a dose-dependent manner to various concentrations of conditioned medium obtained by incubating confluent cells in serum-free medium, an indication that the motility factor is derived from the cell. Motility was measured by the modified Boyden chamber procedure. Using this assay and the "checkerboard" analysis [11], we have also found that the conditioned medium factor has both chemotactic (directional) and chemokinetic (randomly motile) properties.

Isolation and Characterization of a Human Melanoma Autocrine Motility Factor

Conditioned protein-free medium which elicited both large (10%–15% cell migration), dose-dependent chemotactic responses and randomly motile responses (checkerboard analysis) was used to isolate AMF. After concentration (Amicon), the conditioned medium was subjected to molecular sieve chromatography. AMF emerged as a broad major peak between 40 000 and 65 000 daltons (data not shown). The AMF was further isolated by fast-performance liquid chromatography.

The AMF activity was iodinated and found to comprise a single major component (on electrophoresis) of approximately 55 000 daltons without reduction of disulfide bonds. Upon reduction with 5 mM dithiothreitol, the migration of this component on the gel became slower, indicating the existence of interchain disulfide bonds. Amino acid analysis of AMF revealed a high content of glycine, serine, glutamic acid, and aspartic acid residues. Both tyrosine and cysteine are present, the latter being concordant with the existence of interchain disulfide bonds, as indicated by the altered electrophoretic mobility of AMF after treatment with dithiothreitol.

Transduction of the Chemical Signal in the Motile Response of Tumor Cells

Because some cells require ongoing protein synthesis to develop a motile response, we determined whether inhibition of protein synthesis affected the response of the melanoma cells to the melanoma autocrine factor. We found that concentrations of cycloheximide that eliminate de novo protein synthesis had no effect on stimulated cell motility; therefore, the cell protein components required for development of a motile response appear to be stable for the duration of migration (4 h).

Studies with leukocytes [12, 13] have implicated a G protein in the receptor-mediated initiation of a motile response in these cells. There is convincing evidence that the locomotion of certain tumor cells also directly involves a G protein [14]. Pertussis toxin, known to inhibit action of the Gi protein of the adenylate cyclase pathway [15], profoundly and rapidly inhibited the AMF-stimulated migration of A2058 melanoma cells [4] and two breast cancer cell lines in vitro (Guirguis et al., submitted). In the melanoma cell line, pertussis toxin (0.5 μg/ml) completely blocked motility without affecting growth in culture (M.L. Stracke, unpublished results). However, the adenylate cyclase pathway does not appear to be directly involved in the motility response since agents which selectively modulate or have a role in this pathway, e.g., cholera toxin, forskolin, the cyclic AMP analogue 8-bromoadenosine-3',5'-cyclic monophosphate, and the cyclase inhibitor 2',5'-dideoxyadenosine, all had minor effects on cell migration. It is likely, then, that effector systems other than that of adenylate cyclase are mediated by a G protein in producing tumor cell motility.

G proteins have been shown to act in a variety of second-messenger pathways, including phospholipase A$_2$ [16] and phospholipase C [17], and in the activation of calcium channels [18]. In the neutrophil, pertussis toxin inhibits both lipase enzymes and cell motility [19, 20]. Evidence that suggests a role for phospholipase A$_2$ in tumor cell locomotion has been obtained with the melanoma cell. Quinacrine, an agent that inhibits phospholipase A$_2$, markedly reduced AMF-stimulated migration. Additionally, deaza-adenosine, an inhibitor of biological methylation [21], was found to reduce markedly both membrane phospholipid methylation and AMF-stimulated motility, whereas AMF itself caused a sustained increase in the methylation of phosphatidyl choline (Ptd Cho) in melanoma cells. Since Ptd Cho is the major substrate for phospholipase A_2, these findings are consistent with a role for this enzyme in tumor cell motility. Studies with a murine tumor cell line, BU-L, suggest that metabolism of arachidonic acid, a product of the lipase reaction, may play a role in tumor cell motility [22]. Lipoxygenase inhibitiors such as quercetin, nordihydroguaretic acid, and nafazatrom signficantly reduced stimulated motility, but indomethacin, a cyclooxygenase–blocking agent, had no effect; calmidazolium also substantially inhibited motility. Collectively, these results are in accord with both the lipoxygenase pathway for arachidonate metabolism and a calmodulin-mediated mobilization of calcium participating in migration of certain tumor cells; however, a role for the cyclo-oxygenase pathway cannot be ruled out.

It has been reported that phorbol myristate acetate and laminin-stimulated motility in murine fibrosarcoma cells are inhibited by prostaglandins of the E series [23]. Preliminary studies (M. Stracke, unpublished work) with human melanoma cells indicate that calcium channel-blocking agents partially inhibit AMF-stimulated motility. On the other hand, calcium ionophores were found to stimulate motility. These results are consistent with the participation of phosphodiesterase (PDE), and the generation of inositol-1,4,5-triphosphate (IP_3) in the initiation of motility. Preliminary experiments clearly demonstrate that lithium, an inhibitor of the IP_3 pathway, significantly reduces AMF-induced motility (Kohn et al., in preparation).

From these considerations, it is likely that the generation of a motile response in tumor cells initially involves a direct role for a G protein which interacts with an activated receptor and then transduces the signal to an effector system such as the PDE IP_3 pathway and phospholipase A_2. The subsequent production of arachidonate and its metabolism via lipoxygenase may contribute to the mobilization of calcium by IP_3 and diacyl glycerol (DAG), which could also be required for changes in the cytoskeleton that are essential for locomotion. With respect to a role for cathepsin B, it is conceivable that AMF may stimulate its activity within the membrane to cause a specific cleavage of a proenzyme whose active form, e.g., protein kinase C [24], is required for the motile response.

Early events in migration may involve pseudopodia protrusion. During the course of invasion, the same tumor cell must interact with a variety of extracellular matrix proteins as it traverses each tissue barrier. For example, the tumor cell encounters laminin and type IV collagen when it penetrates the basement, and type I collagen and fibronectin when it crosses the interstitial stroma. It has recently been shown that cells express specific cell surface receptors which recognize extracellular matrix proteins. The first example of such a receptor is the laminin receptor, which binds to laminin with nanomolar affinity. Laminin receptors have been shown to be augmented in actively invading tumor cells, and they may play an important role in tumor cell interaction with the basement membrane. The integrins are another class of cell surface proteins which bind extracellular matrix components recognizing the protein sequence Arg-Gly-Asp (RGD) [8]. Such proteins include fibronectin, collagen type I, and vitronectin. The process of cell migration undoubtedly requires a series of adhesion and detachment steps resulting in traction and propulsion. Studies using the AMF-stimulated motility as a model system have revealed an important function of pseudopodial protrusion in this process. AMF stimulates motility on a variety of different substrata; therefore, its action is independent of the mchanism of attachment. Furthermore, AMF induces the rapid protrusion of pseudopodia in a time- and dose-dependent manner [25]. Isolation of the induced pseudopodia reveals that they are highly enriched in their content of laminin and fibronectin matrix receptors. Since cell pseudopodia formation is known to be a prominent feature of actively motile cells, we can now set forth a working hypothesis to explain the early events in cell motility. Cytokines such as AMF which stimulate intrinsic motility may induce exploratory pseudopodia prior to cell translocation. Such pseudopodia may express augmented levels of matrix receptors (and possibly proteinases). The protruding pseudopodia may serve multiple functions, including acting as "sense organs" to interact with the extracellular matrix proteins and thereby locate directional cues, providing propulsive traction for locomotion, and even inducing local matrix proteolysis to assist the penetration of the matrix.

Laminin Receptors

Cell surface receptors for the basement membrane glycoprotein laminin mediate adhesion of tumor cells to the basement membrane prior to invasion [4, 26]. Laminin as visualized by rotary shadowing electron microscopy has a distinctive cruciform shape with three short arms (35 nm) and one long arm (75 nm). All arms have globular end regions. The specialized structure of the laminin molecule may contribute to its multiple biologic functions. Laminin plays a role in cell attachment, cell spreading, mitogenesis, neurite outgrowth, morphogenesis, and cell movement. Many types of neoplastic cells contain high-affinity cell surface binding sites (laminin receptors) for laminin with a dissociation constant (Kd) in the nanomolar range. The molecular weight of the isolated receptor is 65 000 daltons [25]. The laminin receptor binds to the "B" chain (short-arm) region of the laminin molecule. Laminin receptors may be altered in number or degree of occupancy in human carcinomas. This may be the indirect result of defective basement membrane organization in the carcinomas. Breast carcinoma and colon carcinoma tissue contains a higher number of exposed (unoccupied) receptors than benign lesions. The laminin receptors of normal epithelium may be polarized at the basal surface and occupied with laminin in the basement membrane. In contrast, the laminin receptors on invading carcinoma cells are amplified and may be distributed over the entire surface of the cell. The laminin receptor can be shown experimentally to play a role in hematogenous metastases. Treating tumor cells with the receptor-binding fragment of laminin at very low concentrations markedly inhibits or abolishes lung metastases from hematogenously introduced tumor cells. The mechanism of action involves blocking the adhesion of circulating tumor cells to the subendothelial basement membrane (Table 1).

391

Effect of Antilaminin Receptor Antisera on Laminin-Mediated Haptotaxis

A2058 human melanoma cells migrate in response to a gradient of laminin, as assayed in a modified Boyden chamber with laminin-coated nucleopore filters. In this system, the tumor cells are placed on one side of a nucleopore (8 μm pore size) filter and the opposite face of the filter is coated with laminin (10 μg/ml). In the presence of a solid phase laminin gradient, tumor cells migrate through the pores and attach to the laminin-coated side of the filter facing the lower part of the chamber. In this manner, the laminin receptor function associated with migration on laminin substrata could be separated from its effect on primary attachment. The polyclonal antiserum against the natural laminin receptor and the polyclonal antisera against the synthetic peptides derived from the receptor cDNA clone all inhibited the laminin haptotaxis of A2058 cells in a dose-dependent manner compared with preimmune controls. The A2058 cells also exhibited a significant haptotactic response to a gradient of fibronectin. Anti-laminin antiserum abrogated haptotactic response to laminin but not to fibronectin. In contrast, the integrin recognition peptide, GRGDS (50 μg/ml), significantly inhibited haptotaxis on fibronectin. The control peptide GRGES, which is not an active binding sequence of fibronectin, did not have an inhibitory effect on fibronectin haptotaxis. There was no inhibition of laminin haptotaxis with these fibronectin peptides. Furthermore, the antilaminin receptor antisera did not significantly inhibit fibronectin haptotaxis compared with controls. These results support the concept that different receptors are involved in laminin versus fibronectin haptotaxis.

Correlation Between In Vivo Expression of Laminin Receptor in Human Tumors and Invasive and Migratory Capacities

Bearing in mind the in vitro results, we next investigated the possibility that the laminin receptor might also be preferentially associated with cells involved in in vivo invasion and migration. Invading trophoblasts of decidua basalis in early human pregnancy, which are characterized by invasive and migratory properties, exhibited a prominent cytoplasmic laminin receptor immunoreactivity. In the malignant human tumors investigated, the tumor cells aggressively invading the extracellular matrix also exhibited intense cytoplasmic staining with the polyclonal antilaminin receptor antisera. The identical topographic distribution pattern was found using antiserum against the natural laminin receptor or synthetic peptide antisera. Surrounding normal tissues had little immunoreactivity, except for some proliferating blood vessels. Metastatic carcinoma cells in liver were strongly immunoreactive, whereas the surrounding parenchyma was essentially nonreactive with these antisera. There appeared to be a correlation between the degree of differentiation and the level of laminin receptor-positive cytoplasmic immunos'aining. The moderately or poorly differentiated carcinomas (33 of 48 cases studied) had more abundant and intense laminin immunoreactivity than the well-differentiated carcinomas (15 of 48 cases). The observation that laminin receptor expression in vivo might be augmented in highly malignant tumor cells which are involved in invasion and migration is also supported by our finding that metastatic tumor tissue is a successful source for biochemical purification of the laminin receptor.

RGD Recognition Receptors

A family of cell surface glycoproteins, termed *integrins*, has been identified which bind with low affinity (micromolar Kd) to a variety of adhesion proteins, including fibronectin, von Willebrand factor, fibrin, vitronectin, type I collagen, and thrombospondin [27]. The integrins are a complex of alpha (140 000-dalton) and beta (95 000-dalton) subunit proteins. The functions of several of the integrins are inhibited by peptides related to the Arg-Gly-Asp (RGD) sequence of fibronectin. RGD sequences present on a wide variety of proteins may serve as the recognition site for binding of the integrins. It is likely that specific ligand sequences adjacent to the RGD site may confer preferential recognition of one type of adhesion protein by certain members of the integrin family. Integrin proteins are thought to align adhesion proteins such as fibronectin on the cell surface with cytoskeletal components such as talin and actin, thus altering cell shape. Integrin-type proteins may play an adhesive role in platelet-tumor cell interactions; the binding of lymphoid cells to endothelium; and the interaction of circulating tumor cells with endothelial surfaces, fibrin, von Willebrand factor, or thrombospondin. In keeping with this concept, it has been reported that coinjection of tumor cells with large quantities of RGD peptides will inhibit metastases formation in animal models. The RGD peptides may interfere with the adhesion of tumor cells to the endothelial surface, which may directly or indirectly be mediated through integrin proteins.

Tumor Cell Proteinases

In vitro studies of tumor cell invasion of the extracellular matrix have shown that cell proliferation is not absolutely required. Invasion of the matrix is not merely due to passive growth pressure, but requires active biochemical mechanisms. Inhibitors of protein synthesis or inhibitors of proteinases block invasion of the matrix [4]. Many research groups have proposed that invasive tumor cells secrete matrix-degrading proteinases. Collagen is an important substrate because it constitutes the structural scaffolding upon which the other components of the matrix are assembled. Tumor-derived collagenases which degrade interstitial collagen types I, II, and III have been characterized by a number of investigators. They are metal ion (calcium and zinc)-dependent enzymes which function at neutral pH. Classic collagenase produces a single cleavage in the collagen molecule (interstitial collagen types I, II and III), producing three-quarter- and quarter-size fragments (75% of the distance from the NH_2 terminal). Tumor cells can degrade both collagenous and noncollagenous components of the basement membrane [4, 5, 28]. Basement membrane-specific collagen types IV and V are *not* susceptible to classic collagenase, which degrades collagen types I, II, and III. A separate family of collagenolytic enzymes (type IV collagenase) [4, 28] cleave the type IV collagen chain a quarter of the distance from the NH_2 terminal. Type IV collagenases are augmented in highly metastatic tumor cells and in endothelial cells during angiogenesis. Antibodies prepared against type IV collagenase react with invading breast carcinoma cells and breast carcinoma lymph node metastases by immunohistology. Amplification of type IV collagenase production is biochemically linked to the genetic induction of metastases in experimental models [28].

Molecular Genetics of Metastasis

It is apparent that interactions in the complicated metastatic process involve multiple gene products. A cascade or coordinated group of gene products expressed above a certain threshold level may be required for a tumor cell to successfully traverse the successive steps in the metastatic process. The crucial gene products may regulate host immune recognition of the tumor cells, cell growth, attachment, proteolysis, locomotion, and differentiation. The specific family of gene products necessary for metastasis may be different for each histologic type of tumor.

The evidence linking oncogenes to the induction or maintenance of human malignancies has become increasingly compelling. In the past, oncogenes have been linked to unrestrained tumor growth. Recently, two different types of experimental approaches [5, 28, 29] have indicated that certain classes or combinations of oncogenes may play a role in the metastatic behavior of tumors. In the first type of experimental approach, human tumor DNA samples are surveyed for the level of oncogene expression, and this is correlated with disease stage. In the second type of approach, tumor DNA or isolated oncogenes are transfected into recipient cells. The transfected cells are then studied for their metastatic propensity. Notable examples of these two approaches are work with the *HER-2/neu* oncogene in human breast cancer [29] and transfection of the *ras* oncogene in rodent systems [28].

The *HER-2/neu* (*neu*) oncogene (also termed *c-erbB-2* and *HER-2*) encodes a

394

protein which is a member of the tyrosine kinase family, and it is related to, but distinct from, the epidermal growth factor (EGF) receptor gene. At the time of writing, the ligand for the *neu* oncogene-encoded receptor protein has not yet been identified. A significant increase in the incidence of *neu* gene amplification is noted in breast cancer patients with more than three axillary lymph nodes positive for metastases. Amplification of *neu* is also highly correlated with disease relapse (actuarial survival), as well as tumor size. Thus, even though the function of *neu* is unknown, its level of expression may provide important prognostic information for breast cancer.

Transfection of members of the *ras* oncogene family into suitable rodent recipient cells, including diploid rat embryo fibroblasts, can induce these cells to progress rapidly to express the complete metastatic phenotype [5, 28]. Other oncogenes—including *myc*, *src*, and *fos*—failed to induce metastases in rodent cells. Furthermore, when *ras* was transfected in combination with the adenovirus type 2 *E1A* oncogene, the recipient cells became very tumorigenic but totally nonmetastatic [28]. Thus, some genes can suppress the ability of *ras* to induce metastases. The current working hypothesis is that induction of the metastatic phenotype requires at least two (and possibly more) complementary genes or gene products. In the correct rodent cells, one of these genes may be the activated form of the *ras* oncogene. When these genes interact in the correct fashion, a cascade of specific gene products which confer the metastatic phenotype is elaborated.

New Strategies for Metastasis Diagnosis and Therapy

The elucidation of the biochemical and genetic mechanisms which play a role in cancer metastasis (Table 1) have led to new strategies for cancer diagnosis and therapy. Obviously, normal host parenchymal cells do not invade and metastasize. Thus the biochemical changes which are expressed in the malignant phenotype may provide a target for strategies which are more selective for tumor cells compared to conventional cytotoxic agents.

The most immediate application of these basic research findings is in the area of tumor diagnosis and prognosis. The clinical aggressiveness of a patient's individual tumor could be more accurately predicted by the measurement of genes or gene products functionally associated with the phenotype of invasion and metastases. These include oncogenes such as *ras*, *myc*, *neu*, newly discovered genes which may be associated with suppression of the metastatic phenotype [30], and genes which encode receptors, proteinases and motility factors associated with invasion. The average levels of such metastasis markers could be measured in a sample of the patient's tumor tissue. On the other hand, antibodies or genetic probes for the markers could be applied to a histologic section of the tumor to study the tumor cell population distribution of the marker. In this manner the proportion of tumor cells reacting with the marker could be used as an index of the aggressiveness of the tumor. Application of antibodies to metastasis-associated antigens by the surgical pathologist may provide increased accuracy in the identification of micrometastases in lymph nodes. Furthermore, immunohistological applications are not limited to tumor associated antigens. Host antigens may also be altered in the vicinity of the tumor. This is the case for host basement membranes which are locally fragmented or lost in the area of tumor cell invasion [4]. Loss of basement membrane antigens has already proved to be very useful for the detection of breast cancer microinvasion and in the grading and staging of colorectal tumors [31].

Some of the proteins associated with invasion and metastasis are secreted by the tumor cell. Examples are degradative enzymes such as type IV collagenase and heparanase, or hormone-like proteins such as tumor autocrine motility factors and growth factors. Following secretion by the tumor cell, the proteins (whole or as fragments), may accumulate in the blood or urine of the patient. Measurement of the level of the proteins by sensitive immunoassay procedures may be a means to a) detect the existance of occult metastases, b) estimate the body burden of metastatic disease, and c) detect local tumor recurrence. Furthermore, in the case of bladder cancer, the level of the marker in the urine may reflect the invasive stage of the transitional cell carcinoma.

Tumor cell proteins functionally associated with the metastatic phenotype may be quantitatively augmented in tumor cells composing the metastatic foci. Systemically administered antibodies or synthetic ligands which bind to the tumor cell proteins may preferentially accumulate in the metastatic foci, compared to other body sites. This could be of use in the radioscintigraphic detection of clinically occult metastases. Furthermore, if the antibody or ligand is coupled to a toxic agent it may selectively kill the tumor cells in the metastatic foci.

An increased understanding of the mechanisms of tumor cell invasion may lead to the development of pharmacologic agents or strategies which block tumor cell metastasis [32]. In theory, blocking any of the necessary steps for invasion listed in Table 1 could prevent tumor cell invasion and metastasis formation. Tumor angiogenesis may depend on mechanisms similar to cancer invasion, including proteolysis. Consequently an anti-invasion agent may also block tumor angiogenesis. Chronic systemic treatment or local administration with an anti-invasion agent may be clinically useful in the following settings. a) Preventing the transition from in situ to invasive cancer in high risk patients. b) Reduction of local tumor recurrence and invasion following surgical removal of primary tumors. c) Inhibition of metastasis formation by circulating tumor cells disseminated from inoperable primary tumors, metastases, or released during surgical manipulation of the primary tumor.

The ultimate goal of metastasis research would be to develop strategies to selectively eradicate established metastases. This could be based on the targeting of toxic agents to the metastatic foci. However actual killing of the tumor cells in the metastatic foci may not be necessary to prevent the clinical outcome of metastatic disease. Inhibition of the growth of metastases by chronic treatment regimens may achieve the same end. This is a hopeful area for therapy strategies since it has been found that common cellular pathways may be derranged by genetic events, such as increased *ras* expression, in such a way as to increase both the growth and invasion of tumor cells. An example of a common pathway is the inositol phosphate cascade operating through phospholipase C. This pathway may be altered by a number of oncogenes. Agents which normalize this pathway in tumor cells may act to suppress both growth and invasion.

References

1. Sugarbaker EV (1981) Patterns of metastasis in human malignancies. Cancer Biol Rev 2: 235
2. Weiss L, Gilbert HA (1981) Bone metastases. Hall, Boston
3. Schirrmacher V (1985) Cancer metastasis: experimental approaches, theoretical concepts, and impacts for treatment strategies. Adv Cancer Res 43: 1–73
4. Liotta LA (1986) Tumor invasion and metastases—role of the extracellular matrix: Rhoads memorial award lecture. Cancer Res 46: 1–7
5. Nicolson GL (1987) Tumor cell instability, diversification, and progression to the metastatic phenotype: from oncogene to oncofetal expression. Cancer Res 47: 1473
6. Furcht LT (1986) Critical factors controlling angiogenesis: cell products, cell matrix, and growth factors (Editorial). Lab Invest 55: 505
7. Lam WC, Delikatny JE, Orr FW, Wass J, Varani J, Ward PA (1981) The chemotactic response of tumor cells: a model for cancer metastasis. Am J Pathol 104: 69–76
8. McCarthy JB, Basara ML, Palm SL, Sas DF, Furcht LT (1985) Stimulation of haptotaxis and migration of tumor cells by serum spreading factor. Cancer Metastasis Rev 4: 125–152
9. Anzano MA, Roberts AB, Smith JM, Sporn MB, De Larco JE (1983) Sarcoma growth factors from conditioned media of virally transformed cells composed of both type α and type β growth factors. Proc Natl Acad Sci USA 80: 6264–6268
10. Liotta LA, Mandler R, Murano G, Katz DA, Gordon RK, Chiang PK, Schiffmann E (1986) Tumor cell autocrine motility factor. Proc Natl Acad Sci USA 83: 3302–3306
11. Zigmond SH, Hirsch JC (1973) Leukocyte locomotion and chemotaxis. New methods for evaluation, and demonstration of cell-derived chemotactic factor. J Exp Med 137: 387–410
12. Bokoch GM, Gilman AG (1984) Inhibition of receptor-mediated release of arachidonic acid by pertussis toxin. Cell 39: 301–308
13. Smith CD, Cox CC, Snyderman R (1986) Receptor-coupled activation of phosphoinositide-specific phospholipase C by an N protein. Science 232: 97–100
14. Stracke ML, Guirguis R, Liotta LA, Schiffmann E (1987) Pertussis toxin inhibits stimulated motility independently of the adenylate cyclase pathway in human melanoma cells. Biochem Biophys Res Commun 146: 339–345
15. Katada T, Ui M (1982) Direct modification of the membrane adenylate cyclase system by islet-activating protein due to ADP-ribosylation of a membrane protein. Proc Natl Acad Sci USA 79: 3129–3133
16. Okajima F, Ui M (1984) ADP-ribosylation of the specific membrane protein by islet-activating protein, pertussis toxin, associated with inhibition of a chemotactic peptide-induced arachidonate release in neutrophils. A possible role of the toxin substrate in Ca^{2+}-mobilizing biosignaling. J Biol Chem 259: 13863–13871
17. Kikuchi A, Kozawa O, Kaibuchi K, Katada T, Ui M, Takai Y (1986) Direct evidence for involvement of a guanine nucleotide-binding protein in chemotactic peptide-stimulated formation of inositol bisphosphate and trisphosphate in differentiated human leukemia (HL-60) cells. Reconstitution with Gi or Go of the plasma membranes ADP-ribosylated by pertussis toxin. J Biol Chem 261: 11558–11562

18. Hescheler J, Rosenthal W, Trautwein W, Schultz G (1987) The GTP-binding protein, Go, regulates neuronal calcium channels. Nature 325: 445–447
19. Molski TF, Naccache PH, Marsh ML, Kermode J, Becker EL, Sha'afi RI (1984) Pertussis toxin inhibits the rise in the intracellular concentration of free calcium that is induced by chemotactic factors in rabbit neutrophils: possible role of the "G proteins" in calcium mobilization. Biochem Biophys Res Commun 124: 644–650
20. Lad PM, Olson CV, Grewal IS, Scott SJ (1985) A pertussis toxin-sensitive GTP-binding protein in the human neutrophil regulates multiple receptors, calcium mobilization, and lectin-induced capping. Proc Natl Acad Sci USA 82: 8643–8647
21. Guranowski A, Montgomery JA, Cantoni GL, Chiang PK (1981) Adenosine analogues as substrates and inhibitors of S-adenosylhomocysteine hydrolase. Biochemistry 20: 110–115
22. Boike GM, Sloane BF, Deppe G, Stracke M, Schiffmann E, Liotta LA, Honn Kv (1987) The role of calcium and arachidonic acid metabolism in the chemotaxis of a new tumor line. Am Assoc Cancer Res 28: 82
23. He XM, Fligiel SE, Varani J (1986) Modulation of tumor cell motility by prostaglandins and inhibitors of prostaglandin synthesis. Exp Cell Biol 54: 128–137
24. Pontremoli S, Melloni E, Michetti M, Sacco O, Salamino F, Separatore B, Horecker BL (1986) Biochemical responses in activated human neutrophils mediated by protein kinase C and a Ca^{2+}-requiring proteinase. J Biol Chem 261: 8309–8313
25. Guirguis R, Margulies I, Taraboletti G, Schiffmann E, Liotta L (1987) Cytokine-induced pseudopodial protrusion is coupled to tumour cell migration. Nature 329: 261–263
26. Wewer UM, Liotta LA, Jaye M, Ricca GA, Drohan WN, Claysmith AP, Rao CN, et al. (1986) Altered levels of laminin receptor mRNA in various human carcinoma cells that have different abilities to bind laminin. Proc Natl Acad Sci USA 83: 7137–7141
27. Hynes RO (1987) Integrins: a family of cell surface receptos. Cell 48: 549
28. Garbisa S, Pozzatti R, Muschel RJ, Saffiotti U, Ballin M, Goldfarb RH, Khoury G, Liotta LA (1987) Secretion of type IV collagenolytic protease and metastatic phenotype: induction by transfection with c-Ha-ras but not c-Ha-ras plus Ad2-E1a. Cancer Res 47: 1523–1528
29. Slamon DJ, Clark GM, Wong SG, et al. (1987) Human breast cancer: correlation of relapse and survival with amplification of the HER-2/neu oncogene. Science 235: 177
30. Steeg PS, Bevilacqua G, Kopper L, Thorgeirsson UP, Talmadge JE, Liotta LA, Sobel ME (1988) Evidence for a novel gene associated with low metastatic potential. J Natl Cancer Inst 80: 200–204
31. Forster SJ, Talbot IC, Critchley DR (1984) Laminin and fibronectin in rectal adenocarcinoma: Relationship to tumour grade, stage and metastasis. Br J Cancer 50: 51–59
32. McCarthy J, Skubitz A, Palm S, Furcht L (1988) Metastasis inhibition of different tumor types by purified laminin fragments and a heparin-binding fragment of fibronectin. J Natl Cancer Inst 80: 108–116

21. Prospects for the Development of Antineoplastic Therapy Based on Molecular Pathology

I.T. Magrath

The Genetic Basis of Neoplasia

It is only in recent years that it has become apparent that neoplasia is frequently, and perhaps invariably, a consequence of somatic genetic aberrations [1–3]. The earliest evidence for this was provided by the demonstration of chromosomal abnormalities in hemopoietic neoplasms, which are more readily subjected to karyotypic analysis than other neoplasms [4]. With improvements in the methodology of cytogenetics, neoplasms of all kinds have been shown to be associated with non-random chromosomal abnormalities. Cytogenetic analysis can detect, however, only gross structual changes in chromosomes, and the presence of multiple karyotypic abnormalities can sometimes obscure the primary genetic abnormality. In such circumstances, if the molecular consequences of the karyotypic abnormalities have been identified (e.g., in 14;18 translocations [5]), molecular analysis may increase the likelihood of detecting genetic changes. Knowledge of the molecular changes associated with specific cytogenetic abnormalities is, of course, essential to the elucidation of the functional results of the genetic rearrangements. Moreover, many relevant genetic changes may be sufficiently subtle not to be detectable by cytogenetic analysis (e.g., mutation in a gene such as may occur in Wilms' tumor or retinoblastoma). This new discipline, molecular pathology, is likely to become of increasing value in establishing a diagnosis. In fact, it seems entirely appropriate that definitions of individual tumors should ultimately be based upon structural genetic changes or their functional consequences. This is fast becoming a reality for chronic myeloid leukemia and Burkitt's lymphoma, both of which are associated with chromosomal translocations which have been analyzed in detail, and which can be further subdivided according to the position of the chromosomal breakpoints, ascertained by molecular biological techniques [6, 7].

Whereas the concept of neoplasia as a cellular disorder caused by structural genetic changes is useful, a further level of refinement is necessary and, once again, insights presently come almost exclusively from the lympho-hematopoietic system. Since the genetic changes must involve relevant cellular processes, namely proliferation and/or differentiation, they must also cause a degree of functional change in the cell itself that minimizes or nullifies the normal external mechanisms of control of these vital processes (i.e., growth and differentiation factors produced by other cells). In circumstances where

399

such mechanisms are intrinsically dysfunctional, e.g., in immunodeficiency syndromes, inappropriate cellular proliferation (of specific classes of lymphoid cells in the example given) may occur in the absence of a genetic defect. A conceptually intermediate situation is that in which viral infection of a cell increases its proliferative potential. Technically, virus infections can cause structural genetic changes (in as much as integration of viral or proviral genomes into cellular DNA occurs) and may induced cellular proliferation. This occurs in Epstein–Barr virus (EBV) and HTLV I infection, both of which are associated with benign, self-limited proliferations of lymphocytes (B and T cells respectively). Normally EBV infection does not cause neoplasia (although it may predispose to it in special circumstances), but in the presence of an impairment of the mechanisms responsible for the regulation of B-cell proliferation, B cells carrying EBV genomes may escape from control and give rise to a localized or generalized lymphoproliferative process which may be sufficiently severe as to cause death, e.g., fatal infectious mononucleosis [8]. Whether or not such cellular proliferations are considered to be truly neoplastic is a semantic debate, but there are important consequences of these differences in pathogenesis. For example, genetically normal cellular proliferation is likely to be polyclonal and can, theoretically, be reversed if the regulatory defect can be corrected. Neoplasia arising as a consequence of a genetic change, on the other hand, is almost always monoclonal, occasionally oligoclonal, and so far, with rare exceptions, has appeared to be irreversible (i.e., deletion of the neoplastic clone must be accomplished if cure is to be achieved). Although the mechanisms leading to cellular proliferation are very different—respectively extrinsic and intrinsic to the cell in question—the development of monoclonal tumors from initially polyclonal lymphoproliferative processes has been observed [9]. This suggests that deregulated, but not truly neoplastic cellular proliferation may predispose to the development of specific genetic abnormalities in an individual cell in the population, giving rise to a monoclonal neoplasm. In fact, many neoplasms are preceded by hyperplasia or metaplasia of the target cell population, a finding consistent with this possibility. Immunoblastic lymphomas occur with increased frequency (as much as several hundredfold) in immunodeficiency syndromes (including AIDS), immunoblastic lymphadenopathy and α-heavy chain disease, in all of which there is lymphoid hyperplasia [10]. Environmental stimuli may also induce lymphoproliferation which predisposes to lymphoma. For example, EBV and malaria, both polyclonal B-cell activators, appear to increase the likelihood of Burkitt's lymphoma developing in African children [11]. Pre-existing hyperplasia or metaplasia, often a consequence of chronic inflammation, usually precedes colon cancer (superimposed upon polyps or ulcerative colitis), bilharzial bladder cancer, uterine cervical cancer, hepatoma, mouth, esophageal and possibly stomach cancers [12, 13].

Factors Influencing the Location of Chromosomal Breakpoints

Although the reason for the predisposition of hyperplastic cell populations towards cancer is not known, it seems probable that it is a result of an increased likelihood of a genetic change occurring during DNA replication as a consequence either of the increased mitotic rate or greater number of replication cycles of a specific cell subpopulation. The role played in pathogenesis by decreased genomic stability (i.e., the frequency of occurrence of cytogenetic abnormalities), which appears to be a general feature of cancer cells, is unclear, although defective DNA repair systems appear to predispose to cancer in some circumstances, e.g., murine plasmacytoma and several inherited disorders in humans [8, 14]. To a degree, genetic changes may occur at random. However, chromosomal regions have been identified at which breaks are more likely to occur (so-called "fragile sites") and which are the sites of breakpoints in neoplastic cells bearing translocations or deletions much more often than is explicable on the basis of a totally random process [15]. It also appears that "active areas" of the genome, i.e., regions where transcription is occurring, are at greater risk for chromosomal breakage. In such areas, altered chromatin structure (i.e., an alteration in the location of bound histones and nonhistone proteins as well as a change in the "packaging" of DNA within the nuclear matrix) occurs in order for RNA polymerases to have access to promoter regions. This may well greatly increase the possibility of DNA breakage at these sites. The general relationship between active regions of the chromosome and fragile sites has not been definitively demonstrated, although for individual genes these sites are known to coincide.

Cell differentiation, with consequent expression (and even rearrangement) of specific genes and essentially permanent suppression of others, probably influences quite markedly the likelihood of genetic changes occurring at specific locations in the DNA, so that particular cell lineages may be predisposed towards breakpoints occurring at specific chromosomal sites. Only some of these genetic changes, however, will give rise to neoplastic growth, and this may well be the explanation for the finding of a limited number of chromosomal regions at which breakpoints are observed in cancer cells. These regions probably include genes involved in proliferation, differentiation, or cellular migration.

Involvement of Lineage-Associated Genes

Another factor which influences the location of chromosomal breakpoints is operative in lymphoid cells, which undergo rearrangement of their antigen receptor genes as a part of normal differentiation, a process whereby antigen receptor diversity is generated. The frequency with which immunoglobulin genes are involved in the specific translocations observed in B-cell tumors [4, 11, 16] and T-cell antigen receptor genes in T-cell lymphoid neoplasms [17–19] is unlikely to be a chance phenomenon. While these genetic loci may simply be more fragile, due to their obligate activity, an additional potentially contributory factor is that during the process of antigen receptor gene recombination, the DNA molecule must be broken and religated. At least some translocations probably arise as a consequence of mistakes occurring during this process, and hence are probably mediated by the recombinases which normally control antigen receptor gene recombination. This is supported by the finding that some of the translocations occurring in B-cell and T-cell neoplasms have been shown to have breakpoints in regions where site-specific recombinations occur during normal cell differentiation, namely adjacent to the signal sequences (heptamers and nonamers separated by 12 or 23 nucleotides) known to be necessary for normal VJ and VDJ joining [20].

Oncogenes

Another group of genes frequently (possibly invariably) involved in the cytogenetic aberrations associated with neoplasia are the proto-oncogenes. These genes are conserved throughout evolution, sometimes with a surprising degree of precision, and appear to be involved in essential cellular processes such as proliferation and differentiation [21, 22]. Proto-oncogene products may be growth factors, growth factor and other cell surface receptors (which often encode a specific protein kinase activity which phosphorylates tyrosine residues), and molecules involved in the transmission (transduction) of signals from the cell surface to the cell nucleus. It is not surprising, therefore, that evidence of the "activation" of proto-oncogenes has been obtained in a variety of neoplasms. Activation in this context implies altered regulation, a modification of function or increased expression of the gene compared to the normal counterpart cells of the neoplasm (which in many cases have not been identified). The mechanisms whereby this may be brought about are numerous, including mutation, translocation, and amplification (Table 1).

Table 1. Mechanisms of proto-oncogene activation in human tumors

Mechanism	Consequence	Examples	Oncogene
Translocation	Structural/functional change and/or altered regulation	Burkitt's lymphoma	c-*myc*
		Chronic myeloid leukemia (CML)	c-*abl*
Mutation	Functional change	Bladder cancer	H-*ras*
		Lung cancer	K-*ras*
		Breast cancer	N-*ras*
		Stomach cancer	
		Liver cancer	
Insertional mutagenesis	Activation of transcription	T-cell leukemia	Il-2[a]
Amplification	Elevated mRNA level	Lung cancer	*myc*[b]
		Breast cancer	*neu*
		Neuroblastoma	N-*myc*
Recessive mutations	Loss of function Lack of suppression?	Retinoblastoma	?
		Osteosarcoma	
		Wilms' tumor	
		Bladder cancer	
		Acoustic neuroma	

[a] Il-2 is not normally considered to be an oncogene, but is a growth factor. Enhanced expression in T-cell leukemias and lymphomas is induced by transactivating factors rather than cis activation of a nearby gene. This may be a premalignant rather than truly malignant lesion
[b] This includes N-*myc*, c-*myc* and L-*myc*

Chromosomal translocations in hemopoietic cells often involve a lineage specific gene (e.g., an immunoglobulin or T-cell receptor gene), or at least a gene which is obligately expressed in the cell lineage, and a proto-oncogene, each being initially on a different chromosome, but brought into proximity by the chromosomal translocation. The best examples of this are Burkitt's lymphoma and chronic myeloid leukemia [11, 23, 24]. In each case, although the mechanisms differ, the translocation appears to result in the regulation of a proto-oncogene (respectively c-*myc* and c-*abl*) as if it were a lineage-specific or associated gene (respectively an immunoglobulin gene and *bcr*).

In a number of neoplasms (e.g., retinoblastoma, osteosarcoma, Wilms' tumor, rhabdomyosarcoma, bladder carcinoma, acoustic neuroma, and possibly one form of acute lymphoblastic leukemia) where nullizygosity (i.e., complete absence) for a specific gene locus appears to be of pathogenetic significance, it has been suggested that the missing gene function is normally responsible for suppressing a second gene (presumptively a proto-oncogene). Nullizygosity or two mutations causing absence of function of both alleles would therefore permit over-expression or inappropriate expression of the second (onco-) gene [22, 25–27]. Frequently, reduplication of the allelic chromosome which lacks the repressor gene occurs, so that the loss of the normal chromosome may be masked. If nullizygosity or mutation in both alleles does result in the loss of repressor genes, there is no a priori reason to believe that the involved chromosomal region bears lineage-specific genes. Since, however, constitutive chromosomal abnormalities which predispose to neoplasia tend to be associated with neoplasms of specific organs (e.g., the eye or the kidney), it has been suggested that the involved chromosomal regions are concerned with the growth and development of the organ in question. While this may be so, it seems unlikely that such genes are relevent to only a single tissue. Patients with the familial form of retinoblastoma, for example, are also predisposed towards other neoplasms, particularly osteosarcoma [22, 28], in which identical genetic findings have been observed, although the latter tumor occurs at an older age.

Significance of Molecular Pathogenesis to Therapy

Until now, all approaches to cancer therapy have focused upon the eradication of neoplastic cells. Furthermore, the methods utilized in this process of eradication have taken no account of how the neoplasm arose. Clearly, knowledge of etiology and pathogenesis can lead to the development of preventive measures, e.g., avoidance of tobacco—perhaps the greatest single environmental cause of cancer in the world. It is less obvious how a knowledge of etiology and pathogenesis can lead to new approaches to therapy. Nonetheless, knowledge of the molecular mechanisms of oncogenesis is likely to provide otherwise inaccessible insights into potential approaches to overcoming the effects of the genetic abnormality, or to provide a target for therapeutic measures. It is worth nothing that the presence of the genetic abnormality in the neoplastic cells confers a unique characteristic upon them. As such, this could be the key to the development of highly specific therapy.

At the present time the enormous potential of approaches aimed at the biochemical abnormalities of cancer cells cannot be realized. Much more information needs to be obtained regarding the mechanisms and regulation of normal cellular differentiation and proliferation and the nature of the abnormalities of these process in cancer cells. Yet it seems inevitable that future approaches to cancer treatment will be derived more and more from a knowledge of pathogenetic mechanisms, i.e., the disorders of oncogene expression associated with specific types of cancer. It is therefore worth considering, albeit of necessity from an inadequate vantage point, what kinds of new approaches to cancer treatment can be contemplated at the present time or in the future, utilizing available information regarding the molecular pathogenesis of neoplasia.

The Possibility of Reversal of the Malignant Phenotype

The concept of correcting or bypassing a cellular abnormality resulting from a somatic genetic change is not new. Inherited enzyme deficiencies have been corrected by supplying the errant molecule (e.g., adenosine deaminase by blood transfusion), and congenital immunodeficiencies and enzyme deficiencies have been effectively treated by allogeneic bone marrow transplantation, thereby providing a new population of potentially immunocompetent stem cells or enzyme-replete hemopoietic cells. However, the replacement of a missing molecule or cell type is a similar and more readily accomplished objective than the restoration of an extremely complex intracellular biochemical equilibrium, disturbed because of enhanced or reduced function of one or more of the elements of the balance. The probability that neoplasia is the consequence of not one, but several genetic derangements, i.e., that progression from a normal to a highly invasive neoplastic cell takes place in a series of steps, possibly involving different pathways, renders the concept of phenotypic reversal the more daunting. It may not be necessary, however, to correct multiple abnormalities. The possibility exists that one or more of the most crucial changes, such as indefinite proliferation or metastatic potential, can be nullified or bypassed, such that the cell, though possibly not totally normal, is no longer neoplastic. In fact, this objective appears to have been accomplished in vitro already, albeit temporarily, in cells expressing mutated *ras* oncogenes [29, 30].

For the purposes of discussion, it is helpful to consider potential intervention measures at two levels. The first level involves a general approach in which an attempt is made to circumvent abnormalities of differentiation and/or proliferation (under one or both of which headings, it would appear, all neoplasms must fall) and metastasis. The second level includes direct intervention with respect to the abnormal functioning of specific oncogenes.

404

Nonspecific Therapeutic Approaches Directed Towards Molecular Abnormalities

The two quintessential characteristics of malignant neoplasia are abnormal accumulation of a specific cell type and invasiveness—i.e., the spread and subsequent proliferation of the neoplastic cells in locations where normal cell counterparts of the neoplastic cell are not found (e.g., secondary brain metastases). Most hemopoietic neoplasms must be thought of in a somewhat different light, since leukocytes, by virtue of their normal functions, naturally migrate to practically all parts of the body. Therefore, in the context of the hemopoietic system, the characteristic of "invasiveness" is not necessarily peculiar to the neoplastic state. Abnormal accumulation alone may be sufficient to account for the clinical manifestations of leukemias and lymphomas, although the tendency to form solid masses, as opposed to a diffusely infiltrating process, and, possibly, involvement of the meninges, may be the consequences of subtle genetic variations in the neoplastic cells. The development of the attribute of "invasiveness" in solid tumors is probably, at least in some cancers, the result of tumor progression, i.e., the accumulation of additional genetic abnormalities beyond those which are essential to the growth of the tumor locally.

These characteristics—proliferation and invasion—are not totally aberrant forms of cell behavior, but simply misplaced; immature cells, for example, manifest both characteristics (tissue migration is an essential component of embryogenesis), and the special case of hematopoietic cells has already been mentioned. Many other cell types undergo continuous self-renewal throughout the life of the organism. In most circumstances, however, proliferation is incompatible with terminal differentiation, so that tumor cells, or at least the proliferating cells within the tumor, remain in a less differentiated state. It is clear even from a consideration of purely morphological characteristics—and more so when phenotype is also examined biochemically or immunologically—that many neoplasms, particularly those of children, manifest the characteristics of immature ore precursor cells, e.g., embryonal rhabdomyosarcoma, pre-B-cell and immature T-cell leukemias and lymphomas, neuroblastoma, medulloblastoma, etc. In neoplastic cells, the regulation of the processes of proliferation, differentiation, and invasion is defective with respect to their counterpart cells *in their normal tissue environment*. Theoretically, the same genetic change in a cell could sometimes result in neoplastic behavior in one environment, and normal or only slightly abnormal behavior in another. Mouse teratocarcinoma cells implanted into a blastocyst, for example, can differentiate quite normally [31]. This, coupled to the observation that neoplastic cells can be induced to differentiate in vitro [32–34] provides grounds for optimism that it may prove possible to reverse, by biochemical means, the basic attributes of neoplastic cells. The reversal of a block to differentiation, the inhibition of unbounded proliferation, and the prevention of metastases represent treatment strategies which are not conceptually new, but have only recently become realistic beyond an empirical level because of new knowledge of the biochemistry of these processes.

Correction of a Differentiation Defect

New information has become available which indicates that some chemotherapeutic agents may induce differentiation. Ara-C(Cytarabine), anthracyclines, and numerous other compounds, discussed elsewhere in this book, have been shown to have potent differentiation-inducing properties in vitro [32–34]. Further, a number of factors produced by normal cells have been identified to be potent inducers of differentiation, particularly in hemopoietic cells. These include various "colony stimulating" factors, identified through in vitro marrow culture systems, interferons (e.g., γ-interferon) and B-cell differentiation-inducing factor [35, 36]. The induction of differentiation as a therapeutic manipulation therefore holds promise [34], and although empirical attempts to induce differentiation may be successful, such an approach is more likely to succeed when the precise defect in differentiation is known. It is possible that the abnormal maintenance of a proliferative state may inhibit differentiation. The c-*myc* gene, for example, which is necessary for proliferation in most cell types appears to inhibit the differentiation of Friend erythroleukemia [37]. Other possible causes of differentiation failure include lack of one or more differentiation factors (an unlikely event unless the normal counterpart cell produces its own differentiation factor, which the tumor cell fails to do), lack of differentiation factor receptors, a defect in signal transduction from the receptor to the cell nucleus, and altered expression of genes which are responsible for confering the differentiated phenotype on a cell. These various defects could theoretically be replaced by provision of a missing or defective molecule (e.g., by synthesis through recombinant DNA technology), by production of a drug (e.g., a peptide with similar effects on the cell to the missing factor), by means of a monoclonal antibody which binds to and activates the differentiation factor receptor, or even by the raising of an anti-idiotypic antibody against a monoclonal antibody specific for the growth factor. Such anti-idiotypic molecules resemble the structure of the original antigen and may have functional properties [38, 39]. Where the defect lies in the cell itself (e.g., in a receptor or transducing molecule), replacement is a more formidable problem, and a more practicable approach would be to bypass the need for such molecules by means of appropriate drugs capable of interacting within the cell at a step in the biochemical pathway beyond that at which the defect lies, e.g., with protein kinase C. Differentiation in some in vitro systems is believed to be induced by phorbol esters by this route [40], although phorbol esters could not be used clinically because of their tumor-promoting activity. A more exotic approach might be to consider the use of recombinant molecules which mimic activated differentiation factor receptors. This is similar in concept to the causation of neoplastic proliferation by molecules such as the *erb*-B oncogene, which is a truncated epidermal growth factor receptor (EGFR) lacking the ligand binding region and probably represents a permanently activated growth factor receptor [41]. A potential difficulty, but not necessarily an insurmountable problem with such an approach would be the need to ensure intracellular penetration.

In spite of the potential problems associated with the use of differentiation-inducing agents, a number of attempts to induce differentiation in human tumors—mostly leukemias—have been made. Retinoids, for example, have induced remission in patients with acute promyelocytic leukemia, and reports of low-dose Ara-C inducing remission in acute myeloid leukemia or pre-leukemia have been published [42]. One difficulty with interpreting these results is the inability to determine whether remission was truly induced by virtue of differentiation induction, or whether some other mechanism led to the destruction of neoplastic cells [43]. However, in view of its potential importance, the induction of differentiation in neoplastic cells as a therapeutic modality is discussed further by Glazer (this volume).

Prevention of Neoplastic Proliferation

Another approach to the correction of neoplastic behavior is to directly influence the ability of the cell to proliferate. Inhibition of proliferation is one objective of a number of empirical clinical trials currently underway and discussed elsewhere in this book, listed generally under the title of "biological response modification." Such approaches utilize "cytokines" such as interferons and tumor necrosis factor which may inhibit growth or even cause cell death. In general, however, the use of cytokines is not directed towards recognized cellular pathology relevant to oncogenesis. The possible strategies which could be employed, other than the use of cytokines, are very similar to those discussed in the context of differentiation induction, since proliferation similarly involves the binding of growth factors to surface receptors followed by activation and signal transduction to the cell nucleus (Fig. 1). The fact that different tissues appear to utilize at least some factors and receptors specific to the tissue may permit the achievement of selectivity. Antibodies directed towards a growth factor or its receptor (with the goal of using such antibodies to prevent binding of the growth factor to its receptor) can be either highly nonspecific, e.g., via transferrin receptor-specific antibodies [44] or much more specific, as in the use of bombesin-specific antibodies in small-cell lung cancer [45]. Perhaps the most specific approaches which can be envisaged are those directed towards oncogenes relevent to proliferation which have been activated in specific cancers (see below).

Prevention of Metastasis

The complex process whereby a malignant cell spreads from its original location is discussed in detail by Liotta et al. (this volume). Knowledge of the biochemistry of this process permits the consideration of several approaches directed to-

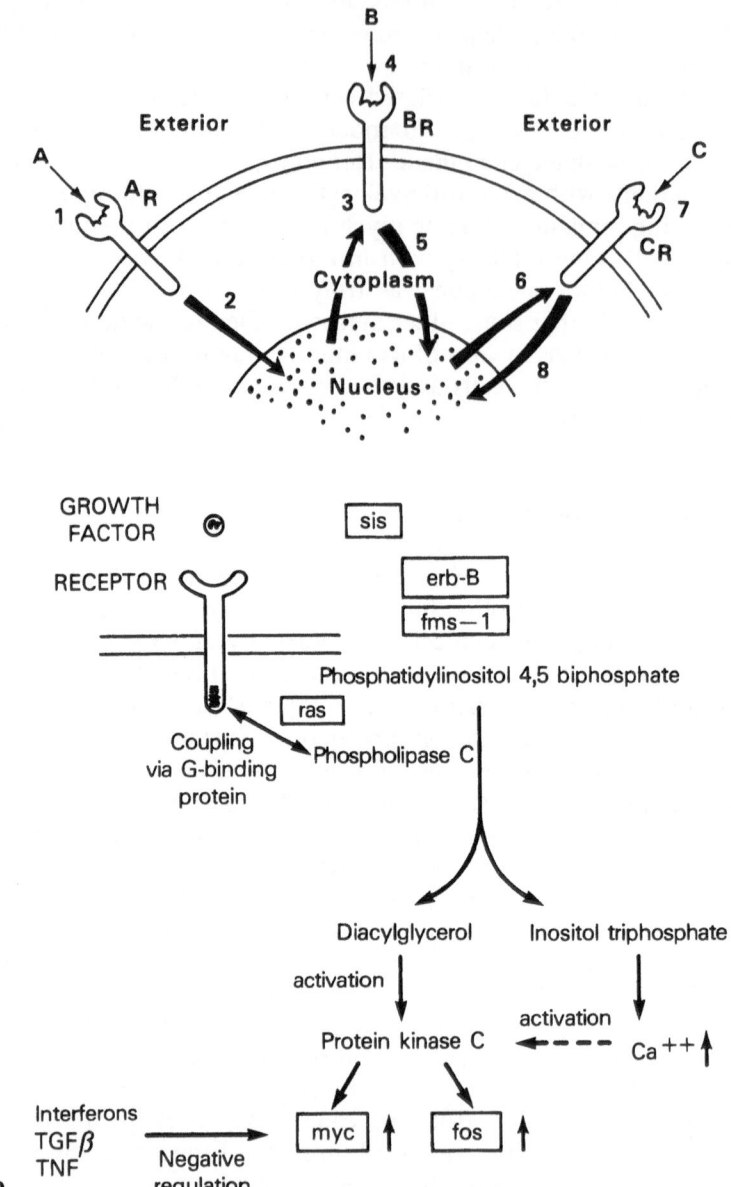

Fig. 1. a Schematic depiction of the proliferation receptor cascade. For a resting cell to enter a proliferative phase (i.e., pass from G0 to G1 and S phase), a sequence of events (1 through 8) is necessary. The binding of ligand *A* to its receptor (A_R) results in the expression of a new receptor B_R, to which ligand *B* will bind, stimulating the expression of receptor C_R. In this illustration, the binding of ligand *C* to C_R is the final initiating event for passage from G0 to G1. In normal T-lymphocytes, for example, antigen binding to the antigen receptor complex triggers the expression of a series of activation antigens, including interleukin-2 receptor. Interleukin-2 binding in turn stimulates the expression of other receptors, including that for transferrin, with the ultimate consequence being cellular proliferation. Similar cascades have been described in other cell types, including B-

408

wards the specific pathways involved, including the prevention of the binding of tumor cells to basement membrance or impairment of their ability to lyse intercellular matrix. The relationship of amplification of the HER-2/*neu* oncogene to axillary lymph node metastasis in human breast cancer, and *ras* oncogenes to the development of the metastatic phenotype in rodent cells, provides optimism that in the future it may be possible to direct antimetastatic therapy towards specific cancers. The HER-2/*neu* gene is a member of the tyrosine kinase family which includes a number of cell surface receptors, raising the possibility that inhibition of tyrosine kinase activity may, in some tumors, impair metastatic potential. It will clearly be critically important to elucidate the precise actions of this gene in breast cancer cells if more specific therapy is to be employed. Therapy targeted towards the *ras* family of oncogenes is discussed below.

The prevention of metastases could have a therapeutic role in localised tumors or tumors with limited spread; it would justify exhaustive efforts to deal with all known sites of disease by local measures and could limit the appearance of subsequent metastases to those already present subclinically.

Therapeutic Approaches Directed Against Specific Oncogenes

It seems highly probable, as information accumulates regarding the specific actions of oncogene products and the precise disorders of oncogene expression associated with various types of cancer, that therapeutic measures directed towards individual oncogenes or their products may become a reality (Table 2). At the present time it is not possible to envision in any detail the form that such future therapeutic interventions will take, nor whether they can provide primary treatment or will be ancillary to other treatment approaches. In some cases it is not even certain that the observed changes in oncogenes are of primary pathogenetic importance [45]. However, it is difficult to escape the conclusion that altered oncogene expression is of primary importance in some tumors (e.g., Burkitt's lymphoma, chronic myeloid leukemia), and for the purposes of this

---

lymphocytes. **b** Schematic depiction of one of several possible sequences of events which result from binding of a ligand to a receptor, and probable roles of some oncogenes. Ligand binding permits a G protein to bind transiently to the receptor, and thus itself be activated by binding guanosine triphosphate. Activation of phospholipase C generates inositol triphosphate and diacyglycerol from phosphatidylinositol-4,5-biphosphate. Inositol triphosphate leads to the release of intracellularly stored calcium ions, while diacylglycerol activates protein kinase C. Calcium ions may also directly activated protein kinase C. The latter may have, as at least one of its functions, the alteration of Na+/H+ exchange, causing an increase in intracellular pH. Several of these pathways can lead to c-*myc* and c-*fos* expression, as can direct stimulation of protein kinase C by phorbol esters, vasopressin etc. Platelet-derived growth factor seems also to activate c-*myc* expression by a pathway other than that involving diacylglycerol and protein kinase C. Interferons, transforming growth factor β (TGFβ), and tumor necrosis factor (*TNF*) provide negative regulation of c-*myc*. c-*myc* and c-*fos* expression is necessary for the proliferation of most somatic cells.

Table 2. Some potential therapeutic measures directed against oncogenes

Reduction of Transcription
Use of drugs or cloned, biologically produced molecules (BRMs)
Induction of differentiation or impairment of proliferation

Reversal of amplification
Removal of factors selecting for amplification
Use of drugs or BRMs which impair transcription from amplified genes or reverse the process of amplification

Inhibition of translation
Use of antisense oligonucleotides

Inhibition of function of oncogene products
Monoclonal antibodies directed towards specific proteins, including abnormal protein products
Development of drugs designed to inhibit GTP binding to *ras* proteins
Development of anti-tyrosine kinases

Bypass or inhibition of a deranged cellular function
Induction of differentiation by drugs or BRMs
Blockade of growth factor receptors by drugs or monoclonal antibodies
Use of monoclonal antibodies against growth factors to inhibit binding to receptor

Gene therapy (?)
Insertion of appropriate surface receptors (for growth inhibitory or differentiation factors) into tumor cells
Continuous production of antisense oligonucleotides
Insertion of negative regulator of proliferation or specific oncogene expression into tumor cells

---

discussion, it will be assumed that all modifications in oncogene structure, expression, or function are of pathogenetic significance. Although there is much to be learnt, enough information is already available to begin to define at least the general stratagems which might be considered in the future.

As listed in Table 1, several different mechanisms have been identified whereby proto-oncogenes become "activated." Where activation involves sequence alterations in the proto-oncogene leading to an altered gene product, it is difficult to envisage how, short of genetic repair by homologous recombination (see below), such a process could be reversed—not simply in one cell, but in all the cells of a neoplasm. In such circumstances, the oncogene function may need to be blocked, bypassed, or counteracted. On the other hand, increased expression of a normal gene product—in some cases consequent upon gene amplification, as occurs in small-cell carcinoma of the lung, squamous carcinoma, some gliomas, and neural tumors, including retinoblastoma and neuroblastomas [47–49]—may prove, in some cases, to be a reversible phenomenon.

Therapeutic Approaches Directed Towards Amplified Oncogenes

Amplification of chromosomal domains occurs during the life cycles of many different organisms [50] but is rare in mammalian cells, although it may be rel-

410

evant to the evolution of gene families, i.e., genes which are structurally related and appear to have evolved from a single parent gene, presumably by a process of duplication. Examples include the hemoglobins and the immunoglobulin supergene family, encompassing a large number of surface receptors on both T- and B-lymphocytes [51–54]. Some genes, e.g., ribosomal RNA genes, are present in multiple copies in the genome. Gene amplification was first observed in mammalian cells which acquired resistance to methotrexate, by amplification of the enzyme dihydrofolate reductase (DHFR) [55]. It appears that in the case of drug resistance, increased transcription precedes gene amplification, and that the degree of amplification and the associated increases in transcription are dependent upon the degree of selective pressure to which the cell is exposed (see Fojo, this volume). Amplification may, however, be reversed once the selective pressure is removed.

The presence of amplified chromosomal regions encompassing oncogenes in a variety of tumors is likely to have etiological significance in some cases, but may also be associated with tumor progression, as appears to be the case with amplification of HER-2/*neu* in breast cancer [47]. Similarly, in neuroblastoma, amplification correlates with clinical stage and prognosis and is absent in most patients with early-stage disease [49]. It will be important to determine in more detail the similarities and differences between, for example, amplification of the DHFR gene in methotrexate resistance or the multi-drug resistance (MDR) gene in pleiotropic drug resistance and amplification of the N-*myc* oncogene in neuroblastoma or small-cell lung carcinoma. Is there some kind of demonstrable selective pressure in vivo in the latter case? There would appear to be so, since the degree of amplification is stable in multiple tumors in the same patient [56]. Alternatively, might it prove possible, once more is known of the mechanism of amplification, to chemically reverse the process, or alternatively to reduce transcription specifically from genes in an amplified chromosomal region? If the methods developed were specific for newly amplified genes, they would presumably be essentially specific for the tumor cells, because the rapidity and degree of amplification of localized regions of the genome appear to be attributes of tumor cells rather than normal cells [57].

Reduction of the expression of amplified genes is a realistic possibility since it has been shown that in neuroblastoma cell lines bearing amplified N-*myc* genes, levels of N-*myc* messenger RNA are markedly reduced by the induction of differentiation with retinoic acid [58]. A similar observation has been made in the case of the HL60 promyelocytic leukemia cell line, in which an amplified c-*myc* gene is shut off when differentiation is induced [59]. Whether a reduction in the expression of amplified oncogenes in cancer cells, even if it could be readily achieved in vivo, would result in a reversion to a nonmalignant state, or perhaps to a less invasive one, must await the results of further experimental observations. It is of interest, however, as demonstrated in the experiments described above, that amplified genes appear to retain at least some responses to normal regulatory signals. This could prove to be a disadvantage from the perspective of developing specificity to the regulation of oncogenes involved in cancer.

In the case of other oncogenes, a broad variety of mechanisms, frequently involving structural changes, are involved in the altered expression or function

411

of these genes. This provides the potential to develop therapeutic methods specifically targeted towards these structural abnormalities. At present, detailed information regarding the molecular abnormalities involving specific oncogenes is available for only a small number of tumors. These neoplasms will hopefully provide paradigms for the ultimate development of similar approaches in other tumors.

Therapeutic Approaches Directed Towards the Molecular Abnormalities in Burkitt's Lymphoma

Burkitt's lymphoma provides a good example of a neoplasm in which an essential component of pathogenesis is believed to be altered regulation of a protooncogene, in this case c-*myc*. In Burkitt's lymphoma cells the c-*myc* allele on the normal chromosome 8 is not expressed (except to a limited degree in a small number of exceptional Burkitt's lymphoma cell lines), but the translocations which occur in this disease result in the gene involved in the translocation being juxtaposed to an immunoglobulin-constant region (Fig. 2) and inappropriately expressed [7]. The breakpoint on chromosome 8 varies considerably and may be some distance upstream of c-*myc* or actually within the gene itself, although never within the protein coding region for the major gene product (the second

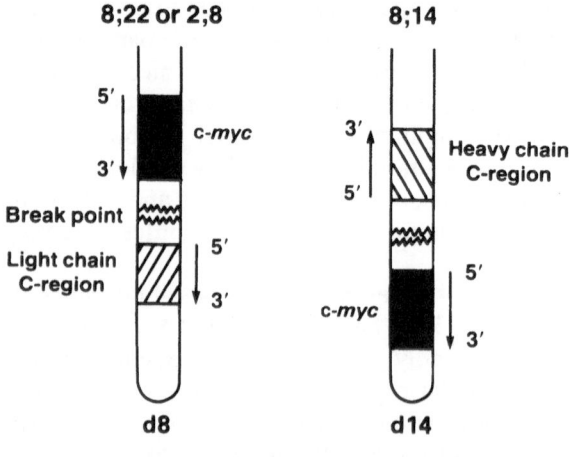

Fig. 2. Schematic depiction of the common feature of the chromosomal translocations in Burkitt's lymphoma. d8 represents the derivative chromosome 8 in 2;8 and 8;22 translocations (the less common "variant" translocations), in which c-*myc* remains on chromosome 8 while light-chain immunoglobulin constant region sequences are translocated distal (3') to c-*myc* from chromosomes 2 (*K*) or 22 (λ). Note that the c-*myc* and translocated immunoglobulin region genes are in the same transcriptional orientation. d14 represents the derivative chromosome 14 in 8;14 (the most common) translocations. Here the c-*myc* gene is translocated from chromosome 8 to a location distal (3') to the heavy chain immunoglobulin sequences which remain on the chromosome (a part of the immunoglobulin heavy-chain sequence is reciprocally translocated to the distal end of chromosome 8)

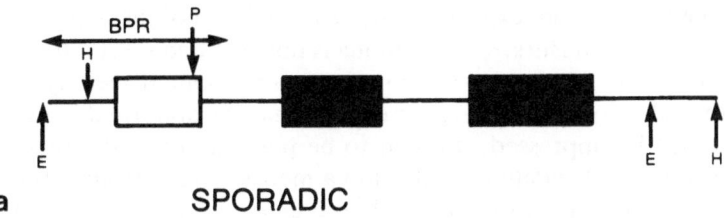

a   SPORADIC

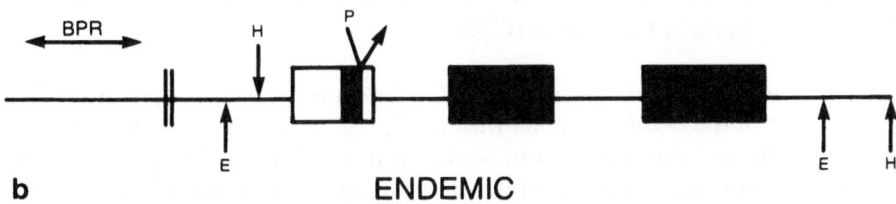

b   ENDEMIC

Fig. 3. Schematic representation of the c-*myc* gene in Burkitt's lymphoma. The exons (i.e., sequence regions represented in cytoplasmic mRNA) of the gene are shown as rectangles, intervening sequences as horizontal lines. The second and third exons are shaded black. Lettered arrows indicate target sequences for restriction endonucleoses (E = ECoRI, H = HindIII, P = PvuII). **a** shows the regions of the gene or its 5′ flanking sequences in which breakpoints occur predominantly in Burkitt's tumor in North America; **b** shows the region upstream of the gene in which the breakpoints occur predominantly in African Burkitt's lymphoma, and the nucleotide sequence abnormalities within the first exon which frequently result in failure of the restriction enzyme PvuII to cut at its target sequence in the first exon. The 5′ flanking region of the gene, and its first exon are believed to be involved in regulation of expression of c-*myc*

and third exons), which is nearly always normal. When the breakpoint is outside the gene there are mutations in the first exon, a region believed to be involved in the regulation of the gene (Fig. 3). It seems probable that these genetic changes result in the gene's being regulated as if it were an immunoglobulin gene, and highly expressed in a cell type in which it should be expressed to a limited extent or not at all. Since c-*myc* is believed to be involved in the proliferation of somatic cells, it is not difficult to envisage how inappropriate expression of c-*myc* can result in or be an integral component of neoplasia. Moreover, if this is the case, inhibition of the expression of c-*myc* in Burkitt's lymphoma could well cause reversion to a nonneoplastic state.

It might be presumed that the abnormal c-*myc* is constitutively expressed and cannot be down-regulated in Burkitt's lymphoma. However, it has been shown that treatment of Daudi cells with various interferons inhibits c-*myc* expression by reducing the half life of c-*myc* messenger RNA [60]. In addition, in somatic cell hybrids between some Burkitt's lymphoma cell lines (but not others) and EBV transformed lymphoblastoid cell lines of normal origin, the translocated c-*myc* gene is not expressed even though the Burkitt's lymphoma cell immunoglobulin genes are expressed [61]. Thus, control of the expression of the abnormal c-*myc* gene in Burkitt's lymphoma is possible and must ultimately have a biochemical basis. Moreover, since in some of the somatic cell hybrids mentioned, the normal c-*myc* allele is expressed, whereas the abnormal c-*myc* gene (of Burkitt's origin) is suppressed, it ought to be possible, once the regulatory mechanisms have been elucidated, to develop a means of specifically influencing the regulation of the expression of the altered c-*myc* gene in Burkitt's lymphoma without affecting the c-*myc* gene of normal cells.

Therapeutic Approaches Directed Towards the Molecular Abnormalities of Chronic Myeloid Leukemia (CML)

The 9;22 chromosomal translocation of CML results in the juxtaposition of most of the exons of the c-*abl* oncogene with the *bcr* gene such that a hybrid transcript initiated at the normal promoter of *bcr* is produced (Fig. 4). This provides potential opportunities for cancer treatment. Although the function of the *bcr* gene is not known, the altered c-*abl* gene in CML is regulated exactly as though it were the *bcr* gene. Moreover, its tyrosine kinase activity appears to have been activated by the structural alterations. Potential therapeutic approaches in CML based on a knowledge of molecular pathology would thus include modification of the transcription of *bcr*, inhibition of the translation of the hybrid *bcr/abl* protein, inhibition of tyrosine kinase activity, or the development of drugs which bind specifically with the fusion protein present in CML, but not with the normal gene product.

Antisense Regulation of Translation

The role of antisense (anticodon) nucleotide sequences, which prevent translation by binding to complementary regions of RNA messages, is worthy of consideration as a potential cancer therapy. This method of gene regulation is used in some bacteria, e.g., to regulate plasmid replication [62], and has been shown to be feasible as a means of altering gene expression in a number of mammalian, including human systems [62–64]. Small oligonucleotides which are readily synthesized can enter viable cells, but relatively inefficiently. Methods of enhancing cell entry will need to be devised if total abrogation of oncogene expression is to be achieved. Liposome encapsulation is one method under exploration. It might also prove possible to couple antisense oligomers to other molecules to increase cell penetration and prevent degradation. Such molecules could also, if appropriately selected, confer a degree of specificity on the system (e.g., the use of molecules, such as monoclonal antibodies, which bind only to B cells). Another approach to increasing the specificity of antisense oligomers is to synthesize them against sequences present only in the transcripts of structurally altered oncogenes. This should be possible for a subset of Burkitt's lymphomas and for the abnormal *bcr/abl* fusion gene resulting from the 9;22 translocation of

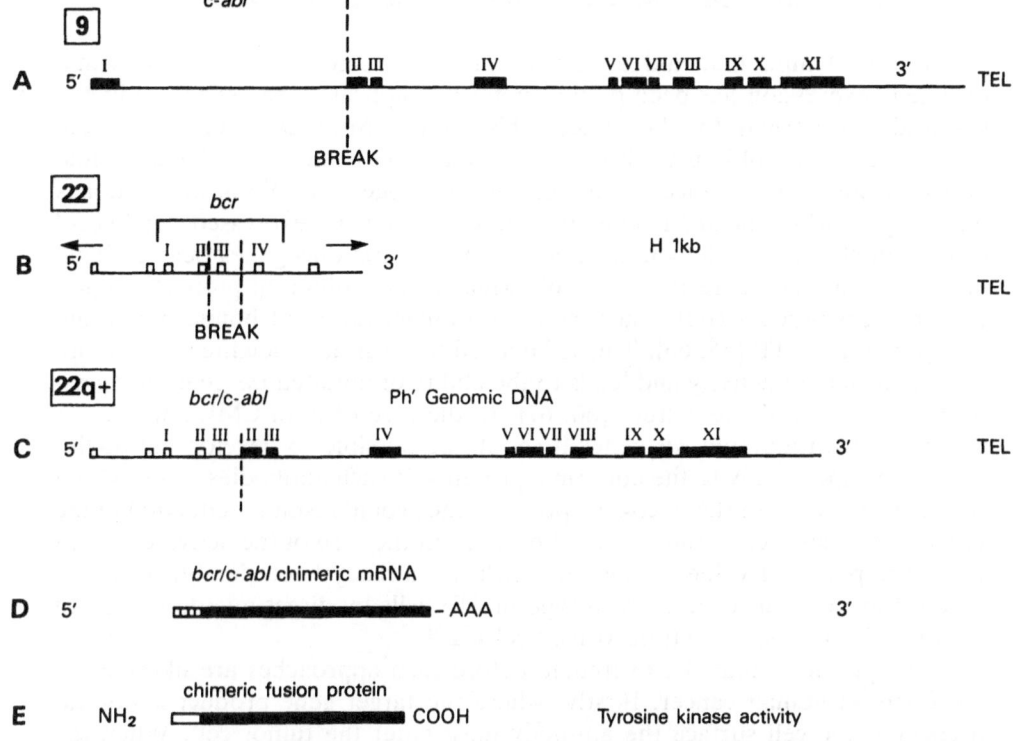

Fig. 4. A Schematic representation of the c-*abl* gene, normally situated on chromosome 9. The vertical interrupted line indicates the most 3′ limit of the breakpoint within the gene. The breakpoint may be anywhere within the first intron, or even within the first exon, without a change in the fusion-gene product since 3′ first exon and first intron sequences will be spliced out in the mature messenger RNA. **B** Part of the gene in the '*bcr*' region on chromosome 22. Breaks occur within the limited region bounded by the interrupted lines. **C** Breakpoint region on the derivative chromosome 22 resulting from the 9;22 translocation. Note creation of a *bcr/abl* fusion gene. **D** The chimeric messenger RNA species resulting from transcription of the *bcr/abl* fusion gene. **E** The chimeric protein, which has tyrosine kinase activity, resulting from the translocation

chronic myeloid leukemia. Another problem to be surmounted with antisense therapy is that continuous exposure to antisense is necessary if translation is to be persistently impaired. Since RNA synthesis is not impaired, a single dose of antisense will ultimately be overwhelmed. This could possibly be overcome by inserting antisense sequences into tumor cells by means of a retrovirus vector (see below).

Even if therapy with antisense oligomers proves to be impractical, these molecules provide a powerful tool with which to dissect the role of any given gene product in the genesis of neoplasia. Reversion of the neoplastic phenotype with antisense oligomers, even if only accomplished in vitro, would also serve to emphasize the principle that the pathogenetically relevant genetic abnormality of the neoplastic cell is both the cause of the cancer and the potential Achilles heel that could lead to the development of truly specific anticancer therapy.

Therapeutic Approaches Directed Towards Mutated *ras* Genes

In Burkitt's lymphoma, and a number of other tumors in which abnormal oncogene expression has been pathogenetically implicated, the gene product is believed to be normal. In other cancers this is not so. Mutated *ras* genes, capable of transforming fibroblasts in vitro, for example, have been detected in a cell line derived from bladder cancer, although their pathogenetic role in this tumor is unclear [65], while the *abl* gene is structurally altered and expressed as a hybrid protein in chronic myelocytic leukemia [23]. The *ras* oncogenes bear a single mutation, generally at residue 12 or 61, which confers different properties upon their protein product (p21), such as reduced inactivation of bound guanosine triphosphatase GTP [65, 66]. This is believed to result in a heightened or more persistent state of activity and leads to the ability of mutated *ras* genes to transform cell lines in tissue culture [66, 67]. In the case of both CML and tumors associated with mutated *ras* genes it should be possible to develop antibodies which bind specifically to the abnormal proteins. If such antibodies were to bind to "active regions" of the oncogene product, they could result in reduction of the functional properties of the activated protein. In the case of the activated H-*ras* gene, the potential value of this approach has already been demonstrated by reversal of the transformed phenotype in 3T3 cells by direct microinjection of p21-specific antibody into transformed cells [29].

Many problems must be overcome before such approaches are likely to be successful in human cancer. Firstly, where the target gene product is not expressed at the cell surface the antibody must enter the tumor cell. When the oncogene product is a membrane protein, the exposed portion must differ from the normal counterpart protein if tumor specificity is to be achieved. Further, continuous exposure of the tumor cells to the antibody would presumably be necessary, since new protein is being continuously made. Some of these formidable difficulties may ultimately be surmounted. Entry into the cell, for example, could theoretically be accomplished by linkage to another molecule (possibly another antibody molecule) which will bind to a surface receptor and be internalized, although this in itself contains its own set of problems: the fate of the antibody depends upon the intracytoplasmic path of ligand/receptor complexes. Intracellular penetration of all cells depends upon many factors including the variability of expression of the chosen surface target molecule. Finally, the problems common to all therapeutic attempts using monoclonal antibody therapy apply (see Byers Baldwin, this volume). There is, however, one potential advantage to the use of antibodies directed towards oncogene products rather than immunotoxins or radionuclide-coupled antibodies directed towards other antigens. Since the target (if properly selected) is one of the abnormalities, perhaps the quintessential abnormality, responsible for the neoplastic state, the cell is not able to modulate (reduce) expression of the antigen, and thereby escape from the effect of antibody therapy.

An alternative and possibly more promising approach to the use of monoclonal antibodies is to alter the function of the oncogene product by means of anti-oncogene drugs. For example, there is good evidence that the *ras* products (p21) are activated when bound to GTP [67, 68]. It might prove possible to synthesize GTP analogues which bind avidly to the protein but do not activate it. Alternatively, synthetic polypeptides could be developed which bind to p21 at its substrate acceptor site. This is likely to become a realistic possibility when the substrate(s) of p21 are identified. The effect of such drugs on normal cells cannot be predicted, but if tumor cells have an excess of p21 activity they may be preferentially affected. Further, drugs which bind more readily to the mutated p21 of cancer cells than to normal p21 may be developed to enhance the tumor selectivity still further. Some compounds which affect the function of G proteins (inhibitors and stimulators of adenyl cyclase and probably other intracellular second messenger systems) to which the *ras* genes are structurally related [69, 70] are already known (e.g., pertussis and cholera toxins) and could provide a basis for the development of such drugs [71].

It can be seen, using the *ras* genes as an example, that the identification of abnormal oncogene products can lead to new treatment approaches, one of the more promising of which is the development of drugs specific for structurally altered oncogene products. Naturally, a prerequisite for the success of this approach is that the identified abnormality must be of major pathogenetic importance, although in the case of the *ras* and HER-2/*neu* genes, and others yet to be identified, reversal of some of the consequences of tumor progression such as metastatic potential may also prove to be possible. Oncogene-directed therapy may thus have an alternative role as adjunctive, rather than primary therapy.

Therapeutic Approaches Directed Towards Tyrosine Kinase Activity

As shown in Fig. 1, molecular abnormalities in cancer frequently involve the cascade of events which result in cell proliferation. It appears that the specificity of the signal to proliferate resides in the ligand-binding portion of the relevant cell surface receptors, which will bind only the appropriate ligands. A number of cell surface receptors, however, (e.g., insulin receptor, epidermal growth factor receptor, and platelet-derived growth factor receptor) possess a common region in the intracytoplasmic portion of the molecule which contains a particular protein kinase activity capable of phosphorylating tyrosine residues [72–74]. The tyrosine kinase moiety is activated when the appropriate ligand binds to the extracellular portion of the receptor molecule and results in autophosphorylation of the receptor molecule itself and phosphorylation of other protein substrates, including, in the case of epidermal growth factor receptor, *ras* proteins, with resultant stimulation of guanine nucleotide binding [73]. Whether different receptors phosphorylate different proteins or whether this part of the pathway is "common" to several different receptors remains unknown. Protein phosphorylation, however (of tyrosine, serine, or threonine), is a critically important means by which enzyme reactions are regulated, and tyrosine phosphorylation, in particular, appears to be an integral component of one pathway whereby signals are transduced from the exterior of the cell to the nucleus. Perhaps not surprisingly, with so essential a cellular function, a number of oncogenes have been shown to encode molecules which contain a tyrosine kinase activity and some, e.g., c-*abl*, have been implicated in human neoplasia [22, 74]. There is also evidence that there is an increased level of *src*-specific tyrosine kinase activity in a number of human tumors. Thus, enhanced tyrosine phosphorylation may be an important feature of several human neoplasms and represents a potential biochemical target for therapeutic approaches.

In principle, such approaches would be similar to those discussed in the section on *ras* genes. The tyrosine kinase portion of normal growth factor receptors and oncogenes is remarkably similar at a structural level and it has proved possible to develop antibodies specifically directed towards the tyrosine kinase region of several different molecules [75], and to synthesize peptides or tyrosine analogues which inhibit tyrosine kinase activity (see also Glazer, this volume) [76]. The inhibition of tyrosine phosphorylation is likely to be more specific for tumor cells if differences in the substrates phosphorylated in tumor cells and in normal cells could be found; an area where, at present, little information exists. Nonetheless, the development of molecules (e.g., synthetic peptides) able to specifically prevent phosphorylation of the substrates for tyrosine kinase in specific neoplasms provides an attractive goal for experimental therapeutics.

Potential Role of Gene Therapy in Cancer

The possibility of incorporating drug-resistance genes into normal bone marrow cells in order to permit the administration of higher doses of myelosupressive agents has been briefly mentioned elsewhere in this book. In this section, the theoretical possibility of using gene therapy the genetic abnormalities present in cancer cells directed toward themselves will be discussed.

In any form of gene-therapy a number of problems, some of which at this time appear to be insurmountable, must be overcome. These include (a) the isolation (cloning) of the chosen gene or genes in functional form—a relatively straight forward matter today; (b) the introduction of the gene(s) into the tumor cell—a much more difficult problem, particularly since entry into *all* tumor cells (or at least all clonogenic cells) must be effected; (c) the introduction of the gene, if necessary, into a specific chromosomal location; (d) ensuring that the gene is expressed at an appropriate level; and (e) the provision for amelioration of the possible harmful effects of entry of the gene(s) into normal cells (which could include the induction of a second malignancy). Perhaps the most difficult problem of all, however, is the development of sufficient knowledge of the cellular derangements leading to neoplasia in any given tumor to permit the design of a therapeutic approach utilizing gene therapy. At most, we can consider here some potential stratagems based on our current, rather limited knowledge of pathogenetic mechanisms, and then explore the practical possibilities and major problems which must be surmounted if gene therapy of neoplasia is to become a realistic proposition.

One reason for believing that gene therapy is at least a potentially effective approach is the very close resemblance of neoplastic cells to their normal counterparts in tumors where the normal counterpart cells are known. This suggests that neoplasia is the consequence of a limited number of genetic changes, the reversal of any one of which may be sufficient to partially or completely reverse the malignant phenotype. Since in all known biological systems there are both positive and negative regulators, overexpression of a particular cellular function ought to be reversible either by direct inhibition of the relevant overexpressed gene(s) (at the transcriptional, post-transcriptional, or translational level), or by activating or inserting a second gene which is inhibitory for the function in question. For this form of therapy to become a reality, a means of developing specificity for tumor cells would be needed. Some approaches worthy of consideration, if only at a very general level at present, are discussed below, followed by a consideration of possible methods of affecting cell entry.

Insertion into Tumor Cells of Genes Coding for Cell Surface Receptors for Differentiation Factors or Growth Inhibitory Factors

For this approach to be successful, the cell must possess intracellular systems capable of insuring correct positioning of the receptor in the surface membrane and transducing the signal, generated by ligand binding, to the cell nucleus. As such, success would be more likely in neoplastic cells which lack normal receptors or express abnormal receptors as a component of pathogenesis, but have a normal transduction system. In spite of the major difficulties apparent in this approach, its feasibility was recently demonstrated by the insertion and expression of a cloned gene for human insulin receptor into chinese hamster ovary cells [77].

Insertion of Genes Coding for Regulator Molecules Involved in Signal Transduction

An example of this method would be the insertion of genes coding for molecules inhibiting the transmission of signals from an inappropriately activated growth factor receptor. Interestingly, it is possible that certain oncogenes such as the *ras* genes may be useful therapeutically, by virtue of their effect on the transduction of receptor-generated signals. This possibility is borne out by a recent report of the induction of differentiation in a rat pheochromocytoma cell line by infection with a retrovirus containing a *ras* oncogene [78]. A similar effect has been observed after infection with the oncogene-bearing (*src*) Rous sarcoma virus [79], while the *fos* oncogene has been shown to promote differentiation in teratocarcinoma cells [80].

Insertion of Genes Coding for Molecules which Directly Influence the Expression of Other Genes

Some genes, such as *myc*, *myb*, E1A of adenovirus, the transactivation genes of the HTLV viruses, genes involved in development, and many others, are known to regulate the expression of other genes [81–84]. Several of the products of these genes, including those of *myc* and *myb*, are known to be DNA-binding

419

proteins which could directly regulate the transcription of other genes. The incorporation, into the genome of a neoplastic cell, of functional genes which have an inhibitory effect on other genes which are overexpressed in the neoplasm, may have application in some circumstances. In tumors in which loss of function of an inhibitory gene is of pathogenetic significance, provision of the missing gene function could result in reversion or prevention of the neoplastic state. Wilms' tumor and retinoblastoma, which are associated with deletion or inactivation of a gene or genes residing on bands 11p13 and 13q14 respectively, are tumors to which this may apply [25–28]. The insertion of a normal gene into the offspring of families susceptible to these tumors (possibly as many as 40% of cases belong to such families in retinoblastoma) is possibly within the bounds of presently available technology, particularly if recent reports that the retinoblastoma gene has been cloned prove correct [85]. In theory, the cloned gene could be inserted into a human embryo after in vitro fertilization—a technique which has been used repeatedly to create "transgenic" mice but has not so far been used in humans. Obviously, numerous ethical and moral issues would need to be resolved before attempting such a controversial experiment.

Insertion of Synthetic Genes Expressing Antisense Sequences

The possibility of preventing translation by means of antisense oligonucleotides was discussed above. If continuous inhibition is to be achieved, one approach would be to insert into the tumor cell genome a DNA sequence, complete with regulator regions such as viral promoter and termination sequences, which is identical to the nontranscribed DNA strand of the gene in question (i.e., contains antisense information). Plasmids of this kind (e.g., pSP64 and pSP65, or more recent derivatives pGEM) which contain the strong bacteriophage promoters SP6 or T7, or both, are already in frequent use for the generation of both sense and antisense RNA probes [86]. Not only is this approach already within the capabilities of current recombinant DNA technology, but the experimental demonstration of its feasibility has been accomplished—for example in mouse cells transfected with a plasmid expressing an antisense RNA complementary to the normal thymidine kinase transcript. Marked inhibition of the thymidine kinase gene occurred [64].

Gene Repair and Gene Destruction

The repair of mutated genes has already been accomplished in vitro by inserting the correct sequences into the correct location in the genome by a process of homologus chromosomal recombination [87]. At present, the process is relatively inefficient, but it is likely that efficiency will be increased in the future. This method could possibly be applicable to tumors like Burkitt's lymphoma and chronic myeloid leukemia, although not in the near future. An alternative approach, also requiring the insertion of molecules of specific sites, would be to destroy a gene by inserting "non-sense" sequences into it. This would have the effect of preventing transcription of an oncogene, although the results would be somewhat unpredictable. Whereas gene repair may not necessarily adversely influence normal cells, even if the same sequences are inserted, gene destruction could be deleterious in nontumor cells, as shown by the chance insertion of c-*myc* sequences into a transgenic mouse which resulted in a recessively inherited limb deformity [88]. Ideally, homologous recombination should therefore be aimed at sequences specific to the abnormal gene. Clearly, this approach is presently far from human experimentation, but it is currently feasible in in vitro systems. Site-specific mutagenesis is frequently employed to study genetic structure/functional relationships [89].

Gene Vectors and Gene Insertion

Where a convincing case for further exploration of the possibility of gene therapy for neoplasia can be made, the enormous problem of the method of gene insertion must next be broached. Standard transfection methods used in vitro, such as calcium precipitation, are clearly not feasible therapeutically because of the very low efficiency and the fact that gene therapy must be done in vivo, since all tumor cells must receive the gene. This also requires a quite different approach from the use of gene therapy to render marrow cells resistant to a cytotoxic drug such in vitro transfected cells could be infused, then selected for in vivo by treatment of the patient with the appropriate drug. Perhaps the most promising approach to in vivo transfection would be the utilization of a gene vector consisting of an artificially constructed virus particle [89]. This approach, which has already been successfully used to insert genes into mouse embryos, cell lines, and hemopoietic precursor cells [90–92] would have several advantages. Firstly, virus infections represent natural means of inserting genes into both prokaryotic and eukaryotic cells. Secondly, not only could a degree of specificity for tumor cells be incorporated into the construction of the vector (e.g., by choosing viruses which infect specific cell types or by using coat or envelope proteins of such viruses in the vector to confer the same specificity), but a very high proportion of tumor cells—theoretically, all—could be infected with multiple high-multiplicity exposures. At present, practically 100% of target cells can be infected in vitro. Whether or not this could be achieved in vivo remains speculative, although there is no reason to believe that efficacy, in terms of the proportion of cells penetrated, would differ from that in currently employed drug or biological therapy. If the artificial virus construct were replication-defective, the potentially hazardous spread of the virus to other individuals would not occur, but a replication-competent particle would have the advantage of replication within the patient and a higher chance of infecting all tumor cells. Methods may be found of limiting virus replication to within the patient, or even to tumor cells. Indeed, if it proved possible to construct the virus vector such that it could only replicate in, or only infect tumor cells, the virus infection would be self-limited by patient cure. This possibility is presently remote, but there are precedents for its becoming a reality in the future.

Control of Transcription of Genes Artificially Inserted into Other Cells

For a gene inserted into a foreign genome to be expressed at all, appropriate enhancers or promoters must be linked to it. Some of these are tissue-specific and will only function in a limited range of cell types [93]. Thus, in the transgenic mice constructed by Adams et al. [92], since an immunoglobulin enhancer with tissue specificity was linked to the inserted c-*myc* gene only B-cell tumors developed, even though all mouse cells contained the c-*myc* gene artificially inserted into the mouse embryo. Since some promoters or enhancers respond to hormonal or other influences, e.g., the hormone-responsive mouse mammary tumor virus promoter, or the metallothianine gene promoter, the linkage of this type of sequence to the gene of interest would make it possible to control the expression of the gene after insertion. Such techniques are used frequently in experimental systems. Ultimately, it might even prove possible to use a promoter or enhancer responsive only to a chemical compound not normally encountered in humans, which could be administered to the patient to induce expression of the transfected gene. Alternatively, if a method could be devised whereby promotion or enhancement occurred as a consequence of the binding of a molecule present only in tumor cells (e.g., an abnormal protein resulting from a somatic genetic change), the expression of the gene or possibly viral replication could be rendered truly tumor specific.

Doubts and Hazards

Although gene therapy is an exciting concept and will almost certainly eventually become commonplace for the treatment of a number of human deficiency diseases, the use of this approach to deal with cancer involves several more orders of magnitude of complexity, such that at present it appears to be quite unrealistic. It is, of course, even possible that successful gene therapy directed towards the modification of tumor cell behavior may never be accomplished. The approach presents formidable technical problems, and until the genetic derangements leading to specific neoplasms have been defined precisely, such approaches must remain purely theoretical. Except in the cases of Burkitt's lymphoma and chronic myeloid leukemia, such knowledge is currently almost totally lacking. Further, potentially serious hazards, both to the patient and, in some cases, to other individuals, are associated with gene therapy, raising numerous ethical concerns [94]. These include the mutation of a vector with unexpected consequences and the insertion of genes or viral sequences, (such as the long terminal repeat (LTR) region which contains promoter and enhancer functions), into normal cells with possibly serious consequences—even the induction of a new neoplasm. The latter problem may well have already been overcome, however, by the development of "clipped wing" retrovirus vectors which have mutations in the enhancer sequences of the viral LTR regions [95]. Infection of germ cells and potential harmful effects on offspring is an additional theoretical hazard. Methods of minimizing these risks must be developed alongside the primary strategy. If replication-competent viruses were to be used as gene vectors, a series of safety measures would need to be taken to eliminate risks to the normal population before such methods could be contemplated in a clinical setting. Nevertheless, in spite of these legitimate questions, the fact that genomic engineering is now frequently performed in cell lines and animals indicates that such approaches must be taken seriously, and are worthy of continued exploration in in vitro and animal systems.

Conclusions

In this overview of the potential therapeutic relevance of knowledge of the pathogenetic mechanisms leading to neoplasia, only a few examples from the best understood tumors have been provided and much speculation has been indulged in. Some of this will doubtless prove unrealistic, while new approaches, inconceivable in our present state of knowledge, will surely be devised in the future. A short while ago, however, it would not have been possible to write a chapter of this kind because of the absence of any information. Today, with detailed pathogenetic information available from several tumors—notably Burkitt's lymphoma, chronic myeloid leukemia and, to a lesser extent, retinoblastoma and Wilms' tumors—a number of new approaches to therapy can be explored. Perhaps the most immediately accessible of these is the development of new drugs designed to inhibit enzymes or other proteins known to be involved in the pathway which has been altered pathologically in the tumor in question. In the cases of Burkitt's lymphoma and chronic myeloid leukemia, there is already sufficient understanding of the molecular pathogenesis to initiate preclinical studies of the feasibility of circumventing or correcting the observed cellular abnormalities.

It is hoped that this chapter has demonstrated that there is indeed hope that, in the future, highly selective cancer therapy based upon knowledge of molecular pathogenetic mechanisms may be possible and that the unravelling of mechanisms whereby cells become malignant may prove to have both practical as well as purely intellectual value.

References

1. Mitelman F (1984) Restricted number of chromosomal regions implicated in aetiology of human cancer and leukaemia. Nature 310: 325–327
2. Yunis J (1983) The chromosomal basis of human neoplasia. Science 221: 227–236
3. Yunis JJ (1981) Specific fine chromosomal defects in cancer: an overview. Hum Pathol 12: 503–515
4. Bloomfield CD, Arthur DC, Frizzera G, Levine EG, Peterson BA, Gajl-Peczalska KJ (1983) Non-random chromosome abnormalities in cancer. Cancer Res 43: 2975–2984

5. Bakhshi A, Jensen JP, Goldman P, Wright JJ, McBride OW, Epstein AL, Korsmeyer SJ (1985) Cloning the chromosomal breakpoint of t(18;14) bearing human lymphomas: clustering around JH on chromosome 14 and near a transcriptional unit on 18. Cell 41: 899–906

6. Shtivelman E, Lifshitz B, Gale RP, Canaani E (1985) Fused transcript of abl and bcr genes in chronic myeloglouus leukemia. Nature 315: 550

7. Pellici P–G, Knowles D, Magrath I et al. (1986) Chromosomal breakpoints and structural alterations of the c-myc locus differ in endemic and sporadic forms of Burkitt lymphoma. Proc Natl Acad Sci USA 83: 2984

8. Magrath IT (1987) Infectious mononucleosis and malignant neoplasia. In: Schlossman D (ed) Infectious mononucleosis. Praeger, New York, pp 225–227

9. Hanto DW, Frizzera G, Gail-Peczalskakj et al. (1982) Epstein–Barr virus induced B-cell lymphoma after renal transplantation, acyclovir therapy and transition from polyclonal to monoclonal B-cell proliferation. N Engl J Med 306: 913–918

10. Magrath IT (1982) Malignant lymphomas. In: Levine As (ed) Cancer in the young. Masson, New York, pp 473–574

11. Magrath IT (1986) Burkitt's lymphoma as a human tumor model: New concepts in etiology and pathogenesis. In: Pochedly C (ed) Pediatric hematology oncology reviews. Praeger, New York, p 1

12. El-Bolkainy MN (1983) The pathology of cancer of the bilharzial bladder. Bladder Cancer 1: 83–120

13. Correa P (1982) Precursors of gestric and esophageal Cancer. Cancer 50 [Suppl 11]: 2554–2565

14. Sanford KK, Parshad R, Potter M et al. (1986) Chromosomal radiosensitivity during G2 phase and susceptibility to plasmacytoma induction in mice. Curr Top Microbiol Immunol 132: 202–208

15. Yunis JJ, Soreng AL (1984) Constitutive fragile sites and cancer. Science 226: 1199–1203

16. Tsujimoto Y, Finger LR, Yunis J, Nowell PC, Croce C (1984) Cloning the chromosome breakpoint of neoplastic B cells with the t(14;18) chromosome translocation. Science 226: 1097–1099

17. Erikson J, Williams DL, Finan J, Nowell PC, Croce C (1985) Locus of the alpha-chain of the T-cell receptor is split by a translocation in T-cell leukemias. Science 229: 784–786

18. Croce CM, Isobe M, Palumbo A, Puck J, Ming J, Tweardy D, Erikson J (1985) Gene for alpha-chain of human T-cell receptor involved in T-cell neoplasms. Science 227: 1044–1047

19. McKeithan TW, Shima EA, Le Beau MM et al. (1986) Molecular cloning of the breakpoint junction of a human chromosomal 8:14 translocation involving the T cell receptor alpha-chain gene and sequences on the 3' side of MYC. Proc Natl Acad Sci USA 83: 6636–6640

20. Finger LR, Harvey RC, Moore RCA, et al. (1986) A common mechanism of chromosomal translocation in T and B cell neoplasia. Science 234: 982–985

21. Weinberg RA (1985) The action of oncogenes in the cytoplasm and nucleus. Science 230: 770–776

22. Bishop JM (1987) The molecular genetics of cancer. Science 235: 305–311

23. Bartram CR et al. (1983) Translocation of c-abl oncogene correlates with the presence of a Philadelphia chromosome in chronic myelocytic leukemia. Nature 306: 277–280

24. Ben Neriah Y, Daley GQ, Mes-Masson AM et al. (1986) The chronic myelogenous leukemia-specific p210 protein is the product of the bcr/abl hybrid gene. Science 233: 212–214

25. Murphree AL, Benedict WF (1984) Retinoblastoma: clues to human oncogenesis. Science 223: 1028–1033

26. Fearon ER, Vogelstein B, Feinberg AP (1984) Somatic deletion and duplication of genes on chromosome 11 in Wilms' tumors. Nature 309: 176–178

27. Koufos A, Hansen MF, Copeland NG, et al. (1985) Loss of heterozygosity in three embryonal tumors suggests a common pathogenetic mechanism. Nature 316: 330–334

28. Draper GJ, Sanders BM, Kingston JE (1986) Second primary malignant neoplasms in patients with retinoblastoma. Br J Cancer: 53: 661–171

29. Drebin JA, Link VC, Stern DF et al. (1985) Down-modulation of an oncogene protein product and transformed phenotype by monoclonal antibodies. Cell 41: 695–706

30. Feramisco JR, Clark R, Wong G et al. (1985) Transient reversion of ras oncogene-induced antibodies specific for amino-acid 12 of ras protein. Nature 314: 639–642

424

31. Stewart TA, Mintz B (1981) Successive generations of mice produced from an established culture line of euploid teratocarcinoma cells. Proc Natl Acad Sci USA 78: 6314–6318
32. Bodner AJ, Ting RC, Gallo RC (1981) Induction of differentiation of human promyelocytic leukemia cells (HL60) by nucleosides and methotrexate. JNCI 67: 1025–1030
33. Griffin J, Munroe D, Major P, Kufe D (1982) Induction of differentiation of human myeloid leukemia cells by inhibitors of DNA synthesis. Exp Hematol 10: 774–781
34. Sartorelli AC (1985) Malignant cell differentiation as a potential therapeutic approach. Br J Cancer 52: 293–302 (The Walter Hubert Lecture)
35. Schlick E, Ruffman R, Hartung K, Chirigos MA (1985) Modulation of myelopoiesis by CSF or CSF-inducing biological response modifiers. J Immunopharmacol 7: 141–166
36. Matsui T, Takahashi R, Mihara K et al. (1985) Cooperative regulation of c-*myc* expression in differentiation of human promyelocytic leukemia induced by recombinant gamma-interferon and 1,25-dihydroxy vitamin D3. Cancer Res 4545: 4366–4371
37. Prochownik EV, Kukowska J (1986) Deregulated expression of c-*myc* by murine erythroleukemia cells prevents differentiation. Nature 322: 848–850
38. Farid NR, Briones-Urbina R, Islam MN: Anti-idiotypic antibodies as probes for hormone-receptor interaction.
39. Kennedy RC, Melnick JL, Dreesman GR (1984) Antibody to hepatitis B virus induced by injecting antibodies to the idiotype. Science 223: 930–931
40. Nishizuka Y (1984) The role of protein kinase C in cell surface signal transduction and tumor promotion. Nature 308: 693–698
41. Ullrich A, Coussens L, Hayflickjs et al. (1984) Human epidermal growth factor receptor cDNA sequence and aberrant expression of the amplified gene in A431 epidermoid carcinoma cells. Nature 309: 418–425
42. Baccarani M, Zaccaria A, Bandini G, Cavazzini G, Fanin R, Tura S (1983) Low dose arabinosyl cytosine for treatment of pre-leukemia and acute myeloid leukemia. Leuk Res 7: 539–545
43. Castaigne S, Daniel MT, Tilly H et al. (1983) Does treatment with Ara-C in low dosage cause differentiation in leukemic cells? Blood 62: 85–86
44. Lesley JF, Schulte RJ (1985) Inhibition of cell growth by monoclonal anti-transferrin receptor antibodies. Mol Cell Biol 5: 1814–1821
45. Carney DN, Cuttitta F (1986) Interruption of small cell lung cancer (SCLC) growth by a monoclonal antibody to bombesin (Abstr). 5th NCI-EORTC Symposium on New Drugs in Cancer Therapy, October 22–24, 1986, Amsterdam
46. Duesberg PH (1985) Activated proto-oncogenes: sufficient or necessary for cancer? Science 228: 669–676
47. Nau MM, Carney DN, Battey J et al. (1984) Amplification, expression and rearrangement of c-*myc* and N-*myc* oncogenes in human lung cancer. Curr Top Microbiol Immunol 113: 172–177
48. Libermann TA, Nusbaum HR, Razon N et al. (1985) Amplification, enhanced expression and possible rearrangement of EGF receptor gene in primary human brain tumors of glial origin. Nature 313: 144–147
49. Seeger RC, Brodeur GM, Sather H et al. (1985) Association of multiple copies of the N-*myc* oncogene with rapid progression of neuroblastomas. N Engl J Med 313: 1111–1116
50. Stark GR, Wahl GM (1984) Gene amplification. Annu Rev Biochem 53: 447
51. Efstratiadis A, Posakony JW, Maniatis T et al. (1980) Structure and evolution of the human beta-globin gene family. Cell 21: 653–668
52. Nakauchi H, Nolan C, Hsu H et al. (1985) Molecular cloning of Lyt-2, a membrane glycoprotein present on mouse T lymphocytes: molecular homology to its human counterpart, Leu-2/T8, and to immunoglobulin variable regions. Proc Natl Acad Sci USA 82: 5126–5130
53. Williams A (1984) The immunoglobulin superfamily takes shape. Nature 308: 12–13
54. Maddon PJ, Littman DR, Godfrey M et al. (1985) The isolation and nucleotide sequence of a cDNA encoding the T cell surface protein T4: a new member of the immunoglobulin gene family. Cell 42: 93–104
55. Shimpke RT, Brown PC, Johnston RN et al. (1983) Gene amplification and methotrexate resistance in cultured animal cells. In: Murphy SB, Gilbert JR (eds) Leukemia research: advances in cell biology and treatment. Elsevier, New York, pp 121–134

56. Brodeur GM, Hayer FA, Green AA et al. (1987) Consistent n-*myc* copy number in simultaneous or consecutive neuroblastoma samples from sixty individual patients. Cancer Res 47: 4248–4253

57. Sager R, Gader IK, Stephens L, Grabowy CT (1985) Gene amplification: an example of accelerated evolution in tumorigenic cells. Proc Natl Acad Sci USA 82: 7015–7019

58. Thiele CJ, Reynolds CP, Israel M (1985) Decreased expression of N-*myc* precedes retinoic acid-induced morphological differentiation of human neuroblastoma cells. Nature 313: 404–406

59. Matsui T, Takahashi R, Mihara K, et al. (1985) Cooperative regulation of c-*myc* expression in differentiation of human myelocytic leukemia induced by recombinant gamma-interferon and 1,25 dihydroxyvitamin D3, Cancer Res 45: 4366–4371

60. Knight E Jr, Anton ED, Fahey D et al. (1985) Interferon regulates c-*myc* gene expression in Daudi cells at the post transcriptional level. Proc Natl Acad Sci USA 82: 1151–1154

61. Croce C, Erikson J, Bar-Rushdi A et al. (1984) Translocated c-*myc* oncogene of Burkitt lymphoma is transcribed in plasma cells and repressed in lymphoblastoid cells. Proc Natl Acad Sci USA 81: 3170–3174

62. Green P, Pines O, Masayori I (1986) The role of antisense RNA in gene regulation. Annu Rev Biochem 55: 569–597

63. Izant JG, Weintraub H (1984) Inhibition of thymidine kinase gene expression by anti-sense: a molecular approach to genetic analysis. Cell 36: 1007–1009

64. Heikkila R, Schwag G, Wickstrom F et al. (1987) A c-*myc* antisense oligodeoxynucleotide inhibits entry into S phase but not progress from G_0 to G_1. Nature 328: 445–449

65. Reddy EP, Reynolds RK, Santos E, Barbacid M (1982) A point mutation is responsible for the acquisition of transforming properties by the T24 human bladder carcinoma oncogene. Nature 300: 149–152

66. Tabin CJ, Bradley SM, Barsmann CI et al. (1982) Mechanism of activation of a human oncogene. Nature 300: 143–149

67. McGrath JP, Capon DJ, Goeddel DV, Levinson A (1984) Comparative biochemical properties of normal and activated human *ras* protein. Nature 310: 644–649

68. Papageorge A, Lowy D, Scolnick EJ (1982) Comparative biochemical properties of p21 *ras* molecules coded for by viral and cellular *ras* genes. J Virol 44: 509–519

69. Broek D, Samiy N, Fasano O et al. (1985) Differential activation of yeast adenylate cyclase by wild-type and mutant ras proteins. Cell 41: 763–769

70. Breckner SK, Hattori S, Shih TY (1985) The *ras* oncogene product p21 is not a regulatory component of adenylate cyclase. Nature 317: 71–72

71. Spiegel AM, Gierschik P, Levine MA, Downs RW Jr (1985) Clinical implications of guanine nucleotide-binding proteins as receptor effector couplers. N Engl J Med 312: 26–33

72. White MF, Maron R, Kahn CR (1985) Insulin rapidly stimulates tyrosine kinase phosphorylation of a Mr-185,000 protein in intact cells. Nature 314: 183–186

73. Kamata T, Feramisco JR (1984) Epidermal growth factor stimulates guanine nucleotide binding activity and phosphorylation of *ras* oncogene proteins. Nature 310: 147–150

74. Hunter T, Alexander CB, Cooper JA (1985) Protein phosphorylation and growth control. Ciba Found Symp 116: 188–204

75. Lax I, Bar-Elim, Yarden Y et al. (1984) Antobodies to two defined regions of the transforming protein pp 60 *src* interact specifically with the epidermal growth factor receptor kinase system. Proc Natl Acad Sci USA 81: 5911–5915

76. Casnellie JE, Krebs EG (1984) The use of synthetic peptides for defining the specificity of tyrosine protein kinases. Adv Enzyme Regul 22: 501–515

77. Ebina Y, Edery M, Leland E et al. (1985) Expression of a functional human insulin receptor from a cloned cDNA in chinese hamster ovary cells. Proc Natl Acad Sci USA 82: 8014–8018

78. Noda M, Ko M, Ogura O et al. (1985) Sarcoma viruses carrying *ras* oncogenes induce differentiation associated properties in a neuronal cell line. Nature 318: 73–75

79. Alema S, Casalbore P, Agostini E, Tato F (1985) Differrentiation of PC 12 phaeochromocytoma cells induced by v-*src* oncogene. Nature 316: 557–559

80. Muller R, Wagner EF (1984) Differentiation of F9 teratocarcinoma stem cells after transfer of c-*fos* proto-oncogenes. Nature 311: 438–442

426

31. Stewart TA, Mintz B (1981) Successive generations of mice produced from an established culture line of euploid teratocarcinoma cells. Proc Natl Acad Sci USA 78: 6314–6318
32. Bodner AJ, Ting RC, Gallo RC (1981) Induction of differentiation of human promyelocytic leukemia cells (HL60) by nucleosides and methotrexate. JNCI 67: 1025–1030
33. Griffin J, Munroe D, Major P, Kufe D (1982) Induction of differentiation of human myeloid leukemia cells by inhibitors of DNA synthesis. Exp Hematol 10: 774–781
34. Sartorelli AC (1985) Malignant cell differentiation as a potential therapeutic approach. Br J Cancer 52: 293–302 (The Walter Hubert Lecture)
35. Schlick E, Ruffman R, Hartung K, Chirigos MA (1985) Modulation of myelopoiesis by CSF or CSF-inducing biological response modifiers. J Immunopharmacol 7: 141–166
36. Matsui T, Takahashi R, Mihara K et al. (1985) Cooperative regulation of c-*myc* expression in differentiation of human promyelocytic leukemia induced by recombinant gamma-interferon and 1,25-dihydroxy vitamin D3. Cancer Res 4545: 4366–4371
37. Prochownik EV, Kukowska J (1986) Deregulated expression of c-*myc* by murine erythroleukemia cells prevents differentiation. Nature 322: 848–850
38. Farid NR, Briones-Urbina R, Islam MN: Anti-idiotypic antibodies as probes for hormone-receptor interaction.
39. Kennedy RC, Melnick JL, Dreesman GR (1984) Antibody to hepatitis B virus induced by injecting antibodies to the idiotype. Science 223: 930–931
40. Nishizuka Y (1984) The role of protein kinase C in cell surface signal transduction and tumor promotion. Nature 308: 693–698
41. Ullrich A, Coussens L, Hayflickjs et al. (1984) Human epidermal growth factor receptor cDNA sequence and aberrant expression of the amplified gene in A431 epidermoid carcinoma cells. Nature 309: 418–425
42. Baccarani M, Zaccaria A, Bandini G, Cavazzini G, Fanin R, Tura S (1983) Low dose arabinosyl cytosine for treatment of pre-leukemia and acute myeloid leukemia. Leuk Res 7: 539–545
43. Castaigne S, Daniel MT, Tilly H et al. (1983) Does treatment with Ara-C in low dosage cause differentiation in leukemic cells? Blood 62: 85–86
44. Lesley JF, Schulte RJ (1985) Inhibition of cell growth by monoclonal anti-transferrin receptor antibodies. Mol Cell Biol 5: 1814–1821
45. Carney DN, Cuttitta F (1986) Interruption of small cell lung cancer (SCLC) growth by a monoclonal antibody to bombesin (Abstr). 5th NCI-EORTC Symposium on New Drugs in Cancer Therapy, October 22–24, 1986, Amsterdam
46. Duesberg PH (1985) Activated proto-oncogenes: sufficient or necessary for cancer? Science 228: 669–676
47. Nau MM, Carney DN, Battey J et al. (1984) Amplification, expression and rearrangement of c-*myc* and N-*myc* oncogenes in human lung cancer. Curr Top Microbiol Immunol 113: 172–177
48. Libermann TA, Nusbaum HR, Razon N et al. (1985) Amplification, enhanced expression and possible rearrangement of EGF receptor gene in primary human brain tumors of glial origin. Nature 313: 144–147
49. Seeger RC, Brodeur GM, Sather H et al. (1985) Association of multiple copies of the N-*myc* oncogene with rapid progression of neuroblastomas. N Engl J Med 313: 1111–1116
50. Stark GR, Wahl GM (1984) Gene amplification. Annu Rev Biochem 53: 447
51. Efstratiadis A, Posakony JW, Maniatis T et al. (1980) Structure and evolution of the human beta-globin gene family. Cell 21: 653–668
52. Nakauchi H, Nolan C, Hsu H et al. (1985) Molecular cloning of Lyt-2, a membrane glycoprotein present on mouse T lymphocytes: molecular homology to its human counterpart, Leu-2/T8, and to immunoglobulin variable regions. Proc Natl Acad Sci USA 82: 5126–5130
53. Williams A (1984) The immunoglobulin superfamily takes shape. Nature 308: 12–13
54. Maddon PJ, Littman DR, Godfrey M et al. (1985) The isolation and nucleotide sequence of a cDNA encoding the T cell surface protein T4: a new member of the immunoglobulin gene family. Cell 42: 93–104
55. Shimpke RT, Brown PC, Johnston RN et al. (1983) Gene amplification and methotrexate resistance in cultured animal cells. In: Murphy SB, Gilbert JR (eds) Leukemia research: advances in cell biology and treatment. Elsevier, New York, pp 121–134

425

22. Differentiation of Malignant Cells as a Strategy for Cancer Treatment

R.I. Glazer

Introduction

Recent developments in the fields of cell and molecular biology have contributed greatly to our understanding of the intricacies of the biological processes underlying the differentiation and proliferation of the malignant cell. The purpose of this chapter is to give an overview of some of the model cell systems that are being utilized to study differentiation and growth, the biochemical processes associated with these processes, and the areas that may be exploited for the design of new chemo- or biotherapeutic agents.

Differentiation of Leukemic Cells in Vitro

The study of differentiation of leukemic cells has been facilitated greatly by the use of several human leukemia cell lines. The promyelocytic leukemia HL-60 [1] is a pluripotent cell line with the ability to differentiate along either the myeloid or monocyte/macrophage pathways. The histiocytic lymphoma U937 [2] and myelogenous leukemia K562 [3] can be induced to express phenotypic characterisitics of macrophage- and erythroid-like cells, respectively. Among the various differentiating agents used in vitro, the most widely employed compound is 12-O-tetradecanoylphorbol-13-acetate (TPA) (Fig. 1). This agent induces HL-60 and U937 cells to undergo phenotypic changes akin to macrophage-like cells [2, 4–6]. Although the differentiated cells resemble morphologically mature macrophages, they do not appear to be identical either functionally [4, 9] or antigenically [7, 8]. The phenotypic changes observed in established leukemia cell lines are similar to those found after TPA treatment of leukemic cells from patients. Thus, TPA in vitro induces macrophage differentiation of leukemia cells from patients with acute and chronic myelogenous leukemia [10, 11]. TPA also induces the appearance of lymphoblastoid and plasmacytoid cells in cultures of chronic lymphocytic leukemia cells [12], the induction of cell adherence in hairy cell leukemia cells [13], alterations in cell surface markers of chronic lymphocytic leukemia cells [14], and the induction of B cell antigens in non-T acute lymphoblastic leukemia [15].

428

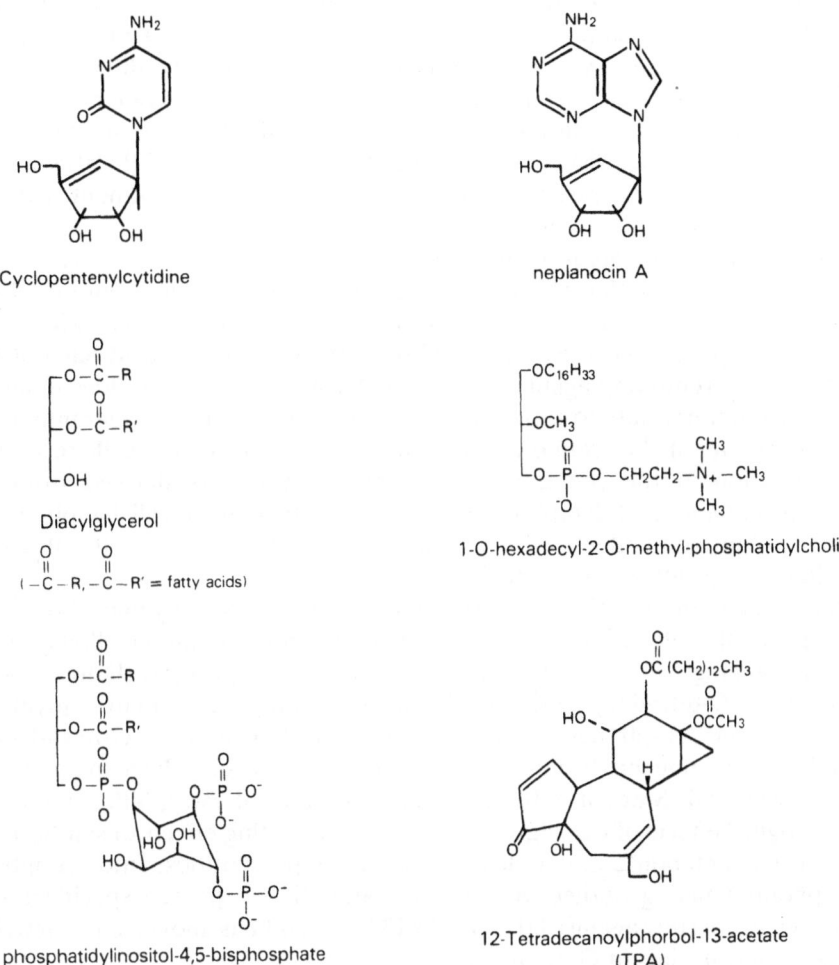

Fig. 1. Structures of differentiation-related drugs, chemicals and metabolites

Functional alterations also result from the treatment of established leukemia cell lines with phorbol esters. The T-cell lymphoblastoid cell lines MOLT-3 and Jurkat were induced to "differentiate" along the normal T-cell pathway by TPA as assessed by an increase in erythrocyte binding ability and the loss of deoxynucleotidyl terminal transferase with an accompanying arrest in proliferation without loss of viability [16, 17]. Similarly, B-cell function such as immunoglobulin secretion was partially restored and proliferation inhibited in six of twelve B-cell lymphoblastic leukemia cell lines following treatment with TPA [18].

Unfortunately, phorbol esters are tumor promoters and not, therefore, suitable for clinical use. Other agents which are not tumor promoters have, however, been used to induce differentiation in leukemia cells. A promising candidate for clinical use is the metabolite of vitamin D, 1,25-dihydroxyvitamin D_3 [1,25(OH)$_2$D$_3$]. This compound induced phagocytosis and C3 rosette formation in HL-60 cells [19], and was subsequently found to induce the differentiation of HL-60 cells to a monocytic phenotype as characterized by increased Mac-1 and OKM-1 antigen expression and enhanced nonspecific esterase activity [7, 20–22]. The latter characteristics are similar to those expressed in HL-60 cells which develop a morphologic resemblance to macrophages after treatment with TPA [5, 7].

One of the most potent agents which induces differentiation of HL-60 cells along the myeloid pathway is all-*trans* retinoic acid [23]. This compound is an analog of vitamin A and has differentiation-inducing characteristics akin to those of polar compounds such as DMSO [24]. Although retinoic acid has not been used as a differentiating agent in vitro as extensively as TPA, it does induce U-937 cells to differentiate to a monocyte phenotype [25]. Of particular importance is the observation that retinoic acid primes HL-60 and U-937 cells to undergo differentiation in the presence of differentiation factors derived from conditioned medium of T-lymphocytes [26] or a cutaneous T-cell lymphoma [1]. Similar potentiating effects on differentiation were noted in HL-60 cells treated simultaneously with these agents [27].

Induction of differentiation in HL-60 cells is also induced by phospholipid and diacylglycerol analogs (Fig. 1). Honma et al. [28] showed that the alkyl lysophospholipid analogs, 1-*O*-octadecyl-2-*O*-methyl-3-glycerophosphocholine and the analogous 1-*O*-tetradecyl derivative induced formation of the mature myelocytic phenotype in HL-60 cells. The alkylglycerol derivative, 1-*O*-hexadecyl-*O*-acetylglycerol induced formation of the monocyte-macrophage phenotype in HL-60 cells [29]. Since it is believed that the phorbol ester, TPA, mimics the physiological effects of diacylglycerol, the differentiating effects of synthetic analogs of this metabolite may indicate therapeutic possibilities. Interestingly, the phospholipid analog studied by Honma et al. [28] does possess specific antiproliferative properties against HL-60 cells [30–32] and has shown some activity in phase I clinical trials in Germany [33].

Apart from the more commonly used differentiating agents such as DMSO, TPA, 1,25-dihydroxyvitamin D_3, and retinoic acid, a diverse spectrum of other compounds elicit morphologic changes in HL-60 cells [1]. In general, the more cytotoxic the drug, the less differentiation occurs, and the narrower the dose-response relationship. Antimetabolite drugs such as the nucleoside analogs 5-azacytidine [34] and neplanocin A (Fig. 1) [35, 36], which preferentially inhibit the methylation of DNA and RNA respectively, induce a partial differentiation response in HL-60 cells mainly because of their potent cytocidal activities (Fig. 2). Cell cycle specificity also plays a role in differentiation. The agents DMSO and retinoic acid generally produce an accumulation of cells in the G_0/G_1 phase of the cell cycle [37, 38], an event which accompanies or precedes differentiation. The cytidine analog, cyclopentenyl cytidine (cCyd) (Fig. 1) produces a rapid induction of mature myeloid cells upon treatment of HL-60 cells due to its ability to inhibit cytidine triphosphate synthesis, rapidly inhibit DNA synthesis, and inhibit cells from traversing S phase (Fig. 2) [39, 40]. The latter effect on HL-60

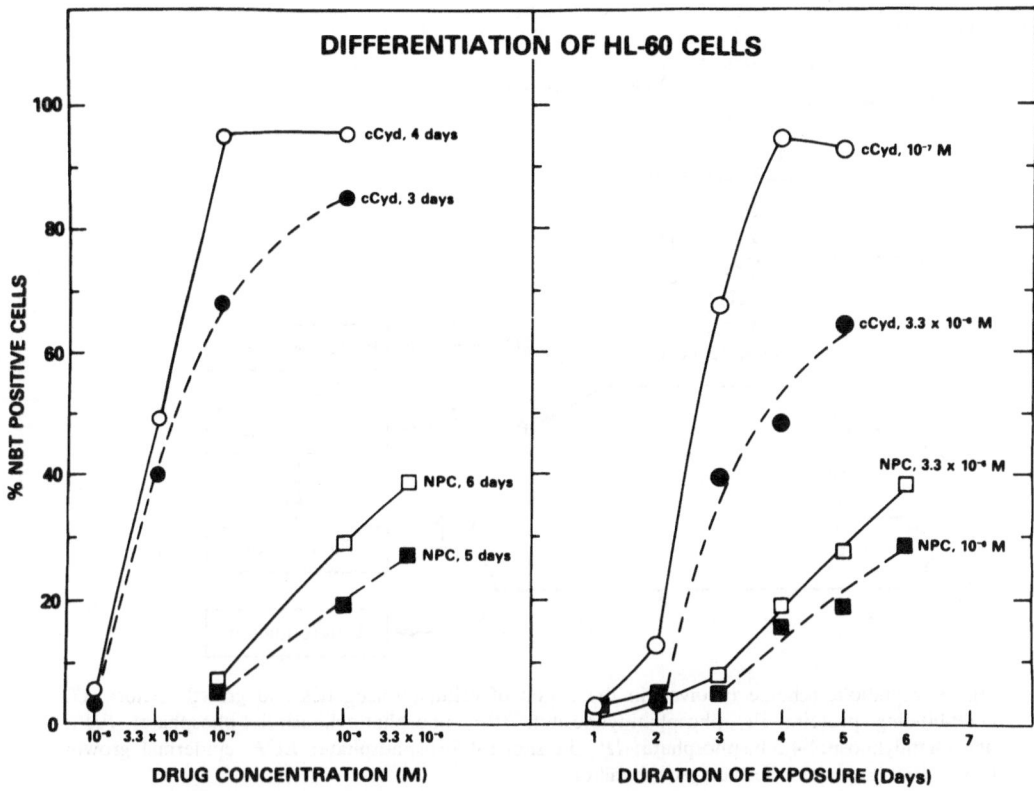

Fig. 2. Differentiation of HL-60 promyelocytic leukemia cells by neplanocin A and cyclopentenyl-cytidine. *NBT*, nitrotetrazolium blue. Differentiation was monitored by the cytochemical reduction of NBT to formazan [35, 39]

cells is also expresed by other inhibitors of CTP synthetase such as carbodine [39] and 3-deazauridine [41], and by pyrazofurin, an inhibitor of orotidylate decarboxylase [41]. Drugs which inhibit purine synthesis de novo such as the inosine monophosphate dehydrogenase inhibitors tiazofurin and mycophenolic acid appear to be less effective inducers of myeloid differentiation in HL-60 cells [41, 42].

Biochemical Processes Associated with the Action of Differentiating Agents

The process of cellular differentiation has been predominantly phenomenologi-cal rather than mechanistic. It is known that several marker enzymes and cell surface antigens correlate with morphologic changes in HL-60 cells induced to

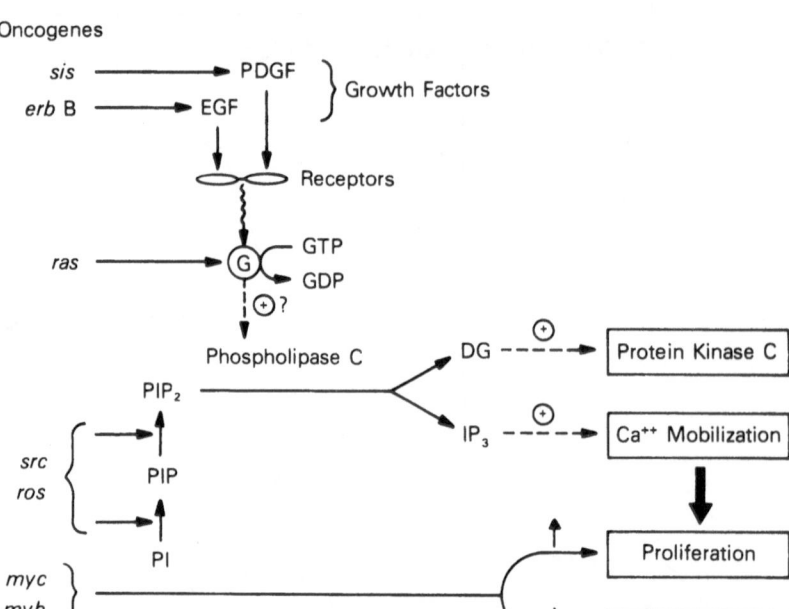

Fig. 3. Metabolic scheme involved in the action of cellular oncogenes and growth factors. *G*, GTP-binding protein; *PI*, phosphatidylinositol; *PIP*, phosphatidylinositol-4-phosphate; *PIP₂*, phosphatidylinositol-4,5-bisphosphate; *IP₂*, inositol-1,4,5-trisphosphate; *EGF*, epidermal growth factor; *PDGF*, platelet-derived growth factor

differentiate along the myelocytic or monocytic pathways in response to a variety of agents. However, among all these descriptive studies are very few dealing with the key signaling events responsible for initiating the differentiative response. At present, cell biologists are addressing this problem and several major developments in this field are rapidly being examined. Among these areas are: (a) the role of cellular oncogenes in cell proliferation and differentiation, (b) the role of inositol triphosphate as a second messenger in signal transduction, and (c) the role of protein kinase C in cellular proliferation and function (Fig. 3). One of the important points concerning the metabolic processes encompassing these areas is that with the exception of the cellular oncogenes c-*myc* and c-*myb*, they all are associated with the plasma membrane of the cell. Thus, they provide a mechanism for regulating the growth and differentiation of the cell at an entirely different level from the approaches exploited in the past in traditional cancer chemotherapy. In the following sections, I will highlight some of the major findings related to the aforementioned processes and cellular differentiation.

Protein kinase C (or phospholipid- and Ca^{++}-dependent protein kinase) was discovered by Nishizuka et al. [43]. This enzyme, isolated from rat brain, showed a striking dependence on Ca^{++} as well as specific phospholipids, viz. phosphatidylserine or phosphatidylinositol. Since this initial study, numerous reports have appeared regarding the regulation of protein kinase C activity [44, 45]. Perhaps the most striking development with respect to the regulatory influence of protein kinase C on other metabolic processes was the discovery that this enzyme bound phorbol esters such as TPA with high affinity [46–49]. The association of this enzyme with HL-60 cells [50] has led to speculation that it may be involved in TPA-induced maturation of these cells along the monocyte-macrophage pathway. In biological terms, TPA acts as a metabolically stable analog of diacylglycerol which activates protein kinase C in the presence of low (micromolar) concentrations of Ca^{++} [51]. It is this unique TPA-binding property of protein kinase C which has been exploited experimentally to infer the consequences of activation of this enzyme on various metabolic processes. Thus, TPA or diacylglycerol activation of phosphorylation of a 40-kd protein in platelets has been used as a biological response indicative of protein kinase C-mediated phosphorylation [52–54]. Similarly, the protein kinase C activating property of TPA led to the deduction that this enzyme mediated early changes (within 1 h) in specific phosphoproteins in HL-60 cells treated with the phorbol ester [55–57]. However, it should be noted that TPA-mediated stimulation of protein phosphorylation may not always result from its direct effect on protein kinase C. In U-937 cells, TPA promotes tyrosine phosphorylation [58], an effect not directly attributable to protein kinase C. In the human epidermoid carcinoma cell line A431, which overexpresses the epidermal growth factor (EGF) receptor and its associated tyrosine kinase activity [59, 60], TPA and diacylglycerol inhibit EGF binding to the EGF receptor and enhance serine and threonine phosphorylation with a resultant loss in phosphotyrosine [61–64]. However, the relationship between enhanced tyrosine phosphorylation of the EGF receptor by EGF vs. enhanced serine and threonine phosphorylation of the receptor by TPA and cell proliferation still remains a mystery, since both EGF and TPA inhibit cell growth in A431 cells [57, 65].

Thus, the role of protein kinase C in cell growth and differentiation has not been clearly defined. It is probable that phosphorylation of specific targets will differ in various cell systems according to whether their growth is inhibited or stimulated by protein kinase C activators such as diacylglycerol and TPA [57]. Alternatively, it is likely that other metabolic processes are affected by TPA, and thus not every effect of TPA should be attributed to protein kinase C. Preliminary evidence suggests that the response of HL-60 cells to DMSO, retinoic acid, and 1,25-dihydroxyvitamin D_3 is associated with changes in phospholipid- and Ca^{++}-dependent phosphorylation patterns in vitro which are related to the respective morphologic changes produced by these agents [66]. However, the treatment of HL-60 cells with TPA results in the disappearance of protein kinase C activity, and, thus, it is not clear how this enzyme functions during the differentiation of these cells to the macrophage phenotype [66].

One of the most rapidly expanding fields in cell biology is the study of the metabolism of phosphatidyl inositides to inositol phosphates which act as second messengers mediating singal transduction from receptors [67, 68]. The hydrolysis of phosphatidylinositol(4,5)-bisphosphate (PIP_2) to yield inositol(1,4,5) triphosphate (IP_3) produces a multitude of pharmacological effects, most of which are presumed to be associated with the mobilization of Ca^{++} from intracellular storage sites in the endoplasmic reticulum by IP_3 [69–71] (Fig. 3). The exact roles of Ca^{++} and IP_3 in cellular proliferation and differentiation is not clear. Calcium may stimulate protein kinase C in the absence of diacylglycerol [43, 51] or affect the activity of phosphatidylinositol polyphospate phosphodiesterase (phospholipase C) [72], which mediates the breakdown of PIP_2 to yield IP_3 and diacylglycerol (Fig. 3). Evidence has been presented for a role of IP_3 in mediating the receptor-coupled pathway produced by chemoattractant peptide in HL-60 cells differentiated with DMSO [73]. IP_3 directly elevates and mobilizes Ca^{++} in this cell line permeabilized with saponin [74], suggesting a direct role of IP_3-mediated Ca^{++} release in eliciting the stimulus-receptor response. IP_3 also directly stimulates phosphorylation of a 62-kd protein in cell lysates of fibroblasts and bovine brain in a Ca^{++}-independent manner [75]. However, in permeabilized platelets, IP_3 stimulated phosphorylation of presumably the same 40-kd protein which is the endogenous substrate of protein kinase C [76]. This effect was attributed to release of Ca^{++} since phosphorylation was increased by diacylglycerol at low but not at high Ca^{++} concentrations. Thus, most experimental evidence suggests that IP_3 may influence phosphorylation either by mobilizing Ca^{++} or by stimulating phosphorylation directly, and that the alternate product of PIP_2 hydrolysis, diacylglycerol, may function additively with Ca^{++} or IP_3 in promoting protein kinase C-mediated phosphorylation.

One of the more revolutionary developments in the last few years has been the elucidation of cellular oncogene expression in normal cellular differentiation, proliferation and transformation [77–79]. Cellular oncogenes are DNA sequences in normal cells which are very similar to retroviral DNA sequences originally picked by the virus from the host during the course of infection. Since the structures of cellular oncogenes are very closely conserved throughout evolution, it is presumed that they have an essential role in cell differentiation and in the regulation of cell division. Recent studies have determined that several cellular oncogene products are closely related to growth factors or growth factor receptors (Fig. 3). The v-*sis* oncogene product resembles platelet-derived growth factor (PDGF) which plays an important role in wound healing [80, 81]. Similarly, the human EGF receptor is closely related to the product of the v-*erb* B oncogene. In the latter instance, the overproducing epidermoid carcinoma cell line A431 has been used almost exclusively to study the EGF receptor tyrosine kinase [59–65] and the messenger RNAs [82–84] encoding the normal and aberrant EGF receptor in these cells. This cell line is also the only one, thus far, possessing amplified receptor gene sequences and an aberrant truncated form of the EGF receptor which is devoid of tyrosine kinase activity [85]. Although the latter mutant EGF receptor can be considered a result of a rearrangement and amplification in the gene, its presence has not provided any clue to the neoplastic properties of this cell line.

The role of growth factors in cellular differentiation is only beginning to be explored. HL-60 cells secrete a number of hemoregulatory peptides after induction of differentiation by retinoic acid [86] and secrete PDGF-related peptides during normal growth [87]. The fact that many growth factor receptors such as the EGF receptor, as well as that for PDGF [88], possess tyrosine kinase activity suggests that this enzymatic activity may play a crucial role in regulating proliferation and differentiation. This hypothesis has received support by several recent studies showing the increased expression of c-*fms* and c-*src* tyrosine kinases during monocytic and granulocytic differentiation of HL-60 cells [89–91], and by the elevated activities of total cellular tyrosine kinase and phosphotyrosine phosphatase with the onset of differentiation in HL-60 cells induced by DMSO or phorbol ester [92]. The induction of the monocytic phenotype in HL-60 cells by immune interferon and tumor necrosis factor was also associated with the appearance of a new membrane-associated form of tyrosine kinase recently found to be c-*fes* [93].

It is believed that for malignant transformation to take place, at least two oncogenes must be activated in a concerted manner. One oncogene required for malignant transformation is H-*ras* [94]. Microinjection of the H-*ras* gene product, a 21-kd GTP-binding protein associated with the inner surface of the plasma membrane, results in proliferation of normally quiescent fibroblasts [95]. A recent report has shown that EGF enhances the GTP-binding activity of H-*ras* p21 [96], which suggests a direct link between growth factors and their receptors and the GTP-binding protein, which itself may be related to the GTP-binding regulatory proteins controlling adenylate cyclase [97] and PIP_2 phosphodiesterase [98] (Fig. 3). Therefore, it is possible that the elevation of IP_3 from PIP_2 hydrolysis mediated by *ras* p21 is an intermediate event in cell proliferation and perhaps, in a sustained form, cell transformation. Such a mechanism may explain why EGF enhances PI turnover in A431 cells [99]. In this context, it might be expected that a second oncogene with the ability to elevate PIP_2 levels would enhance the ability of the *ras* p21 to mediate proliferation. Such is the case for the tyrosine kinase products of v-*src* and v-*ros* [100,101]. These kinases were originally reported to phosphorylate PI and PIP, thus generating PIP_2 and its resultant hydrolysis product, IP_3 (Fig. 3), although there is recent evidence that the phosphorylation of tyrosine and PI in v-*src* and Moloney leukemia virus transformed cells are catalyzed by different kinases [102].

Among the cellular oncogenes associated with cell division are c-*myc* and c-*myb*. The c-*myc* gene is amplified in HL-60 cells [103–105] as well as in a human breast carcinoma [105], gastric adenocarcinoma [106], and small-cell lung carcinoma [107] cell lines. Expression of c-*myc* mRNA correlates with an early G_1 event and is elevated in concert with the proliferative response of cells to mitogens or growth factors [108]. It is believed that the synthesis of c-*myc* mRNA is growth-related, as shown in a B-cell lymphoma cell line stimulated with anti-IgM [109], in Daudi lymphoma cells inhibited by interferon [110], and in peripheral lymphocytes from patients with systemic lupus erythematosus [111]. Reduced c-*myc* expression has also been reported to be an early event which precedes retinoic acid-induced morphologic changes in neuroblastoma cells [112] and in HL-60 cells treated with DMSO, TPA, retinoic acid, or 1,25-dihydroxyvitamin D_3 [113–115]. The cellular function of the c-*myc* protein was

435

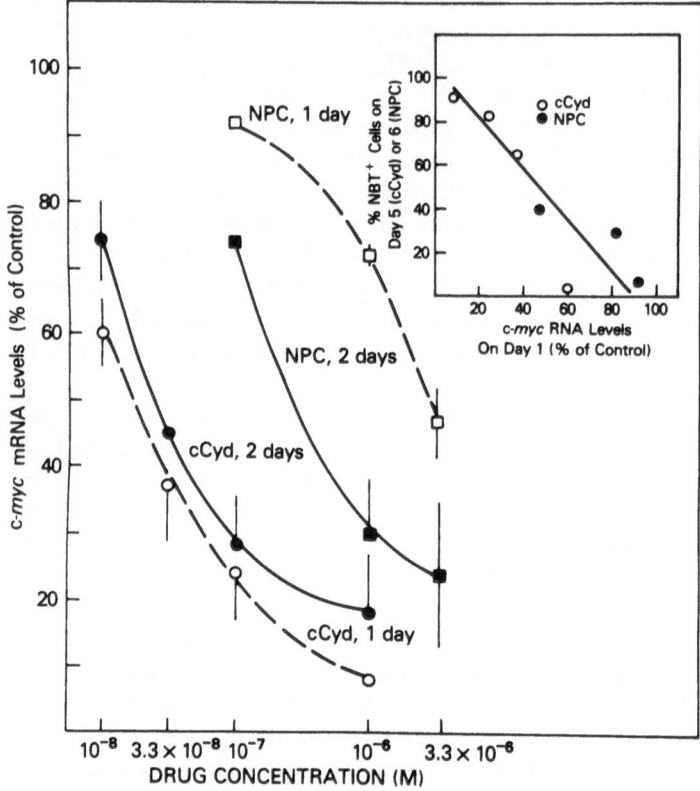

Fig. 4. Cellular *myc* mRNA expression in HL-60 cells treated with neplanocin A and cyclopentenyl cytidine. c-*myc* mRNA levels were monitored by dot-blot hybridization and differentiation by the percentage of NBT+ cells, [35, 39]

recently elucidated, and it appears to be associated with the stimulation of DNA polymerase activity [116]. Thus, its reduced synthesis in cells undergoing differentiation and its elevation in various tumors suggests a direct role for this cellular oncogene in the regulation of proliferation. Recent studies in this laboratory have documented a striking correlation between the reduction in c-*myc* mRNA levels and the increase in myelocytic differentiation induced in HL-60 cells by the carbocyclic analogs neplanocin A and cyclopentenyl cytidine [35, 39] (Fig. 4). The decrease in c-*myc* mRNA in this instance appears to be an early indication of the ability of these nucleoside analogs to reduce the progression of cells through S phase. Similar results have been obtained for the related cellular oncogene, c-*myb*, in the myeloblastic cell line ML-1 preceding its differentiation to monocyte-macrophage-like cells by TPA [117].

Future Drug Development

There are many points of intervention in the metabolic sequences presented in Fig. 3 which may be exploitable therapeutically in the future to differentiate or inhibit the proliferation of tumors. The first obvious point of attack is the growth factor receptor and its associated tyrosine kinase activity. If the latter proves essential for the transduction of the growth factor signal to the nucleus of the cell, then specific inhibitors of the kinase may prove therapeutically useful in the treatment of growth factor-dependent neoplasms. The possible utility of this approach was reported by Braun et al. [118], who synthesized a series of polytetrapeptides containing (Tyr-Glu-Ala-Gly)$_4$ as potent inhibitors of several tyrosine kinases. This approach may not be useful in tumors with mutated receptors such as the truncated EGF receptor lacking the tyrosine kinase domain in A431 cells, but would be useful in cells containing receptors with tyrosine kinase activity.

A second approach might be to understand in more detail the functioning of the *ras* gene product, p21 GTP-binding protein, and its postulated ability to regulate phosphatidylinositide hydrolysis [98]. The generation of IP$_3$ from PIP$_2$ is a key process in the mediation of not only proliferation but several autonomic pharmacological processes as well. Drugs such as the dialkylether phosphatidylcholine analogs, which show effective antitumor activity against HL-60 cells [30–33], may possibly mediate their effects via inhibition of phospholipase C activity or disruption of phosphatidylinositol metabolism. Moreover, little is known about the importance of Ca^{++} mobilization by IP$_3$ in the growth and differentiation of cells. Perhaps specific blockers of the effect of IP$_3$ on Ca^{++} mobilization, such as inositol analogs, will prove of utility for inhibiting cell proliferation or effecting differentiation.

A third avenue for chemotherapeutic intervention might be either the stimulation or inhibition of protein kinase C. Diacylglycerol analogs, which stimulate this enzyme, also induce differentiation in some cell lines [29]. However, it has also been reported that some phospholipid analogs, which induce differentiation in HL-60 cells, inhibit protein kinase C activity in vitro [28]. Thus, it is important to establish the relevance of this enzyme to the pathway of differentiation vs. growth inhibition in order to assess the usefulness of this target enzyme in differentiation therapy.

Finally, the products of most cellular oncogenes are not well defined as to their role in cellular differentiation and proliferation. The ability of the c-*myc* product to regulate DNA polymerase [116] suggests that analogs of the 64-kd nuclear phosphoprotein [119, 120] may be good therapeutic agents to either reduce proliferation or induce differentiation. The inhibitory role of c-*myc* expression on cellular differentiation has been demonstrated in transfection experiments with erythroleukemia cells where the continued synthesis of the c-*myc* gene dramatically inhibited differentiation [121, 122]. Obviously, other cellular oncogene products, or perhaps the genes themselves, will prove to be therapeutically exploitable targets for future strategies in the treatment of cancer.

References

1. Hiromichi H, Breitman TR (1984) Induction of differentiation of the human promyelocytic cell line HL-60 and primary cultures of human leukemia cells: a model for clinical treatment. In: Glazer RI (ed) Developments in cancer chemotherapy. CRC, Boca Raton, FL, pp 247–280
2. Larrick JW, Fischer DG, Anderson SJ, Koren HS (1980) Characterization of a human macrophage-like cell line stimulated in vitro: a model of macrophage functions. J Immunol 125: 6–12
3. Lozzio BB, Lozzio CB (1979) Properties and usefulness of the original K-562 human myelogenous leukemia cell line. Leuk Res 3: 363–370
4. Kimberly RP, Ralph P (1983) Endocytosis by the mononuclear phagocyte system and auto-immune disease. Am J Med 74: 481–493
5. Rovera G, Santoli D, Damsky C (1979) Human promyelocytic leukemia cells in culture differentiate into macrophage-like cells when treated with a phorbol ester. Proc Natl Acad Sci USA 76: 2779–2783
6. Lotem J, Sachs L (1979) Regulation of normal differentiation in mouse and human leukemic cells by phorbol esters and the mechanism of tumor promotion. Proc Natl Acad Sci USA 76: 5158–5162
7. Murao S, Gemmell MA, Callaham MF, Anderson NL, Huberman E (1983) Control of macrophage cell differentiation in human promyelocytic HL-60 leukemia cells by 1,25-dihydroxyvitamin D_3 and phorbol-12-myristate-13-acetate. Cancer Res 43: 4989–4996
8. Rovera G, Ferrero D, Pagliardi GL, Vartikar J, Pessano S, Bottero L, Abraham S, Lebman D (1982) Induction of differentiation of human myeloid leukemias by phorbol diesters: phenotypic changes and mode of action. Ann NY Acad Sci 397: 211–220
9. Newberger PE, Baker RD, Hansen SL, Duncan RA, Greenberger JS (1981) Functionally deficient differentiation of HL-60 promyelocytic leukemia cells induced by phorbol myristate acetate. Cancer Res 41: 1861–1865
10. Koeffler HP, Bar-Eli M, Terito M (1980) Phorbol diester-induced macrophage differentiation of leukemic blasts from patients with human myelogenous leukemia. J Clin Invest 66: 1101–1108
11. Fibach E, Rachmilewitz EA (1981) Tumor promoters induce macrophage differentiation in human myeloid cells from patients with acute and chronic myelogenous leukameia. Br J Haematol 47: 203–210
12. Totterman TH, Nilsson K, Sundstrom C (1980) Phorbol ester-induced differentiation of chronic lymphocytic leukaemia cells. Nature 288: 176–178
13. Lockney MW, Dawson G, Golomb HM (1984) Effect of phorbol ester tumor promotors on hairy cell leukemic cells. Semin Oncol 11: 433–438
14. Shawler DL, Glassy MC, Wormsley SB, Royston I (1984) Alterations in cell surface phenotype of T- and B-cell chronic lymphocytic leukemia cells following in vitro differentiation by phorbol ester. JNCI 72: 1059–1063
15. Nadler LM, Ritz J, Bates MP, Park EK, Anderson KC, Salan SE, Schlossman SF (1982) Induction of human B cell antigens in non-T cell acute lymphoblastic leukemia. J Clin Invest 70: 433–442
16. Nagasawa K, Howatson A, Mak TW (1981) Induction of human malignant T-lymphoblastic cell lines MOLT-3 and Jurkat by 12-O-tetradecanoylphorbol-13-acetate: biochemical, physical, and morphological characterization. J Cell Physiol 109: 181–192
17. Hu AD, Ma DDF, Price G, Hoffbrand AV (1983) Effect of thymosin and phorbol ester on purine metabolic enzymes and cell surface phenotype in a malignant T-cell line (MOLT-3). Leuk Res 7: 779–786
18. Ralph P, Kishimoto T (1981) Tumor promoter phorbol myristic acetate stimulates immunoglobulin secretion correlated with growth cessation in human B lymphocyte cell lines. J Clin Invest 68: 1093–1096
19. Miyaura C, Abe E, Kuribayashi T, Tanaka H, Konno K, Nishii Y, Suda T (1981) 125-

Dihydroxyvitamin D$_3$ induces differentiation of human myeloid leukemia cells. Biochem Biophys Res Commun 102: 937–943

20. McCarthy DM, San Miguel JF, Freake HC, Green PM, Zola H, Catovsky D, Goldman JM (1983) 1,25-Dihydroxyvitamin D$_3$ inhibits proliferation of human promyelocytic leukemia (HL-60) cells and induces monocyte-macrophage differentiation in HL-60 and normal human bone marow cells. Leuk Res 7: 51–55

21. Bar-Shavit Z, Teitelbaum SL, Reitsma P, Hall A, Pegg LE, Trial J, Kahn AJ (1983) Induction of monocytic differentiation and bone resorption by 1,25-dihydroxyvitamin D$_3$. Proc Natl Acad Sci USA 80: 5907–5911

22. Mangelsdorf DJ, Koeffler HP, Donaldson CA, Pike JW, Haussler MR (1984) 1,25-Dihydroxyvitamin D$_3$-induced differentiation in a human promyelocytic leukemia cell line (HL-60): receptor-mediated maturation to macrophage-like cells. J Cell Biol 98: 391–398

23. Breitman TR, Selonick SE, Collins SJ (1980) Induction of differentiation of the human promyelocytic leukemia cell line (HL-60) by retinoic acid. Proc Natl Acad Sci USA 77: 2936–2940

24. Collins SJ, Ruscetti FW, Gallagher RE, Gallo RC (1978) Terminal differentiation of human promyelocytic cells induced by dimethyl sulfoxide and other polar compounds. Proc Natl Acad Sci USA 75: 2458–2462

25. Olsson IL, Breitman TR (1982) Induction of differentiation of the human histiocytic lymphoma cell line U-937 by retinoic acid and cyclic adenosine 3′:5′-monophosphate-inducing agents. Cancer Res 42: 3924–3927

26. Olsson IL, Breitman TR, Gallo RC (1982) Priming of human myeloid leukemic cell lines HL-60 and U-937 with retinoic acid for differentiation effects of cyclic adenosine 3′:5′-monophosphate-inducing agents and a T-lymphocyte-derived differentiation factor. Cancer Res 42: 3928–3933

27. Tomida M, Yamamoto Y, Hozumi M (1982) Stimulation by interferon of induction of differentiation of human promyelocytic leukemia cells. Biochem Biophys Res Commun 104: 30–37

28. Honma Y, Kasukable T, Hozumi M, Tsushima S, Nomura H (1981) Induction of differentiation of cultured human and mouse myeloid leukemia cells by alkyl-lysopholipids. Cancer Res 41: 3211–3216

29. McNamara MJC, Schmitt JD, Wykle RL, Daniel LW (1984) 1-O-Hexadecyl-2-acetyl-sn-glycerol stimulates differentiation of HL-60 human promyelocytic leukemia cells to macrophage-like cells. Biochem Biophs Res Commun 122: 824–830

30. Hoffman DR, Stanley JD, Berchtold R, Snyder F (1984) Cytotoxicity of ether-linked phytanyl phospholipid analogs and related derivatives in human HL-60 leukemia cells and polymorphonuclear neutrophils. Res Commun Chem Pathol Pharmacol 44: 293–306

31. Hoffman DR, Hajdu J, Snyder F (1984) Cytotoxicity of platelet activating factor and related akyl-phospholipid analogs in human leukemia cells, polymorphonuclear neutrophils, and skin fibroblasts. Blood 63: 545–552

32. Tidwell T, Gusman G, Vogler WR (1981) The effects of alkyl-lysophospholipids on leukemia cell lines. I. Differential action on the two human leukemic cell lines, HL-60 and K562, Blood 57: 794–797

33. Berdel WE, Schlehe H, Fink U, Emmerich B, Maubach PA, Emslander HP, Daum S, Rastetter J (1982) Early tumor and leukemia response to alkyl-lysophospholipids in a phase I study. Cancer 50: 2011–2015

34. Christman JK, Mendelsohn N, Herzog D, Schneiderman N (1983) Effect of 5-azacytidine on differentiation and DNA methylation in human promyelocytic leukemia cells (HL-60). Cancer Res 43: 763–769

35. Linevsky J, Cohen MB, Hartman KD, Knode MC, Glazer RI (1985) Effect of neplanocin on differentiation, nucleic acid methylation and c-myc mRNA expression in human promyelocytic leukemic cells. Mol Pharmacol 28: 45–50

36. Glazer RI, Knode MC (1984) Neplanocin A: a cyclopentenyl analog of adenosine with specificity for inhibiting RNA methylation. J Biol Chem 259: 12964–12969

37. Yen A (1945) Control of HL-60 differentiation. Evidence of uncoupled growth and differentiation control, S-phase specificity, and two-step regulation. Exp Cell Res 156: 198–212

38. Blair OC, Carbone R, Sartorelli AC (1985) Differentiation of HL-60 promyelocytic leukemia cells monitored by flow cytometric measurement of nitro blue tetrazolium (NBT) reduction. Cytometry 6: 54–61

39. Glazer RI, Cohen MB, Hartman KD, Knode MC, Lim M-I, Marquez VE (1986) Induction of differentiation in human promyelocytic leukemia cell line HL-60 by the CTP synthetase inhibitor, cyclopentenyl cytidine analogue. Biochem Pharmacol 35: 1841–1848

40. Glazer RI, Knode MC, Lim M-I, Marquez VE (1985) Cyclopentenyl cytidine analogue: an inhibitor of cytidine triphosphate synthesis in human colon carcinoma cells. Biochem Pharmacol 34: 2535–2539

41. Bodner AJ, Ting RC, Gallo RC (1981) Induction of differentiation of human promyelocytic leukemia cells (HL-60) by nucleosides and methotrexate. JNCI 67: 1025–1030

42. Lucas DL, Webster HK, Wright DG (1983) Purine metabolism in myeloid precursor cells during maturation. J Clin Invest 72: 1889–1900

43. Takai Y, Kishimoto A, Iwasa Y, Kawahara Y, Mori T, Nishizuka Y (1979) Calcium-dependent activation of a multifunctional protein kinase by membrane phospholipids. J Biol Chem 254: 3692–13695

44. Nishizuka (1984) Protein kinases in signal transduction. Trends Biochem Sci 9: 163–166

45. Kuo JF, Schatzman RC, Turner RS, Mazzei GJ (1984) Phospholipid-sensitive Ca^{2+}-dependent protein kinase: a major protein phosphorylation system. Mol Cell Endocrinol 35: 65–73

46. Castagna M, Takai Y, Kaibuchi K, Sano K, Kikkawa U, Nishizuka Y (1982) Direct activation of calcium-activated, phospholipid-dependent protein kinase by tumor-promoting phorbol esters. J Biol Chem 257: 7847–7851

47. Kikkawa K, Takai Y, Tanaka Y, Miyake R, Nishizuka Y (1983) Protein kinase C as a possible receptor protein of tumor-promoting phorbol esters. J Biol Chem 258: 11442–11445

48. Ashendel CL, Staller JM, Boutwell RK (1983) Solubilization, purification, and reconstitution of a phorbol ester receptor from the particulate protein fraction of mouse brain. Cancer Res 43: 4327–4332

49. Ashendel CL, Staller JM, Boutwell RK (1983) Protein kinase activity associated with a phorbol ester receptor purified from mouse brain. Cancer Res 43: 4333–4337

50. Vandenbark GR, Kuhn LJ, Niedel JE (1984) Possible mechanism of phorbol diester-induced maturation of human promyelocytic leukemia cells. J Clin Invest 73: 448–457

51. Mori T, Takai Y, Yu B, Takahashi J, Nishizuka Y, Fujikura T (1982) Specificity of the fatty acyl moieties of diacylglycerol for the activation of calcium-activated, phospholipid-dependent protein kinase. J Biochem (Tokyo) 91: 427–431

52. Kajikawa N, Kaibuchi K, Matsubara T, Kikkawa U, Takai Y, Nishizuka Y (1983) A possible role of protein kinase C in signal-induced lysosomal enzyme release. Biochem Biophys Res Commun 116: 743–750

53. Yamanishi J, Takai Y, Kaibuchi K, Sano K, Castagna M, Nishizuka Y (1983) Synergistic functions of phorbol ester and calcium in serotonin release from human platelets. Biochem Biophys Res Commun 112: 778–786

54. Lapetina EG, Reep B, Ganong BR, Bell RM (1985) Exogenous sn-1,2-diacylglycerols containing fatty acids function as bioregulators of protein kinase C in human platelets. J Biol Chem 260: 1358–1361

55. Feuerstein N, Cooper HL (1983) Rapid protein phosphorylation induced by phorbol ester in HL-60 cells. Unique alkali-stable phosphorylation of a 17,000-dalton protein detected by two-dimensional gel electrophoresis. J Biol Chem 258: 10786–10793

56. Feuerstein N, Cooper HD (1984) Rapid phosphorylation-dephosphorylation of specific proteins induced by phorbol ester in HL-60 cells. Further characterization of the phosphorylation of 17-kilodalton and 27-kilodalton proteins in myeloid leukemic cells and human monocytes. J Biol Chem 259: 2782–2788

57. Feuerstein N, Sahai A, Anderson WB, Salomon DS, Cooper HL (1984) Differential phosphorylation events associated with phorbol ester effects on acceleration versus inhibition of cell growth. Cancer Res 44: 5227–5233

58. Grunberger G, Zick Y, Taylor SI, Gorden P (1984) Tumor-promoting phorbol ester stimulates tyrosine phosphorylation in U-937 monocytes. Proc Natl Acad Sci USA 81: 2762–2766

59. Wrann MM, Fox CF (1979) Identification of epidermal growth factor receptors in a hyperproducing human epidermoid cell line. J Biol Chem 254: 8083–8086
60. Hunter T, Cooper JA (1981) Epidermal growth factor induces rapid tyrosine phosphorylation of proteins in A431 human tumor cells. Cell 24: 741–752
61. McCaffrey PG, Friedman BA, Rosner MR (1984) Diacylglycerol modulates binding and phosphorylation of the epidermal growth factor receptor. J Biol Chem 259: 12502–12507
62. Iwashita S, Fox CF (1984) Epidermal growth factor and potent phorbol tumor promoters induce epidermal growth factor receptor phosphorylation in a similar but distinctively different manner in human epidermoid carcinoma A431 cells. J Biol Chem 259: 2559–2567
63. Cochet C, Gill GN, Meisenhelder J, Cooper JA, Hunter T (1984) C-kinase phosphorylates the epidermal growth factor receptor and reduces its epidermal growth factor-stimulated tyrosine protein kinase activity. J Biol Chem 259: 2553–2558
64. Davis RJ, Ganong BR, Bell RM, Czech MP (1984) sn-1,2-Dioctanoyl-glycerol. A cell-permeable diacylglycerol that mimics phorbol diester action on the epidermal growth factor receptor and mitogenesis. J Biol Chem 260: 7761–7766
65. Kawamoto T, Mendelsohn J, Le A, Sato GH, Lazar CS, Gill GN (1984) Relation of epidermal growth factor receptor concentration to growth of human epidermoid carcinoma A431 cells. J Biol Chem 259: 7761–7766
66. Zylber-Katz E, Glazer RI (1985) Phospholipid- and Ca^{++}-dependent protein kinase activity and protein phosphorylation patterns in the differentiation of human promyelocytic leukemia cell line HL-60. Cancer Res 45: 5159–5164
67. Nishizuka Y (1984) Turnover of phospholipids and signal transduction. Science 225: 1365–1370
68. Berridge MJ, Irvine RF (1984) Inositol trishosphate, a novel second messenger in cellular signal transduction. Nature 312: 315–321
69. Burgess GM, Godfrey PP, McKinney JS, Berridge MJ, Irvine RF, Putney JW Jr (1984) The second messenger linking receptor activation to internal Ca release in liver. Nature 309: 63–66
70. Thomas AP, Alexander J, Williamson JR (1984) Relationship between inositol polyphosphate production and the increase of cytosolic free Ca^{2+} induced by vasopressin in isolated hepatocytes. J Biol Chem 259: 5574–7784
71. Streb H, Irving RF, Berridge MJ, Schulz I (1983) Release of Ca^{2+} from a nonmitochondrial intracellular store in pancreatic acinar cells by inositol-1,4,5-trisphosphate. Nature 306: 67–69
72. Downes PC, Michell RH (1981) The polyphosphoinositide phosphodiesterase of erythrocyte membranes. Biochem J 198: 133–140
73. Dougherty RW, Godfrey PP, Hoyle PC, Putney JW Jr, Freer RJ (1984) Secretagogue-induced phosphoinositide metabolism in human leucocytes. Biochem J 222: 307–314
74. Burgess GM, McKinney JS, Irvine RF, Berridge MJ, Hoyle PC, Putney JW Jr (1984) Inositol 1,4,5-triphosphate may be a signal for f-Met-Leu-Phe-induced intracellular Ca mobilization in human leucocytes (HL-60 cells). FEBS Lett 176: 193–196
75. Whitman MR, Epstein J, Cantley L (1984) Inositol 1,4,5-trisphosphate stimulates phosphorylation of a 62,000-dalton protein in monkey fibroblast and bovine brain cells. J Biol Chem 259: 13652–13655
76. Lapetina EG, Watson SP, Cuatrecasas P (1984) myo-Inositol 1,4,5-trisphosphate stimulates protein phosphorylation in saponin-permeabilized human platelets. Proc Natl Acad Sci USA 81: 7431–7435
77. Land H, Parada LF, Weinberg RA (1983) Cellular oncogenes and multistep carcinogenesis. Science 222: 771–778
78. Slamon DJ, de Kernion JB, Verma IM, Cline MJ (1984) Expression cellular oncogenes in human malignancies. Science 224: 256–262
79. Pimentel E (1985) Oncogenes and human cancer. Cancer Genet Cytogenet 14: 347–368
80. Doolittle RF, Hunkopiller MW, Hood LE, Devare SG, Robbins KC, Aaronson SA, Antoniades HN (1983) Simian sarcoma virus onc gene, v-sis, is derived from the gene (or genes) encoding a platelet derived growth factor. Science 221: 275–277
81. Waterfield A, Scrace GT, Whittle N, Stroobant P, Johnsson A, Wasteson A, Westermark B, Heldin C-H, Huang JS, Devel T (1983) Platelet derived growth factor is structurally related to the putative p28 sis of simian sarcoma virus. Nature 304: 35–39

82. Ullrich A, Coussens L, Hayflick JS, Dull TJ, Gray A, Tam AW, Lee J, Yarden Y, Libermann TA, Schlessinger J, Downward J, Mayes ELV, Whittle N, Waterfield MD, Seeburg PH (1984) Human epidermal growth factor receptor cDNA sequence and aberrant expression of the amplified gene in A431 epidermoid carcinoma cells. Nature 309: 418–425

83. Lin CR, Chen WS, Kruiger W, Stolarsky LS, Weber W, Evans RM, Verma IM, Gill GN, Rosenfeld MG (1986) Expression cloning of human EGF receptor complementary DNA: gene amplification and three related messenger RNA products in A431 cells. Science 224: 843–848

84. Xu Y-H, Ishii S, Clark AJL, Sullivan M, Wilson RK, Ma DP, Roe BA, Merlino GT, Pastan I (1984) Human epidermal growth factor receptor cDNA is homologous to a variety of RNAs overproduced in A431 carcinoma cells. Nature 309: 806–810

85. Xu Y-H, Richert N, Ito S, Merlino GT, Pastan I (1984) Characterization of epidermal growth factor receptor gene expression in malignant and normal human cell lines. Proc Natl Acad Sci USA 81: 7308–7312

86. Paukovits JB, Paukovits W-R, Laerum OD (1986) Identification of a regulatory peptide distinct from normal granulocyte-derived hemoregulatory peptide produced by human promyelocytic HL-60 leukemia cells after differentiation induction by retinoic acid. Cancer Res 46: 4444–4448

87. Pantazis P, Lanfrancone L, Pelicci PG, Dalla-Favera R, Antoniades HN (1986) Human leukemia cells synthesize and secrete proteins related to platelet-derived growth factor. Proc Natl Acad Sci USA 83: 5526–5530

88. Bishayee S, Ross AH, Womer R, Scher CD (1986) Purified human plateletderived growth factor receptor has ligand-stimulated tyrosine kinase activity. Proc Natl Acad Sci USA 83: 6756–6760

89. Rettenmier CW, Sacca R, Furman WL, Roussel MF, Holt JT, Nienhuis AW, Stanley ER, Sherr CJ (1986) Expression of the human c-*fms* proto-oncogene product (colony-stimulating factor-1 receptor) on peripheral blood mononuclear cells and choriocarcinoma cell lines J Clin Invest 77: 1740–1746

90. Gee CE, Griffin J, Sastre L, Miller LJ, Springer TA, Piwnica-Worms H, Roberts TM (1986) Differentiation of myeloid cells is accompanied by increased levels of pp60[c-src] protein and kinase activity. Proc Natl Acad Sci USA 83: 5131–5135

91. Barnekow A, Gessler M (1986) Activation of the pp60[c-src] kinase during differentiation of monomyelocytic cells in vitro. EMBO J 5: 701–705

92. Frank DS, Sartorelli AC (1986) Regulation of protein phosphotyrosine content by changes in tyrosine kinase and protein phosphotyrosine phosphatase activities during induced granulocytic and monocytic differentiation of HL-60 leukemia cells. Biochem Biophys Res Commun 140: 440–447

93. Glazer RI, Chapekar MS, Hartman KD, Knode MC (1986) Appearance of membrane-bound tyrosine kinase during differentiation of HL-60 leukemia cells by immune interferon and tumor necrosis factor. Biochem Biophys Res Commun 140: 908–915

94. Land H, Parada LF, Weinberg RA (1983) Tumorigenic conversion of primary embryo fibroblasts requires at least two cooperating oncogenes. Nature 304: 596–602

95. Feramisco JR, Gross M, Kamata T, Rosenberg M, Sweet RW (1984) Microinjection of the oncogene form of the human H-*ras* (T-24) protein results in rapid proliferation of quiescent cells. Cell 38: 109–117

96. Kamata T, Feramisco JR (1984) Epidermal growth factor stimulates guanine nucleotide binding activity and phosphorylation of *ras* oncogene proteins. Nature 310: 147–150

97. Gilman AG (1984) G proteins and dual control of adenylate cyclase. Cell 36: 577–579

98. Cockcroft S, Gomperts BD (1985) Role of guanine nucleotide binding protein in the activation of polyphosphoinositide phosphodiesterase. Nature 314: 534–536

99. Sawyer ST, Cohen S (1981) Enhancement of calcium uptake and phosphatidylinositol turnover by epidermal growth factor in A-431 cells. Biochemistry 20: 6280–6286

100. Macara IG, Marinetti GV, Balduzzi PC (1984) Transforming protein of avian sarcoma virus UR2 is associated with phosphatidyl inositol kinase activity: possible role in tumorigenesis. Proc. Natl. Acad. Sci. U.S.A. 81: 2728–2732

101. Sugimoto Y, Whitman M, Cantley LC, Erikson RL (1984) Evidence that the Rous sarcoma

virus transforming gene product phosphorylates phosphatidylinositol and diacylglycerol. Proc Natl Acad Sci USA 81: 2117–2121

102. MacDonald ML, Kuenzel EA, Glomset JA, Krebs EG (1985) Evidence from two transformed cell lines that the phosphorylation of peptide tyrosine and phosphatidyl inositol are catalyzed by different proteins. Proc Natl Acad Sci USA 82: 3993–3997

103. Dalla-Favera R, Wong-Staal F, Gallo RC (1982) *onc* Gene amplification in promyelocytic leukaemia cell line HL-60 and primary leukaemic cells of the same patient. Nature 299: 61–63

104. Collins S, Groudine M (1982) Amplication of endogenous *myc*-related DNA sequences in a human myeloid leukaemia cell line. Nature 298: 679–681

105. Kozbor D, Croce CM (1984) Amplification of the c-*myc* oncogene in one of five breast carcinoma cell lines. Cancer Res 44: 438–444

106. Shibuya M, Yokota J, Ueyama Y (1985) Amplification and expression of a cellular oncogene (c-*myc*) in human gastric adenocarcinoma cells. Mol Cell Biol 5: 414–418

107. Saksela K, Bergh J, Lehto V-P, Nilsson K, Alitalo K (1985) Amplification of the c-*myc* oncogene in a subpopulation of human small cell lung cancer. Cancer Res 45: 1823–1827

108. Kelly K, Cochran BH, Stiles CD, Leder P (1983) Cell-specific regulation of the c-*myc* gene by lymphocyte mitogens and platelet-derived growth factor. Cell 35; 603–610

109. McCormack JE, Pepe VH, Kent RB, Dean M, Marshak-Rothstein A, Sonenshein GE (1984) Specific regulation of c-*myc* oncogene expression in a murine B-cell lymphoma. Proc Natl Acad Sci USA 81: 5546–5550

110. Jonak GJ, Knight EJ (1984) Selective reduction of c-*myc* mRNA in Daudi cells by human β interferon. Proc Natl Acad Sci USA 81: 1747–1750

111. Boumpas DT, Tsokos GC, Mann DL, Eleftheriades EG, Harris CC, Mark GE (1985) Increased oncogene expression in peripheral lymphocytes from patients with systemic lupus erythematosus. Fed Proc 44: 600

112. Thiele CJ, Reynolds CP, Israel MA (1985) Decreased expression of N-*myc* precedes retinoic acid-induced morphological differentiation of human neuroblastoma. Nature 313: 404–406

113. Westin EH, Wong-Staal F, Gelmann EP, Dalla-Favera R, Papas TS, Lautenberger JA, Eva A, Reddy EP, Tronick SR, Aaronson SA, Gallo RC (1982) Expression of cellular homologues of retroviral *onc* genes in human hematopoietic cells. Proc Natl Acad Sci USA 79: 2490–2494

114. Reitsma PH, Rothberg PG, Astrin SM, Trial J, Bar-Shavit Z, Hall A, Teitelbaum SL, Kahn AJ (1983) Regulation of *myc* gene expression in HL-60 leukaemia cells by a vitamin D metabolite. Nature 306: 492–494

115. Grosso LE, Pitot HC (1984) Modulation of c-*myc* expression in the HL-60 cell line. Biochem Biophys Res Commun 119: 473–480

116. Studzinski GP, Brelvi ZS, Feldman SC, Watts RA (1986) Participation of c-*myc* protein in DNA synthesis of human cells. Science 234: 467–470

117. Craig RW, Bloch A (1984) Early decline in c-*myb* oncogene expression in the differentiation of human myeloblastic leukemia (ML-1) cells induced with 12-*O*-tetradecanoyl-13-acetate. Cancer Res 44: 442–446

118. Braun S, Raymond WE, Racker E (1984) Synthetic tyrosine polymers as substrates and inhibitors of tyrosine-specific kinases. J Biol Chem 259: 2051–2054

119. Beimling P, Beuter T, Sander T, Moelling K (1985) Isolation and characterization of the human cellular *myc* gene product. Biochemistry 24: 6349–6355

120. Watt RA, Shatzman AR, Rosenberg M (1985) Expression and characterization of the human c-*myc* gene product. Biochemistry 24: 6349–6355

121. Prochownik EV, Kukowska J (1986) Deregulated expression of c-*myc* by murine erythroleukemia cells prevent differentiation. Nature 322: 848–850

122. Dmitrovsky E, Kuehl WM, Hollis GF, Kirsch IR, Bender TP, Segal W (1986) Expression of a transfected human c-*myc* oncogene inhibits differentiation of a mouse erythroleukemia cell line. Nature 322: 748–750

Therapeutic Trends
in Specific Neoplasms

23. Malignant Brain Tumors

D.C. Wright

Current Results and Therapeutic Issues

Malignant gliomas account for approximately 45% of all brain tumors, with 60%–70% of this group belonging to the highly malignant category (glioblastoma multiforme and anaplastic astrocytoma). These tumors represent a significant epidemiologic fraction (8%–10%) of malignant disease, with 12000 new cases per year and 10200 estimated deaths annually in the United States [7]. In terms of overall prevalence, malignant gliomas are largely a disease affecting adults in their 5th–7th decades, although they also account for a significant fraction of childhood cancers. Glioblastoma multiforme (GBM) represents the most malignant of the group, with fully developed pathologic features, while the anaplastic astrocytoma (AA), anaplastic ependymoma and anaplastic oligodendroglioma complete the pathologic spectrum of malignant gliomas in roughly decreasing order of malignancy. These tumors, while capable of metastatic spread within the central nervous system (CNS), tend to be regionally confined, and rarely metastasize outside the CNS. Ninety percent of patients in whom treatment fails have local recurrence rather than develop diffuse or multicentric metastases. This chapter will *not* consider the well-differentiated astrocytomas ("grades I–II") of lower malignant potential with variable clinical behavior, though approximately 20% of these lesions may undergo malignant degeneration and develop the pathologic characteristics which constitute the criteria for the highly malignant glioma group [10].

Toxicity of Therapy

In many of the available therapies directed against brain tumors, the limiting factor is local (neural) injury rather than systemic side effects. Surgery, radiation therapy, and chemotherapy all have toxic effects on brain function. Mechanical distortion, direct destruction or interruption of connecting neural pathways can arise secondary to surgery. Radiation can induce or aggravate brain edema, and cerebral radionecrosis accompanies conventional teletherapy doses exceeding 55–65 Gy (Gy = gray, or 100 rads), depending on the length of survival, age of the patient, and other factors. Chemotherapy has neurotoxic and myelotoxic effects, particularly in patients receiving combination therapy.

Clinical Resistance

Multiple factors are involved in the clinical resistance of malignant gliomas. Despite similarities in pathologic classification criteria, wide differences are found in tumor cell kinetics, in abnormalities in chromosomal number and DNA content, in morphologic and cytologic appearance, in expression of biochemical and immunologic markers, and in biologic behaviour in terms of physiology and in vitro and in vivo growth. Therapeutic failure can be attributed to at least three separate problems: heterogeneity of tumor cell populations, cell kinetics, and inadequate drug delivery [1, 2, 9, 10]. Future therapeutic strategies must address these problems in order to exceed currently achieved results.

Current Results

The completion of several large-scale multicenter cooperative studies identified prognostic variables, established optimal teletherapy radiation doses, and examined several combination therapy groups. Current optimal therapy of malignant brain tumors includes surgery, radiation therapy, and chemotherapy (nitrosoureas and other drugs). The median survival in these trials was 51 weeks, with an 18-month survival of 27% [7, 10, 12]. These studies confirmed that surgery alone (16 weeks) and surgery plus radiation therapy (36 weeks) were less successful than triple therapy, but in addition showed those patients treated with higher radiation doses (>50 Gy) had an increased median survival. Prognostic variables correlating with increased survival were (a) good neurologic condition (Karnofsky score) prior to treatment, (b) age less than 45 years, and (c) histopathologic characteristics of the tumor. Minor variables included sex, duration of symptoms, blood type, cognitive dysfunction, occurrence of seizures, motor symptoms, and multicentricity. Patients with favorable prognostic characteristics (e.g. age < 45, Karnovsky > 70, non-GBM, and long duration of symptoms) who received combination therapy had a 24-month survival of 46%. Specialized brain tumor treatment centers currently achieve a median survival of approximately 66 weeks, using aggressive multimodality therapy in selected patients [9].

Current Approaches Under Study

Surgery

The development of microsurgical techniques, preoperative and intraoperative location of tumors with high resolution scanning (transmission X-ray, magnetic resonance, ultrasound) neuroanesthesia, perioperative care, and a variety of surgical instrumentation advances (laser resection, ultrasonic aspiration, CT-

448

directed stereotaxis, etc.) have decreased the risk inherent in surgical procedures while increasing the potential for more extensive resection in many patients. Currently, surgical goals for malignant brain tumors are to:

—Establish a diagnosis and classify patients' disease according to pathologic characteristics
—Reduce the number of tumor cells (cytoreduction)
—Relieve symptoms arising from mechanical distortion or obstruction of CSF pathways
—Gain time to institute other forms of therapy
—Alter the kinetics of quiescent cells, thereby increasing their susceptibility to therapy [13]

Radiation Therapy

Radiation is the most effective adjunctive therapy for primary malignant brain tumors. Since the highest tolerated dose delivered to the smallest possible post-surgical treatment volume results in the greatest cell kill, investigations have focused on means of safely increasing the total dose or quality of radiation and potentiating the biologic effects of the delivered dose. Two current therapeutic strategies with promising preliminary results reflecting these concepts involves the use of (true) radiation sensitizers (halogenated pyrimidines), combined with conventional or double fractionated teletherapy, and local radiation approaches (interstitial radiation).

In a recently completed phase I-II study [4], 60 patients with malignant brain tumors (50 GBM, 8 AA) matched for the known prognostic variables underwent systemic infusion of bromo- or iodo-deoxyuridine (BUdR or IUdR) while receiving conventional or double fractionated radiation doses (65–70 Gy). The median survival for the entire group was 12 months, with a 18-month survival of 24%. Those patients with favorable prognostic characteristics had a median survival of 15 months, versus 9.4 months for the group with poor prognostic characteristics. Such a study, with variations in drug dose from suboptimal to toxic, is not designed to determine efficacy, but represents a promising therapeutic approach, particularly in view of the results achieved in such a patient group dominated by glioblastoma multiforme.

A number of regional (local) approaches under current study are attractive since one may potentially limit the neurotoxicity associated with increasing radiation doses. The interstitial radiation approach is a means of increasing the total treatment dose without exceeding normal tissue tolerance. Toxicity is dependent on the total dose, the treatment volume, and the time over which the radiation is deposited. Positioning a radioactive source or a multiple source array within a treatment volume (tumor plus an arbitrary margin) delivers continuous low dose rate radiation (0.4–1.5 cGy/min) over time (days to weeks) and delivers high local doses (80–150 Gy). Conventional fractionated teletherapy utilizes intermittent high dose rate radiation (200–300 cGy/min) delivered over 4–6 weeks, and the total dose is limited by neurotoxicity to 55–65 Gy (or equivalent dose). The rationale for low dose rate radiation is to *just* exceed a certain (and variable) "critical dose rate" for neoplastic tissue, at which cell proliferation is arrested and the absorbed dose per cell cycle exceeds the tumor's capacity to repair radiation damage. Normal tissue is thought to have a superior capacity to repair sublethal damage, and further sparing of normal tissue is achieved by placing the radiation sources within the boundaries of the tumor, attenuation of radiation being inversely related to the square of the distance from the source. The theoretic advantages of interstitial radiation over conventional teletherapy are thus (a) focal delivery of low dose rate radiation to high total doses (b) a differential capacity of normal tissue to repair sublethal radiation damage, and (c) prolongation of cell cycle time by mitotic arrest, increasing the dose absorbed per cell cycle.

The recent renaissance in low dose rate therapy was triggered by the introduction and clinical use of computers for radiation dosimetry algorithms, high resolution images of the brain and the brain–tumor interface (contrast-enhanced computed tomography), and stereotactic surgical systems able to utilize directly the CT localization of a tumor for preoperative dosimetry planning and subsequent placement of radioactive sources to prescribed coordinates. Figure 1 is a CT scan showing a stereotactically placed multiple array of ^{125}I sources to a previously specified treatment volume in a patient harboring a glioblastoma. In a recent review [3], 43 patients with recurrent malignant gliomas achieved a

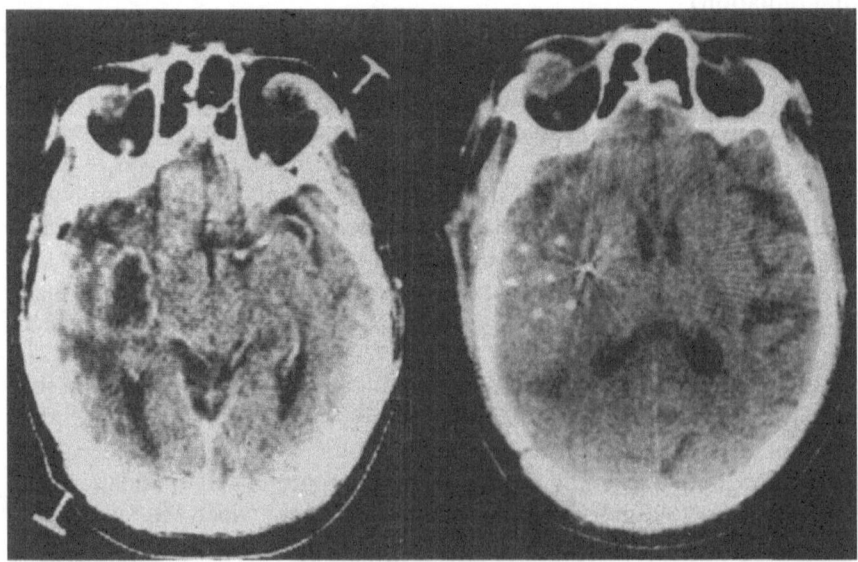

Fig. 1. CT scan showing a temporal lobe glioblastoma prior to therapy (*left*), and following an interstitial implant (*right*). Note the stereotactically placed multiple catheter array bearing the ^{125}I radioactive sources, which cause a metallic scatter artifact on the CT scan. Such an implant approach can position sources to an accuracy of 1 mm

450

median survival of 18 months after implantation. There was a 51% response rate (response was defined as a decrease in tumor volume or increase in the patient's neurologic performance). Stabilization of the disease occurred in 16% of patients, while in 37% symptoms prgressed despite therapy. The notable toxic complications observed were symptomatic radiation necrosis, requiring surgical exploration to determine the pathology (necrosis, recurrent tumor, or admixture) or for control of mass effect. Extended survivals were achieved in patients undergoing such reoperation following brachytherapy. The remaining clinical problems include determining the optimal dose rate for highly malignant tumors, accurately localizing the tumor–brain interface and minimizing neurotoxicity and radiation-induced brain edema. This form of therapy represents the most promising advance in the treatment of malignant brain tumors under current investigation.

Chemotherapy

Chemotherapy has traditionally been a strategy for malignant disease that has spread beyond its site of origin. As previously noted, malignant gliomas are largely a regional problem and not ideally suited to a systemic chemotherapeutic approach. In a systemic (intravenous) approach, tumor and normal tissue are exposed to equal doses of drug in multiple passes through the capillary bed. Therapeutic effect depends on biochemical and cytokinetic differences between the target and normal tissues. The available cytotoxic agents have a narrow therapeutic index and response is usually transient. The intra-arterial route has a delivery advantage of 3–5 times the exposure over the intravenous route for the same drug, and means of increasing the exposure can be accomplished which will increase intra-arterial drug delivery by a log order (≥ 10 times) over the intravenous route. Regional infusions of drugs have had limited trials, but the overall impact of chemotherapy in the treatment of malignant brain tumors has been disappointing despite 30 years' experience with various drug regimens and routes of administration. Thus, for brain tumors, chemotherapy is a palliative modality and employed as an adjunct to surgery and radiation [9].

Two regional chemotherapy approaches showing promise are under current investigation. The first makes use of intra-arterial delivery, with novel catheter systems, drugs, and means of reducing systemic toxicity. The second combines an intra-arterial and intravenous administration of drugs with modification of the blood–brain barrier (this topic is discussed in Chapter 13), which transiently increases regional permeability to allow the use of water-soluble drugs which would otherwise have limited transcapillary passage.

In a representative intra-arterial study [6], 13 patients with malignant gliomas underwent intra-arterial infusion of two agents [BCNU (carmustine), cisplatin] via a selective catheter placed in the supraophthalmic carotid artery to avoid ocular toxicity. The median survival was 11 months and a response rate of 83% was reported, response being defined as a decrease in the volume of tumor as measured by CT scan. The treatment had significant neurotoxicity, 15% of patients having a permanent deficit. One patient died due to nephrotoxicity. The response of patients and the toxicity was directly related to the total dose administered. Although no conclusions regarding efficacy are possible from the initial studies, large scale cooperative trials are under way investigating this question. Focal toxicity arising from selective arterial catheterization and infusions of cytotoxic drugs are the major obstacles to the widespread use of this approach.

Future Approaches

The poor results of brain tumor therapy have encouraged the development of a number of alternate therapeutic strategies, the majority of which involve a regional approach. The most promising are still years away from reaching the clinic and making a notable impact in the treatment of this group of tumors.

Immunotherapy as applied to brain tumors has had limited success in the past. The recent development of technology for the production of large amounts of specific monoclonal antibody (MAb) has significant promise for the characterization, localization, and treatment of malignant gliomas [1]. Potentially, identification of specific target antigens present in the majority of malignant gliomas will permit passive serotherapy (administration of specific MAb) to be used as a primary treatment against malignant gliomas. Problems of target antigen identification, tumor heterogeneity, and delivery of MAb to the tumor remain. Possibly, individualized therapy will be necessary, using a panel of MAb reacting with specific tumor antigens.

An adoptive immunotherapy approach already in phase I trials is the use of lymphokine factors to stimulate T-lymphocytes to attack glial tumors [5]. In this approach, recombinant IL-2, a T-cell growth factor, is given by systemic or local administration to stimulate the patient's own lymphocytes against a tumor. A further step employing these lymphokine-activated killer cells (LAK cells) is the in vitro stimulation of autologous lymphocytes collected (by plasmapheresis and differential centrifugation) from a patient by incubation with IL-2, and subsequent re-infusion of these cells directly into the tumor. The initial reports do not address efficacy, but have demonstrated minimal toxicity over a range of IL-2 doses. The combination of IL-2 with infused LAK cells did not appear to increase toxicity in this study, although subsequent studies with higher doses of IL-2 and LAK cells have noted reactive brain edema. Despite these problems, the future of monoclonal antibodies and lymphokine-mediated cytolysis of tumor as therapy appears promising.

Hyperthermia, used primarily as an adjunct in combination with radiation therapy, has also shown some promise. The approach is attractive since it is effective against hypoxic cells and dividing cells during the S phase (DNA synthesis) of mitosis; both conditions are highly resistant to ionizing radiation—hence the adjunctive combination of hyperthermia and radiation. Technical problems with production and precise control of thermal fields, a narrow therapeutic index (normal tissue damage occurs at 44°C) and variable tumor sensitivity to thermal injury remain, but a phase I trial has been completed showing the feasibility and relative safety of this approach [12].

Photoradiation utilizes the property of certain molecules to fluoresce when stimulated with appropriate wavelength radiation (laser light). Hematoporphyrin and related compounds incorporate into actively dividing cells and liberate hydroxyl or superoxide radicals when stimulated. A phase I trial demonstrated the feasibility and limitations of such an approach in brain tumors [8]. Patients are given a bolus dose of a hematoporphyrin derivative (HpD), normally excluded by an intact blood–brain barrier, but incorporated into actively dividing brain tumors. Stereotactic placement of a small fiberoptic cable or similar device to transmit energy to the intracranial target is then performed, and laser energy is delivered to the target, stimulating the HpD incorporated by neoplastic cells. Cutaneous photosensitivity appears to be a toxic manifestation of HpD but was easily minimized. The technique has some promise, but technical problems with totally implantable light transmission systems has hindered therapeutic trials.

The successful clinical management of malignant gliomas will likely be the culmination of a sustained incremental improvement in results, rather than a sudden and dramatic therapeutic "breakthrough." Future therapy must place a larger fraction of patients with malignant brain tumors in prolonged periods of clinical remission as a necessary prelude to achieving a biologic cure. The most promising approaches appear to be on the threshold of attaining this goal.

References

1. Bullard DE, Bigner DD (1985) Applications of monoclonal antibodies in the diagnosis and treatment of primary brain tumors (review article). J Neurosurg 64: 2–16
2. Groothuis DR, Blasberg RG (1985) Rational brain tumor chemotherapy. The interaction of drug and tumor. Neurol Clin 3: 801–816
3. Gutin PH, Leibel SA (1985) Stereotaxic interstitial irradiation of malignant brain tumors. Neurol Clin 3: 883–892
4. Jackson D, Kinsella T, Rowland J, Wright D, Katz D, Main D, Collins J, Kornblith P, Glatstein E (1987) Halogenated pyrimidines as radiosensitizers in the treatment of glioblastoma multiforme. Am J Clin Oncol 10: 437–443
5. Jacobs SK, Wilson DJ, Kornblith PL, Grimm EA (1986) Interleukin-2 and autologous lymphokine-activated killer cells in the treatment of malignant glioma. Preliminary report. J Neurosurg 64: 743–749
6. Kapp JP, Vance RB (1985) Supraophthalmic carotid infusion for recurrent glioma: rationale, technique, and preliminary results for cisplatin and BCNU. J Neurooncol 3: 5–11
7. Kelly KA, Kirkwood JM, Kapp DS (1984) Glioblastoma multiforme: pathology, natural history and treatment. Cancer Treat Rev 11: 1–26
8. Laws ER, Cortese DA, Kinsey JH, Eagan RT, Anderson RE (1981) Photoradiation therapy in the treatment of malignant brain tumors: A phase I (feasibility) study. Neurosurgery 9: 627–678
9. Levin VA (1985) Chemotherapy of primary brain tumors. Neurol Clin 3: 855–866

10. McComb RD, Bigner DD (1984) The biology of malignant gliomas—a comprehensive survey. Clin Neuropathol 3: 93–106
11. Neuwelt EA, Howieson J, Frenkel EP, Specht HD, Weigel R, Buchan CG, Hill SA (1986) Therapeutic efficacy of multiagent chemotherapy with drug delivery enhancement by blood-brain barrier modification of glioblastoma. Neurosurgery 19: 573–582
12. Salcman M (1985) The morbidity and mortality of brain tumors. A perspective on recent advances in therapy. Neurol Clin 3: 229–257
13. Shapiro WR (1982) Neurological progress. Treatment of neuroectodermal brain tumors. Ann Neurol 12: 231–237

24. Head and Neck Cancer

C. Jacobs

Current Results and Therapeutic Issues

Squamous cancers of the head and neck are a heterogeneous group of cancers which have variable presenting symptoms, staging, therapy, and outcome [1]. Although they account for only 5% of neoplasms in the United States, head and neck cancers and their treatment are associated with significant morbidity. In contrast to many cancers, most head and neck sites are highly associated with an etiologic agent—tobacco.

Therapeutic plans are based on tumor stage (International Union Against Cancer TNM Staging System) and site, since these two factors significantly affect outcome. Most T1 and T2 cancers can be treated with either surgery or radiotherapy with equivalent outcome [2–4]. The decision whether to electively treat an N0 neck cancer is based on the whether or not occult disease is expected to be found. Most T3 and resectable T4 cancers are best treated with combined surgery and radiation. Some small T3 glottic cancers and all nasopharynx cancers are treated with radiation alone. Chemotherapy has been added to the primary treatment program in patients with advanced disease in attempts to improve curability (a) prior to initial therapy, (b) as a radiosensitizer, (3) following standard therapy as adjuvant treatment. Althouth some trials have shown a modest improvement in disease-free survival for selected subgroups, most have not shown improvement in survival [5–7].

Two-thirds of recurrences are local and one-third distal. Chemotherapy is palliative in less than half of the patients, but is rarely curative. The best single agents are cisplatin, methotrexate, bleomycin, 5-fluorouracil (5-FU). Combinations appear superior, but randomized trials do not demonstrate a survival advantage.

Current therapy is unsatisfactory for many reasons, including the following:

1. Therapy is based on clinical staging which is often inaccurate. Better radiologic techniques are needed to assess tumor extent.
2. For stage I and II disease the cure rate is acceptabe—70%–90%—but morbidity can be significant. Radiation toxicities include xerostomia, mucositis, chronic otitis media, osteoradionecrosis, laryngeal edema. Lhermitte's syndrome, and hypothyroidism. Long-term surgical complications include cosmetic deformities, aspiration, pneumonia, speech impediments, and shoulder droop from accessory nerve dysfunction.

3. For stages III and IV disease, not only are there the above toxicities, but cure rates range from 10% to 45%, depending on site. (Glottic cancer—75%).
4. For patients with recurrent disease, results from salvage surgery are poor (except salvage laryngectomy for glottic cancers). Less than half of the patients treated with chemotherapy will derive benefit, and that is usually short-lived.
5. Even for the patient who is cured, second primary tumors, predominantly at lung, esophagus, or other head and neck sites, occur in up to 10% of patients.

Current Approaches Under Study

Radiation Therapy

Radiotherapy for most head and neck squamous cancers consists of 1.8–2.0 Gy fractions for 5 days per week. Deviations from this have been tried in attempts to increase tumor dose or decrease toxicity. Hyperfractionated radiotherapy refers to the use of more than one fraction per day in smaller than conventional doses. Several trials of advanced head and neck cancer have suggested improvement in loco-regional control with similar acute toxicities [3]. Brachytherapy, or interstitial implantation of radioactive sources, has also been used as a means to deliver higher doses to the tumor while minimizing damage to normal tissues. ^{125}I seeds are used for permanent implants, primarily for positive surgical margins, particularly in the neck or base of skull [3]. Removable implants using ^{192}Ir or ^{137}Cs have been used in the oral cavity, oropharynx, laryngopharynx, skin, and cervical nodes. The results with base tongue cancer and tonsillo-platine cancers have been excellent.

High linear energy transfer radiation (fast neutrons)has been investigated because of potentially superior radiobiologic properties [2]. Neutrons have been combined with photon irradiation for "mixed beam" treatment. In a randomized trial from the Radiation Therapy Oncology Group (RTOG) results were superior for a trial of patients with neck node metastases. Hyperthermia to a temperature of 42°C or higher, as delivered by radiofrequency, microwave, and ultrasound systems, has been shown to be cytotoxic to cancer cells. Hyperthermia has shown activity for recurrent disease, and responses are enhanced by concurrent chemotherapy [2]. Chemical agents have been used during radiotherapy as sensitizers, many by acting as oxygen mimics. Misonidazole has not produced any major therapeutic advantages, and a new agent, SR-2508, is now in clinical trials [2].

Surgery

Efforts in surgical therapy have included improvement in functional and cosmetic disabilities through modification of conventional surgical procedures, reconstruction, and rehabilitation [1, 3]. the necessity for a radical neck dissection is currently being debated, and in many situations a modified neck dissection may be appropriate. Extended partial laryngeal surgery is being refined to allow for normal voice without reduction in cure rate. Innovative new techniques in reconstructive surgery, such as mandibular reconstruction and surgical restoration of the voice after laryngectomy, have improved quality of life. Laser surgery, particularly with the carbon dioxide laser, provides excellent results with early glottic and oral cavity cancers.

Chemotherapy

Chemotherapy has been added to radiation and surgery in combined modality programs in attempts to improve cure. Chemotherapy has been used as a radiosensitizer in controlled trials for patients with advanced, unresectabe disease [2]. Bleomycin and 5-fluorouracil (5-FU) have both been shown to improve local control and survival in individual trials. Benefit, however, is marginal.

Chemotherapy used prior to standard therapy (induction chemotherapy) produces response rates of up to 90% with 50 to 60% complete clinical responses. The most commonly used regimen is cisplatin (100 mg/m^2) on day 1 and 5-FU (1 gm/m^2) on days 1 through 5 by continuous infusion [6]. Although response to induction chemotherapy may predict for improved overall survival, no study to date has shown improvement in disease-free survival or survival of patients receiving induction chemotherapy vs. controls [5, 7]. The potential advantage of adjuvant chemotherapy has been studied mostly following induction chemotherapy and standard therapy. Results to date are conflicting but are suggestive that adjuvant chemotherapy may reduce the incidence of distant metastases and perhaps improve disease-free survival. Most groups have found it difficult to deliver adjuvant chemotherapy to this particular patient population. The Head and Neck Intergroup is currently studying the use of three cycles of cisplatin plus 5-FU sandwiched between surgery and radiation, compared to standard therapy.

A further role of chemotherapy may be to reduce morbidity by acting as a substitute for surgery. In a pilot trial, in which surgery was not performed in patients whose disease responded completely to induction chemotherapy as documented by endoscopy and biopsy, results were as good as with standard therapy. This concept is being studied in a randomized trial by the Veterans Administration Cooperative Group.

New approaches for recurrent disease have included creative combinations of chemotherapeutic agents, use of high-dose chemotherapy, investigational drugs such as carboplatin and CHIP, intra-arterial chemotherapy, and interferon [2]. None to date has proven to be superior to conventional single-agent chemotherapy, but trials are still in progress.

Future Approaches

The role of chemotherapy and the newer techniques in radiation therapy have not yet been fully developed or explored. In the future, combinations of these new approaches may significantly enhance outcome. More effective chemotherapeutic agents and biologic modifiers are needed to enhance combined modality programs. The use of highly sensitive imaging techniques, such as magnetic resonance imaging, or monoclonal antibody to determine residual disease may be helpful in selecting those patients who would benefit from more aggressive programs while sparing unnecessary toxicity to others. Retinoids have been used to treat preneoplastic lesions, and they have a potential role in chemoprevention for high-risk groups, including the prevention of second primary tumors [8].

Innovative approaches in head and neck squamous cancer will come from the laboratory or from pilot studies. However, randomized trials are necessary to to establish the superiority of any new approach over standard therapy. The current morbidity and mortality from this disease continues to stimulate basic science and clinical research.

References

1. Cummings CW, Fredrickson JM, Harker LA, Krause CJ, Schuller DE (1986) Otolaryngology—head and neck surgery. Mosby, St Louis
2. Wolf GT (ed) (1984) Head and neck oncology, 1st edn. Nijhoff, Boston
3. Jacobs C (ed) (1987) Head and neck oncology, 2nd edn. Nijhoff, Boston
4. Arrigada R, Eschwege F, Cachin Y, Richard JM (1983) The value of combining radiotherapy with surgery in the treatment of hypopharyngeal and laryngeal cancers. Cancer 51: 1819–1825
5. Tannock IF, Browman G (1986) Lack of evidence for a role of chemotherapy in the routine management of locally advanced head and neck cancer. J Clin Oncol 4: 1121–1126
6. Weaver A, Fleming S, Ensley J, Kish JA, Jacobs J, Kinzie J, Crissman J, Al-Sarraf M (1984) Superior clinical response and survival rates with initial bolus of cisplatin and 120 hour infusion of 5-fluorouracil before definitive therapy for locally advanced head and neck cancer. Am J Surg 148: 525–529
7. Taylor SG, Applebaum E, Showell JL, Norusis M, Holinger LD, Hutchinson JC, Murthy AK, Caldarelli DD (1985) A randomized trial of adjuvant chemotherapy in head and neck cancer. J Clin Oncol 3: 672–679
8. Hong WK, Itri L, Endicott J et al. (1986) The effectiveness of 13-cis retinoic acid (13-CRA) in the treatment of premalignant lesions in the oral cavity. N Engl J Med 315: 1501–1505

25. Lung Cancer

R.L. Comis

Current Results and Therapeutic Issues

In the United States alone there will be approximately 140 000 cases of lung cancer during 1987. Functionally, these diseases are divided into tumors of the non-small cell (NSCL) and small cell (SCLC) varieties. The former category includes squamous cell adenocarcinoma and large cell anaplastic tumors and the latter includes small cell anaplastic carcinoma, all defined by light microscopy. This functional classification is based upon each category's distinctive clinical biology, i.e., (a) the potential for surgical curability of NSCL; (b) the propensity of SCLC to widespread dissemination; and (c) the relative responsiveness or unresponsiveness of SCLC and NSCL to existing cytotoxic modalities.

During the last decade tremendous advances have been made in understanding the biology of certain types of lung cancer. Particularly, the ability to culture SCLC in liquid, non-serum containing media has led to establishing the neuroendocrine nature of the disease, the importance of various autocrine growth factors in sustaining its growth, and the potential role of specific chromosome abnormalities in the 3p region of chromosome 3 in the genesis of the disease [1]. A similar approach is now being taken with non-small cell tumors with interesting preliminary results. It is anticipated that these laboratory efforts will led to novel clinical strategies in the future.

Non-Small Cell Lung Cancer

Recently a new staging system for NSCL has been proposed. The critical features of this system include TNM stages: including only T1-T2, N0 disease as stage I; defining stage II as T1-T2, N1 disease; dividing stage III into an A and a B category to accommodate the potential role for surgery with or without radiation in selected T3 cases, and including stage IV disease for patients with distant metastases [2].

Surgery remains the primary curative modality for 20% of patients with resectable tumors. Meticulous mediastinal lymph node dissection has become an integral part of the accepted surgical approach to NSCL. This approach has yielded apparent increases in survival, particularly for stage I and II patients, but also for patients with microscopically positive ipsilateral mediastinal nodes. These shifts are more a function of the new approach to staging than an increase in the ability of surgery to cure.

A recent trial re-evaluating the role of radiation therapy in patients with clinically detectable N2 disease has shown a reduction in local recurrence in patients with squamous cell carcinoma, without a significant impact on survival. Although the same group has reported an advantage for adjuvant chemotherapy with cyclophosphamide, adriamycin (doxorubicin), and cis-platinum (CAP) in high-risk groups, this singular result has appropriately not become the standard until it, or other similar approaches, have been shown to be reproducibly effective.

The evaluation of cytotoxic therapy has progressed from the study of single drugs, to nitrosourea/alkylating agent-based combinations, to plant alkaloid/ cisplatin-based programs [3]. The latter has yielded somewhat more consistent objective response rates and modest, but detectable, advantages in median survival. To date, however, no treatment can be viewed as standard.

Small Cell Lung Cancer

SCLC represents approximately 25% of all cases of lung cancer. Between 5% and 8% of patients present with stage I–II disease (TNM system), 35%–40% present with classically defined limited disease, and 55%–60% have extensive disease at presentation. During the last two decades the development of moderately effective aggressive combination chemotherapy programs have significantly altered the clinical course of SCLC [4]. A small but significant proportion of patients with limited disease are cured with combined modality treatment, and the majority of patients with extensive disease derive substantial palliation from therapy.

During the 1970s the role of radiotherapy for patients with limited disease was questioned. Recent studies have shown that simultaneous radiation therapy combined with chemotherapy is superior to chemotherapy alone [5]. A more drug-oriented approach in limited disease has been evaluated by the Southeastern Cancer Study Group. This trial built upon the potential noncross-resistance of etoposide and cisplatin (VP-DDP) with the combination of cyclophosphamide, adriamycin, and vincristine (CAV) [6]. After six cycles of CAV therapy, patients were randomly assigned to two cycles of consolidation with VP-DDP. The addition of VP-DDP yielded a doubling in median survival from the time of randomization. Confirmatory trials are now underway.

The role of surgery combined with aggressive combination chemotherapy has recently been re-evaluated, yielding an apparent increase in disease-free survival. These preliminary results are now being evaluated in a randomized, controlled national group study.

Recent trials in extensive disease have evaluated the role of VP-DDP alternating with CAV. A study by the National Cancer Institute of Canada has indicated a modest shift in median survival with the alternating approach [7]. It should be noted, however, that a similar shift in median survival has been found in all studies which have used etoposide early in the treatment of patients with extensive disease.

460

Current Approaches Under Study

Non-small Cell Lung Cancer

Combination chemotherapy prior to the use of radiation and/or surgery is being employed in non-small cell lung cancer. These trials are directed towards selected stage III patients with T3 and/or ipsilateral N2 disease. Three phase 2 studies which employed *Vinca* alkaloid/cisplatin-based chemotherapy prior to surgery or radiation therapy have provided some interesting leads. Such studies have shown that approximately 50% of patients develop a response to chemotherapy; approximately 10%–15% have no histologically detectable disease in the resected specimen. The impact of this approach on survival remains to be determined. It is possible that this and other approaches combining local modalities with aggressive platinum-based chemotherapy may provide advances in the future.

Laboratory-based programs have reported that approximately 10% of patients with histologically confirmed NSCL will harbor neuroendocrine markers. Preliminary data indicate that patients with such tumors respond better to chemotherapy than those without such markers. Further studies are being designed to address this issue.

Small Cell Lung Cancer

There are several studies which are evaluating increased dose intensity in SCLC. Pilot studies in patients with extensive disease have not yielded substantial evidence for increased survival [4]. On the other hand, preliminary data from certain limited-disease trials may indicate that high-dose therapy with autologous bone marrow support may be of some benefit in patients who have achieved a complete remission. Such studies evaluating dose intensity are now taking two different angles. On the one hand, increasingly intensive treatment with autologous bone marrow support is being pursued by certain groups. In addition, the availability of colony-stimulating factors has led to the initiation of early trials combining them with high-dose chemotherapy. It is possible that such approaches may increase not only the objective response but also survival in limited-disease patients.

Future Approaches

Biologic approaches to the treatment of lung cancer are in the initial phases of development. The United States National Cancer Institute/Navy Medical Oncology Branch has initiated the first trials with an anti-bombesin monoclonal

461

antibody. This approach is designed to exploit the critical role of bombesin in sustaining the growth of SCLC. Also, trials are now being designed to employ substances such as the interferons or interleukin-2 in programs designed for patients in complete remission with limited disease.

As mentioned earlier, it is anticipated that during the next decade there will be substantially more trials directed by laboratory investigations. These investigations may be based on further studies relating to the autocrine growth of small cell or non-small cancers. In addition, disease-site directed drug development programs will hopefully lead to the development of new compounds, while the explosion of information relating to drug resistance may yield new trials directed towards altering the inherent or acquired resistance which is the bane of the chemotherapeutic treatment of lung cancer.

References

1. Carney DN, Broder L, Edelstein M et al. (1983) Experimental studies of the biology of human small cell lung cancer. Cancer Treat Rep 67: 27
2. Mountain CF (1986) A new international staging system for lung cancer. Chest 89: 225S
3. Greco FA (1986) Rationale for chemotherapy for patients with advanced non-small cell lung cancer. Semin Oncol 13: 92
4. Comis RL (1987) Chemotherapy of small cell lung cancer. In: DeVita VT, Hellman S, Rosenberg SA (eds) Principles and practice of oncology update, vol 1. Lippincott, Philadelphia, p 7
5. Perry MC, Eaton WL, Propert KJ et al. (1987) Chemotherapy with or without radiation therapy in limited small cell carcinoma of the lung. N Engl J Med 316: 912
6. Einhorn L, Greco FA, Cohen H, Birch R (1987) Late consolidation with cisplatin plus VP-16 (PVP$_{16}$) following induction chemotherapy with cyclophosphamide, adriamycin and vincristine (CAV) in limited small cell lung cancer (SCLC): a Southeastern Cancer Study Group (SECSG) random prospective study. Proc Am Soc Clin Oncol 6: 166
7. Feld R, Evans WK, Coy P et al. (1987) Canadian multicenter randomized trial comparing sequential and alternating administration of two noncross-resistant chemotherapy combinations in patients with limited small-cell carcinoma of the lung. J Clin Oncol 5(9): 1401

26. Breast Cancer

G. Wilding and M.E. Lippman

Current Results and Therapeutic Issues

Breast cancer is diagnosed in more than 120000 women in the United States each year. Although 90% of these women will present with disease limited to the breast and axillary lymph nodes, one third of all patients with breast cancer will eventually develop metastases and succumb to their disease. From 1976 to 1981, a 20% decline in mortality in breast cancer patients below age 50 occurred. One of the major causes of this decline in mortality in premenopausal women was the widespread use of adjuvant chemotherapy.

Early-Stage Disease

Reports of prospective studies by the National Surgical Adjuvant Breast Project (NSABP) using melphalan [4] and by the Cancer Institute of Milan using combination chemotherapy [2] demonstrated, after nearly 10 years of follow-up, a statistically significantly improved relapse-free survival, most prominent in premenopausal women with metastases in 1–3 lymph nodes. Numerous subsequent trials have focused on defining which subsets of women would benefit most from adjuvant therapy and which forms of adjuvant therapy are most efficacious. A consensus development conference report formulated at the National Institutes of Health (NIH) in 1985 summarizes the findings of these trials [7]. Currently, for premenopausal women with metastases in axillary nodes (premenopausal node-positive women), adjuvant chemotherapy with established drug regimens is the recommended care regardless of estrogen receptor status. In premenopausal women without lymph node metastases (node-negative women), a number of factors can be used to identify subsets of women who are at greater risk of developing metastatic disease. The high risk factors include lack of estrogen and progesterone receptors in the tumor sample evidence for high growth rate in the form of either a high S-phase fraction or high thymidine labeling index, lack of tumor differentiation, and age under 35. Several studies show chemotherapy to have a major treatment advantage in these women [7]. Therefore, women with these high risk factors should be seriously considered for adjuvant chemotherapy, preferably as part of prospective clinical trials.

Adjuvant therapy for postmenopausal women shows great promise but again it is difficult to draw firm conclusions from the data available. Postmenopausal women with axillary node metastases comprise one subset of women most likely to benefit from adjuvant therapy. The NIH consensus development conference recommended that postmenopausal women with estrogen receptor-positive tumors and lymph node metastases receive adjuvant tamoxifen therapy. However, chemotherapy is the adjuvant treatment of choice for women with estrogen receptor-negative tumors and should not be ruled out as a treatment option for women with estrogen receptor-positive tumors. Recent studies have indicated that intensity is an important factor in determining the effectiveness of adjuvant chemotherapy [6]. Investigations at the Cancer Institute of Milan demonstrated that patients receiving 85% of the planned chemotherapy dose had a 77% relapse-free survival at 5 years, compared to the 48% relapse-free survival of those patients receiving 65% of their planned therapy [1]. Clearly, the optimal adjuvant therapy for postmenopausal node-positive women has not been determined. These women should be treated as part of prospective trials designed to resolve this therapeutic question.

Equally perplexing questions can be raised in determining when and how to give adjuvant therapy to node-negative postmenopausal women. The NIH consensus development panel concluded that there was no indication for routine adjuvant therapy in these women except in those subsets with a high risk of recurrence [7]. However, analysis of the tamoxifen trials showed a 30% improvement in recurrence-free survival in women with no nodal metastases, a figure equivalent to the improvement seen in node-positive women. In addition, analysis of chemotherapy results as a function of node involvement failed to demonstrate any differences in benefit for women who had no nodes involved versus women who did. For these reasons, the usefulness of adjuvant therapy in node-negative postmenopausal patients must be considered; definition of optimal therapy awaits prospective trial results.

Significant advances in the local management of breast cancer have also been achieved. In one study, life table estimates based on data from 1843 women with stage I or II breast cancer indicated that treatment by segmental mastectomy with or without breast irradiation resulted in disease-free, distant disease-free, and overall survival at 5 years that was no worse than that after total breast removal [5]. This observation has been substantiated by the early results of Veronesi et al. [9] and the National Cancer Institute, USA [3]. Remaining issues include the relative merits of the various conservative surgical procedures, optimal radiation technique, cosmesis, and the psychological aspects of breast preservation and reconstruction.

Locally Advanced Disease

Patients with locally advanced disease (stage III) at presentation have a poor prognosis, with 5-year survival rates of about 30%. Chemotherapy for a fixed number of cycles prior to local therapy has achieved improved local control in approximately 80% of patients and modest improvements in survival of 10–20%. However, many patients (about 50%) continue to develop metastases by 5 years and die of disseminated disease. Considering the poor prognosis of these patients, more aggressive approaches and the evaluation of chemohormonal therapy are clearly warranted.

Metastatic Disease

Approximately 10% of patients present with disseminated disease and one-third of all breast cancer patients will die from disseminated disease. Nearly half of the patients with metastases will respond to chemotherapy, and one-third of those will achieve complete remissions. While survival has improved, the duration of response is only from 6 months to 1 years. For those patients with hormone-responsive tumors (about one-third of all patients), hormonal manipulations, either additive or ablative, produce responses of 12–18 months' duration. Effective therapy against hormone-independent tumors is desperately needed.

Current Approaches Under Study

The gains made in the therapy of breast cancer have been substantial. To continue to add to our understanding of breast cancer and improve on existing therapy, all patients should be strongly encouraged to participate in ongoing and future controlled trials aimed at improving the therapy of breast cancer. A number of issues are currently under investigation and require further attention. These include refining the division of patients into prognostic subgroups by assessing the limits of pathological, biochemical, cytokinetic, and immunological variables in determining patient outcome and assessing the need for adjuvant therapy. In particular, the question of treatment of node-negative women with adjuvant therapy needs considerably more attention.

The recent observation that dose intensity and scheduling substantially influence treatment outcome suggest that even with current treatment modalities improvements in overall results can be achieved [6]. Endocrine treatment and chemotherapy can be combined, but the optimal combination of these two modalities remains to be defined. Should these therapies be given sequentially or simultaneously, and for how long? Should therapy be administered before or after surgery? These are all questions which need to be answered by well-controlled clinical trials.

Studies at the National Cancer Institute are addressing some of these questions. In patients with locally advanced disease (stages III_A and III_B), combination chemotherapy is given to the point of maximal objective clinical response, in efforts to (a) maximally reduce the tumor bulk prior to definitive local therapy and (b) destroy occult micrometastatic disease. Endocrine therapy is used with chemotherapy by giving tamoxifen and Premarin (conjugated estrogenic hormones) sequentially before administration of cell cycle-specific agents, in an attempt to synchronize DNA synthesis in a proportion of these tumor cells and, thus, make them more susceptible to cytotoxic chemotherapy. Thus far the rate of objective response to chemotherapy has been 90%, with 52% achieving complete clinical responses. The median time to disease progression and median survival time have not been reached by the 51 patients studied thus far [8].

A number of studies have shown that significant tumor responses can be achieved using high-dose chemotherapy followed by autologous bone marrow transplantation (ABMT). Since high-dose therapy might be of greater benefit if used in patients in complete remission but at risk of early relapse, patients with inflammatory breast cancer who achieve complete responses with chemo-hormonal therapy and local treatment are now being randomized to either observation or high-dose melphalan therapy with ABMT at the National Cancer Institute.

The approaches described above are also being applied in patients with metastatic disease (stage IV). In addition, the problems of drug resistance and hormone independence are being addressed. As described by Fojo in this volume, a molecular approach to the phenomenon of multiple drug resistance has provided insight into the mechanisms of drug resistance. Recent advances in the ability to culture primary and metastatic human breast cancer have enabled investigators to evaluate drug sensitivity in vitro on biopsy specimens. Finally, multiple hormonal manipulations are being applied simultaneously in efforts to optimize response to hormonal therapy.

Future Approaches

Future advances in breast cancer therapy will depend on expansion of our current basic research data base. Findings in the general disciplines of molecular biology, pharmacology, genetics, and cell biology alone or in concert could substantially alter our understanding of ways to disrupt the growth of breast cancer in a therapeutically beneficial sense. As outlined by Wilding and Lippman (this volume), investigations into the nature of the cellular response to hormones have provided us with a glimpse into the future. The discovery of autocrine growth loops, driven by steroids in hormone-dependent tumor cells and constitutively active in hormone-independent tumor cells, has provided a variety of targets through which cell growth could be disrupted in both hormone-dependent and hormone-independent tumor cells. Disruption of these growth loops by immunologic, pharmacologic, and gene transfer techniques is already underway using in vitro and in vivo laboratory models.

References

1. Bonadonna G, Valagussa P (1981) Dose-response effect of adjuvant chemotherapy in breast cancer. N Engl J med 304: 10
2. Bonadonna G, Valagussa P, Rossi A et al. (1985) Ten-year experience with CMF-based adjuvant chemotherapy in resectable breast cancer. Breast Cancer Res Treat 5: 95
3. Findlay P, Lippman M, Danforth D et al. (1986) A randomized trial comparing mastectomy to radiotherapy in the treatment of stage I–II breast cancer: a preliminary report. Am Soc Clin Oncol 5: 246
4. Fisher B, Carbone P, Economou SG et al. (1975) L-phenylalanine mustard (L-PAM) in the management of primary breast cancer: a report of early findings. N Engl J Med 292: 117
5. Fisher B, Bauer M, Margolsese R et al. (1985) Five year results of a randomized clinical trial comparing total mastectomy and segmental mastectomy with or without radiation in the treatment of breast cancer. N Engl J Med 312: 665
6. Hryniuk W, Bush H (1984) The importance of dose intensity in chemotherapy of metastatic breast cancer. J Clin Oncol 2: 1281
7. Lippman ME (ed) (1986) Proceedings of the NIH Consensus Development Conference on adjuvant chemotherapy and endocrine therapy for breast cancer. NCI Monogr 1
8. Sorace RA, Lippman ME, Bagley CS, Lichter AS, Danforth DW, Wesley MN, Young RC (1985) The management of nonmetastatic locally advanced breast cancer using primary induction chemotherapy with hormonal synchronization followed by radiation therapy with or without debulking surgery. World J Surg 9: 776
9. Veronesi U, Saccozzi R, Del Vecchio M et al. (1981) Comparing radical mastectomy with quadrantectomy, axillary dissection and radiotherapy in patients with small cancers of the breast. N Engl J Med 305: 6

27. Renal Cell Carcinoma

C.N. Robertson and W.M. Linehan

Current Results and Therapeutic Issues

There are 12 000–17 000 new cases of renal cell carcinoma in the United States per year. Renal cell carcinoma is responsible for 7000 to 9000 deaths annually. Approximately 56% of the cases are localized, 14% are locally advanced, and 30% of patients present with metastatic disease. The main occurrence of renal cell carcinoma is in the age range 40–70 years. While the youngest reported age of occurrence is 6 months, there are less than 100 reported cases in children under 10. The most commonly used staging system for renal cell carcinoma is the one devised by Robson, in which stage I is tumor confined within the capsule, stage II denotes tumor invasion of perinephric fat (confined to Gerota's fascia); in stage III there is tumor involvement of the regional lymph nodes and/or renal vein and vena cava, and in stage IV there is adjacent organ involvement or distant metastasis. The 5-year survival rate for stages I and II renal cell carcinoma is approximately 80% [1]. The 5-year survival for stage III is 40%–50%; only 8%–12% of patients with stage IV renal cell carcinoma survive 2 years. Involvement of the regional lymph nodes in renal cell carcinoma (stage IIIB) is associated with decreased survival—only 20% at 5 years. Renal cell carcinoma can be either clear-cell, granular-cell, or sarcomatoid-type. The sarcomatoid-type renal cell carcinoma carries a worse prognosis than either the clear or granular histologic types. Renal cell carcinoma often spreads to the lungs, skeletal system, or to lymph nodes. Less often involved are the brain, liver, or skin/subcutaneous tissue.

The current treatment for stage I or stage II renal cell carcinoma is radical nephrectomy. Radical nephrectomy most often involves the removal of the entire contents of Gerota's fascia including the ipsilateral adrenal gland. Many surgeons include regional lymphadenectomy in radical nephrectomy, although this is not universally performed and it is not clear that it improves survival.

Some have advocated the use of nephrectomy in patients with stage IV renal cell carcinoma in order to induce spontaneous regression of metastases. In nine series reviewed by Montie et al. [2] in which nephrectomy had been performed in patients with metastatic renal cell carcinoma, only 4 or 474 (0.8%) had evidence of regression of metastatic foci. Angioinfarction of the kidney has often been used in patients with metastatic renal cell carcinoma. In a series of 100 patients with metastatic renal cell carcinoma treated with angioinfarction, Swanson et al.

[3] found no improvement in survival with this technique over patients treated with nephrectomy alone. Angioinfarction and/or nephrectomy can, however, play an important role in decreasing or preventing the occurrence of local or systemic symptoms in patients with metastatic renal cell carcinoma.

Surgical resection of metastatic foci in conjunction with nephrectomy may play a role in management of selected patients with metastatic renal cell carcinoma. Up to a 30% 5-year survival has been reported in selected patients in whom solitary metastatic foci are surgically resected.

Hormonal therapy has for a number of years been frequently used in the treatment of patients with metastatic renal cell carcinoma, on the basis of work in which kidney tumors were induced in male hamsters with estrogen and the growth of such tumors inhibited with estrogen antagonists. However, the use of hormonal therapy in humans with metastatic renal cell carcinoma is associated with a very low response rate. The reported results with progesterone therapy in patients with metastatic renal cell carcinoma demonstrate only a 10% (31/299) response rate, results with testosterone a 9% (9/115) response rate, and those with estrogen antagonists a 6% (10/162) response rate [4].

The response of renal cell carcinoma to chemotherapy also has been disappointing. Numerous single-agent and multi-agent chemotherapy trials have been performed in patients with metastatic renal cell carcinoma. In a review by Harris [4] of the reported response rates using single chemotherapeutic agents from a number of published reports, there was an overall 9% response rate. The response to combinations of agents may be higher than that to single agents and there are some complete responses reported. The response to combination chemotherapeutic agents seems to be highest with vinblastine-containing regimens. However, the toxicity of combination agents is higher than for single agents and a significant impact on survival has yet to be demonstrated.

Current Approaches Under Study

A number of trials have been performed evaluating the effect of interferon on metastatic renal cell carcinoma. The first trials were with human leukocyte α-interferon, followed by trials with purified human lymphoblastoid α-interferon. Purified recombinant α-, β-, and γ-interferon are now available and trials are currently under way with each of these agents as well as with combinations of these agents. The most active agent seems to be α-interferon. The response rates for natural interferons have been reported to be 14%; the response rates for the recombinant interferons are 12%–20% [5]. Post-nephrectomy patients who have had no other treatment and, who do not have bony metastases, but have disease at other sites respond the best to this type of therapy.

Since the description of monoclonal antibody production in 1975, the potential for specific tumor-associated antigen binding and its use for imaging and therapy has been recognized. To date a small number of clinical trials using monoclonal antibodies to renal cell carcinoma have been initiated, evaluating both imaging and therapeutic potential, which are currently at an early stage.

A therapeutic approach to the treatment of metastatic renal cell carcinoma by adoptive immunotherapy using lymphokine-activated killer (LAK) cells and recombinant interleukin-2 (IL-2) has been recently developed by Rosenberg et al. [6, 7]. The goal of this therapy is to develop a method for mediating the rejection of established human tumors by the adoptive transfer of lymphoid cells with anti-tumor reactivity. The properties of recombinant IL-2, previously called T-cell growth factor, have been determined by Rosenberg [6]. The lymphokine-activated killer phenomenon is seen in the incubation of lymphocytes in IL-2, which results in the generation of cells capable of lysing fresh tumor cells in short-term chromium-51 release assays. It has been shown in the murine model that: (a) IL-2 alone can reduce established pulmonary and hepatic metastases, (b) LAK cells can reduce the number of established metastases, and (c) therapy with LAK cells plus IL-2 is more effective than either agent alone in reducing the number of established metastases [6].

Clinical trials are now under way exploring combined therapy with LAK cells and IL-2 in patients with advanced cancer. Over 100 patients with advanced renal cell carcinoma have been treated with either IL-2 alone or IL-2 plus LAK cells. A recent report of 157 patients with advanced cancer treated with LAK cells and IL-2 or IL-2 alone by Rosenberg et al. included 57 patients with advanced renal cell cancer. Of the 36 patients with renal cell carcinoma treated with LAK cells plus IL-2, 12 (33%) underwent a complete or partial response. Of the 21 patients treated with IL-2 alone, 1 had a complete response [7]. Although this regimen is currently cumbersome to administer and has toxic side effects [7], it has induced significant response in diseases for which there are no standard, effective therapies. Trials are currently under way to evaluate whether IL-2 or IL-2 plus LAK cell therapy is more effective in renal cell carcinoma and to study this therapy in patients with smaller tumor burdens, i.e., completely or partially resected in locally advanced renal cell carcinoma.

Another approach currently under study is the use of tumor-infiltrating lymphocytes. In murine studies, tumor-infiltrating lymphocytes have been found to have specificity and to be more effective than LAK cells in reduction of established 3-day micrometastases [8]. Tumor-infiltrating lymphocytes have also been grown from surgical specimens containing renal cell carcinoma that are capable of being grown and subsequently expanded in media containing IL-2 [9]. Clinical trials in the Surgery Branch of the National Cancer Institute are now under way to evaluate the effect of treatment with IL-2 and tumor-infiltrating lymphocytes in patients with metastatic renal cell carcinoma.

Future Approaches

Future directions with adoptive immunotherapy will include studies to further increase the effectiveness of therapy and to decrease the toxicity. Lower-dose regimens with IL-2 and regimens with prolonged, maintenance administration of

IL-2 will be studied. Combinations of agents such as IL-2 with or without LAK cells, with or without tumor-infiltrating lymphocytes, plus IL-1, IL-4, tumor necrosis factor (TNF), interferon, chemotherapeutic agents or radiation, or combinations of these agents could also be evaluated. The possibility exists of cloning an even more active LAK cell or tumor-infiltrating lymphocyte which would be more specific and/or require less IL-2.

Studies of the paracrine, endocrine, and, particularly, autocrine effects of renal cell carcinoma-produced growth factors are in progress. In a significant number of patients with renal cell carcinoma there is evidence for a paracrine and/or endocrine effect from tumor-produced factors, such as hypercalcemia. Transforming growth factor (TGF-)α and epidermal growth factor (EGF) have been shown to be capable of inducing bone resorption and increasing serum calcium levels in rodents when administered systemically [10]. Message levels for TGF-α, TGF-β and the EGF receptor have recently been shown to be increased in renal cell carcinoma, cell lines, and solid tumors [11]. This raises the possibility that TGF-α, for example, could have an autocrine role in the initiation or progression of renal cell carcinoma. Potential therapeutic strategies to block this potential autocrine mechanism include use of such agents as monoclonal antibodies or modified EGF-binding peptides to block the EGF receptor.

New molecular techniques are providing greater insight into chromosomal abnormalities in this disease. It has recently been reported by Zbar et al. [12] that, by use of restriction fragment length polymorphism analysis, an interstitial deletion in the short arm of chromosome 3 could be identified in tumor tissue from patients with renal cell carcinoma. The potential significance of the identification of a chromosomal deletion lies in the fact that it may localize a critical gene which, when it loses normal function, may result in malignant transformation. It is possible that such a gene could code for a repressor protein which inhibits the expression of growth factor genes or other genes capable of cell transformation. Alternatively if the corresponding allele to a deleted "wild-type" allele contained a mutated gene, this mutated gene could code for an altered protein which could result in transformation. Identification of this altered protein and/or an understanding of its role in transformation could lead to new therapeutic strategies in the treatment of this disease.

References

1. Boxer RJ, Waisman J, Lieber MM, Mampaso FM, Skinner DG (1979) Renal carcinoma: computer analysis of 96 patients treated by nephrectomy. J Urol 122: 598–601
2. Montie JE, Stewart BH, Straffon RA, Banowsky LHW, Hewitt CB, Montague DK (1977) The role of adjunctive nephrectomy in patients with metastatic renal cell carcinoma. J Urol 117: 272
3. Swanson DA, Johnson DE, von Eschenbach AC, Chuang VP, Wallace S (1983) Angioinfarction plus nephrectomy for metastatic renal cell carcinoma—an update. J Urol 130: 449–452
4. Harris DT (1983) Hormonal therapy and chemotherapy of renal-cell carcinoma. Semin Oncol 10(4): 422–430
5. Neidhart JA (1986) Interferon therapy for the treatment of renal cancer. Cancer 57: 1696–1699

6. Rosenberg SA (1986) Adoptive immunotherapy of cancer using lymphokine activated killer cells and recombinant interleukin-2. In: DeVita VT, Hellman S, Rosenberg SA (eds) Important advances in oncology. Lippincott, Philadelphia, pp 55–91

7. Rosenberg SA, Lotze MT, Muul LM, Chang AE, Avis FP, Leitman S, Linehan WM, Robertson CN, Lee RE, Rubin JT, Seipp CA, Simpson CG, White DE (1987) Clinical experience with the treatment of 157 patients with advanced cancer using lymphokine-activated killer cells and interleukin-2 or high-dose interleukin-2 alone. N Engl J Med 316(15): 889–905

8. Rosenberg SA, Spiess P, Lafreniere R (1986) A new approach to the adoptive immunotherapy of cancer with tumor-infiltrating lymphocytes. Science 223: 1318–1321

9. Belldegrun A, Linehan WM, Robertson CN, Rosenberg SA (1986) Isolation and characterization of lymphocytes infiltrating human renal cell cancer: possible application for therapeutic adoptive immunotherapy. Surg Forum 37: 671–673

10. Tashjian AH, Voelkel EF, Lloyd W, Derynck R, Winkler ME, Levine L (1986) Actions of growth factors on plasma calcium: epidermal growth factor and human transforming growth factor-alpha cause elevation of plasma calcium in mice. J Clin Invest 78: 1405–1409

11. Derynck R, Goeddel DV, Ullrich A, Gutterman JU, Williams RD, Bringman TS (1987) Synthesis of messenger RNAs for transforming growth factors alpha and beta and the epidermal growth factor receptor by human tumors. Cancer Res 47: 707–712

12. Zbar B, Brauch H, Talmadge C, Linehan WM (1987) Loss of alleles of loci on the short arm of chromosome 3 in renal cell carcinoma. Nature 327: 721–724

28. Carcinoma of the Pancreas

W.F. Sindelar

Carcinoma of the pancreas is an aggressive visceral malignancy which results in the death of over 99% of the patients who develop the disease. In the United States approximately 25 000 lives are claimed yearly by carcinoma of the pancreas. Survival expectations with this disease are quite limited, with a median survival of only approximately 6 months from the time of diagnosis and an overall 5-year survival rate of under 1%. The treatment of pancreatic cancer has been difficult and largely unsuccessful, with surgical resection offering only a limited opportunity for cure and with radiation therapy, chemotherapy, or other modalities resulting at best in only modest expectations of prolonged survival or temporary palliation of symptoms.

Current Therapy

Surgery

Surgical resection of pancreatic carcinoma provides the only current therapeutic modality with any potential for cure. Unfortunately, resection is possible in only the few patients with disease localized to the pancreas. In most series, fewer than 15% of patients who are brought to surgery with the intention of performing a resection are found to have a tumor at a stage early enough to permit complete extirpation [1].

For patients with tumors confined to the pancreatic parenchyma, the conventional surgical treatment is pancreaticoduodenectomy, or Whipple's operation. Whipple's procedure is a technically difficult operation that requires removal of the distal stomach, entire duodenum, distal bile duct, and head of the pancreas. Total pancreatectomy with resection of the entire pancreas along with the duodenum, distal stomach, and regional lymph nodes has been advocated by some surgeons. Pancreatic resections carry an operative mortality in most series that averages 20% and an overall surgical complication rate of more than 50%. Various series of resections performed for carcinoma of the pancreas have shown disappointing salvage rates, with 3-year survivals averaging less than 15% and 5-year survivals of 10% or less [1].

473

Radiation Therapy

Radiation therapy has chiefly been used for pancreatic cancer in patients with large local tumors. Typically, up to 60 Gy radiation is administered in 1.5–2.0 Gy daily fractions to the upper abdomen, with coned-down volumes to the tumor taken to high dose. Radiosensitive organs in the upper abdomen, such as stomach and small intestine, limit the dose of radiation that can be delivered. Although radiation therapy can help control local disease and may provide palliation of pain or obstruction, radiation has not been convincingly demonstrated to prolong survival.

Chemotherapy

Chemotherapy has been used in the treatment of pancreatic carcinoma in attempts to palliate symptoms or to prolong survival in patients with advanced disease. A variety of drugs have been shown to have activity in pancreatic carcinoma, typically showing evidence of clinical benefit in approximately 20% of patients treated. Drugs with activity include 5-fluorouracil (5-FU), doxorubicin, mitomycin-C, and streptozotocin. When used in combination, various cytotoxic drug regimens have demonstrated clinical responses in approximately 35% of patients treated. The overall prognosis for patients with advanced pancreatic cancer treated with chemotherapeutic agents is poor, with a survival expectation of less than 6 months following the initiation of treatment.

Combined Modality Treatment

Chemotherapy combined with radiation therapy is the most frequently utilized current modality for the treatment of pancreatic cancer. In a prospectively randomized clinical trial, the Gastrointestinal Tumor Study Group [2] showed that combined radiation and chemotherapy was superior to radiation treatment alone and resulted in a median survival of approximately 1 year.

New Therapeutic Strategies Under Study

Extended Surgical Resections

Disease recurrence is common following surgical resection for pancreatic cancer. The lack of complete extirpation of regional tissues and lymph node groups in Whipple's operations or total pancreatectomies has been considered by some to be a reason for disease failure after resection. Extended or regional pancreatic resections have been advocated in an attempt to improve upon the surgical results in pancreatic carcinoma. Extended resections are designed to remove all tissues in the region of the pancreas which potentially harbor malignant cells, including the entire pancreas with duodenum and distal stomach, peripancreatic and retroperitoneal lymph nodes, retroperitoneal soft tissues, and major blood vessels such as the portal vein in the vicinity of the pancreas.

Fortner [3] initially described regional pancreatectomy and reported on 61 patients who had undergone extended resections. The resectability rate among patients explored was 30%, and the perioperative mortality was 23% overall. The median survival of 35 patients resected for adenocarcinomas of the pancreatic parenchyma was 15 months, while the median survival of 21 patients undergoing resection for periampullary or islet cell tumors was 40 months. Five patients had resections for benign disease.

Proponents of regional pancreatectomy have advocated the procedure as a method of prolonging survival in selected patients by providing good local control of disease in the region of the pancreas. Although a technically demanding procedure, in experienced hands a regional pancreatectomy can be performed with morbidity comparable to a Whipple's operation or a total pancreatectomy and can result in a modest improvement in survival expectation. Critics of regional pancreatectomy have suggested that the procedure is a technical exercise that does little to prolong overall survival, since patients requiring extended resections probably have disease too extensive to expect a cure [4]. It must be concluded at present that the experience with extended pancreatectomy is limited and has been confined to small numbers of selected patients. Further evaluations of the effectiveness of extended resections is necessary in order to determine whether regional pancreatectomy should play in a role in the surgical treatment of pancreatic carcinoma.

Intraoperative Radiotherapy

Intraoperative radiotherapy (IORT) is a technique of delivering therapeutic doses of radiation to areas of malignant disease during surgical procedures. Tumors can be exposed operatively and treated directly with large single doses of radiation. Radiosensitive and potentially dose-limiting normal organs and tissues may be surgically displaced from the beam path or may be physically shielded to prevent exposure within the radiation treatment volume. The rationale of IORT has been to allow the radiation dose to be maximized to areas of malignancy and to minimize the possibility of radiation damage to normal tissues [5].

IORT has been utilized in carcinoma of the pancreas by various institutions. Abe and Takahashi [6] reviewed 100 patients with unresectable pancreatic carcinoma who were treated with IORT at doses ranging 15–40 Gy. IORT did not have an important impact on overall survival, which averaged less than 6 months, but did provide a significant palliative benefit by producing pain relief in 80% of the patients treated. The Massachusetts General Hospital (MGH) has employed IORT (typically 15 Gy) in conjunction with external beam irradiation delivered both preoperatively and postoperatively (50 Gy total external beam dose). The MGH experience with 29 patients with unresectable pancreatic carcinoma revealed a median survival of 17 months, a 1-year actuarial local disease control rate of 64%, and a 50% rate of complete pain relief [7]. The MGH experience has suggested that IORT improves survival in selected patients. Experience with using IORT in unresected pancreatic cancer has been accumulated at Howard University and at the Mayo clinic with suggestions of prolonged survival and improved local disease control [5].

Evidence currently exists that suggests that IORT may represent a technical advance in the treatment of pancreatic carcinoma. It is necessary, however, to critically examine the efficacy and toxicity of IORT in prospectively randomized clinical trials to determine whether IORT actually offers significant advantages over conventional radiation therapy, either in terms of enhanced disease control or in terms of diminished radiation toxicity [8]. The National Cancer Institute, USA, has conducted a randomized trial in patients with unresectable pancreatic carcinoma who undergo external beam radiation therapy and 5-FU chemotherapy. Patients are randomized to receive or not to receive IORT boost at the time of laparotomy. Preliminary findings in the study suggest that IORT significantly enhances disease control and may provide a survival advantage. Further trials are required to establish any definitive role for IORT in the treatment of pancreatic cancer.

Adjuvant Therapy

Adjuvant therapy is treatment administered after resectional surgery in an attempt to eradicate systemic micrometastatic disease or locally persistent microscopic residual tumor and thereby diminish the likelihood of local or systemic recurrent disease. In pancreatic cancer, therapies that reduce the chance of recurrence are desirable since the failure rate after attempted resection is high. The adjuvant treatment of carcinoma of the pancreas after resection is currently experimental, but limited studies have suggested that adjuvant therapy may be of benefit.

Some centers have used radiation therapy in combination with resection to improve local disease control in pancreatic cancer [1]. The National Cancer Institute has studied adjuvant radiation therapy for resected pancreatic carcinomas where patients with positive regional lymph nodes or extrapancreatic tumor extension received radiation therapy to the resection bed. Patients were randomly assigned to receive either intraoperative radiation therapy or conventional postoperative external beam radiation. Of 25 patients placed in the study, the median survival in the group receiving IORT was 13 months and the survival of those receiving conventional external beam radiation was 9 months. Patients receiving IORT showed an actuarial 2-year survival of 38% and a local disease control rate of 35%. Patients receiving conventional radiation therapy had a 0% 2-year survival, and no patients achieved long-term control of local disease.

Chemotherapy as an adjuvant to resection has not been used extensively for pancreatic carcinoma, although some centers occasionally have given chemotherapy after pancreatic resection and have claimed some survival benefit [1].

Experience with combined modality therapy in resectable pancreatic cancer is small but suggestive of therapeutic benefit. The Gastrointestinal Tumor Study Group conducted a prospectively randomized clinical trial evaluating the role of combined radiation and 5-FU chemotherapy for resectable pancreatic cancer [9]. Patients with localized carcinomas of the pancreas who underwent pancreatectomy were prospectively randomly assigned to receive resection alone or to receive adjuvant combined modality therapy consisting of 40 Gy radiation therapy and 5-FU chemotherapy (500 mg/m^2) weekly. Of 43 patients entered into the study over an 8-year period, the patients who underwent surgery alone had a median survival of 11 months and a 15% 2-year survival, while the combined modality adjuvant group had a superior median survival of 20 months and a 42% 2-year survival rate. The disease-free interval was 11 months for the combined modality therapy arm and 9 months for the surgery alone arm. Disease eventually recurred in 86% of surgery alone patients and in 71% of the combined modality patients. Although the advantage of adjuvant therapy may be small, combined modality therapy following pancreatectomy appears to have promise for improving therapeutic efficacy in patients with localized disease amenable to surgical resection.

Future Approaches

Monoclonal Antibodies

A variety of monoclonal antibodies with reactivity against carcinomas of the pancreas have been discovered. Monoclonal antibody CO17-1A was originally generated against a colorectal carcinoma cell line and was found to have the ability to inhibit the growth of xenografts of human gastrointestinal tumors in nude mice. In a pilot clinical trial, CO17-1A was administered without significant toxicity to 20 patients with advanced gastrointestinal cancer and resulted in tumor regressions in three patients, including one patient with carcinoma of the pancreas [10].

Several institutions initiated pilot therapies using CO17-1A in patients with advanced pancreatic carcinoma. In a symposium on CO17-1A held at the Wistar Institute in 1986, it was reported that 115 patients were treated with CO17-1A administered at various doses either alone or in combination with activated mononuclear cells. No clinically significant toxicity was reported. It was felt that 23 out of 115 patients (20%) showed some clinical evidence of benefit from monoclonal antibody immunotherapy. Three patients were felt to have no clinical evidence of disease following treatment and were considered to be complete responders. Six patients were considered partial responders, with a measurable 50% decrease in the size of selected sites of tumor. An additional 14 patients were considered to have minor responses or stable disease over prolonged periods which were longer than would be expected from conventional therapy. The preliminary conclusion was that CO17-1A has some therapeutic efficacy in pancreatic carcinoma. Additional studies are ongoing and further investigations will be necessary to assess the potential utility of monoclonal antibodies in the treatment of pancreatic carcinoma.

Biological Response Modifiers

There is considerable current interest in various biological response modifiers in the treatment of malignant disease. Biological response modifiers include interferons, interleukins, tumor necrosis factors, colony stimulating factors, and various lymphokines and cytokines. At present there has been little utilization of biological response modifiers in patients with pancreatic carcinoma. Based on early reports of activity of biological response modifiers in a variety of diseases, it appears reasonable to suggest that patients with pancreatic carcinoma be investigated for possible therapeutic effects.

References

1. Sindelar WF, Kinsella TJ, Mayer RJ (1985) Cancer of the pancreas. In: DeVita VT, Hellman S, Rosenberg SA (eds) Cancer: principles and practice of oncology, 2nd edn. Lippincott, Philadelphia, pp 691–739
2. Moertel GC, Frytak S, Hahn RG, O'Connell MJ, Reitemeier RJ, Rubin J, Schutt AJ, Weiland LH, Childs DS, Holbrook MA, Lavin PT, Livstone E, Spiro H, Knowlton A, Kalser M, Barkin J, Lessner H, Mann-Kaplan R, Ramming K, Douglas HO, Thomas P, Nave H, Bateman J, Lokich J, Brooks J, Chaffey J, Corson JM, Zamcheck N, Novak JW (1981) Therapy of locally unresectable pancreatic carcinoma: a randomized comparison of high dose (6000 rads) radiation alone, moderate dose radiation (4000 rads + 5-fluorouracil), and high dose radiation + 5-fluorouracil. The Gastrointestinal Tumor Study Group. Cancer 48: 1705–1710
3. Fortner JG (1984) Regional pancreatectomy for cancer of the pancreas, ampulla, and other related sites. Tumor staging and results. Ann Surg 199: 418–425
4. Moossa AR, Scott MH, Lavelle-Jones M (1984) The place of total and extended total pancreatectomy in pancreatic cancer. World J Surg 8: 895–899
5. Kinsella TJ, Sindelar WF (1985) Newer methods of cancer treatment. Intraoperative radiotherapy. In: DeVita VT, Hellman S, Rosenberg SA (eds) Cancer: principles and practice of oncology, 2nd edn. Lippincott, Philadelphia, pp 2293–2304
6. Abe M, Takahashi M (1981) Intraoperative radiotherapy: the Japanese experience. Int J Radiat Oncol Biol Phys 7: 863–868
7. Shipley WU, Wood WC, Tepper JE, Warshaw AL, Orlow EL, Kaufman SD, Battit GE, Nardi GL (1984) Intraoperative electron beam irradiation for patients with unresectable pancreatic carcinoma. Ann Surg 200: 289–296
8. Sindelar WF, Kinsella T, Tepper J, Travis EL, Rosenberg SA, Glatstein E (1983) Experimental and clinical studies with intraoperative radiotherapy. Surg Gynecol Obstet 157: 205–219
9. Kalser MH, Ellenberg SS (1985) Pancreatic cancer. Adjuvant combined radiation and chemotherapy following curative resection. Arch Surg 120: 889–903
10, Sears HF, Herlyn D, Steplewski Z, Koprowski H (1984) Effects of monoclonal antibody immunotherapy on patients with gastrointestinal adenocarcinoma. J Biol Response Mod 3: 138–150

29. Hepatocellular Carcinoma

J.S. Macdonald

Current Results and Therapeutic Issues

The curative therapy of hepatocellular carcinoma is surgical resection of the tumor [1]. Although it is important to consider every patient with hepatocellular carcinoma as a potential candidate for surgical cure, it should be understood that the vast majority of patients will not benefit from surgery and will be candidates for palliative treatment only. One of the major problems with attempting surgical resection in patients with liver carcinoma is that this disease develops most frequently in individuals with cirrhosis. A major hepatic resection in a cirrhotic patient is not feasible since the cirrhosis will inhibit regeneration of the liver after resection. Hepatic regeneration is depended upon to provide adequate liver function after resection. Another confounding problem in the surgery of hepatocellular cancer is the fact that in many instances hepatomas will be multi-focal. Thus, hepatic lobectomy, for example, can hardly be expected to be curative if multiple tumors exist throughout the liver.

There are however some patients with hepatocellular cancer who are good candidates for surgical resection for cure. These include patients with a unifocal lesion on the background of a non-cirrhotic liver, patients with fibrolamellar or encapsulated varieties of hepatoma, or hepatoblastoma, a rare lesion seen in infants and very young children. In these groups of patients, surgical resection should follow an evaluation which includes obtaining a tissue diagnosis. Hemorrhage is a risk with percutaneous or peritonoscopy-directed liver biopsy, but tissue confirmation of hepatic neoplasm is essential in planning therapeutic approaches. Hepatic arteriography to define the extent and location of the tumor is important pre-operatively. Bleeding is a major operative complication of liver resection and it is essential that a skilled hepatic surgeon undertake such surgical procedures. Care must be taken to obtain wide operative exposure, and careful dissection of hepatic vascular structures for ligation must occur before transection of the liver parenchyma is performed. In patients with hepatoma undergoing complete resection, the 5-year disease-free survival varies between 12% and 30%.

There are some palliative surgical approaches which may be helpful to the patient with unresectable hepatocellular carcinoma [1]. For example, hepatic dearterialization may be palliative in patients with hepatocellular carcinoma by causing necrosis of vascular tumors. This procedure may be performed surgically

479

or by percutaneous angiographic techniques. However, patients with cirrhosis and portal vein hypertension cannot be considered candidates for either hepatic artery ligation or percutaneous dearterialization procedures, since the hepatic artery in these patients is critical for oxygenation of normal liver tissue. Normally, the hepatic parenchyma receives adequate oxygenation through the portal venous system. However, in cirrhotic patients this is not the case and the hepatic arterial circulation provides oxygen and metabolic substrates for the liver.

Both radiation and chemotherapy have been used in the treatment of patients with unresectable hepatocellular carcinoma. Although radiation dosages of 20–35 Gy may result in regression of tumor in as many as 50% of the cases, median survivals are still in the range of 6 months and long-term survivors are very uncommon [2]. Radiation has been combined with chemotherapy, including the use of external beam radiation with hepatic artery infusion of drugs such as adriamycin (doxorubicin) and 5-fluorouracil (5-FU). Radiation doses of 15–24 Gy combined with 5-FU/adriamycin by hepatic artery catheterization have resulted in objective regression of tumor in as many as 50% of patients. However, complete regression and long-term survival is not attained with this approach [3].

Systemic chemotherapy both by single agents or combinations of drugs has not been an effective modality of treatment in patients with hepatocellular cancer. Response rates for single agents in the more recent studies performed by Cooperative Oncology Groups have been very poor, with less than 20% objective regressions. Combinations of drugs have been reported to produce response rates as high as 38% with 5-FU + mitomycin-c [1] but there have been no studies that have suggested long-term regression or cure of hepatocellular carcinoma by systemic chemotherapy.

Current Approaches Under Study

A significant current approach in the treatment of hepatocellular cancer is the use of high energy radionuclides bound to antibodies relatively specific for hepatocellular cancer cells. Order et al. [4, 5] have recently reported an update of work performed at Johns Hopkins University using this technique. Anti-ferritin polyclonal antibodies, which are relatively specific for hepatocellular carcinoma, have been developed by these workers. Ferritin is an iron storage protein synthesized and secreted by hepatocellular cancers and is found in significantly higher concentration in liver cancers than in normal liver [5]. In vivo imagine has demonstrated that anti-ferritin antibodies are highly specific for hepatocellular cancer [5] and ^{131}I-labelled anti-ferritin antibodies (polyclonal and monoclonal) have been developed by Order et al. ^{131}I-labelled polyclonal antibody may be directly administered intravenously and has been shown to localize with specificity in hepatoma and not in normal liver. It appears that tumor neovascularity is important for the antibody to localize successfully in the hepatoma. Hepatomas not exhibiting significant neovascularity do not take up the radiolabelled antibody nearly as well as tumors with high orders of neovascularity. Such tumors will demonstrate a large tumor blush on hepatic arteriography.

To date, clinical trials of ^{131}I-labelled anti-ferritin antibody have been of considerable interest. The group at Johns Hopkins, in cooperation with other investigators [5], have treated 105 patients with hepatocellular carcinoma. In this group of patients, there was a 48% overall response rate (41% partial responses and 7% complete responses). Although follow-up is short, there have been some 2-year survivors after therapy with ^{131}I-labelled anti-ferritin. Currently a randomized trial comparing ^{131}I-labelled anti-ferritin antibody to chemotherapy for hepatocellular cancer is being carried out by a consortium of universities under the auspices of the Radiation Therapy Oncology Group. Results of this study will be awaited with interest.

Future Development

The future developments in the treatment of hepatocellular cancer will depend upon our ability to integrate and expand upon several avenues of investigation. For example, the early results with radionuclide-labelled antibodies are certainly of interest. It may be possible to develop studies in which selective dearterialization, radionuclide-labelled antibodies, and perhaps, hepatic vascular infusion of drugs or biologic response modifiers may be carried out. Attempts to define and refine the maximum potential for radiolabelled antibodies also need to be performed. For example, studies are being performed to evaluate the role of chemotherapy combined with radionuclide-labelled antibody [5]. Also, external beam radiation to the liver is being evaluated with ^{131}I-labelled antiferritin treatment in an attempt to increase, either in an additive or a synergistic fashion, the cytotoxicity of the radiolabelled antibody to hepatoma. Hopefully, the approaches described above will result in an aggressive combined modality approach to the management of individuals with hepatocellular carcinoma that will provide significant palliation and prolongation of survival for these patients.

References

1. Cady B, Macdonald JS, Gunderson LL (1985) Cancer of the hepatobiliary system. In: DeVita VT, Hellman S, Rosenberg SA (eds) Cancer: principles and practice of oncology. Lippincott, Philadelphia, p 741
2. Phillips R, Murikami K (1960) Primary neoplasms of the liver: results of radiation therapy. Cancer 13: 714
3. Friedman MA, Volberding PA, Cassidy MI et al. (1979) Therapy for hepatocellular cancer with

intrahepatic arterial adriamycin and 5-fluorouracil combined with whole liver radiation: an NCOG Study. Cancer Treat Rep 63: 1885
4. Order SE, Stillwagon GB, Klein JL et al. (1985) Iodine[131] antiferritin, a new treatment modality in hepatoma: a radiation therapy oncology group study. J Clin Oncol 3: 1573
5. Order SE, Klein JL, Leichner PK (1987) Hepatoma: model for radiolabeled antibody in cancer treatment. NCI Monogr 3: 37

30. Esophageal Carcinoma

J.S. Macdonald

Current Results and Therapeutic Issues

Esophageal cancer will affect approximately 10 000 Americans in 1987 [1]. Although not as common as other major gastrointestinal cancers (gastric, pancreatic, and colorectal adenocarcinomas), squamous cell carcinoma of the esophagus is highly lethal. Over 90% of patients with this diagnosis will die.

The standard therapy of esophageal cancer is surgical resection. Obtaining valid estimates of the effectiveness of surgery in patients with carcinoma of the esophagus is difficult. The likelihood of a favorable surgical outcome clearly varies with the local extent of cancer. For example, survival rates as high as 20%–30% [2] have been reported for patients with distal esophageal lesions and no paraesophageal lymph node involvement who underwent surgery. If the nodes are involved, the survival rate decreases by at least 50%, so that patients with nodal involvement have at best a less than 10% probability of 5-year survival. Also, one should be aware that some patients reported upon in surgical series have been operated on merely for palliation and not with curative intent. Finally, surgery for esophageal cancer is fraught with complications resulting in postoperative morbidity and mortality. As many as 50% of the patients undergoing esophagectomy have major postoperative complications and the operative mortality for esophageal resection generally varies between 5% and 30% [2].

Radiation as a single modality may also be used in the treatment of esophageal cancer. Patients with lesions smaller than 5 cm in size are potentially curable with radiation alone [3]. There are also indications that patients with squamous cell carcinoma of the cervical esophagus may be more curable with radiation than patients with distal or midesophageal lesions. Patients with large lesions of the esophagus may receive palliation from radiation but are not curable with this technique. In general, the curative radiation approach for esophageal cancer requires a field of irradiation encompassing the lesion and lymph node drainage areas. The dosage varies between 50 Gy and 65 Gy over a 5- to 7-week period [2]. Radiation also has been combined with surgery in the treatment of esophageal cancer. Patients have been treated with preoperative irradiation followed by surgical resection of the lesion. The value of this approach remains undefined and randomized studies of preoperative radiation versus surgery only have generally shown no significant differences in survival or morbidity between the irradiated and operated groups [2].

Chemotherapy has not been widely used as a single modality of treatment for primary esophageal cancer. The activity of chemotherapeutic agents in esophageal cancer has been defined in patients with established metastatic disease. Agents such as 5-fluorouracil (5-FU), cisplatin and methotrexate have been shown to be active in causing regression of disease. Platinum-based combination chemotherapy regimens in patients who have had no previous chemotherapy result in approximately 40%–60% response rates, with as many as 20% of the patients evidencing complete regression of the disease [2].

Current Approaches Under Study

Esophageal cancer is of interest to the clinical oncologist because it is a disease where neoadjuvant therapy is being explored and may have significant benefit. The neoadjuvant approach uses combination chemotherapy along with irradiation followed by esophagectomy. Combination chemotherapy regimens in neoadjuvant studies of esophageal cancer are 5-FU plus mitomycin and 5-FU plus cisplatin [4]. A study performed by the Southwest Oncology Group in which patients with stage I and II esophageal cancer were treated with neoadjuvant therapy is of interest. In this trial, patients received a combined irradiation chemotherapy program consisting of continuous infusion of 5-fluorouracil at 1000 mg/m^2 per day, days 1–4 and days 29–32; cisplatin 75 mg/m^2 on day 1 and on day 29; and radiation 30 Gy administered over days 1–19. Of the 71 patients in this phase II study who underwent surgical resection after neoadjuvant therapy, 18 (25%) had no pathologic evidence of disease in the resected specimen [5]. Median postsurgical survival for all 71 patients was 14 months and was 32 months for those who attained complete remission from neoadjuvant therapy. It should be emphasized that, although it is encouraging that 25% of patients achieved complete pathologic regression of disease from combined chemotherapy and radiation, neoadjuvant therapy remains an investigational approach. There is no evidence at present documenting survival benefit with this technique. There is currently a randomized phase III study being performed in the United States in which patients with early esophageal cancer will be randomly allocated to neoadjuvant therapy as tested by the Southwest Oncology Group study versus 64 Gy radiation therapy only. This study will accrue in excess of 100 patients and will be very useful in defining the value of the neoadjuvant approach compared to standard radiation therapy.

Another approach that is of considerable interest in esophageal cancer is the use of endoscopic laser therapy for cytoreduction [6, 7]. This approach will allow the palliation of obstruction lesions to the esophagus and thus will allow patients to aliment themselves and improve their nutrition. It has been shown that laser cytoreduction results in good palliation of patients with esophageal cancer causing luminal obstruction. Mellow et al. [7] demonstrated that all patients with obstructing esophageal cancer treated with endoscopic laser cytoreduction, using a Nd:YAG laser, had rapid palliation of their symptoms. Also 8/11 patients had improvement in performance status. A Southwest Oncology Group study is being performed which will test whether or not laser cytoreduction followed by a neoadjuvant approach of chemotherapy and radiation will provide effective palliation for patients with advanced esophageal cancer. The results of this study are awaited with interest.

Future Approaches

The future approaches in the treatment of esophageal cancer will certainly entail further investigations of combined modality therapy. The use of laser cytoreduction of the primary tumor along with neoadjuvant irradiation and chemotherapy may make more patients candidates for either combined modality approaches or surgical approaches carried out with curative intent.

References

1. American Cancer Society (1987) Cancer facts and figures 1987. American Cancer Society, New York, p 17
2. Rosenberg JC, Roth JA, Lichter AS, Kelsen DP (1983) Cancer of the esophagus. In: DeVita VT, Hellman S, Rosenberg SA (eds) Cancer: principles and practice of oncology. Lippincott Philadelphia, p 621
3. Beatty JD, DeBoer G, Rider WD (1979) Carcinoma of the esophagus—pretreatment assessment, correlation of radiation treatment parameters with survival and identification and management of radiation treatment failure. Cancer 43: 2254
4. Pazdur R, Baker L (1987) Anal canal and esophageal squamous cell carcinomas: the role of combined modality therapy. In: MacDonald JS (ed) Gastrointestinal oncology: basic and clinical aspects. Nijhoff, Boston (in press)
5. Poplin E, Fleming T, Leichman L et al. (1987) Combined therapy for squamous cell carcinoma of the esophagus, a Southwest Oncology Group study (SWOG 8037). J Clin Oncol 5: 622
6. Fleischer DE (1983) Endoscopic ND:YAG laser therapy for disease of the esophagus. In: Joffe SN (ed) Neodymium-YAG laser in medicine and surgery. Elsevier, New York
7. Mellow MH, Pinkas H et al. (1984) Endoscopic therapy for esophageal carcinoma with ND:YAG laser: prospective evaluation of efficacy, complications, and survival. Gastrointest Endosc 30(6): 34

31. Gastric Cancer

R.G. Gray and P.V. Woolley

Current Results and Therapeutic Issues

While the incidence of gastric cancer has fallen dramatically in the United States in the past 50 years, it remains an important problem worldwide, accounting for approximately 30% of the malignancies occurring in males in Chile and Japan. However, incidence is also dropping in these areas. Possible etiologic factors in the development of gastric carcinoma include nitrosamines and nitrosamides, which can be formed in the food or in the stomach by the nitrosation of secondary amines by nitrite, and also carcinogenic hydrocarbons and asbestos. Changes in food preparation and storage, as well as increases in dietary ascorbic acid which can inhibit the nitrosation reaction, may be partly responsible for this decreasing incidence.

Surgery remains the only therapy with curative potential. Unfortunately, while the 5-year survival of patients with disease localized to the stomach wall is 85%–90%, less than 20% of the cases diagnosed in the United States present in this manner. The much poorer survival of patients presenting with local or distant spread accounts for the overall 10%–15% 5-year survival seen in the USA. The use of combined radiographic, endoscopic, and cytologic screening, as is currently practiced in Japan, can increase the detection of early stage disease. However, this is not cost-effective in areas with a lower incidence of disease.

The treatment of gastric carcinoma with radiation therapy is limited by (a) the intrinsic radiation resistance of gastric carcinoma; (b) the relatively low radiation tolerance of the tissues of the upper abdomen, and (c) peritoneal and distant metastatic spread. While newer techniques, including intraoperative therapy with or without hyperthermia and effective radiosensitizers, may improve local control, significant increases in long-term survivorship will depend upon advances in systemic therapies.

5-Fluorouracil (5-FU), doxorubicin, mitomycin-C, and cisplatin are active drugs in the treatment of advanced gastric carcinoma, but they produce short responses that do not affect survival. Drug combinations have produced response rates of 20%–55% and response durations of 4–11 months [1]. However, complete responses and long-term survivors are infrequent, and the effect of combination chemotherapy on overall survival remains controversial.

Progress in the management of gastric cancer could result from research in both prevention and treatment. The greatest need in clinical management is for new effective drugs and the means of delivering them selectively to the tumor. Many of the ideas mentioned in the section on colon cancer might also apply to gastric cancer, since they are both resistant gastrointestinal neoplasms.

Current Approaches Under Study

While empiric testing of new drugs emerging from developmental screening programs has been an inefficient mechanism for identifying active agents for gastric cancer, new methods of in vitro drug sensitivity testing could improve the selection process. Many assays are available, but one that depends upon reduction of nitrotetrazolium blue dye in living cells is of interest because it can be automated [2]. In vitro sensitivity testing using multiple gastric carcinoma cell lines could identify new active agents as well as optimized combination regimens for individual patients. In vitro drug sensitivity testing could also be used to help develop new chemotherapy combinations with true synergy.

Optimum scheduling of existing chemotherapeutic agents could also improve the treatment of gastric carcinoma. The prolonged in vitro exposure of colon cancer cells to 5-FU greatly increases the cytotoxicity of the drug and a recent clinical trial has shown that continuous infusion 5-FU produces a greater response rate and longer survival than weekly bolus administration of the drug in advanced colon cancer [3]. The integration of continuous infusion of 5-FU into chemotherapy combinations could improve their efficacy. For example, the current protocol for advanced gastric cancer at Georgetown University utilizes intermittent infusions of cisplatin, mitomycin C, and doxorubicin with a continuous infusion of 5-FU.

Some drug interactions produce favorable pharmacomodulatory or synergistic effects. PALA, thymidine, and folinic acid, for instance, can all increase the intracellular accumulation of 5-FU metabolites or increase the in vitro incorporation of 5-FU into RNA. However clinical trials have yet to show that such combinations increase the therapeutic activity of 5-FU [4]. 5-FU and cisplatin have in vitro and clinical synergy against various tumors, and identification of other synergistic drug combinations could improve treatment of gastric cancer.

Future Approaches

A particularly promising route of future investigation is to attempt to understand the multifactorial process of drug resistance in gastric cancer to the extent that tumor cells could be sensitized by pharmacologic inhibitors of specific resistance mechanisms [5]. A few examples of such mechanisms include multidrug resistance, cytoplasmic thiol synthesis, and DNA repair. Multidrug or pleiotropic resistance is cross-resistance to drugs of different structures, mediated by membrane-associated protein efflux pumps that reduce intracellular drug concentration. Some drugs such as quinidine are known to antagonize this process in vitro, and other inhibitors could be designed. Cytoplasmic glutathione is an important defense against free radical damage and its synthesis can be blocked by buthionine sulfoximine, thereby potentiating the effects of drugs that produce intracellular free radicals. Rapair of single strand breaks in DNA that is mediated by poly(ADP-ribose) polymerase can be inhibited by nicotinamide analogues such as 3-aminobenzamide. This short list of examples of biochemical processes that could be inhibited to sensitize the cell could be expanded as knowledge increases.

Selective delivery of both cytotoxic drugs and drug sensitizers to gastric cancer cells is an important aspect of designing an overall therapeutic strategy. The transport medium of a drug can affect its pharmacokinetics and tissue distribution, and either increase drug concentrations in tissues frequently involved with metastatic disease, e.g., liver or lymph nodes, or decrease toxicity by decreasing drug concentrations in other tissues such as heart or bone marrow. The oral administration of a water-in-oil fat emulsification of N1-(2-tetrahydrofuryl)-5-FU increases 5-FU concentrations in the gastric wall and regional lymph nodes, as compared with the oral administration of a nonemulsified preparation of the same agent [6].

The entire field of drug encapsulation by liposomes and biodegradable polymers offers opportunities for delivery of high concentrations of cytotoxic agents to gastric tumors either by intravenous or regional administration. Investigators at Georgetown are studying liposome-encapsulated doxorubicin, which produces less cardiotoxicity than free doxorubicin [7]. Biodegradable polymers of various composition are also under development and liposome technology could be extended to include many combinations of drugs and/or cell sensitizers. Such systems might be most effective if antibodies to specific tumor cell antigens were incorporated into their structure.

Monoclonal antibodies could contribute to treatment of gastric cancer by the targeting of carrier systems, by direct coupling of drugs to the antibody, or by inhibiting specific oncogene products and growth factors. Although antigens truly specific for gastric carcinoma have yet to be identified, quantitative differences may exist in the expression of antigens such as carcinoembryonic antigen (CEA) between normal and neoplastic tissues. Antibodies to surface glycolipid antigens preferentially expressed by gastric neoplasms have been developed, and have demonstrated antitumor activity in nude mice implanted with human tumors. The mechanisms include antibody-dependent macrophage-mediated cytotoxicity. Antibody-mediated isotopic or drug therapy for gastric carcinoma is a logical extension of radioimmunodetection studies, which have shown that ^{131}I-labelled antibodies to CEA can localize to both the primary and metastatic lesions of gastric carcinomas [8]. Successful antibody-mediated therapy will have to circumvent problems of nonspecific antibody uptake and attachment, loss of antibody specificity from in vivo antigen modulation, dissociation of the antibody–drug complex, and heterogeneous antigen expression by different cells

488

within a single tumor. The last problem might require using antibody mixtures for therapeutic application.

Detailed understanding of the cellular biochemistry of gastric cancer could also lead to improvements in therapy. DNA sequences with transforming activity have been isolated from several gastric carcinomas, and the activation and/or amplification of *ras* and c-*erb*-B-2 [9, 10] has been demonstrated in gastric adenocarcinoma. If the overproduction or increased activity of the protein product of a specific oncogene(s) were causally related to neoplastic proliferation, then specific inactivators of that product could have antitumor activity. These could include monoclonal antibodies to growth factors, to growth factor receptors, or to oncogene products. An example of this phenomenon is the in vitro growth inhibition of small-cell lung cancer cells by antibombesin antibodies. Possible gastric tumor growth factors include gastrin, somatostatin, VIP, histamine, and epidermal growth factor [11].

Cellular immune functions can be altered both in vivo and in vitro in patients with disseminated gastric neoplasms. In vitro studies suggest that tumor antigens or immune complexes associated with increasing tumor burdens can activate some suppressor T-lymphocyte populations, in turn causing decreased lymphocyte mitogen responsiveness and antibody production. The suppressor cells could also directly inhibit cell-mediated antitumor activity, thus promoting tumor progression. Although these abnormalities might be a consequence rather than a cause of gastric carcinoma, their existence suggests a rationale for immunotherapy and biological response modifiers in treatment. To date, trials of immunomodulators such as various interferon species have demonstrated little activity in disseminated gastric neoplasms. OK-432, a penicillin and heat-treated derivative of *Streptococcus pyogenes*, stimulates in vitro lymphocyte and macrophage cell-mediated immunity, and at high concentrations is directly cytotoxic to gastric tumor cells [12]. The intraperitoneal administration of OK-432 to patients with gastric cancer and malignant ascites increased the number of T-lymphocytes and activated macrophages in the ascitic fluid. The amount of ascites and the number of malignant cells in the ascitic fluid also decreased. This therapy also increased the number of circulating T-lymphocytes, the serum total protein concentration, and skin test reactivity. Other, newer strategies for the use of lymphokines, including interleukin-2, lymphokine-activated killer cells, and tumor necrosis factor, both alone, in combination with each other, and in combination with chemotherapeutic agents, are currently under investigation. The most forseeable uses of these therapies are as adjuvant therapy of minimal disease and in combination with monoclonal antibodies, where they could serve to enhance antibody-dependent cell-mediated cytotoxicity. It is likely that overall therapeutic progress in gastric cancer will come from a multifaceted approach that combines several of these areas.

References

1. Goldberg R, Woolley PV (1986) Nonsurgical treatment of gastric cancer. In: Moosa AR, Robson MC, Schimpff SC (eds) Comprehensive textbook of oncology. Williams and Wilkins, Baltimore, pp 1042–1051
2. Alley MC, Scudiero DA, Monks A, Czerwinski MJ, Shoemaker RA, Boyd MR (1986) Validation of an automated microculture tetrazolium assay (MTA) to assess growth and drug sensitivity of human tumor cell lines. Proc Am Assoc Cancer Res 27: 389
3. Lokich J, Ahlgren J, Gullo J, et al. (1987) A randomized trial of standard bolus 5-FU vs. protracted infusional 5-FU in advanced colon cancer. Proc ASCO 6: 81
4. Chiuten DF, Valdivieso M et al. (1985) Sequential administration of thymidine, 5-fluorouracil and PALA. Am J Clin Oncol 8: 332–335
5. Woolley PV, Kumar S, Monks TJ, Ortiz JE (1987) Colon cancer as a model for resistance to neoplastic drugs. In: Woolley PV, Tew KD (eds) Mechanisms of drug resistance in neoplastic cells. Academic, New York
6. Nanaue H, Kurasawa T et al. (1986) N1-(2 Tetrahydrofuryl)-5-fluorouracil (FT-207) in the postoperative adjuvant chemotherapy of gastric cancer. Cancer 57: 693–698
7. Rahman A, Carmichael D, Harris M, Roh J (1986) Comparative pharmacokinetic of free doxorubicin and doxorubicin entrapped in cardiolipin liposomes. Cancer Res 46: 2295–2299
8. Nelson MO, Deland FH et al. (1983) External imaging of gastric cancer metastases with radiolabeled CEA and CSAp antibodies. N Engl J Med 308: 847
9. O'Hara BM, Oskarsson M, Tainsky MA, Blair DG (1986) Mechanism of activation of human *ras* genes cloned from a gastric adenocarcinoma and a pancreatic carcinoma cell line. Cancer Res 46(9): 4695–4700
10. Yokota J, Yamamoto T, Toyoshima K, Terada M, Sugimura T, Battifora H, Cline JM (1986) Amplification of c-*erb*-B-2 oncogene in human adenocarcinomas in vivo. Lancet 1(8484): 765–767
11. Moyer MP, Armstrong A et al. (1986) Effects of gastrin, glutamine, and somatostatin on the in vivo growth of normal and malignant human gastric mucosal cells. Arch Surg 121: 285–288
12. Torisu M, Kitano M et al. (1983) New approach to management of malignant ascites with a streptococcal preparation, OK-432. I. Improvement of host immunity and prolongation of survival. Surgery 93: 357–364

32. Colon Cancer

N.E. Rothschild and P.V. Woolley

Current Results and Therapeutic Issues

Although colorectal cancer is a common malignancy, we have made little progress in its treatment. Several problems contribute to this situation. First, although 5-fluorouracil (5-FU) is the single most active drug for colon cancer, its effect on patient survival is marginal. Second, extensive experience has failed to show that any drug combinations are better than 5-FU alone. Third, randomized prospective trials of 5-FU alone and with other agents have not altered the natural history of surgically resected colon cancer, although the drugs are theoretically of maximum effectiveness against minimal disease. Finally, empiric testing of drug development has been a very ineffective way of identifying active new agents for colon cancer [1].

We can postulate that the clinical drug resistance of colon cancer drugs is mediated by specific cellular biochemical mechanisms. Colon cancer cells studied in the human tumor stem-cell assay are usually sensitive to cytotoxic drugs in 10%–15% of cases, in contrast to over 40% of lymphomas or small-cell lung cancers [1]. The failure of colon cancer to respond to drugs could then represent the inherent resistance of a slowly cycling population of stem cells. The vascular supply of the tumor may also limit effective drug delivery. However, despite the slow progress in this disease, there are now several promising avenues of research that could lead to improvement in this situation.

Current Approaches Under Study

Empiric Testing of New Drugs

While empiric drug development has been an inefficient approach, it is important to continue clinical testing of new compounds. One agent of current interest is flavone acetic acid, which has entered clinical trials on the basis of its ability to inhibit tumor growth in 60%–80% of mice xenografted with resistant murine colon adenocarcinoma 38 [2]. Improved ability to design drugs may result from better understanding of specific drug resistance mechanisms and the means by which such mechanisms could be inhibited.

Improved Use of Existing Agents

5-FU, given as a single-agent in a variety of schedules, remains the standard treatment of advanced colorectal cancer. In general, approximately 20% of patients treated with this drug experience a regression of disease. To date, controlled trials have failed to demonstrate that intermittent bolus administration of 5-FU can prolong survival in patients with colon cancer. However, the activity of 5-FU could be improved by prolonged infusion, by pharmacologic modulation, by identification of synergistic drug combinations, or by regional infusion.

Both laboratory and clinical evidence suggest that tumoricidal effects of the fluorinated pyrimidines can be augmented by prolonging exposure time [3]. 5-FU has a plasma half-life in humans of approximately 10 min and is predominantly cell-cycle specific. Thus, the clinical resistance to bolus 5-FU may represent a failure to expose slowly cycling tumor cells to its cytotoxic effect. Drewinko and Yang [3] have demonstrated that low but therapeutically achievable concentrations of 5-FU maintained over extended periods result in profound cytotoxicity in colon carcinoma cell lines. In a recent clinical trial, continuous infusion of 5-FU delivered by portable external infusion pump for a period of 12 weeks produced a response rate of 30% compared to 7% in patients given the conventional 5-FU loading dose schedule [4]. Preliminary analysis also indicates a survival benefit for the continuous infusion arm of the study.

In the presence of hepatic metastases, hepatic arterial infusion selectively delivers high drug concentrations to the tumor capillary bed, while hepatic extraction minimizes systemic toxicity. Most of the experience with this technique is with 5-FU, its analogue 5-FUdR, and mitomycin C. Recent randomized trials indicate that higher response rates can be achieved with intrahepatic infusion than with systemic infusion, but overall survival with both modalities is essentially equivalent [5]. Recipients of intrahepatic infusional therapy have a high rate of extrahepatic relapse and can develop chemical cholangitis and gastroduodenal ulceration.

There is less experience with intraperitoneal 5-FU. Direct instillation of 5-FU into the peritoneal cavity produces a 2–3 log concentration advantage over the systemic circulation method. Because of physical limitations on drug penetration into tumor tissues, the major applications of this approach are probably in adjuvant treatment or in those patients with minimal residual peritoneal disease. Sugarbaker compared intraperitoneal administration of 5-FU to intravenous infusion in 66 colon cancer patients at high risk for developing recurrence [6]. Although the relapse rate and overall survival were comparable in both groups, the incidence of peritoneal carcinomatosis was lower in those treated intraperitoneally. Intraperitoneal therapy could ultimately be part of a multimodality approach to the prevention of recurrence.

5-FU may have synergistic interactions with other agents. There is laboratory evidence that folinic acid, methotrexate, and cisplatin can pharmacomodulate the effects of 5-FU therapeutic advantage. Thus far the results of clinical studies have been mixed, although some responses have been reported in patients who were previously refractory to 5-FU alone. In a recent randomized trial, three other putative pharmacomodulatory agents, N-(phosphonacetyl)-L-aspartic acid

(PALA), high-dose thymidine, and levamisole were examined, but there was no statistically significant advantage of these combinations over 5-FU alone or the MOF-Strep regimen [7]. Other randomized trials are now under way to define the optimum clinical value of various doses and schedules of the leucovorin–5-Fu combination. The analysis of drug synergy itself has undergone recent refinement, and improved mathematical models may be useful in designing clinical strategies based upon laboratory data [8]. The median effect function has been applied to an analysis of 5-FU–cisplatin synergy [8], with the finding that synergy is determined by both the duration of exposure to 5-FU and the ratio of 5-FU to cisplatin.

Radiation Therapy

Photon irradiation has principally been used as an adjunct to surgery in primary colorectal cancer and for the palliation of local complications of advanced disease. The use of sensitizing agents to enhance the effectiveness of radiation is an area of active investigation. N-methylformamide (NMF), for example, appears to potentiate the cytotoxic effect of irradiation on colon cancer cells by its action on intracellular glutathione [9].

Dritschilo et al. [10] at Georgetown University are investigating the treatment of hepatic metastases with high-intensity radiation delivered by a "remote afterloading" iridium-192 source either percutaneously under sonographic guidance or during laparotomy. The technique permits the delivery over a few minutes of radiation doses of 20–50 Gy to each individual metastatic lesion. Conceivably this procedure could be used in conjunction with continuous drug infusion systemically or directly into the hepatic circulation.

Future Approaches

Although some of these developments give cause for optimism, they may produce only incremental progress and newer approaches will be required to significantly alter the course of this disease. The area of biological response modifiers is one of great interest. Various interferon species have been tested clinically but lack single agent activity against colon cancer. However, synergistic interactions between α-interferon and γ-interferon may be valuable. Tumor necrosis factor is now completing phase I testing. Interferon and tumor necrosis factor could be synergistic with each other an potentiate the effects of some cytotoxic drugs as well. Interleukin-2 and lymphokine-activated killer (LAK) cells have been tested in patients with colon carcinoma with some indications of benefit. The treatment is very toxic but is a fundamentally new approach. Many other lymphokines and cytokines have been isolated and are currently undergoing preclinical evaluation.

As discussed elsewhere in this volume, monoclonal antibodies (MAbs) offer opportunities for imaging and tumor marker studies and also for targeted delivery of toxins and radiation. Studies in colon cancer have centered on antibodies that react with carcinoembryonic antigen- (CEA-)related antigens, but problems of tumor cell heterogeneity and cross-reactivity with normal tissues, particularly polymorphonuclear leukocytes, have been encountered. Mixtures of MAbs which react with different CEA epitopes may solve some of the problems related to antigenic heterogeneity. The development of MAbs to non-CEA-related antigens will also be helpful. Finally, more novel applications of MAbs, such as targeting of growth factors and their receptors, may have therapeutic potential.

Biochemical Mechanisms of Drug Resistance

An understanding of the biochemical basis of drug resistance could lead to the identification of pharmacologic inhibitors of specific biochemical protective pathways. We postulate, for example, that the drug resistance of colon cancer is a multifactorial phenomenon that is mediated through a combination of pathways that include, but are not limited to, expression of membrane transport proteins, protection against free radicals by intracellular thiols, effective DNA repair by any of several pathways, stability of the DNA conformation by polyamines or topoisomerases, and/or amplification of particular gene loci. Multiple drug resistance refers to the acquisition of cross-resistance to structurally unrelated drugs with differing mechanisms of action (see Ivy/Ozols/Cowan, this volume). Ling and coworkers have identified a membrane-associated glycoprotein (P170) that plays a role in this process by promoting drug efflux from the cell. The level of expression of the gene coding for this protein correlates with degree of drug resistance in experimental cell lines. Furthermore, high levels of expression have been demonstrated in colon tumors and other resistant neoplasms [11]. Verapamil, quinidine, and other drugs can reverse the multidrug-resistant phenotype in cell culture and clinical trials are under way to examine the significance of this observation.

Attention has also focused on intracellular glutathione metabolism and its relationship to detoxification of free radicals. Interruption of glutathione synthesis by buthionine sulfoximine can sensitize cells to the cytotoxic effects of various drugs. Similarly the repair of DNA damage by specific mechanisms such as poly(ADP-ribose) polymerase can be inhibited by some agents. Further understanding of the biochemical basis and genetic control of these phenomena are important priorities.

Selective Targeting

If problems of preferential delivery of drugs to tumors could be solved it would represent an enormous advance in cancer therapy. Even the effectiveness of currently available drugs would be improved if they could be concentrated in tumor cells. The general application of MAb technology to this problem is a

494

logical approach. These antibodies could be inherently cytotoxic or could be coupled to a drug or toxin. One method could be to incorporate MAbs into the structure of liposomes which in turn encapsulate one or more cytotoxic agents. This would still leave issues of immunogenicity and distribution of liposomes within the body. However, in the specific case of colon cancer, direct perfusion of liposomes into the liver or the peritoneal cavity could be a solution.

References

1. Woolley PV, von Hoff DD, Kyle GW et al. (1986) Biology of colon cancer resistance to treatment. In: Mastromarino AJ (ed) Biology and treatment of colorectal cancer metastasis. Nijhoff, Boston, pp 295–309
2. Plowman J, Narayanan VL, Dykes D et al. (1986) Flavone acetic acid: a novel agent with preclinical antitumor activity against colon adenocarcinoma 38 in mice. Cancer Treat Rep 70: 631–635
3. Drewinko B, Yang L (1985) Cellular basis for the inefficacy of 5-FU in human colon carcinoma. Cancer Treat Rep 69: 1391–1398
4. Lokich J, Ahlgren J, Gullo J et al. (1987) A randomized trial of standard bolus 5-FU vs. protracted infusional 5-FU in advanced colon cancer. Proc ASCO 6: 81
5. Hohn D, Stagg R, Friedman M et al. (1987) The NCOG randomized trial of intravenous vs. hepatic arterial FuDR for colon cancer metastatic to the liver. Proc ASCO 6: 85
6. Sugarbaker PH, Gianola FJ, Speyer JL et al. (1985) Prospective randomized trial of intravenous vs. intraperitoneal 5-FU in patients with advanced primary colon or rectal cancer. Semin Oncol [Suppl 4] 12: 101–111
7. Buroker TR, Moertel, CG, Fleming TR et al. (1985) A controlled evaluation of recent approaches to biochemical modulation or enhancement of 5-fluorouracil therapy in colorectal carcinoma. J Clin Oncol 3: 1624–1631
8. Ortiz JE, Woolley PV (1987) A study of the synergistic effects of 5-fluorouracil and cisplatin on colon cancer cells using median effect analysis. Proc Am Assoc Cancer Res 6: 414
9. Glicksman AS, Lee ES, Leite D, Leith JT (1986) Production of increased cytotoxicity in human colon tumor cells after X-irradiation or drug treatment (cis-platinum, bleomycin, 5-fluorouracil) by pre-exposure to the differentiating agent N-methylformamide (NMF). Proc ASCO 5: 45
10. Dritschilo A, Grant EG, Harter KW et al. (1986) Interstitial radiation therapy for hepatic metastases: sonographic guidance for applicator placement. AJR 146: 275–278
11. Fojo AT, Ueda K, Slamon DJ et al. (1987) Expression of multidrug resistance gene in human tumors and tissues. Proc Natl Acad Sci USA 84: 265–269

33. Bladder Cancer

L.G. Gomella and W.M. Linehan

Current Results and Therapeutic Issues

Carcinoma of the urinary bladder consists of three main histologic types: transitional cell carcinoma, squamous cell carcinoma, and adenocarcinoma. Worldwide, the majority of cases (> 80%) are transitional cell carcinoma. There are a number of areas of the world, such as Northern Africa, where squamous cell carcinoma predominates. In the United States, there are an estimated 40 500 new cases of bladder cancer per year, with 10 600 deaths expected from the disease. The majority of work presented here relates to the treatment of transitional cell carcinoma (TCC)

Treatment options for carcinoma of the bladder depend primarily on the stage of the disease. Bladder cancer is classified as being superficial (TIS, Ta, T1), having muscle invasion (T2, T3a), being locally invasive (T3b, T4), or having nodal or systemic disease (T×N+M+).

Transitional cell carcinoma of the bladder normally arises in the bladder mucosa, usually as a papillary, exophytic mass. However, it can occasionally occur as a flat carcinoma-in-situ (CIS). In the early stages (TIS, Ta, T1) it is often a curable disease, with a greater than 90% 5-year survival for patients presenting with superficial papillary lesions. However, bladder cancer is a disease that requires close follow up of patients because (a) it can be multicentric and (b) patients who undergo surgical excision of a superficial lesion will often develop recurrent tumors. Muscle-invasive disease requires aggressive diagnosis and intervention because, if it is untreated, the 2-year survival rates are low.

Transurethral surgical resection is the primary method of therapy for superficial lesions (Ta, T1). There is often a high recurrence rate for superficial tumors, and emphasis has been placed on the prevention of recurrence. Intravesical chemotherapy is now an accepted measure to reduce the rate of recurrence. It is not used as a primary mode of treatment unless the patient has diffuse field changes such as CIS. Agents that shown to have activity when applied topically in the bladder include mitomycin C, thiotepa (triethylene thiophosphamine), Epodyl (etoglucid: triethylene glycol di-glycerol ether), and adriamycin (doxorubicin hydrochloride). In the United States, mitomycin C and thiotepa are the most frequently employed agents, usually administered intravesically on a monthly basis for up to 1 year if no tumor recurrences are detected. Recurrence rates of 7% are usually seen, with one study reporting a

496

zero recurrence rate [1]. Intravesical cisplatin is no longer used due to the high rate of hypersensitivity reactions.

Intravesical Bacillus Calmette-Guerin (BCG) has been used as a prophylactic agent for superficial transitional cell carcinoma. It is thought by some, however, to be most useful in the treatment of CIS, in which response rates of 65%–71% have been reported [2]. The questionable efficacy and safety of intradermally administered BCG has led to a discontinuation of parenteral administration at most centers.

External beam radiotherapy (6–70 Gy) has been used as definitive treatment of muscle invasive transitional cell carcinoma. However, only about 20% of tumors undergo a significant regression with this therapy and a number of patients treated with external beam radiotherapy will require a "salvage cystectomy". Overall, 15%–35% survival at 5 years has been reported with this modality, and although it is used infrequently, it may play a role in the management of selected patients with invasive bladder carcinoma [3].

Muscle-invasive transitional cell carcinoma (T2, T3a) is most often treated with radical cystectomy and total urinary diversion. In well-selected patients, less radical extirpation, such as partial cystectomy, may be employed. A major issue is the preservation of bladder function without sacrificing treatment efficacy.

Once the carcinoma has spread beyond the bladder, 5-year survival decreases significantly. Even in patients who undergo radical cystectomy, over 50% will develop metastatic disease within 2 years. Response rates of up to 40% have been reported for some single-agent chemotherapy regimens, but the tumor tends to recur after a short duration. Single agents that have shown some activity include cisplatin (42%), cytoxan (27%), methotrexate (28%), 5-fluorouracil (5-FU; 17%), mitomycin C (23%), and adriamycin (19%) [4].

Very encouraging results have been reported with the use of multiagent regimen chemotherapy. Recently, MVAC (methotrexate, velban, adriamycin, and cisplatinum) has shown response rates greater than 65%, and it is currently the most active regimen for metastatic bladder cancer [5].

Current Approaches Under Study

Large-scale, prospective, randomized trials are under way to determine the role of preoperative radiation therapy in the management of invasive bladder cancer. Previously published treatment regimens using 16–50 Gy preoperative irradiation followed by cystectomy have 5-year survival rates of 30%–50% compared to historical controls in which cystectomy alone gave 16% survival at 5 years. Local recurrence rates were decreased from 37% to 24% when preoperative radiation was used. These comparisons have recently been questioned because of the use of historical controls in the early studies that led to this regimen and hence there is the need for prospective randomized trials.

Photodynamic therapy, which often combines high-energy laser light and a photosensitizer such as hematoporphyrin derivative (HPD), is currently under study at a number of institutions. Laser detected hematoporphyrins may also be used to visualize areas of abnormal bladder mucosa. Technical improvements in the laser systems and photosensitizers are needed (see Delaney, this volume), and current research is also directed towards identifying patients that will benefit most from this new approach. Such patients are likely to include those with CIS, widespread Ta disease, those with a tumor in a diverticulum, and those whose age or medical status makes them poor surgical candidates [6].

Lasers, particularly the neodymium:yttrium-aluminum-garnet (Ng:YAG) laser, also show promise in the treatment of bladder cancer. High recurrence rates for superficial lesions treated by transurethral resection are thought to be secondary to implantation of tumor cells at the time of surgery. Since the Ng:YAG laser destroys by thermal necrosis, an advantage of this form of therapy is that recurrence rates could be less. Laser therapy also has the advantage of a "bloodless" resection and dose not appear to cause contracture of the bladder with healing as transurethral resection may. Studies are being carried out to determine the role of laser therapy in the management of superficial and invasive bladder cancer.

Intraoperative radiation therapy (IORT) offers the advantage of delivering high doses of radiation directly to the tumor while potentially minimizing the radiation effect on normal tissue. IORT is usually often used in conjunction with external beam radiotherapy. The largest published experience with this modality comes from Japan. The tumor is usually removed surgically, the site is sterilized with IORT, and bladder function is maintained. Five-year survival rates of 96% and 61% have been reported for T1 and T2 lesions and 7.3% with T3 and T4 lesions. Most notable is the marked decrease in the local recurrence rate [7]. Work is under way to establish the efficacy of this technique and to study its role as a potential adjunct to radical cystectomy in patients with local residual disease.

Interstitial radiotherapy using either gold grains, iridium wires, tantalum wires, or radium needles is under study at various institutions. Interstitial implantation of superficial and locally invasive bladder carcinomas has been associated with remarkably low recurrence rates. Patients with T2 disease have been reported to have 56% 5-year survival when interstitial radiotherapy was coupled with external beam radiotherapy. A potential advantage of this approach is the control of local disease while maintaining a functional bladder [8]. Intracavitary implantation brachytherapy has been shown to produce promising results; however, it has not gained widespread acceptance, but needs to be compared to established therapies in prospective trials [9].

Systemic treatment to prevent superficial recurrences of bladder cancer is also an area of ongoing investigation. Oral pyridoxine (vitamin B6) may block the excretion of abnormal tryptophan metabolites, which may be associated with bladder cancer. Likewise, retinoids such as vitamin A and etretinate, that reduce proliferation and differentiation of epithelial tissue, show promise in animal studies. Human trials evaluating their usefulness, are currently underway.

Human leuocyte interferon has shown some activity in the bladder. Studies have demonstrated some complete responses of tumor in the bladder when the bladder lesions are injected directly with interferon and the patients are given systemic interferon [10].

Future Approaches

Advances in the quality of life for patients with invasive bladder cancer have been made and will continue to develop with surgical advances. The Kock pouch (continent ileostomy), Camey procedure, and other bladder "substitution procedures" will continue to be refined.

The poor survival of patients with node-positive or metastatic disease should significantly improve with development of new, more effective chemotherapeutic regimens.

Combining modalities such as radiation, neoadjuvant chemotherapy such as cisplatin, and radical surgical excision will be an area of further investigation. This approach may decrease the treatment failures seem with muscle-invasive disease after the primary tumor is removed by eliminating micrometastatic disease. Early studied show that combining modalities can downstage and even totally eradicate the primary tumor [11].

The most efficacious regimens to treat superficial recurrences, and the role of biologic response modifiers such as interleukin-2, lymphokine-activated killer cells, tumor-infiltrating lymphocytes, monoclonal antibodies, and interferon await further study in this disease.

References

1. Flanigan RC, Ellison ME, Butler KM, Gomella LG, McRoberts JW (1986) Trial of prophylactic mitomycin C or thiotepa intravesical chemotherapy in patients with recurrent or multiple superficial bladder cancers. J Urol 136: 38
2. Herr HW, Pinsky CM, Whitmore WF et al. (1983) Effect of intravesical BCG on carcinoma in situ of the bladder. Cancer 51: 1323
3. Klimberg IW, Wajsmanz (1986) Treatment for muscle invasive carcinoma of the bladder. J Urol 136: 1169
4. Yagoda A (1983) Chemotherapy in advanced urothelial cancer. Semin Urol 1: 60
5. Sternberg CN, Yagoda A, Scher HI et al. (1985) M-VAC: update of methotrexate (MTX), vinblastine (VLB), adriamycin (ADM) and cisplatin (DDP) for urothelial tract cancer. Proc Am Soc Clin Oncol 4: 105
6. Benson RC (1984) Endoscopic management of bladder cancer with hematoporphyrin derivative therapy. Urol clin North Am 11: 637
7. Abe M, Takahashi M (1981) Intraoperative radiotherapy: The Japanese experience. Int J Radiat Oncol Biol Phys 7: 863

8. van der Werf-Messing B, Menon RS, Hop WCJ (1983) Carcinoma of the urinary bladder category T3NXMO treated by the combination of radium implant and external irradiation: second report. Int J Radiat Oncol Biol Phys 9: 177
9. Hewitt CB, Babiszewski JF, Antunez AR (1981) Update on intracavitary radiation in the treatment of bladder tumors. J Urol 126: 323
10. Ikik D, Maricic Z, Oresic V et al. (1981) Application of human leukocyte interferon in patients with urinary bladder papillomatosis, breast cancer and melanoma. Lancet 1: 1022
11. NCOG Study (1986) Effect of preoperative cisplatin (CDDP) and radiation therapy (XRT) on downstaging for invasive bladder cancer. Proc Am Soc Clin Oncol 5: 103

34. Prostate Cancer

G. Wilding and M.E. Lippman

Current Results and Therapeutic Issues

Prostate cancer, the most prevalent cancer among American men, kills approximately 25 000 each year. Current therapy, while effective in early stages, achieves only palliation of poor durability in advanced disease. Clearly, the status quo is not acceptable. By stage, the current therapy of prostate cancer and its deficiencies are as follows.

Stage A1: Focal disease usually found on transurethral prostatectomy specimens. This stage of disease, in the past, was considered unlikely to progress to metastatic disease. In fact, although the incidence of progression in older patients is low (<5%), young patients, who are less likely to die of intercurrent disease, show a progression rate of 16% after 8 years of follow-up [4]. Treatment beyond close follow-up is clearly mandated in a subset of patients with stage A1 disease. Radical prostatectomy would guarantee the removal of all of the tumor. The dilemma is how to determine which men are at high risk of recurrence, and thus would benefit from surgery, and spare the remaining majority from the morbidity of surgery.

Stages A2 and B1: Patients with these stages of disease, anatomically, are ideal candidates for local forms of therapy. As a consequence of advances in surgical technique, nerve-sparing procedures for radical prostatectomy result in the maintenance of potency in more than 80% of patients [1]. Alternatively, radiotherapy has achieved results comparable to radical prostatectomy in terms of survival. Unfortunately, 13%–25% of patients with clinical A2 or B1 disease will prove on lymphadenectomy to have positive lymph nodes, which upstages them to stage D1. Therefore, if radical prostatectomy is a therapeutic consideration, pelvic lymphadenectomy should be performed first. The choice between prostatectomy and radiotherapy should be determined by the experience of the surgeons and therapists involved, as well as the medical condition of the patient.

Stages B2 and C: Patients with these clinical stages of disease may be upstaged to D1 disease with lymphadenectomy in 30% and 42% of the cases, respectively. When D1 disease is not present, radiotherapy is the treatment of choice in these patients. Ultimately, 25% of all stage B patients and 35% of stage C patients will die of metastatic prostate cancer within 5 years of their initial diagnosis. Efforts to improve survival with adjuvant hormonal therapy or chemotherapy have failed. Since stage B and C patients represent two-thirds of all prostate cancer patients at diagnosis, effective adjuvant therapies would have a great impact. Future research efforts should focus on extending the disease-free survival of these patients. The development of less toxic, effective hormonal therapy such as the luteinizing hormone releasing hormone (LHRH) agonists e.g., Leuprolide, now make this problem a little more approachable [3]. However, the eventual breakthrough of hormone-independent clones will require the development of nonhormonal treatment strategies.

Stage D1: Traditionally, metastatic disease limited to the pelvic lymph nodes has been followed until symptoms warranted palliative hormonal therapy. Recent results from the Mayo Clinic suggest a more aggressive approach may improve survival [10]. Combining radical prostatectomy with orchiectomy, a marked improvement in disease-free survival was observed. A re-evaluation of early therapy and the determination of selection criteria for patients with this stage of disease who will benefit from such therapy are needed.

Stage D2: Despite the development of new hormonal therapies, the systemic treatment of metastatic prostate cancer has not progressed beyond palliative hormonal manipulations. Chemotherapy, though palliative in some cases, is not generally effective [2]. The most active agents, adriamycin (doxorubicin) and cisplatin, show objective responses of 10% or less in patients with hormone refractory disease. Combination therapies are no more effective than single agents. One of the major causes of difficulty in evaluating new agents for activity has been the almost exclusive use of patients with advanced, refractory disease in phase II trials. The recent observations of Seifter et al. [9] at the National Cancer Institute (NCI), USA, suggest that patients initially treated with chemotherapy still showed the expected response to hormonal manipulation given upon subsequent disease progression. Evaluation of new agents in previously untreated patients with metastatic disease at a time when their tumor burden is smaller in volume and they are more able to tolerate higher doses of therapy will allow a more accurate assessment of the potential efficacy of new agents.

Current Approaches Under Study

Current investigations of prostate cancer have focused on several aspects of the disease. First, with current therapy, the only curable form of disease is that localized to the prostate gland. To determine which patients have localized disease and are, therefore, candidates for aggressive, curative therapy, better forms of noninvasive anatomical evaluation are needed. Refinements in several diagnostic modalities hold promise for improved sensitivity in the evaluation of the prostate gland and its surrounding soft tissue structures for the presence of tumor. Using the transrectal and transurethral approaches, ultrasound can provide a better assessment of the prostatic parenchyma. This approach in combination with transabdominal ultrasound-guided biopsy, increases the accuracy of prostatic examination and provides a reasonable diagnostic modality to judge whether or not prostate cancer is present. Once a carcinoma is diagnosed, evaluation by magnetic resonance imaging (MRI) for local tumor extension appears to be more accurate (83%) than computed tomography (CT; 65%) [5]. However, the accuracy of ultrasound, CT, and MRI are not sufficient to replace lymph node biopsies in the evaluation of lymphatic spread.

With regard to radiotherapy, the combination of external beam irradiation with interstitial implants, high energy proton or neutron irradiation, and/or radiosensitizers may improve local control of the primary site and decrease the incidence of positive prostatic biopsies following radiation therapy. The improved efficacy and the decreased morbidity of both surgical and radiation treatment modalities now provide the opportunity to approach current clinical problems via controlled trials. For example, in young men with stage A1 disease and otherwise long-term life expectancy, radical prostatectomy would ensure the removal of all tumor and maintain potency in many men. However, this would represent overtreatment in other men who would never develop metastases. With new diagnostic techniques and refined treatment modalities, we may now be able to determine which men would benefit from aggressive prophylactic therapy.

The use of total androgen blockade—the inhibition of both testicular androgen production and adrenal androgen function—has been proposed and implemented by Labrie et al. [6], who have achieved impressive improvements in rate of response and survival in men with stage C and D prostate cancer by combining LHRH agonists and the antiandrogen flutamide. His results, though promising, were not compared to a suitable control group and they await confirmation by randomized studies such as the recently closed trial by the Collaborative Study Group.

The confirmation that the LHRH agonists are as effective but less toxic than diethylstilbestrol has several important implications [7]. First, the LHRH agonists are more acceptable agents for introduction earlier in the course of a patient's disease and in a variety of adjuvant settings. As suggested by Torti, there is urgent need for a randomized trial to determine whether early hormonal therapy will improve survival in patients at high risk of tumor progression and death. In addition, the less toxic the hormonal therapy, the easier it will be to evaluate combination chemohormonal therapies as the first treatment of metastatic disease [8].

The development of effective chemotherapy in prostate cancer has been slow and difficult. The observation by workers at the NCI, showing that hormone response is not diminished by prior treatment with chemotherapy, will allow, without fear of jeopardizing the response to subsequent standard therapy, the evaluation of new drugs earlier in a patient's course at a time when the tumor burden is lower, the ability of the patient to tolerate chemotherapy is higher, and the chance of resistant clones being present is lower.

Future Approaches

Current hormonal therapy, though effective, lacks durability, and it inevitably fails when hormone-resistant tumor clones emerge and predominate. As outlined by Wilding and Lippman (this volume), hormone-stimulated growth may be achieved through the activation of autocrine growth pathways. Hormone-independent growth may be achieved by constitutively activating these pathways in the absence of hormones. Future therapies will focus on the alteration of these autocrine pathways to inhibit the growth of both hormone-dependent and hormone-independent tumor cells. The tools needed to achieve growth inhibition through the disruption of autocrine growth loops are already being evaluated in in vitro and in vivo model systems. With time these therapies will undoubtedly play a vital role in the management of prostate cancer in humans.

References

1. Catalona WJ, Dresner SM (1985) Nerve-sparing radical prostatectomy: extraprostatic tumor extension and preservation of erectile function. J Urol 134: 1149
2. Eisenberger MA, Simon R, O'Dwyer PJ, Wittes RE, Friedman MA (1985) A reevaluation of nonhormonal cytotoxic chemotherapy in the treatment of prostatic carcinoma. J Clin Oncol 3: 827
3. Eisenberger MA, O'Dwyer PJ, Friedman MA (1986) Gonadotropin hormone-releasing hormone analogues: a new therapeutic approach for prostatic carcinoma. J Clin Oncol 4: 414
4. Epstein JI, Paull G, Eggleston JC, Walsh PC (1986) Prognosis of untreated stage A1 prostate carcinoma: a study of 94 cases with extended follow-up. J Urol 136: 837
5. Hricak H, Dooms GC, Jeffrey RB, Avallone A, Jacobs D, Benton WR, Naragans P, Tanagho EA (1987) Prostatic carcinoma: diagnosing and staging by magnetic resonance imaging and computerized tomography. J Urol (in press)
6. Labrie F, DuPont A, Belanger A (1985) Complete androgen blockade for the treatment of prostate cancer. In: DeVita VT, Hellman S Jr, Rosenberg SA (eds) Important advances in oncology. Lippincott, New York, pp 193–217
7. The Leuprolide Study Group (1984) Leuprolide versus diethylstilbestrol for metastatic prostate cancer. N Engl J Med 311: 1281
8. Torti FM (1984) Hormonal therapy for prostate cancer. N Engl J Med 311: 1313
9. Seifter EJ, Bunn PA, Cohen MH, Makuch RW, Dunnick NR, Javadpour N, Bensimon H, Eddy JL, Minna JD, Ihde DC (1986) A trial of combination chemotherapy followed by hormonal therapy for previously untreated metastatic carcinoma of the prostate. J Clin Oncol 4: 1365
10. Zincke H, Utz DC (1983) Radical surgery for stage D1 prostate cancer. Semin Urol 1: 252

35. Advanced Germ Cell Tumors*

G.J. Bosl

Current Treatment and Therapeutic Issues

Germ cell tumors (GCT) in men, most commonly presenting in the testis and less commonly in the mediastinum and retroperitoneum, are highly curable. High doses of cisplatin (≥ 100 mg/m^2 per cycle of therapy), added to drug combinations which include vinblastine and bleomycin (with or without cyclophosphamide and dactinomycin), and with adjunctive surgical resection of apparent residual sites of disease, will cure 70%–80% of patients with advanced metastatic GCT. Serum tumor markers play a vital role in patient management. α-fetoprotein (AFP) and human chorionic gonadotropin (HCG) are highly specific and sensitive markers, and radioimmunassays for both are routinely available. Lactate dehydrogenase (LDH) is another GCT marker and although less specific than AFP and HCG, it is equally valuable in patient management. Salvage chemotherapy with etoposide + cisplatin (EP) will cure 15%–25% of patients relapsing from complete remission and possibly a few patients with primarily refractory disease.

Despite these outstanding results, about 20% of patients still die of their disease. Considerable effort has been expended in trying to identify those prognostic variables which would distinguish between those patients most likely ("good risk") and least likely ("poor risk") to be cured. If poor-risk patients could be identified prior to therapy, then alternative treatment strategies could be designed in an attempt to improve treatment outcome. A few generalizations are possible. Patients with extragonadal nonseminomatous GCT do less well than those with tumors of testicular origin. Multivariate analyses of clinical variables in patients with testicular GCT have usually shown that the pretreatment level of HCG and some measure of extent of disease are independent prognostic variables. Values of LDH and AFP and tumor cell type have been less consistently found to be independent variables.

Treatment toxicity constitutes an opposing problem. Fatal bleomycin pneumonitis and septicemia during neutropenia still occur. Late vascular toxicity has been reported, including Raynaud's phenomenon (the most common),

*Work supported in part by grant CA-05826 and contract CM-07337 from the National Cancer Institute, USA.

malignant hypertension, myocardial infarction, and transient ischemic attacks. Hyperreninemia, hyperaldosteronemia, and hypomagnesemia have been reported long after cessation of treatment, indicating chronic renal toxicity. Practically all patients develop compensated hypogonadism, with recovery in some. The retroperitoneal lymph node dissection (RPLND) is standard therapy for patients with clinical stage I and early clinical stage II nonseminomatous testicular GCT and is often needed after chemotherapy when residual tumor masses are present, but infertility is a frequent consequence. Thus, possible gains in efficacy must be weighed against the potential acute and chronic toxicities.

A dilemma exists in the treatment of patients with GCT: how can toxicity be minimized in good risk patients but efficacy be increased in poor-risk patients? Separate trials have evolved for each group.

Current Approaches Under Study

The goal in good-risk patients is to maintain efficacy but decrease toxicity. Treatment may be made less toxic either by decreasing the number of drugs, or the number of cycles of therapy, or substituting new drugs.

Three randomized studies are comparing two-drug regimens to regimens containing either three or five drugs. In two of these studies, EP is being compared with either bleomycin + EP (BEP) or cyclophosphamide + cisplatin + bleomycin + actinomycin D + vinblastine (VAB-6). The third study compares vinblastine + cisplatin against vinblastine + cisplatin + bleomycin (PVB). In early reports, the proportion of complete response is not compromised by the reduction in the number of drugs, but the median follow-up is so far too short to allow evaluation of the frequency of late relapses.

Etoposide and carboplatin are new drugs being studied. In a preliminary report, PVB and BEP were equally efficacious and BEP was less toxic and possibly more efficacious in poor-risk patients. However, toxic deaths were reported with both programs. At Memorial Sloan-Kettering Cancer Center, a randomized trial comparing EP with etoposide + carboplatin, a cisplatin analog, has been started. Carboplatin is less nephrotoxic than cisplatin and can be administered as an outpatient procedure. Thus, both toxicity and financial cost may be decreased. Fewer cycles of therapy are being studied at the University of Indiana, with four cycles of BEP being compared to three cycles of the same regimen.

For poor-risk patients, more intensive therapy has generally been studied. Alternating two cisplatin-based regimens has not improved treatment outcome. Combination chemotherapy including ultrahigh doses of cisplatin (200 mg/m^2 per cycle) has been examined, but it is unclear whether or not these higher cisplatin doses improve the response rate, although the early results were promising. Carboplatin has also been used in poor-risk patients on the basis of studies suggesting non-cross-resistance, but the results do not show an improved response rate.

Other new drugs are being studied. The most promising is ifosfamide, an analog of cyclophosphamide. A phase II trial showed a 23% response rate, and in combination with EP, cures have been reported in the third-line setting. These results, however, have yet to be confirmed.

Future Approaches

In a disease in which about 70% of patients with advanced disease and 95% of patients with early stage disease are cured, improvement in treatment outcome depends upon identifying patients who are unlikely to do well. Even the most sensitive and specific models using clinical prognostic factors will select some patients for more intensive therapy who in fact only require standard therapy. The criteria for poor risk are inconsistent between studies and in an analysis of several criteria, the proportion of complete responders with poor risk features was dependent upon the criteria, not the treatment. Another study has shown that "stage migration" affects GCT clinical trials results. Thus, better markers of treatment failure are needed.

The phenomenon of differentiation observed in GCT has not been exploited. In both murine and human GCT cell lines, differentiation can be induced by 13-*cis*-retinoic acid [1]. In one murine cell line, the neuronal differentiation process was accompanied by the expression of an altered c-*src* product [2]. Expression of c-*myc* has also been reported in some human GCT cell lines [3]. Since oncogenes are involved in the control of normal differentiation and growth, the study of human GCT cell lines and fresh tumor may lead to information implicating specific oncogenes.

Advances in immunohistochemistry may also provide new tools for determining patient subgroups. Patterns of blood group antigen expression and secretor status may be important prognostically, as they are in patients with transitional cell carcinoma of the bladder [4]. Ongoing studies are attempting to characterize these patients in GCT. Using monoclonal antibodies, distinct cell surface antigens have been described which may be characteristic of GCT. Neuroectodermal antigens seem to be the most common [5].

Studies of drug resistance in GCT may prove valuable not only for GCT but also other malignancies. Unlike most other human tumors, GCTs are sensitive to a variety of drugs with different mechanisms of action. The multidrug resistance genotype conveys relative cross-resistance between actinomycin D, vinblastine, doxorubicin, and etoposide. These drugs are all active against human GCT. The cross-resistance between these drugs is not complete in a given cell line; this is consistent with the clinical observation that patients apparently refractory to regimens containing PVB (with or without actinomycin D) can be cured with EP, despite using equivalent doses of cisplatin. In addition, cisplatin binds with DNA and an inverse correlation has been reported between the ability to form cisplatin–DNA adducts and the degree of resistance to cisplatin. Careful study of currently available cell lines and fresh human tumors may provide clues as to why GCTs are usually so sensitive to a wide variety of chemotherapeutic agents, why they occasionally become resistant, and how resistance can be circumvented.

In parallel, cytogenetic abnormalities should be sought. It is likely that chromosomal rearrangements are important in the pathogenesis of malignancy and therefore lead to patterns of oncogene expression and drug sensitivity and resistance [6]. For example, although primitive neuroectodermal tumors and neuroblastoma are similar histologically, only neuroblastoma overexpresses n-*myc*. However, the former has the same cytogenetic abnormality and drug sensitivity as Ewing's sarcoma [7]. In GCT, an isochromosome of the short arm of chromosome 12 has been found, supporting this direction of research [8]. Since high HCG levels are generally associated with drug resistance and a poor outcome, the excessive production of HCG (and possibly other tumor markers) and drug resistance may be linked, perhaps through gene amplification. Both homogenous staining regions and double minute chromosomes have been observed in GCT cell lines.

References

1. Andrews PA (1984) Retinoic acid induces neuronal differentiation of a cloned human embryonal carcinoma cell line in vitro. Dev Biol 103: 285–293
2. Lynch SA, Brugge JS, Levine JM (1986) Induction of altered c-*src* product during neural differentiation of embryonal carcinoma cells. Science 234: 873–876
3. Sikora K, Evan G, Stewart J, Watson JV (1985) Detection of the c-*myc* oncogene product in testicular cancer. Br J Cancer 52: 171–176
4. Lloyd KO (1987) Blood group antigens as markers for normal differentiation and malignant change in human tissues. Am J Clin Pathol 87: 114–124
5. Fradet Y, Houghton AN, Bosl G, Bronson DL, Whitmore WF (1983) Cell-surface antigens of human teratocarcinoma cell lines identified with monoclonal antibodies. Cold Spring Harbor Conf Cell Prolif 10: 591–595
6. Croce CA (1986) Chromosome translocation and human cancer. Cancer Res 46: 6019–6023
7. Israel MA, Triche TJ, Kinsella TJ, McKeon C, Thiele CJ, Longo D, Steis R, Tsokos M, Horwath K, Belasco J, Buell D, Miser JS (1986) Treatment of peripheral neuroepithelioma (PN) in children and young adults: A genetically determined approach. Proc Am Soc Clin Oncol 5: 18
8. Atkin NB, Baker MC (1983) i (12p): Specific marker in seminoma and malignant teratoma of the testis? Cancer Genet Cytogenet 10: 199–204

36. Ovarian Cancer

R.F. Ozols

Current Results and Therapeutic Issues

The development of more effective therapy for patients with advanced ovarian cancer (FIGO Stages III–IV) represents the major challenge in the management of this disease. In the last decade the use of cisplatin-based combination chemotherapy has led to an increase in complete remission rates, a prolongation of disease-free survival, and an increase in overall survival compared to treatment with single alkylating agents. However, the vast majority of patients with advanced disease die of recurrent ovarian cancer due to the fact that drug-sensitive tumors frequently develop primary resistance to the initial combination, which is accompanied by broad cross-resistance to virtually all classes of antineoplastic drugs. Consequently, only 20%–25% of all patients with advanced stage ovarian cancer are alive 5 years after initiation of chemotherapy.

It has also been recently demonstrated that the dose of cisplatin is a critical factor in obtaining optimum results in the treatment of patients with advanced disease [1]. while cisplatin doses up to 200 mg/m² can be administered without dose-limiting nephrotoxicity by using vigorous saline hydration, the development of peripheral neuropathy has limited the number of cycles of high-dose cisplatin which can routinely be administered. The major areas of clinical and laboratory research in ovarian cancer are therefore focused upon the following issues: (a) identifying mechanisms responsible for the multidrug resistance phenotype and developing therapeutic strategies capable of overcoming this form of drug resistance, (b) developing more effective ways to deliver platinum-based chemotherapy, and (c) determining the role of biological response modifiers in the therapy of patients with advanced disease, since it is unlikely that the mechanisms responsible for drug resistance will influence the cytotoxicity of biologicals.

Current Approaches Under Study

Studies on the mechanisms associated with multidrug resistance in ovarian cancer have been facilitated by the recent development of relevant model systems of human ovarian cancer [2]. A series of human ovarian cancer cell lines have been established from drug-resistant patients as well as cell lines developed with acquired resistance in vitro to adriamycin (doxorubicin), cisplatin, and melphalan. Resistance to cisplatin and alkylating agents is associated with high levels of cellular glutathione levels as well as with increased repair of lethal DNA lesions [3, 4]. In cell lines with acquired resistance to adriamycin there is a decrease in drug accumulation and an increase in expression and amplification of the *mdr*-1 gene associated with the P170 membrane glycoprotein [5]. In some cell lines acquired resistance to adriamycin can be reversed with verapamil. Based upon these observations, a clinical trial of verapamil plus adriamycin has recently been performed in drug-resistant patients [6]. The levels of verapamil required to reverse drug resistance in vitro could be attained in some patients. However, this was associated with an unacceptable degree of transient cardiac toxicity. Future trials of agents capable of reversing resistance by increasing drug accumulation will be performed with less cardiotoxic agents. In addition, clinical trials with agents capable of reversing primary drug resistance and cross-resistance associated with alkylating agents, cisplatin, and irradiation will also soon be initiated (see below).

Clinical studies at the Medicine Branch of the National Cancer Institute, USA, with high dose cisplatin (200 mg/m^2) together with cyclophosphamide and irradiation are currently in progress [7]. While the preliminary complete remission rate in this study of 60% is encouraging, the toxicity of this approach has been substantial, with dose-limiting neurotoxicity occurring in approximately one-third of the patients. The cisplatin analog, carboplatin, has also been evaluated and is of particular interest in the treatment of ovarian cancer due to its lack of neurotoxicity. It recently has been demonstrated that high-dose carboplatin (800 mg/m^2) can produce responses in 27% of patients whose disease is refractory to standard-dose cisplatin therapy [8]. However, while carboplatin is not associated with significant neurotoxicity, it does produce more myelosuppression than cisplatin. Studies are currently in progress with combinations of carboplatin and alkylating agents to determine if carboplatin can replace cisplatin in the treatment of newly diagnosed patients with advanced disease. Furthermore, since the dose-limiting toxicity of carboplatin appears to be myelosuppression, very high dose therapy together with autologous bone marrow support is currently under evaluation.

In addition, recent experimental studies have demonstrated that diethyl-dithiocarbamate (DDTC) can protect against the nephrotoxicity of cisplatin and the myelosuppression of carboplatin without reducing the antitumor effect. Clinical studies have recently been initiated at the National Cancer Institute with DDTC plus high-dose carboplatin or high-dose cisplatin in drug-refractory ovarian cancer patients. If these studies demonstrate that DDTC permits further dose escalations of cisplatin or of carboplatin in previously treated patients with ovarian cancer, it will be possible to explore higher dose intensity induction regimens with reduced toxicity as front-line chemotherapy for patients with advanced disease.

Immunologic approaches to the treatment of ovarian cancer have also recently been initiated [9]. Lymphokine-activated killer (LAK) cells and interleukin-2

(IL-2) have been shown to prolong survival in a nude mouse model system of human ovarian cancer. Based in part upon this observation, a clinical trial of intraperitoneal administration of LAK cells plus IL-2 is currently in progress at the National Cancer Institute in refractory ovarian cancer patients. While clinical activity has been demonstrated, it is clear that additional patients are needed to fully assess the therapeutic potential of this modality, particularly since this form of treatment is associated with considerable peritoneal and systemic toxicity.

Intraperitoneal chemotherapy also has a strong biologic and pharmacologic rationale in ovarian cancer, since the disease remains confined to the peritoneal space virtually throughout its entire clinical course [10]. Recent trials have used large volumes of drug-containing fluid (approximately 2 l) to ensure uniform drug distribution throughout the peritoneal cavity. A series of phase I studies have demonstrated the pharmacologic success of intraperitoneal administration. However, the therapeutic impact of this approach remains to be established. Initial results from trials in patients who have small-volume disease left after induction chemotherapy with cisplatin have demonstrated that approximately 30% of these patients can achieve disease-free status by the intraperitoneal administration of cisplatin. Intraperitoneal chemotherapy has not been shown to be useful in patients with bulky disease, and its role in previously untreated patients is being assessed in a prospective randomized trial.

Future Approaches

Abundant laboratory evidence now indicates that a major mechanism in drug resistance in human ovarian cancer is the increase in intracellular glutathione (GSH). Buthionine sulfoximine (BSO), a synthetic peptide inhibitor of γ-glutamyl cysteine synthetase (a critical enzyme in GSH synthesis), is currently undergoing toxicology testing prior to entering into clinical trials in drug-resistant patients. The rationale for a clinical trial of BSO is based upon studies in model systems of human ovarian cancer [3] which have demonstrated that (a) cisplatin and melphalan resistant human ovarian cancer cell lines have increased glutathione levels, (b) BSO decreases GSH levels and leads to increased cytotoxicity of melphalan and platinum-containing compounds, (c) BSO plus melphalan is superior to melphalan alone in a nude mouse model of transplantable human ovarian cancer. In this system BSO plus melphalan produced a 72% increase in median survival as well as cures in some animals compared to melphalan alone which was not curative, and (d) BSO is essentially nontoxic to mice and does not alter the LD_{10} dose of melphalan.

It also had been demonstrated that human ovarian cancer cell lines with acquired resistance to melphalan or cisplatin have an increased capacity for DNA repair [4]. Inhibition of the enzymes involved in DNA repair enhances the cytotoxicity of cisplatin four-fold. It is likely that clinical trials will be initiated with agents such as aphidicolin (an inhibitor of DNA polymerase) to determine whether cisplatin resistance can be reversed.

An alternate way to overcome cisplatin resistance is to develop noncross-resistant platinum-containing drugs. One such drug is tetraplatin, which is currently undergoing toxicology studies prior to phase I clinical trials. This drug has been shown to have little, if any, cross-resistance to cisplatin in human ovarian cancer cell lines with acquired resistance to cisplatin [4]. In addition, since resistance is in part dose-dependent, protective agents such as DDTC and WR2721, which may decrease or eliminate some of the toxic effects of platinum-containing drugs without altering their antineoplastic activity, may further permit evaluation of the importance of dose intensity in the treatment of patients with ovarian cancer.

Biological therapies for ovarian cancer will also be extensively evaluated in the coming decade [9]. In addition to adoptive cellular immunotherapy with LAK cells plus IL-2, clinical studies with monoclonal antibody toxin conjugates will soon be initiated. Monoclonal antibodies against a human transferrin receptor and monoclonal antibodies against tumor-associated antigens when conjugated to either pseudomonas exotoxin (PE) or the A chain of ricin (RTA) lead to marked in vitro cytotoxicity as well as a prolongation of survival when administered intraperitoneally to nude mice with intraabdominal ovarian cancer. In addition, the efficacy of monoclonal antibodies linked to radioisotopes will also be evaluated in ovarian cancer patients in the near future.

Our understanding of the biology of ovarian cancer and the molecular pharmacology of antineoplastic drugs in this disease has been greatly facilitated by the development of relevant experimental model systems. Human ovarian cancer cell lines and in vivo models of ovarian cancer have been used to unravel the mechanisms associated with the broad cross-resistance that limits the effectiveness of standard combination chemotherapy. Pharmacologic techniques have already been shown to be capable of reversing drug resistance both in vitro and in vivo and these new approaches will be entering clinical trial in the near future. Biologic agents have also shown marked activity in these model systems of human ovarian cancer and the intraperitoneal administration of LAK plus IL-2 as well as immunotoxins are just two examples of exciting new approaches that have been developed on the basis of observations made in these experimental systems. It is not unreasonable to anticipate that at least some of these experimental therapies will prove to be beneficial and lead to a further improvement in the survival of patients with advanced ovarian cancer.

References

1. Levin L, Hryniuk WM (1986) Dose intensity analysis of chemotherapy of advanced ovarian carcinoma. Proc Am Soc Clin Oncol 5: 112
2. Hamilton TC, Young RC, Ozols RF (1984) Experimental model systems of ovarian cancer:

applications to the design and evaluation of new treatment approaches. Semin Oncol 11: 285–298

3. Ozols RF, Louie KG, Plowman J, Behrens BC, Fine RL, Dykes D, Hamilton TC (1987) Enhanced alkylating agent cytotoxicity in human ovarian cancer in vitro and in tumor bearing nude mice by buthionine sulfoximine depletion of glutathione. Biochem Pharmacol 36: 147–153
4. Behrens BC, Hamilton TC, Grotzinger KR, Whang-Peng J, Batist G, Louie KG, Knutsen T, Mckoy WM, Young RC, Ozols RF (1987) Characterization of a cisplatin-resistant human ovarian cancer cell line and its use in evaluation of cisplatin analogs. Cancer Res 47: 414–418
5. Fojo A, Hamilton TC, Young RC, Ozols RF (1987) Drug resistance in ovarian cancer. Cancer 60: 2075–2080
6. Ozols RF, Cunnion RE, Klecker RW Jr, Hamilton TC, Ostchega Y, Parrillo JE, Young RC (1987) Verapamil and adriamycin in the treatment of drug resistant ovarian cancer patients. J Clin Oncol 5: 641–647
7. Young RC, Myers CE, Ostchega Y (1985) CPR (cyclophosphamide, high dose cisplatin irradiation): an aggressive short term induction regimen for advanced ovarian adenocarcinoma. Proc Am Soc Clin Oncol 4: 119
8. Ozols RF, Ostchega Y, Curt G, Young RC (1986) High dose carboplatin in refractory ovarian cancer patients. J Clin Oncol 5: 197–201
9. Hamilton TC, Ozols RF, Longo DL (1987) Biologic therapy for the treatment of malignant common epithelial tumors of the ovary. Cancer, 60: 2054–2063
10. Ozols RF (1985) Intraperitoneal chemotherapy in the management of ovarian cancer. Semin Oncol [Suppl 4] 12: 7–11

37. Trophoblastic Neoplasia

K.D. Bagshawe

Current Results and Therapeutic Issues

Hydatidiform Mole

Hydatidiform mole (HM) carries at least a 1000-fold greater risk of subsequent malignancy than a normal pregnancy, and about 1 in 12 patients with HM require chemotherapy for subsequent invasive mole (IM) or choriocarcinoma (CC). Malignancy is probably associated only with complete (classical) hydatidiform mole (CHM) whereas partial hydatidiform mole (PHM) probably carries no special risk.

Although the genetic distinction between CHM (which is a complete male allograft except for maternally derived mitochondrial DNA) and PHM (usually a triploid conceptus) has been established in the past decade, their morphological classification is sometimes difficult [1–3]. When in doubt many pathologists quite properly play safe and report the mole simply as HM requiring follow-up studies with human chorionic gonadotropin (HCG).

The traditional follow-up of HM patients for 2 years has proven well-founded, but it can impose a severe penalty one patients, and so the aim is to be able to predict soon after evacuation which moles will progress to become a serious invasion of maternal tissues or true malignancy. There is still no proof that PHM gives rise to choriocarcinoma, although radiological metastases have sometimes precipitated the use of chemotherapy. Choriocarcinoma has occurred in patients who have had PHM, but in no case has causation by other pregnancies been excluded.

It is common practice in the United States of America to institute chemotherapy if HCG levels have not fallen to undetectable levels 6–8 weeks after evacuation of HM, and on this basis 20%–36% of patients are treated with chemotherapy [4]. In Europe a more conservative policy of observation is generally followed. Only 7.75% of 5124 patients registered for follow-up under a national scheme in the United Kingdom required chemotherapy [5]. This study also showed that 42% of patients had negative HCG values (<5 IU/l) by 56 days postevacuation, and none of these required chemotherapy. Of those whose HCG values first became negative after 56 days, just over 1% required chemotherapy. If HCG tests were persistently negative for 6 months, there was a 1:286 chance of recrudescence between 6 and 24 months after the mole; a risk which patients keen to start a new pregnancy have to consider. The risk of a second HM was 1:76 for subsequent pregnancies; the risk of a third HM in those at risk was 1:6.5 pregnancies. Of eight patients who had three HM, five had not had a successful pregnancy.

Therapeutic intervention after HM is required for persisting, high HCG levels (>20 000 IU/l at 4–8 weeks post-HM) because of the associated risk of uterine perforation, for persisting blood loss, for rising HCG values, or for any elevated HCG value 4–6 months postevacuation. Evidence of metastatic disease also necessitates chemotherapy unless accompanied by falling HCG values.

Invasive Mole and Choriocarcinoma

Gestational trophoblastic tumors are perhaps the only neoplasms in which it is reasonable to undertake treatment without securing a histological diagnosis. In post-HM patients the lesion may be either invasive mole or choriocarcinoma, and whilst it may not be necessary to determine the histological diagnosis, the use of prognostic factors indicates that even in this group some tumors have a potential for drug resistance and require multidrug therapy.

After pregnancies without HM, persisting evidence of trophoblastic proliferation usually constitutes choriocarcinoma, but it is important to be aware of placental site tumor [6, 7]. This rare tumor arises from the placental bed trophoblast, and currettings shows a predominance of cytotrophoblast and little syncytium. It may also be suspected when HCG values are disproportionately low in comparison with tumor volume. HCG values with advanced disease are rarely more than 3000 IU/l and often much lower. Unlike choriocarcinoma it may be accompanied by nephrotic syndrome, and it is relatively refractory to chemotherapy, although in a recent case at this center remission was achieved with the EMA/CO protocol (see later in this section). In the absence of metastatic disease and possibly even with limited metastases, prompt hysterectomy should be undertaken. In making a diagnosis, it is also necessary to consider ovarian germ cell tumor and metaplastic change in gastric and other carcinomas in the differential diagnosis of gestational trophoblastic neoplasms.

The treatment of gestational trophoblastic tumors is primarily chemotherapy. Radiation therapy has only a limited role in the management of these tumours but may have a role in treating resistant disease. A prognostic scoring system [8, 9] provides a more reliable basis for selecting chemotherapeutic protocols than conventional staging (Table 1). The prognosis in the context of trophoblastic neoplasms depends on an assessment of the propensity of the tumor to become drug resistant. The higher the score, the greater the risk. In all cases it is advisable in the initial stages to aim to identify brain metastases by magnetic resonance imaging (MRI) or computerized tomography (CT) and by measuring the serum CSF:HCG ratio, which is reduced below 60:1 in most patients with CNS metastases. Such patients are potential candidates for neurosurgery (see below).

The protocol most widely used for low-risk trophoblastic tumors (WHO score

Table 1. Scoring system based on prognostic factors

Prognostic factors[a]	Score			
	0	1	2	6[b]
Age (years)	<39	>39		
Antecedent pregnancy	HM	Abortion	Term	
Interval[c] (months)	4	4–6	7–12	12
HCG (IU/l)	10^3	10^3–10^4	10^4–10^5	10^5
ABO groups (female × male)		O × A	B ×–[d]	
		A × O	AB ×–	
Largest tumor, including uterine tumor		3–5 cm	5 cm	
Site of metastases		Spleen, kidney	GI tract, liver	Brain
No. of metastases identified		1–4	4–8	8
Prior chemotherapy			Single drug	Two or more drugs

[a] The total score for a patient is obtained by adding the individual scores for each prognostic factor
[b] The weighting has been increased to 6 from 4 in the original WHO scoring table
[c] Interval between end of antecedent pregnancy and start of chemotherapy
[d] Paternal ABO group has not been shown to have an effect if the maternal group is B or AB

<6) consists of intramuscular methotrexate (MTX) on alternate days × 4 with folinic acid (FA) given 30 h after each MTX dose. Alopecia with this regimen is negligible, mucositis and depression of hemopoiesis are uncommon, but pleuritic pain may occur. Courses are given on alternate weeks until HCG has been undetectable for 6 weeks. At Charing Cross Hospital, London, between 1962 and 1986, 618 cases have been treated with this regimen, and over 70% of low-risk patients have required no other therapy. "Low-risk" patients who do not go into complete remission with the MTX/FA regimen and patients with abnormal liver function may achieve remission with actinomycin D. However, in the nonremitters, unless a response to actinomycin D is seen after two courses, the "high-risk"regimen should be introduced promptly. The only deaths in this series of low-risk patients have been one each from serum hepatitis and intercurrent lymphoma.

Patients with a WHO prognostic score >6 require multidrug therapy from the outset. The introduction of etoposide into treatment protocols [10] has been the main advance in the past decade. Several high-risk regimens have been evaluated in the past 20 years but the EMA/CO (etoposide, methotrexate, actinomycin D on days 1 and 2, 15 and 16, etc., cyclophosphamide and Oncovin on days 8 and 21, etc.) delivers a high dosage with acceptable toxicity and limited hospitalization (Table 2). Any low-risk patients with pulmonary metastases and all high-risk patients should receive intrathecal MTX (10 mg) every 2 weeks for CNS prophylaxis; this is an important component of therapy [11]. Patients with brain metastasis at presentation require careful consideration for neurosurgery or higher doses (1000 mg/m²) of MTX. However, high CNS concentrations of

516

Table 2. EMA/CO Protocol for High Risk Choriocarcinomas

Course 1 EMA	
Day 1	Actinomycin D—0.5 mg IV stat.
	Etoposide 100 mg/m² IV in 250 ml 0.9% NaCl over 30 min
	Methotrexate 100 mg/m² IV stat.
	Methotrexate 200 mg/m² IV 12-h infusion in 1L 0.9% NaCl
Day 2	Actinomycin D—0.5 mg IV stat.
	Etoposide 100 mg/m² in 250 ml NaCl over 30 min
	Folinic acid 15 mg/m² po IM b.d. for four doses starting 24 h after start of MTX
	5-day drug free interval to course 2
Course 2 CO	
Day 1	Vincristine (oncovin) 1.0 mg/m² IV stat. (max 2.0 mg)
	Cyclophosphamide 600 mg/m² IV infusion over 20 min
	6-day drug free interval and, if no mucositis:
Course 1	—As above
	5-day interval and, if no mucositis:
Course 2	—As above

NB Patients normally start each course on the same day of the week each time.

Intervals between courses should not be increased unless *WBC* < 1.5 × 10³/L and platelets are <75 × 10³/L or mucositis develops. If mucositis develops, delay the next course until it has healed.

Continue alternating courses 1 and 2 until the patient completes treatment. Usually complete remission is achieved after 12 weeks, or there is evidence of drug resistance.

Intrathecal methotrexate: See text and ref. 11.

MTX with the first course of therapy may precipitate hemorrhage and should be reserved for the second and subsequent courses of therapy. Surgical removal offers the best chance of eradicating brain metastases which occur during the course of chemotherapy.

Current Approaches Under Study

Failure to achieve complete remission with EMA/CO occurred in about 25% of high-risk patients with a WHO score >8 at this center. (Patients with scores between 6 and 8 were treated with a "middle-risk regimen" which can now be replaced by the high-risk EMA/CO protocol.) Prior chemotherapy increased the risk of failure to remit. *Cis*-platinum as a first agent has disadvantages but, if resistance to EMA/CO occurs, a regimen containing *cis*-platinum or the newer platinum analogue, carboplatin, in combination, sometimes achieves remission. The POMB regimen (*cis*-platinum, Oncovin, methotrexate, and bleomycin) is one such protocol currently being studied [10]. At the same time ultrasound, CT, MRI, and radioimmunolocalization with anti-HCG antibodies are undertaken with a view to identifying sites of persistent disease which can be removed surgically. Collectively, these measures have ensured that >90% of patients with

WHO scores >8 have achieved sustained remission. In the series of >1200 patients treated at this center since 1957 for low- and high-risk tumors, the sustained remission rate overall was 88%, and since 1980 has been 96%.

Future Approaches

One consequence of the high level of success with chemotherapy, in some cases combined with surgery, is the ethical dilemma of introducing new treatment methods in patients other than those with advanced, drug-resistant cancer. Attempts to treat drug-resistant choriocarcinoma by active immunization with non-specific agents such as BCG (bacille Calmette-Guérin), "specific" antigens such as paternal leukocytes, and skin grafts (undertaken between 1955 and 1970) assumed the expression of paternally derived MHC (major histocompatability complex) antigens on the trophoblast. It has long been recognized that mammalian evolution has depended on nonrejection of the trophoblast. It is now generally accepted that choriocarcinoma, like the villous trophoblast from which it arises, does not express class II MHC antigens. Studies of patients, consorts, and offspring antecedent to choriocarcinoma, have shown no major deviation in HLA patterns [12]. But marked effects associated with the ABO system have been described even though ABO substances have not been detected in trophoblast [8].

Interferons were not effective in three drug-resistant patients in the UK series: studies with interleukin-2 have not yet been reported. Expression of c-*myc* oncogene in choriocarcinoma, CHM, and third trimester placenta, but not term placenta, have been described. Similarly, c-*fos* expression has been found in choriocarcinoma cell lines and *sis* proto-oncogene expression in term placenta [13]. Radioimmunolocalization has so far been directed against HCG and placental alkaline phosphatase targets. Localization with anti-HCG has detected tumors (<0.5 cm) in some parts of the body. Therapeutic approaches with radiolabeled monoclonal antibodies and antibodies coupled to metabolite-depleting enzymes have begun [14].

References

1. Szulman AE, Surti U (1978) The syndromes of hydatidiform mole. I. Cytogenetic and morphological correlations. Am J Obstet Gynecol 131: 665
2. Szulman AE, Surti U (1978) The syndromes of hydatidiform mole. II. Morphological evolution of the complete and partial mole. Am J Obstet Gynecol 132: 20
3. Lawler SD (1982) Genetic studies in hydatidiform mole. In: Patillo RA, Hussa RO (eds) Human trophoblastic neoplasms. Plenum Press, New York, pp 147–161
4. Lurain JR, Brewer JI, Torok EE (1983) Natural history of hydatidiform mole after primary evacuation. Am J Obstet Gynecol 145: 591

5. Bagshawe KD, Dent J, Webb J (1986) Hydatidiform mole in England and Wales 1973–1983. Lancet 2: 673
6. Scully RE, Young RH (1981) Trophoblastic pseudotumor: a reappraisal. Am J Surg Pathol 5: 76
7. Eckstein RP, Paradinas FJ, Bagshawe KD (1982) Placental site trophoblastic tumor (trophoblastic pseudotumor): a study of four cases requiring hysterectomy including one fatal case. Histopathology 6: 211
8. Bagshawe KD (1976) Risk and prognostic factors in trophoblastic neoplasia. Cancer 38: 1373
9. WHO (1983) Gestational trophoblastic diseases. WHO Tech rep Ser 692
10. Newlands ES, Begent RHJ, Rustin GJS, Parker D, Bagshawe KD (1983) Further advances in the management of malignant teratomas of the testis and other sites. Lancet 1: 948
11. Athanassiou A, Begent RHJ, Newlands ES, Parker D, Rustin GJS, Bagshawe KD (1983) Central nervous system metastases in choriocarcinoma: twenty-three years experience at Charing Cross Hospital. Cancer 52: 1728
12. Lawler SD (1978) HLA and trophoblastic tumors. Br Med Bull 34: 305
13. Kohorn EI, Sarkar S, Kacinski BM, Blakemore KJ, Merino MJ, Carter D (1985) Oncogene expression in trophoblastic disease. In: Trophoblastic disease. Ichinoe (ed) Igaku-Shoin, Tokyo, pp 35–38
14. Searle F, Bier C, Buckley RG, Newman S, Pedley RB, Bagshawe KD, Melton RG, Alwan SM, Sherwood RF (1986) The potential of carboxypeptidase G2-antibody conjugates as antitumor agents. I. Preparation of anti-human chorionic gonadotrophin-carboxypeptidase G2 and cytotoxicity of the conjugate against JAR choriocarcinoma cells in vitro. Br J Cancer 53: 377

38.   Malignant Adrenal Tumors

S.D. Averbuch

Current Results and Therapeutic Issues

Malignant adrenal tumors are rare neoplasms of glandular tissue that have not been well studied largely due to their low incidence in the population. In the United States of America, adrenocortical carcinomas occur with an estimated annual frequency of two cases per million, while malignancies of chromaffin tissue, which constitutes the adrenal medulla and also exists at extra-adrenal paraganglionic sites, occur one-third to one-half as often [1]. These tumors are of particular interest because they are often functional. Adrenocortical carcinomas may cause hypercorticalism, hyperaldosteronism, adrenogenital syndrome, virilization, feminization, or precocious puberty; and malignant chromaffin tumors (malignant pheochromocytoma) may cause severe hypercortisolism as a manifestation of hypersecretory hormonal function. Treatment results and survival statistics in adrenal tumors are complicated by the lack of specific morphological characteristics or histologic criteria which correlate with malignant behavior. With the exception of anaplastic adrenocortical carcinoma, these tumors often appear extremely well differentiated (accounting for their hormone-producing function) and only in the presence of recurrence, local invasion, or dissemination can the malignancy of the tumor be confirmed. The overall 5-year survival rate for patients following resection of malignant tumors confined to the adrenal gland is approximately 40%. However, the presence of metastatic disease in the majority of patients means a much poorer prognosis with a life expectency of less than 3 years, although some individuals may survive long-term [1].

At present, complete surgical resection is the only curative modality for adrenal malignancies confined to the gland. For locally invasive tumors or for extra-adrenal pheochromocytomas, radical surgical excision may also result in long-term disease-free survival. In the case of more extensive, local disease, or in the presence of disseminated, resectable metastases, complete surgical removal of all disease is usually recommended. Whether this approach offers a survival benefit for these patients is not known; however, effective palliation is often achieved. There is no evidence supporting the use of adjuvant radiation or chemotherapy following complete surgical removal, nor are there any data showing that surgical debulking will favorably influence outcome when applied alone or prior to another therapeutic modality.

There is little information on the use of conventional radiation therapy for the treatment of localized, unresectable disease or for palliation of symptoms caused by metastatic lesions. Generally, this modality is reserved for palliation in special situations such as painful bony metastases or for extradural spinal cord compression.

Pharmacological approaches have proven useful in the management of adrenal tumors. The symptoms and morbidity due to excessive production of adrenal hormones may be effectively treated by specific antihormonal therapies. For patients with functional adrenocortical tumors, inhibitors of steroid biosynthesis, such as orthoparaprime DDD (mitotane), aminoglutethimide, or metyrapone can effectively palliate symptoms due to cortisol overproduction. Similarly, the hypertension and symptoms due to excessive production of catecholamines in patients with pheochromocytoma may be controlled with α-adrenergic (phenoxybenzamine) and β-adrenergic (propranolol) blockade or with the use of an inhibitor of catecholamine synthesis (methyltyrosine).

Mitotane also has proven efficacy as a drug capable of causing tumor regression in patients with adrenocortical carcinoma. When titrated up to a dose of 8–10 g per day, mitotane resulted in objective tumor responses of 34% and 61%, respectively, in two independent studies of over 100 patients each [2, 3]. The mean duration of response was 10 months, and durable complete responses were observed. However disease response was poorly defined in these studies, and the tumor response to this agent may prove to be lower [4, 5]. Furthermore, the effect of mitotane on survival has not been evaluated. Mitotane also has antisteroidal properties, decreasing steroid production, and although multiple gastrointestinal and neurologic toxicities limit its use, the drug may provide useful palliation for patients with functional tumors. There is no proven, effective, specific drug therapy for the treatment of malignant pheochromocytoma.

In addition to the concepts already discussed in this volume, there are several issues that need to be addressed regarding future therapeutic approaches designed to alter the morbidity and mortality resulting from malignant adrenal neoplasms. The first major problem is the lack of specific histological criteria for determining the malignant potential of resectable, well-differentiated disease. Thus, investigations are needed firstly to determine whether there are any biochemical, immunohistologic, or molecular criteria for malignancy that would identify those patients at risk for recurrent or metastatic disease. Secondly, there is a need to develop more specific and less toxic treatments for the palliation of symptoms and morbidity from hormonal excess. Thirdly, the role of conventional cytotoxic therapy or experimental biological agents in adrenal tumors needs to be determined. Finally, because of their highly specialized function, adrenal tumors may serve as particularly good models for the development of novel, specific, targeted antitumor therapy.

Current Approaches Under Study

Recently advances have been made in defining the role of conventional cytotoxic therapy for the treatment of adrenal tumors. Several reports suggest that combination regimens containing cisplatin, etoposide, doxorubicin, or alkylating agents may have an effect against adrenocortical carcinoma [4–6]. Unfortunately, in these studies, patient numbers were small and responses were of brief duration. Results from ongoing multi-institutional trials conducted by the Southwest Oncology and Eastern Cooperative Oncology Groups are expected to provide more definitive guidelines regarding the use of cytotoxic therapy for this disease.

As with adrenocortical tumors, there is little data on the use of chemotherapy in patients with malignant pheochromocytoma, with most results being anecdotal. In a trial recently completed at the National Cancer Institute, USA, 14 patients with advanced malignant pheochromocytoma were treated with a combination of cyclophosphamide, vincristine, and dacarbazine [7]. There were two complete responses, six partial responses, and 79% of patients had a significant biochemical response with the median duration of response in excess of 22 months. Thus, it appears that this combination regimen is effective for the treatment of malignant pheochromocytoma.

Future Approaches

The specialized tissue of the adrenal gland provides a unique target for novel therapeutic approaches. For example, ketoconazole is a new systemic antifungal agent that is capable of blocking adrenal steroid synthesis and therefore may be useful for the palliation of functional adrenocortical tumors [8]. Suramin is an antiparasitic drug with specific adrenocortical toxicity that is currently being evaluated in a clinical trial in patients with unresectable adrenocortical carcinoma [9]. ^{131}I-*Meta*-iodobenzylguanidine is a guanethidine derivative which is selectively taken up by chromaffin tissue; in those patients with adequate radioisotope uptake into tumors, this agent may provide targeted radiotherapy against malignant pheochromocytoma [10]. Further investigations of these approaches as well as studies addressing the issues delineated above are clearly needed to improve the results in the management of malignant adrenal tumors.

References

1. Brennan MF, MacDonald JS (1985) Cancer of the endocrine system. In: DeVita VT, Hellman S, Rosenberg SA (eds) Cancer: principles and practice of oncology, 2nd edn. Lippincott, Philadelphia, p 1179
2. Hutter AM, Kayhoe DE (1966) Adrenal cortical carcinoma: results of treatment with o,p′-DDD in 138 patients. Am J Med 41: 581
3. Lubitz JA, Freeman L, Okun R (1973) Mitotane in inoperable adrenal cortical carcinoma. JAMA 223: 1109

4. Haq MM, Legha SS, Samaan NA, Bodey GP, Burgess MA (1980) Cytotoxic chemotherapy in adrenal cortical carcinoma. Cancer Treat Rep 64: 909
5. Van Slooten H, van Oosterom AT (1983) CAP (cyclophosphamide, doxorubicin, and cisplatin) regimen in adrenal cortical carcinoma. Cancer Treat Rep 67: 377
6. Johnson DH, Greco FA (1986) Treatment of metastatic adrenal cortical carcinoma with cisplatin and etoposide (VP-16). Cancer 58: 2198
7. Averbuch S, Steakley C, Young R, Gelmann E, Goldstein D, Stull R, Keiser H (1988) Malignant pheochromocytoma: effective treatment with a combination of cyclophosphamide, vincristine, and dacarbazine. Ann Intern Med 109: 267
8. Contreras P, Altieri E, Liberman C, Gac A, Rojas A, Ibarra A, Ravanal M, Seron-Ferre M (1985) Adrenal rest tumor of the liver causing Cushing's syndrome: treatment with ketoconazole preceding an apparent surgical cure. J Clin Endocrinol Metab 60: 21
9. Stein CA, La Rocca RV, Thomas R, McAtee N, Myers CE (1988) Suramin: an active agent in adrenocortical carcinoma (Abstr). Pro Am Soc Clin Oncol 7: 91
10. McEwan AJ, Shapiro B, Sisson JC, Beierwaltes WH, Ackery DM (1985) Radio-iodobenzylguanidine for the scintigraphic location and therapy of adrenergic tumors. Sem in Nucl Med 15: 132

39.   Neuroendocrine Tumors

J.S. Macdonald

Current Results and Therapeutic Issues

The treatment of neuroendocrine tumors represents an unusual challenge to the oncologist [1]. In patients with malignant islet cell tumors or carcinoid tumors symptoms may appear for two reasons. As in any patient with a malignant neoplasm, such individuals may be symptomatic due to tumor bulk. Both carcinoid tumors and islet cell tumors frequently metastasize to the liver, for instance, and patients may have painful malignant hepatomegaly. However, in contrast to many other malignant neoplasms, neuroendocrine tumors [1] may also produce symptoms due to the biologically active products (usually peptides) released by these tumors. For example, islet cell tumors producing insulin result in hypoglycemia; gastrin-producing tumors cause the Zollinger-Ellison syndrome and gastric ulceration; somatostatin-producing tumors may result in a syndrome of diabetes, steatorrhea, and cholelithiasis. Glucagon production (glucagonoma) causes a syndrome of carbohydrate intolerance and severe dermatitis (necrolytic migratory erythemia); tumors producing vasoactive intestinal peptide (VIP) may result in a clinical picture characterized by watery diarrhea, hypokalemia, and achlorhydria (WDHA syndrome). Likewise, carcinoid tumors, which are most common in the small bowel and frequently metastasize to the liver but may be seen in many sites throughout the body, may cause a syndrome characterized by diarrhea and flushing due to the production of a wide variety of biologically active compounds. It has been found that other disorders, including cardiac valvular disease, endomyocardial fibrosis, and retroperitoneal fibrosis, may also be present with carcinoid tumors. Mediators [2] including histamine, bradykinin, serotonin, and prostaglandins may be products of carcinoid tumors. The carcinoid syndrome is rarely seen in patients who do not have liver metastases with the exception of patients with bronchial carcinoid, primary gastric carcinoid, and carcinoids of the ovary which drain into the systemic venous circulation and not into the portal circulation [1]. In patients who have liver metastases from carcinoid tumors, the elevation of 5-hydroxyindoleacetic acid (5-HIAA) in the urine is characteristic. The challenge to the clinical oncologist lies in the management both of the hormonally mediated syndromes seen with carcinoid tumors and islet cell tumors and of symptoms that are due to tumor mass.

The most important fact in the treatment of patients with either islet cell tumors or primary carcinoids which have not metastasized is that surgical resection of the tumor is curative [1]. However, in many instances, particularly when a syndrome due to biologically active products of the tumor has already appeared, islet cell tumors or carcinoid tumors will have metastasized, and complete surgical resection is not possible. In this situation the patient may be treated with antihormonal therapy or with antitumor therapy. There are a variety of pharmacologic treatments that may be of value aimed at inhibiting the activity of mediators produced by neuroendocrine tumors. These include H_2 histamine receptor blockers (cimetidine and ranitidine) for patients with the Zollinger-Ellison syndrome [3], diazoxide for patients with insulinomas [3], and various drugs including antiserotonin agents, antihistamines, and corticosteroids for patients with carcinoid syndrome. In patients with symptomatic metastatic neuroendocrine tumors not receiving significant palliation from pharmacological therapy, cytoreductive surgery may produce results. Carcinoid tumors and islet cell tumors usually grow slowly: rapidly developing and rapidly disseminating metastatic disease is unusual. Thus, if a patient has a mass of hormonally active tumor, partial surgical resection of the tumor may be carried out. Cytoreductive surgery decreases the mass of tumor producing biologically active mediators and frequently leads to many months of symptomatic [1, 2] palliation for the patient. It also should be noted that hepatic artery ligation for metastatic liver disease may be palliative, resulting in tumor cytoreduction by causing ischemic necrosis of hepatic metastases. In the Mayo Clinic 18 of 25 patients showed significant remission of symptomatic metastatic carcinoid tumors after this procedure [2].

Cytotoxic chemotherapy also has a role in the management of patients with neuroendocrine tumors. In both the therapy of carcinoid tumors and islet cell tumors streptozotocin has been a drug of major interst [4]. This naturally occurring methyl-nitrosourea produces an approximately 30%–40% response rate in metastatic islet cell carcinoma. Combinations of streptozotocin and 5FU (5-fluorouracil) have been shown to be beneficial, producing response rates as high as 60% in patients with islet cell carcinoma [5]. The Eastern Cooperative Oncology Group has performed a study in which 5FU plus streptozotocin is compared with both doxorubicin plus streptozotocin and to chlorozotocin alone. The results show that the response rate for streptozotocin plus doxorubicin is over 60% (Haller 1987, personal communication).

With carcinoid tumors cytoxic chemotherapy may also be used. The chemotherapy used with carcinoid tumors is similar to that with islet cell carcinomas. Single agents including 5FU and DTIC (dacarbazine) have effect in 15%–25% of patients [2]. The Eastern Cooperative Oncology Group has compared 5FU plus streptozotocin with cyclophosphamide plus streptozotocin, demonstrating that 33% of the patients treated with 5FU plus streptozotocin responded against 27% receiving the cyclophosphamide combination [6].

Current Approaches Under Study

Recently in the management of neuroendocrine tumors, there has been interest in the use of biological agents for therapy. New information suggests that a somatostatin analog may be useful in the treatment of islet cell tumors [7] and carcinoid tumors [8]. The hormone somatostatin is able to decrease hormone release from islet cell tumors and carcinoid tumors. However, the plasma half-life of natural somatostatin is very short so that, aside from approaches using continuous infusion, somatostatin therapy for neuroendocrine tumors would be impractical. Meanwhile, a long-acting somatostatin analog (SMS-201-995) which allows for stable somatostatin plasma levels with intermittent dosing has been evaluated in patients with islet cell [7] and carcinoid malignancies [8]. In patients with the watery diarrhea, hypokalemia, and achlorhydria syndrome—and with the Zollinger-Ellison syndrome—the use of this somatostatin analog has produced significant palliation of symptoms [7]. These results were due to a decrease in the production of biologically active materials by the tumors in the treated patients. There is also some evidence that the somatostatin analog may produce partial objective tumor regression in some patients with islet cell tumors [7].

The somatostatin analog has also been researched as a therapy for carcinoid tumors. One of the risks of treating patients with carcinoid tumors is that surgical intervention and/or chemotherapy may cause a massive release of biologically active mediators from the tumor resulting in a "carcinoid crisis"; in these patients there is intense flushing and hypotension. The hypotension may be refractory to therapy and the carcinoid crisis may be fatal [2]. It was noted that the somatostatin analog could promptly reverse a carcinoid crisis by the prevention of release of mediators from the carcinoid tumor. Investigators at the Mayo Clinic [8] have reported complete regression of symptoms of the carcinoid syndrome in 22 of 25 patients, who were refractory to other therapeutic measures, when treated with the somatostatin analog. In 18 of 25 cases there was a greater than 50% reduction of urinary secretion of the marker for the carcinoid syndrome (5-HIAA). A small number of patients (10%) treated with the somatostatin analog evidenced objective regression of their tumor. Thus, the role of the long-acting somatostatin analog in preventing or reversing the carcinoid crisis has already been established, and the roles that this or similar agents may have in other aspects of the treatment of patients with metastatic carcinoid is being actively investigated.

Another biological which is important in the management of islet cell tumors and carcinoid tumors is α-interferon [9]. Data suggest that α-interferon not only causes amelioration of symptoms in patients with carcinoid syndrome by decreasing the release of biologically active materials but also has a positive effect on syndromes produced by islet cell tumors via the same mechanism. Interferon may also cause objective tumor regression in neuroendocrine tumors, but this antitumor activity is not yet well defined.

Finally a new drug undergoing a phase I trial, Pibenzimol [10], is an agent which has the side effect of inducing insulin dependent diabetes. This drug causes islet cell destruction and may be of significant interest in the future for the treatment of some neuroendocrine tumors.

Future Approaches

The neuroendocrine tumors form an area of oncologic study in which major advances may be expected to occur in the future. We now have good evidence that diverse approaches including cytoreductive surgery, hepatic artery ligation and/or embolization, treatment with cytotoxic chemotherapy, and the use of biological agents including the somatostatin analog and α-interferon may all prove helpful. This important evidence now enables exploration of how these various modalities of treatment may be effectively interfaced for the most successful treatment of patients with neuroendocrine tumors.

References

1. Brennan MF, Macdonald JS (1985) Cancer of the endocrine system In: Devita VT, Hellman S, Rosenberg SA (eds) Cancer: principles and practice of oncology. Lippincott, Philadelphia, pp 1179–1241
2. Moertel CG (1983) Treatment of carcinoid tumors and the malignant carcinoid syndrome. J Clin Oncol 1:727–740
3. Haller DG (1985) Chemotherapeutic management of endocrine-producing tumors of the gastrointestinal tract. In: Cohen S, Soloway RD (eds) Hormone-producing tumors of the gastrointestinal tract. Livingston, New York, pp 129–137
4. Broder LE, Carter SK (1973) Results of therapy with streptozotocin in 52 patients. Ann Intern Med 79:108–118
5. Moertel CG, Hanley JA, Johnson LA (1980) Streptozotocin alone compared with streptozotocin plus fluorouracil in the treatment of advanced islet cell carcinoma. N Engl J Med 303:1189
6. Moertel CG, Hanley JA (1979) Combination chemotherapy trials in metastatic carcinoid tumor and the malignant carcinoid syndrome. Clin Cancer Trials 2:327–334
7. Kvols L, Schutt A, Buck M (1986) Treatment of metastatic islet cell carcinomas with a long acting somatostatin analogue. Proc Am Soc Clin Oncol 5:85
8. Kvols LK, Moertel CG, O'Connell MJ et al. (1986) Treatment of the malignant carcinoid syndrome: evaluation of a long-acting somatostatin analogue. N Engl J Med 315:663–704
9. Oberg K, Eriksson B, Norheim I (1987) Interferon treatment of neuroendocrine gut tumors. Proc ASCO 6:80
10. Kraut EH, O'Dorisio TM, Page JG et al. (1986) Evaluation of the pancreatic toxicity of pibenzimol (NSC322921) in dogs. Proc Am Assoc Canc Res 27:420

40. Soft Tissue Sarcomas in Adults

K.H. Antman

Current Results and Therapeutic Issues

Adults with newly diagnosed soft tissue sarcomas generally seek medical attention for an enlarging mass. Evaluation reveals clinical evidence of metastases in only 5%–15%.

Standard Treatment of the Primary Lesion

A radical surgical resection or a conservative resection preceded or followed by radiotherapy is acceptable. Optimal local control and aesthetic results are usually obtained from conservative resection with clean margins and 6600 Gy radiotherapy when feasible. A shelling out procedure routinely leaves residual microscopic tumor resulting in a higher local recurrence rate. Local recurrence rates for extremity and superficial trunk lesions in centers specializing in the treatment of sarcomas range between 2% and 10%, but in one center which did not utilize radiotherapy, 30% of patients developed local recurrence [1].

Intra-abdominal and retroperitoneal sarcomas tend to be large at diagnosis and to abut or involve vital organs. They are difficult to resect with clean margins, and thus local recurrence rates tend to be high (Table 1).

Prognosis

Despite excellent local control 20% of low-grade tumors and 40%–60% of high-grade lesions eventually metastasize generally between 6 months and 2 years after initial treatment for high-grade lesions. Low-grade lesions may recur considerably later. Doxorubicin-containing regimens result in objective response rates of 25%–55% with median remission durations of 5–8 months. Patients with extremity, trunk, and retroperitoneal primaries generally die of respiratory failure from pulmonary metastases. Gynecological and gastrointestinal sarcomas have a higher incidence of intra-abdominal recurrence and liver metastases.

Table 1. Randomized trials of adjuvant chemotherapy in soft tissue sarcomas [modified from 11]

Author (Ref)	Institution	Drugs	Median F/U (mos)[a]	Observation				Chemotherapy			
				n	%LC	%DFS	%S	n	%LC	%DFS	%S
Extremity Sarcomas											
Benjamin et al. [7], Lindberg et al. [16]	MDA	CAV/Ad	120	20	100	35	36	27	93	54	65
Edmonson [1]	MAYO	VAD/VAdD	64	24	75	67	83	24	67	88	63
Rosenberg et al. [8]	NCI	CAM	60	28	93	54	64	37	100	73	84
Bramwell et al. [12]	EORTC	CVAD	28	85	90	65	81	82	90	65	81
Antman et al. [10]	DFCI/MGH	A	46	16	94	81	81	10	100	90	90
Antman et al. [10]	ECOG	A	60	7	100	71	71	11	100	72	64
Gherlinzoni et al. [6]	RIZZOLI	A	28	35	91	54	NA	24	96	79	NA
Eilber et al. [15]	UCLA	A	28	62	90	52	70	57	90	56	80
Alvegard [14]	SCAND	A	22	71	91	55	44	68	91	52	40
Antman et al. [11]	ISTSS	A	24	17	NA	50	62	24	NA	77	72
Nonextremity Lesions											
Edmonson [1]	MAYO	VAD/VAdD	64	7	NA	43	57	6	NA	17	NA
Glenn et al. [9]	NCI	CAM	60	14	NA	49	58	17	NA	77	68
Bramwell et al. [12]	EORTC	CVAD	28	44	74	36	76	36	74	NA	76
Antman et al. [10]	DFCI/MGH	A	46+	9	NA	56	56	10	NA	60	60
Antman et al. [10]	ECOG	A	59+	6	NA	50	33	6	NA	67	50
Alvegard [14]	SCAND	A	22	11	NA	NA	NA	13	NA	NA	NA
Antman et al. [11]	ISTSS	A	24	23	NA	74	91	14	NA	65	81
Omura et al. [13]	GOG	A	24+	81	NA	47	42	75	NA	59	45

MDA, MD Anderson Cancer Institute, University of Texas; MAYO, Mayo Clinic; NCI, National Cancer Institute; EORTC, European Organization for the Research and Treatment of Cancer; DFCI/MGH, Dana-Farber Cancer Institute/Massachusetts General Hospital; ECOG, Eastern Cooperative Oncology Group; SCAND, Scandinavian Sarcoma Group; ISTSS, Intergroup Soft Tissue Sarcoma Study (South West Oncology Group (SWOG), ECOG, CALGB); GOG, Gynecology Oncology Group; UCLA, University of California, Los Angeles; Rizzoli, Instituto Ortopedico Rizzoli, Bologna Italy. A, doxorubicin; Ad, actinomycin D; C, cyclophosphamide; D, dacarbazine; V, vincristine; M, methotrexate; %LC, % of patients with local control; %DFS, % of patients disease free; %S, % of patients alive at time of median follow-up.
[a] F/U (mos), follow up in months.

529

Table 2. Randomized chemotherapy trials in measurable soft-tissue sarcomas in adults [modified from 11]

Author	Group	Regimen	n	CR	PR	RR%
Omura	GOG [2]	A	80	5	8	16
		AD	66	7	9	24
Borden	ECOG [3]	A	93	6	12	19
		AD	95	4	25	30
Schoenfeld	ECOG [4]	A	66	4	14	27
		ACV	70	3	10	19
Baker	SWOG[a]	AD	79	14	18	32
		ADC	95	13	22	35

A, doxorubicin; C, cyclophosphamide; D, DTIC, dacarbazine; V, vincristine; RR%, combined partial and complete response rate; CCR, complete response; PR, partial response.
GOG, Gynecology Oncology Group; ECOG, East Cooperative Oncology Group; SWOG, South West Oncology Group.
[a] Baker, personal communication

Current Approaches Under Study

Single Agent Doxorubicin Versus a Combination

The optimal regimen for metastatic soft tissue sarcoma is currently controversial. Some investigators advocate single agent doxorubicin, others a combination of doxorubicin, dacarbazine (DTIC), and perhaps cyclophosphamide (Table 2). In two studies doxorubicin with and without DTIC was evaluated [2, 3]. In both studies an approximately 10% higher response rate was observed in patients treated with the combination. The difference was significant in one of the studies [3]. Three randomized trials have failed to show a significant advantage for cyclophosphamide (Baker, personal communication) [4, 5]. In one, doxorubicin alone yielded a significantly higher response rate than a combination of doxorubicin, vincristine, and cyclophosphamide, presumably due to a compromised doxorubicin dose in the three-drug regimen [4]. In the second, the response rates were not significantly different between doxorubicin and dacarbazine with and without cyclophosphamide (Baker, pesonal communication). In the third, doxorubicin with and without cyclophosphamide was studied in gynecologic sarcomas. No differences were observed between the study arms [5].

Adjuvant Chemotherapy for Soft Tissue Sarcomas

While primary drug treatment is now established for embryonal rhabdomyosarcoma (and in Ewing's tumor and osteosarcomas), the results of randomized adult soft tissue sarcomas adjuvant trials have been less clear (Table 1). The Mayo Clinic and Italian trials show a significantly improved disease-free survival for the adjuvant treatment group [1, 6]. However, survival in both arms of the first study was similar because of surgical salvage of those patients who suffered recurrence [5]. Given a choice beween 2 years of chemotherapy and a thoracotomy should there be recurrence, many patients would choose the latter as long as survival were not affected [5]. Survival statistics were not given in the second study of doxorubicin versus observation [6].

Although somewhat questionable from a statistical viewpoint, subset analysis in the two studies revealed significant differences favoring chemotherapy treatment for extremity sarcomas. A difference was observed in disease-free survival in the Anderson study [7] and in both disease-free survival and overall survival in the National Cancer Institute, USA, (NCI) study [8]. However, in several of the other reported trials of adjuvant therapy survival trends which were poorer in the chemotherapy group were observed in subgroups with tumors in extremity or central body locations [1, 9, 10].

The Role of Radiotherapy

The efficacy of radiotherapy in the local control of soft tissue sarcomas is being assessed by the NCI in a randomized trial which includes surgery and adjuvant chemotherapy with or without radiotherapy. A role for radiotherapy is suggested by the comparatively high local recurrence rate in extremity sarcomas at the Mayo Clinic where primary radiotherapy was not given. The lowest local recurrence rate was observed in the UCLA study which included preoperative radiotherapy and intra-arterial doxorubicin. University of California, Los Angeles (UCLA) investigators have experimented with various doses of preoperative radiotherapy. Their data suggest that the dose of radiotherapy correlates positively with complications and inversely with local recurrence rates. An optimal dose of radiotherapy would yield a low local recurrence rate with an acceptable comestic result and a low incidence of subsequent fracture and edema.

The timing of primary radiotherapy is currently being debated. Some authors advocate *pre*operative radiotherapy, theorizing that a shrinking tumor may allow a more conservative resection, that tumor cells released inadvertently during surgery may not then be viable, and that a smaller radiation port may be acceptable since the entire surgical field need not be encompassed. Those who advocate *post*operative radiotherapy note that preoperative radiation results in delayed postoperative wound healing. An unradiated tumor speciman is made available for pathologic assessment, enhancing the identification of small high-grade foci in predominantly low-grade tumors, and finally the entire tumor bed can be included in the radiotherapy ports since the surgeon and pathologist can accurately delineate the area at risk. Results compared grade for grade at institutions advocating either approach appear similar.

Future Approaches

Ifosfamide

European and American investigators have confirmed the significant effect of ifosfamide in sarcomas. Almost double the response rate and less toxicity were observed with ifosfamide 5 g/m² when randomized against cyclophosphamide 1.5 g/m² [17]. However, the response rates for both agents were substantially below those reported by other investigators. Response rates of 30%–50% have been reported for combinations of doxorubicin and ifosfamide with and without DTIC. The Southwestern Oncology Group and the Cancer and Leukemia Group B are currently jointly studying doxorubicin and DTIC with or without ifosfamide. If the three-drug regimen results in a high response rate, a trial of the combination in an adjuvant setting compared to observation without further therapy after surgery would be reasonable.

Autologous Bone Marrow Transplantation

An approach which merits evaluation is the use of high-dose chemotherapy with autologous bone marrow transplantation. Preliminary studies have demonstrated responses in resistant sarcomas, suggesting a dose-response relationship. Autotransplantation is currently hampered by the lack of effective drugs.

Acknowledgement. We are grateful to Beth Doucette for careful preparation of this manuscript.

References

1. Edmonson JH (1985) Systemic chemotherapy following complete excision of nonosseus sarcomas: Mayo Clinic experience. Cancer Treat Symp 3: 89–97
2. Omura GA et al. (1983) A randomized study of adriamycin with and without dimethyl trazenoimidazole carboxamide in advanced uterine sarcomas. Cancer 52: 626–632
3. Borden EC, Amato D, Enterline HT, Lerner H, Carbone PP (1983) Randomized comparison of adriamycin regimens for treatment of metastatic soft tissue sarcomas. Proc ASCO 2: 231
4. Schoenfeld D, Rosenbaum C, Horton J et al. (1982) A comparison of adriamycin versus vincristine and adriamycin, and cyclophosphamide for advanced sarcoma. Cancer 50: 2757–2762
5. Muss HB, Bundy B, DiSaia J et al. (1985) Treatment of recurrent or advanced uterine sarcoma, a randomized trial of doxorubicin versus doxorubicin and cyclophosphamide (A phase III trial of the Gynecologic Oncology Group). Cancer 55: 1648–1653
6. Gherlinzoni F, Bacci G, Picci P et al. (1986) A radomized trial for the treatment of high-grade soft-tissue sarcomas of the extremities: preliminary observations. J Clin Oncol 4: 552–558
7. Benjamin RS, Terjanian TO, Tenoglio CV et al. (1987) The importance of combination chemotherapy for adjuvant treatment of high-risk patients with soft-tissue sarcomas of the extremi-

ties. In: Salmon SE (ed) Adjuvant therapy of cancer V. Grune and Stratton, Orlando, pp 735–746

8. Rosenberg SA, Chang AE, Glatstein E (1985) Adjuvant chemotherapy for treatment of extremity soft tissue sarcomas: review of National Cancer Institute experience. Cancer Treat Symp 3: 83–88

9. Glenn J, Sindelar WF, Kinsella T et al. (1985) Results of multimodality therapy of resectable soft-tissue sarcomas of the retroperitoneum. Surgery 973: 316–325

10. Antman K, Amato D, Lerner H et al. (1985) Adjuvant doxorubicin for sarcoma: data from the ECOG and DFCI/MGH studies. Cancer Treat Symp 3: 109–115

11. Antman K, Amato D, Pipepich M et al. (1987) A radomized intergroup soft tissue sarcoma (STS) adjuvant trial of doxorubicin (DOX) versus observation (OBS) In: Salmon SE (ed) Adjuvant therapy of cancer V. Grune and Stratton, Orlando, pp 725–735

12. Bramwell VHC, Rouesse J, Santoro A et al. (1985) European experience of adjuvant chemotherapy for soft tissue sarcoma: preliminary report of randomized trial of cyclophosphamide, vincristine, doxorubicin, and dacarbazine. Cancer Treat Symp 3: 99–107

13. Omura GA, Blessing JA, Major F et al. (1985) A radomized clinical trial of adjuvant adriamycin in uterine sarcomas: a gynecologic oncology group study. J Clin Oncol 3: 1240–1245

14. Alvegard TA (1986) Adjuvant chemotherapy with adriamycin in high-grade malignant soft tissue sarcoma—a scandinavian randomized study. Proc ASCO 5: C–485

15. Eilber FR, Giuliano AE, Huth JR, Morton DL (1986) Adjuvant adriamycin in high-grade extremity soft-tissue sarcoma—a randomized prospective trial. Proc ASCO 5: C–488

16. Lindberg RD, Murphy WK, Benjamin RS et al. (1977) Adjuvant chemotherapy in the treatment of primary soft tissue sarcomas: a preliminary report. In: The University of Texas System Cancer Center MD (ed) Management of bone and soft tissue tumors. Year Book Medical Publishers, Chicago, pp 343–352 (21st annual clinical conference on cancer of the Anderson Hospital and Institute)

17. Bramwell V, Mourisden H, Santoro G et al. (1985) Cyclophosphamide (DP) versus Ifosfamide (IF): a randomized phase II trial in adult soft tissue sarcoma (STS). Preliminary report of EORTC soft tissue and bone sarcomas group. Proc ASCO 4: 413

41. Melanoma

E.T. Creagan

Current Results and Therapeutic Issues

Malignant melanoma is a potentially curable neoplasm in patients with localized disease amenable to complete surgical resection. Patients with disseminated disease, however, have an extremely poor prognosis in view of the limited efficacy of currently available chemotherapeutic agents (see Table 1 for a summary of prognostic factors). The diagnosis and treatment of this neoplasm is enormously important and has profound public health implications. Its rate of increase is exceeded only by lung cancer, and by the year 2000 an estimated 1 in 100 persons will develop malignant melanoma. Moreover, as many as 4.6 million persons in the United States of America may have already acquired preneoplastic nevi.

Microstaging

The thickness of the primary malignant melanoma is a critical parameter of prognosis. Traditionally, lesions have been classified by Clark's anatomical levels of invasion [I (intraepidermal) to V (subcutaneous tissue)]. However, this is not consistently reliable because of variations in skin thickness and the subjective interpretation in assigning anatomical levels. The Breslow method of measuring the tumor from the granular layer of the epidermis to the deepest penetration of the neoplasm is more prognostically accurate. The 8-year survival rates are 93% ± 2% for lesions <1.69 mm vs 38% ± 6% for lesions >3.6 mm in thickness [1].

Surgery

Regional. Correlations between the thickness of the primary lesion and local recurrence and survival permit a reappraisal of surgical margins. In one review among 1151 patients with lesions <1.0 mm thick, two-thirds had margins of ≤2 cm [2]. The local recurrent rate was only 8%, and the median survival was 3 years. There was no substantive survival advantage realized from excising lesions with a radius >3 cm. However, survival does appear to be compromised if lesions ≥2 mm thick were excised with a margin <2 cm.

534

Table 1. Prognostic factors in disseminated malignant melanoma

	Favorable	Unfavorable
Patient		
Sex	Female	Male
Performance score	Ambulatory	Nonambulatory
Treatment		
Prior chemotherapy	None	Any
Resectable metastases	Complete	Incomplete
Metastases		
Site	Soft tissue	Lung
		Liver
		CNS
		Viscera
Number	1	>1
Disease-free interval	>6 months	<6 months

Nodal. The role of elective lymphadenectomy (EL) for patients with apparently localized (stage I) malignant melanoma is exceedingly controversial [3]. Randomized studies by the Mayo Clinic and the World Health Organization (WHO) have not demonstrated any obvious benefit. The trials have been criticized since relatively few patients had histologically involved nodes in the Mayo study and the WHO report did not include adequate microstaging data on all patients. On the other hand, retrospective analyses, which have well-recognized inherent biases, indicate a possible 5%–10% survival advantage emerging at 5–8 years after EL from lesions 1.5–3.99 mm thick. EL does not appear to offer a discernable advantage for patients with lesions <0.76 mm or ≥4.0 mm thick.

Radiation Therapy

An important factor in the radiosensitivity of malignant melanoma is the dose per fraction rather than the total cumulative dose. In one recent review of 618 irradiated lesions, 59% responded to doses >400 cGy vs 33% to doses <400 cGy [10]. Among 77 patients in whom local control was achieved following surgery and radiation therapy (XRT), the 5-year survival rate was 49% vs 3% among the 54 patients in whom local failure occurred (P <0.0001). However, the impact of large dose fractions on brain metastases is less clear. In one report of 59 patients, 26 received a 1-week scheme consisting of twice daily doses of 300–375 cGy, and 33 received a 2-week program of twice daily doses of 188–240 cGy. Those treated with the 1-week program demonstrated a significant symptomatic and survival advantage over patients receiving the 2-week program. It appears that the shorter overall treatment time (1 week vs 2 weeks) was more important than large fraction size. In other words, there was no survival advantage by increasing the dose per fraction from 300 to 375 cGy in the 1-week group, or from 188 to 240 cGy in the 2-week group.

Metastatic Disease

Selected patients may benefit from the resection of disseminated disease [4]. Discriminants of possible survival benefit include total resection of gross disease, single vs multiple lesions, and the site of the disease (soft tissue vs visceral, osseous). The median survival time was 18 months in 69 patients having a complete resection of all gross disease vs 6 months following unsuccessful resection. A somber caveat: unsuccessful resection of metastatic disease usually portends significant morbidity and prolonged hospitalization.

Current Approaches under Study

Chemotherapy

Systemic. The "Standard" single agent therapy for selected patients with disseminated malignant melanoma is arguably imidazole carboxamide (DTIC). Oral lomustine (CCNU) or intravenous 1,3-bis-(2-chloroethyl)-1-(BCNU) nitrosourea are alternative systemic therapies in a noninvestigational setting. Cytotoxic strategies utilizing investigational and conventional agents have not provided consistently meaningful leads [5]. 1-(2-chloroethyl)-3-(2,6-dioxo-3-peperidyl)-1-nitrosourea (PCNU), a nitrosourea derivative which, in preclinical studies, appeared to be an interesting agent, has been disappointing. Among 42 previously untreated patients receiving detorubicin, a daunorubicin analog, there was a 36% response rate and significant cardiac toxicity. A confirmatory trial is awaited with great interest.

Multi-agent regimens utilizing DTIC have typically combined nitrosoureas and vinca alkaloids. Selected trials involving relatively small numbers of patients have reported response rates of approximately 45%, but few patients demonstrate complete recovery. However, the realistic effectiveness of these potentially toxic regimens has not been substantiated by a randomized trial [6]. The combination vinblastine, bleomycin, and cisplatin (VBP) produced a 71% response rate in a preliminary report. Yet, in a randomized comparison of DTIC vs VBP, the response rate was only 14% for each regimen [6]. Regressions have usually been limited to approximately 3–6 months. A variety of single-agent and combination regimens have been administered postoperatively to patients at high risk of disseminated disease following complete resection. To date, few studies have convincingly documented efficacy in enhancing survival or prolonging the interval to recurrence. Based on currently available data, adjuvant chemotherapy outside the context of an investigational trial cannot be routinely recommended.

Autologous Bone Marrow Transplant with Intensive Chemotherapy. A review of 105 patients who received intensive high-dose cytotoxic regimens and autologous bone marrow transplant (ABMT) indicated a composite response rate of 46% [5]. The results in selected patients appear more promising than conventional chemotherapy, but the limited sample size precludes confident comparison with traditional phase II reports. Lethal complications in some patients have been of particular concern.

Regional. Patients having "in transit" metastases between the primary lesion and regional nodes often present a formidable challenge. As an alternative to aggressive local surgery including amputation, isolation perfusion with or without hyperthermia may be a useful modality. In some series, objective regressions have been produced in up to 70% of patients. Although local control may be achieved in a substantial proportion of patients, the impact on survival remains uncertain [7]. Similarly, intralesional therapy, typically with bacille Calmette-Guérin (BCG), may induce transient local control but little overall enhancement of survival.

Biological Response Modifiers: Interferons

Interferon (IFN)-α has clearly induced objective regressions in about 15% of patients receiving an array of doses and schedules [8]. The overall median time to progression of approximately 3–4 months and survival of around 6 months are generally similar to conventional chemotherapy programs [9]. However, a particularly interesting observation is a high proportion of complete responders with especially durable regression following the discontinuation of therapy [9].

The immunomodulatory potential of IFN-γ appears to be greater than IFN-α. Clinical trials with IFN-γ are underway. Combination regimens of the two forms are conceptually appealing since the effects of each molecule appear to be mediated by distinct cell surface receptors.

Future Approaches

Tumor Necrosis Factor

Tumors necrosis factor (TNF) is an antiproliferative protein initially described in the serum of BCG-primed mice who were exposed to endotoxin. Enormous quantities of TNF are now available through recombinant technology. In cell cultures of human malignant melanoma and in nude mouse models, consistent cytotoxic characteristics have been reported. Initial dose-seeking clinical trials indicate the major toxicities to be rigors and fever, but with little hematologic or hepatorenal sequelae. Phase II trials in malignant melanoma will undoubtedly commence within a year.

Interleukin-2 and Lymphokine-Activated Killer Cells

In early trials of adoptive immunotherapy (AI) some objective regressions in patients with advanced malignant melanoma have been documented. However, the initial reports emphasize the need for sophisticated technical and clinical support facilities. Substantial complications may preclude the large scale application of AI for most patients with advanced malignant melanoma. An intriguing modification of AI involves the incubation of tumor-infiltrating lymphocytes (TIL) obtained from neoplasms with interleukin (IL)-2. TIL are 50–100 times more potent on a per cell basis than is the adoptive transfer of lymphokine-activated killer (LAK) cells. These lymphocytes demonstrate antiproliferative characteristics in animal tumor models unaffected by LAK therapy. Clinical trials with TIL are awaited with great interest.

Combination Regimens

TNF plus IFN-γ. In vitro evidence indicates a striking synergism between these molecules which may reflect the modulation of TNF receptors by IFN-γ. Early clinical trials are assessing dose-limiting toxicities prior to phase II investigations in disseminated malignant melanoma.

Interferons and Chemotherapy. Since biological response modifiers (BRMs) and cytotoxic agents have unique antiproliferative characteristics, it is theoretically attractive to administer these agents concomitantly. Experimental data indicate therapeutic synergism from combinations of selected IFNs and conventional chemotherapy, most notably BCNU and doxorubicin. Pilot studies have documented the feasibility and safety of the concomitant usage of IFN-α plus BCNU or doxorubicin in patients with advanced cancer.

Monoclonal Antibodies

A burgeoning volume of literature focuses on the basic biology and clinical utility of monoclonal antibodies directed against malignant melanoma [8]. In most cases, immunohistochemical analyses have documented selective cellular localization of the antibodies, but clinical responses have been inconsistent. Constitutional side effects have been quite tolerable and easily controllable. Conjugates of monoclonal antibodies with radioisotopes cytotoxic or cytostatic agents, and with BRMs are now being developed which may permit antibody-targeted localization of potential therapeutic agents against melanoma cells.

538

Preventive Surveillance

In view of the potential curability of relatively thin malignant melanomas, early recongition and prompt excision of suspicious lesions are of paramount importance. The following characteristics of a preexisting or de novo skin lesion warrant biopsy:

1. A change in the size, color, or surface characteristics of a nevus. Bleeding, scaling, itchiness, pain, or paresthesias are of special note. A new configuration or increase in growth of a previously existing amelanotic macule or papule should suggest malignant potential.
2. An irregular border which may have a "butterfly" or "notched" shape. Some lesions have pigment which appears to diffuse into the surrounding normal skin.
3. A disorganized array of varigated color involving reds, whites, and blues.
4. Irregular pigmentation in a deformed or intact nail, especially without a history of trauma, should be evaluated by a biopsy of the entire nail bed.

Individuals at particularly high risk for malignant melanoma include:

1. People with light complexions, light eye color (green, gray, blue), and those with a history of sun-sensitivity, especially severe sunburns in childhood and early adulthood
2. People with xeroderma pigmentosum
3. People who live in areas of prolonged sun exposure, e.g., near the equator
4. People who primarily work indoors but have intense, episodic recreational sun exposure
5. People with an increased number of melanocytic nevi as children
6. Those with the dysplastic nevus syndrome. This autosomal dominant or sporadic disorder encompasses the following: large numbers (often >100) of irregularly pigmented, "pebbly," nevi with ill-defined borders, usually >6 mm, and occurrence on sun-protected areas. These lesions may be precursors of malignant melanoma and confer a risk of malignant transformation 7–15 times greater than that of the general population.

References

1. Day CL Jr, Lew RA, Mihm MC Jr et al. (1982) The natural break points for primary-tumor thickness in clinical stage I melanoma. N Engl J Med 305: 1155
2. Urist MM, Balch CM, Soong SJ, Shaw HM, Milton GW, Maddox WA (1985) The influence of surgical margins and prognostic factors predicting the risk of local recurrence in 3445 patients with primary cutaneous melanoma. Cancer 55: 1398–1402
3. Balch CM, Milton GW (eds) (1985) Cutaneous melanoma. Clinical management and treatment results worldwide. Lippincott, Philadelphia

4. Overett TK, Shiu MH (1985) Surgical treatment of distant metastatic melanoma: indications and results. Cancer 56: 1222–1230
5. Rumke PH (1986) Malignant melanoma. In: Pinedo HM, Chabner BA (eds) Cancer chemotherapy, vol 8. Elsevier, Amstesdam, pp 484–494
6. Luikart SD, Kennealey GT, Kirkwood JM (1984) Randomized phase III trial of vinblastine, bleomycin, and cis-dichlorodiammine-platinum versus dacarbazine in malignant melanoma. J Clin Oncol 2: 164–168
7. Cumberln R, De Moss E, Lassus M, Friedman M (1985) Isolation perfusion for malignant melanoma of the extremity: a review. J Clin Oncol 3: 1022–1031
8. Yarbro JW (1986) Biological response modifiers. Semin Oncol XIII(2): 131–258
9. Creagan ET, Ahmann DL, Frytak S, Long HJ, Chang MN, Itri LM (1986) Phase II trials of recombinant leukocyte A interferon in disseminated malignant melanoma: results in 96 patients. Cancer Treat Rep 70: 619–624
10. Overgaard J (1986) The role of radiotherapy in recurrent and metastatic malignant melanoma: a clinical radiobiological study. Int J Radiat Oncol Biol Phys 12: 867–872

42. Basal Cell Carcinoma

D.S. Sarnoff and G.L. Peck

Current Results and Therapeutic Issues

There are many excellent methods for the effective treatment of a primary basal cell carcinoma (BCC), the most common of which are (1) curettage and electrodesiccation (C and D), (2) cryosurgery using liquid nitrogen (3) radiation therapy, and (4) surgical excision with primary closure or resurfacing using skin flaps or skin grafts (1–9). The choice of initial therapy for a BCC depends on numerous factors, including its anatomic location, size, clinical characteristics, histologic features, age and medical condition of the patient, anticipated cosmetic result, previous treatment history, and comfort, duration, and cost of treatment. It has been reported that the cure rates with each of the four standard modalities mentioned above approach 95% for simple, primary BCC. Although all of these methods can effectively destroy BCC, in certain situations one method may be preferable to the others.

C and D is the most common method of treatment. While cure rates as high as 96%–100% have been reported, the overall cure rate is dependent upon the size of the lesion. For example, 38% of BCC with diameters between 1 and 3 cm and 50% of BCC with diameters greater than 3 cm have been shown to recur following C and D. While simple to perform, C and D should be limited to the treatment of selected, small, well-defined, primary lesions and should not be used in dense fibrotic BCC (e.g., morphea-like BCC).

Cryosurgery is the destruction of tissue by the rapid application of intense cold. The indications and advantages of cryosurgery are similar to those for C and D; it should not be used on morphea-like BCC or lesions greater than 3 cm in diameter. It is a relatively simple method of treatment, particularly useful in patients who are poor surgical risks (e.g., patients on anticoagulants, or those sensitive to local anesthetics). Cryotherapy is absolutely contraindicated in patients with abnormal cold intolerance (e.g., cryoglobulinemia or cryofibrinogenemia). Complications of this treatment include marked edema at the treated site, permanent loss of pigmentation, occasional hypertrophic or atrophic scarring, and, infrequently, neuropathy in certain areas, particularly the fingers and elbow.

In selected patients with BCC in particular anatomic regions, radiation therapy offers a unique and valuable therapeutic alternative. Radiation therapy is useful in critical areas where maximal preservation of uninvolved tissue is desirable (e.g., lesions of the eyelids, medial and lateral canthi of the eyes, nose, ears, and lips). In elderly patients, X-ray therapy has proved to be very useful because there is less likelihood of late radiation sequelae; however, whereas surgical scars often improve with time, the resultant scars after radiotherapy tend to worsen over the years.

Electron beam therapy may offer some benefit over conventional superficial X-ray therapy with respect to lesions overlying cartilage or bone due to the reduced risk of radionecrosis. Electron beam therapy is expensive, however, and it is not always available.

C and D, cryosurgery, and radiation therapy all rely on clinical evaluation employing the visual and tactile senses of the physician to determine the full extent of the tumor. When these techniques are used, there is no microscopic confirmation that the tumor has seen completely removed. In contrast to these methods, surgical excision yields a biopsy specimen which, under routine pathologic examination, will confirm tumor-free borders with a high degree of accuracy. Therefore, scalpel excision is widely used today to treat primary BCC.

When the initial treatment for BCC has been unsuccessful, retreatment must then be performed on tumor embedded in scar tissue. This makes the boundaries and distribution of recurrent malignancy more difficult to detect and eradicate. Mohs' surgery, with its microscopically controlled serial excision, offers the best chance of cure in treating these recurrent BCC. Cure rates by the Mohs' technique are 96%–99% for recurrent BCC and 99% for primary BCC. In addition to the treatment of recurrent BCC, Mohs' surgery is indicated in the treatment of primary BCC that is (a) in sites associated with a high rate of treatment failure (e.g., periorbital, periauricular, nasal, and perinasal areas), (b) associated with poorly delineated clinical borders, (c) large in size (>2 cm), (d) morphea-like or sclerosing, (e) in critical locations (e.g., the eyelid) where maximum sparing of uninvolved tissue is desirable. Presently, the availability of Mohs' surgery is limited to large academic centers, since special laboratories and trained personnel are required for this technique.

Metastatic BCC is an extremely rare entity associated with an extremely poor prognosis. When the metastasis is localized, surgery is the treatment of choice. When the metastases are widespread, ionizing radiotherapy may be useful. Systemic chemotherapy (e.g., cisplatin, doxorubicin, bleomycin sulfate, or a combination of fluorouracil, methotrexate, and cyclophosphamide) has been rather disappointing both for metastatic and advanced local disease. At this time, the greatest role for systemic chemotherapy may be as an adjuvant, combined with surgery or radiation in the treatment of advanced lesions of the face to minimize cosmetic or functional disability. Further studies are needed to establish this role.

Current Approaches Under Study

Several techniques have been tried, and others are currently under study, to aid physicians in the preoperative determination of the clinical margins of skin tumors. Liquid crystal thermography (LCT) is a rapidly performed method for determining temperature variations [10]. It has been found that skin is usually warmer over carcinomas than over normal tissue, possibly due to increased blood supply. For BCC of heavy or moderate density, such as the adenoid-cystic or solid tumors, LCT can be used to demonstrate the lateral margins with moderate accuracy. The technique is somewhat unreliable for tumors of low density such as morphea-like BCC. Using LCT to assess the lateral margins of BCC has great potential; further refinements in the liquid crystal products themselves, as well as in the technique, may yield more accurate and reliable results. Although lateral margins may be demarcated with LCT, the depth of a BCC is not demonstrable at present. Ultrasonography, in conjunction with LCT, may prove to be useful in this respect.

Various methods to improve the recognition of the histologic margins of skin tumors are also currently under investigation. During Mohs' surgery, when small islands of tumor cells or individual tumor cells remain in the tissue, they are often difficult to distinguish on frozen sections with conventional hematoxylin-eosin or toluidine blue staining. In these cases, tumor may be confused with nerve or vascular tissue or with inflammatory cells. Immunoperoxidase and indirect immunofluorescence techniques using monoclonal antibodies to keratin proteins have recently been employed to distinguish these keratinizing tumor cells from mesodermal cells. Thus, immunohistochemical methods should theoretically improve the accuracy of microscopically controlled excision and decrease the rate of tumor recurrence. Recently, a new murine monoclonal antibody, VM-1, has been shown to stain BCC cells. A limitation of the VM-1 stain is that in addition to carcinoma cells, the antibody also stains cells of the external root sheath of hair follicles within the dermis. This poses a particular problem in the scalp, which is an area associated with a high recurrence rate for skin cancers, because differentiation of BCC cells from the cells of hair follicles may not be possible by this technique. The future of immunoperoxidase staining of BCC will depend on the discovery of a specific monoclonal antibody that only stains BCC cells, and the development of a rapid and efficient technique which would allow its clinical application.

Another current approach under study involves the use of the laser in cutaneous oncology (10). Superficial BCC has been treated with CO_2 laser vaporization, sometimes in conjunction with curettage, to provide high cure rates with rapid healing and minimal postoperative pain. The CO_2 laser can also be used to excise tissue when focused to a small beam diameter of 0.1–0.2 mm. As the incision is made, small blood vessels, lymphatics, and nerve endings are sealed. Application of the CO_2 laser to Mohs' surgery has recently been described. As in the fresh tissue technique, multiple layers may be excised in one session, histologic detail is preserved, and immediate surgical repair is possible.

Advantages of the CO_2 laser in Mohs' surgery include a virtually bloodless field, even in very vascular tissue or in patients receiving anticoagulants. The current major drawbacks of the CO_2 laser modification of Mohs' surgery are the cost of the laser and the size of the instrument.

A new, experimental alternative for treating patients with BCC is hematoporphyrin derivative (HPD) photoradiation therapy [10]. HPD is a photodynamically active dye that is retained preferentially by malignant cells and initiates a cytotoxic reaction when exposed to red light. This approach uses intravenously administered HPD as the photosensitizer of tumors and focally applied red light (630 nm) as the photoactivating source, emitted from a modified xenon arc photocoagulator or an argon or dye laser. A unique property of HPD appears to be its prolonged affinity for tissues with rapid cellular turnover, such as neoplastic cells, long after it has cleared from the surrounding normal tissue.

The major toxic effects secondary to HPD therapy are pronounced photosensitivity to sunlight for at least 1 month, and skin necrosis over the local treatment site. Lesions that are bulky or ulcerated show only a partial response because of light scattering from the surface, inhibiting maximal light penetration.

Current standard therapy is unsatisfactory for patients with numerous lesions. Patients with xeroderma pigmentosum, nevoid basal cell carcinoma syndrome, or a history of arsenic exposure may develop hundreds of BCC throughout their lives. These patients with multicentric disease most certainly could benefit from effective topical chemotherapy, systemic chemotherapy, or other methods designed to cure or prevent widespread lesions.

Various topical agents, including dinitrochlorobenzene (DNCB), Solcoderm (a solution of organic and inorganic acids and ions containing copper, oxalate, lactate, nitrate, and acetate), and topically applied retinoids have proved capable of producing complete regression of BCC. The efficacy of these topical agents, however, is not comparable to that of the standard modalities.

Topical fluorouracil is an approved cytotoxic treatment for superficial BCC, but not for nodular or invasive BCC. Although many BCC appear to be superficial, they frequently invade the reticular dermis; because these deeper extensions are not regularly reached by topical fluorouracil in its present vehicle, even when used under occlusion, there are likely to be recurrences. One danger in using topical fluorouracil is that, while it may produce the appearance of control with superficial destruction of the tumor, deeper extensions may continue to grow; thus, fluorouracil may, in effect, conceal deep foci of invasive BCC. This is a potential danger of all topical chemotherapeutic agents.

Future Approaches

Recently, interferon has been tested in a variety of skin disorders including skin cancer. Results of a single pilot study, using recombinant α-2 interferon injected intralesionally three times a week for 3 weeks into biopsy-proven BCC have

544

been encouraging, suggesting that additional evaluation is warranted in patients who are not candidates for simple surgical removal, have a nonresectable BCC, or request nonsurgical therapy.

The oral retinoids have been used to treat patients with multiple BCC (11). Since the results of these studies, which have approximately a 10% cure rate, compared unfavorably with standard modalities, the use of oral isotretinoin and oral etretinate as chemotherapeutic agents for BCC was abandoned. Nevertheless, the oral synthetic retinoids seem promising in the prevention of cutaneous malignancy. The chemoprophylactic effect of the retinoids may be secondary to their ability to enhance or promote normal cellular differentiation. Unfortunately, the potential exists for chronic toxicity (skeletal hyperostosis and calcification of tendons and ligaments) from the prolonged systemic therapy that appears necessary to maintain the chemopreventive effect. Hence, the development of an oral synthetic retinoid which is effective as a chemopreventive agent, has minimal side effects, and exhibits no associated chronic toxicity would indeed be a most significant goal for the future.

References

1. Stegman SJ (1986) Basal cell carcinoma and squamous cell carcinoma: recognition and treatment. Med Clin North Am 70(1): 95–107
2. Cottel WI (1986) Skin tumors I: Basal and squamous cell carcinomas. Sel Read Plast Surg 4(6): 6–22
3. Haynes HA, Mead KW, Goldwyn RM (1985) Cancers of the skin. In: DeVita VT Jr, Hellman S, Rosenberg SA (eds) Cancer: Principles and practice of oncology, 2nd edn. Lippincott, Philadelphia, pp 1343–1369
4. Browder JP, Tomsick RS (1983) Basal cell epithelioma: types, treatment methods, and prognosis. Postgrad Med 73(2): 161–168
5. Swanson NA (1983) Basal cell carcinoma. Treatment modalities and recommendations. Prim Care 10: 443–458
6. Witkowski JA, Parish LC (1982) Basal cell cancer: a curable malignancy. Drug Ther 12(11): 159–161, 164–165
7. Albright SD (1982) Treatment of skin cancer using multiple modalities. J Am Acad Dermatol 7: 143–171
8. Casson P (1980) Basal cell carcinoma. Clin Plast Surg 7(3): 301
9. Helm F (ed) (1979) Cancer dermatology. Lea and Febiger, Philadelphia, pp 325–481
10. Epstein E (ed) (1984) Controversies in dermatology. Saunders, Philadelphia, pp 107–133, 163–184
11. Peck GL (1985) Therapy and prevention of skin cancer. In: Saurat JH (ed) Retinoids: new trends in research and therapy. Karger, Basel, pp 345–354

43. Acute Lymphoblastic Leukemia

D.G. Poplack

Current Results and Therapeutic Issues

Acute lymphoblastic leukemia (ALL) is the most common childhood malignancy, occurring with an incidence of approximately 2–4 per 100 000 children below 15 years of age. Each year approximately 2000 cases of childhood ALL occur in the United States; a small number of adults are diagnosed with the disease. In the past 40 years there has been dramatic improvement in the outcome of patients with ALL. Prior to the introduction of effective antineoplastic chemotherapy approximately 40 years ago, ALL was uniformly fatal, most children surviving only 2–3 months from diagnosis. Presently, however, approximately 60% of children with this disease are in continuous complete remission 5 years following their initial diagnosis; the majority of these children are considered to be cured [1]. This treatment success has been the result of the stepwise introduction of a variety of new treatment strategies, beginning with the introduction of effective single-agent chemotherapy in the late 1940s, the development and use of combination chemotherapy and subsequently maintenance chemotherapy during the 1950s and early 1960s, the strategy of CNS-preventive therapy in the late 1960s, and, most recently, the concepts of tailoring therapy according to risk factors and intensification of therapy. Combination chemotherapy, which traces its origins to ALL in children, forms the primary therapeutic modality. Radiation therapy has been employed for CNS-preventive therapy and for treatment of selected forms of extramedullary relapse.

In the past decade, characterization of leukemic lymphoblasts on morphologic, immunologic, biochemical, and cytogenetic bases has led investigators to conclude that ALL is a biologically heterogeneous disorder. In addition, certain clinical features evident at diagnosis have prognostic value and permit delineation of patients into subgroups with relatively favorable or unfavorable prognoses. Most current treatment protocols stratify patients at diagnosis into different risk categories according to the most reliable prognostic factors (e.g., initial white blood cell count, age, cytogenetics, etc.) and tailor treatment accordingly. In general, "high-risk" patients (or those with very high initial white blood cell count, unfavorable age at diagnosis, chromosomal translocations, lymphomatous presentations, etc.) are placed on more intensive treatment regimens [2, 3]. In contrast, patients with clinical features associated with a more favorable prognosis are placed on treatment protocols designed to be equally effective but less intensive, in the hope of avoiding treatment-associated adverse sequelae. Most ALL treatment regimens divide therapy into four main treatment phases: remission induction, CNS-preventive therapy, consolidation, and maintenance therapy. Patients are treated for approximately $2\frac{1}{2}$ years. Patients with so called "good-risk" features usually receive three drug-induction therapy (vincristine, prednisone, and L-asparaginase), CNS-preventive therapy with intrathecal chemotherapy alone, and maintenance therapy consisting of daily 6-mercaptopurine, weekly or biweekly methotrexate, and periodic "pulses" of vincristine and prednisone. Although retrospective analysis permits identification of a group of patients with an extremely favorable treatment outcome (90%–95% long-term disease-free survival), it has become evident that when one prospectively stratifies patients according to these same criteria, the overall results obtained on uniform therapy are less favorable than expected (approximately 75%–80% long-term event-free survival). Why a significant number of "good-risk" patients fail current therapy has become a major topic of current investigation.

Patients with "high-risk" features usually receive induction therapy with four (or more) agents (vincristine, prednisone, L-asparaginase, daunorubicin), intensive consolidation therapy, usually employing multiple agents and frequently repeating induction therapy, and maintenance therapy that often includes late intensification or periodic pulses of intensified therapy. Although the use of more intensive therapy has substantially increased the long-term event-free survival for patients in this group, a substantial proportion of such patients (approximately 1/2 to 1/3) will eventually fail therapy. Thus, a major current priority in ALL treatment is to develop more effective treatment for patients with "high-risk" features.

CNS-preventive therapy has become a vital element of all ALL treatment protocols. CNS "prophylaxis" has reduced the incidence of CNS recurrence from approximately 75%–80% to less than 10%, and, because CNS recurrence frequently heralds systemic relapse, has dramatically improved event-free survival. In the 1970s, the use of cranial radiation (2400 cGy) and intrathecal methotrexate were the accepted, effective form of CNS-preventive therapy. Recognition that this approach may be accompanied by significant adverse CNS sequelae, including CT brain scan abnormalities, altered intellectual and psychological function, and neuroendocrine damage, has prompted the search for alternative CNS-preventive therapy strategies which are equally effective but less neurotoxic. The identification of risk factors for CNS relapse (high initial leukocyte count, T-cell disease, very young age, thrombocytopenia, lymphomatous features, black race) has permitted investigators to modify CNS-preventive therapy accordingly. Although effective CNS-preventive therapy can be achieved in "good-risk" patients utilizing intrathecal chemotherapy alone, the optimal, most appropriate form of CNS-preventive therapy for patients in other risk categories remains a major treatment issue.

Approximately 40% of patients with ALL will suffer disease recurrence. Close to 1/3 of patients with a bone marrow relapse will have a human-leukocyte-antigen matched sibling and may potentially benefit from an allogeneic bone marrow transplant. Long-term disease-free survival can be achieved in over 25% of these individuals. Although conventional chemotherapy will induce complete remissions in the majority of patients who suffer bone marrow relapse, most will eventually succumb to their disease. High priority must be given to identification of more effective chemotherapy for these patients and to increasing the applicability of bone marrow transplantation (e.g., to patients with no matched sibling donors).

Current Approaches Under Study

Current treatment approaches have focused on the concept of tailoring therapy according to risk groups. Significant sophistication is now used to define risk groups. For example, the Children's Cancer Study Group uses an algorithm based on initial leukocyte count, age at diagnosis, sex, FAB morphologic classification, degree or extent of bulk disease, and E-rosette positivity to assign patients to one of five currently recognized risk groups [4]. In addition to good, average, and poor risk categories, specific therapy has been designed for infants less than 1 year of age (the group of ALL patients with the worst prognosis) and for patients who present with lymphomatous features (a subgroup at a high risk of extramedullary relapse, particularly CNS recurrence). Although stratification of this type is complex, it permits identification of patients with a propensity for selective patterns of relapse (e.g., CNS relapse in patients with lymphomatous features), providing the potential for more selective application of both systemic and CNS-preventive therapy. Most centers intensify therapy for high risk patients. Although this approach has resulted in improved overall long-term event-free survival curves (as high as approximately 70% in such patients), it is unclear at present whether further intensification is likely to lead to additional improvement for high-risk patients. Analysis of the results of the last three clinical trials performed by the West German BFM study group indicates no significant difference in the overall event-free survival of patients treated on three successive studies, suggesting that the progressive intensification of therapy which occurred over this time may not have improved overall treatment results [5].

Some attention has focused on alternative modes of therapy, particularly bone marrow transplantation, for patients at an excessively high risk for treatment failure (e.g., patients with certain chromosomal translocations). Whether such an approach will improve the outlook for such patients is unclear. Refinements in bone marrow transplantation, however, have already led to some increase in the applicability of this approach. For example, numerous centers are currently evaluating the feasibility of "partial mismatched" transplants and the use of unrelated, matched donors. Should these approaches be successful, it is possible that the use of bone marrow transplantation for patients in relapse, and possibly for selected very high risk patients during first remission, will be increased.

548

A number of current studies are addressing the question of alternative methods of CNS-preventive therapy. 1800 cGy has been shown to be as effective as 2400 cGy in regimens which utilize cranial radiation. However, concern over the likely contribution of cranial radiation to adverse CNS sequelae has prompted investigators to study a variety of alternatives to the use of cranial radiation, including intermediate and high-dose methotrexate.

Studies indicating low and variable bioavailability of orally administered maintenance chemotherapy agents have focused attention on the possibility of a pharmacologic basis for treatment failure, and have prompted studies aimed at assessing whether suboptimal drug exposure is associated with a higher relapse rate [6]. In a recently initiated study at the St. Jude Children's Cancer Research Hospital patients are treated with identical therapy but randomized to receive either "adjusted" or "unadjusted" drug exposure. Whether pharmacologic drug monitoring will ultimately result in improved ALL therapy remains to be determined.

The application of intensified therapy has significantly improved the outcome of adults with ALL. In one recent study approximately 50% of adults treated with an intensive chemotherapy schedule similar to that used in many childhood ALL protocols achieved prolonged disease-free survival [7].

Future Approaches

Despite the dramatic improvement achieved to date in the treatment of ALL, significant obstacles must be overcome before cure is a reality for all patients with this disease. Several major areas are likely to be the focus for future laboratory and clinical studies.

One vital need is for more sensitive methods of detecting relapse and for a better understanding of the causes of treatment failure. Molecular biological techniques such as assessment of immunoglobulin and T-cell receptor gene rearrangements are currently being used to study ALL. These techniques, possibly together with methodology incorporating "in situ hybridization," may eventually permit identification of residual leukemia in otherwise morphologically normal marrows. Although this possibility has been suggested using current methodology, further technical refinements will be required [8].

Understanding the basis for treatment failure is likely to prove more problematic. Although similar in their refractoriness to current therapy, the group of patients failing on current therapy is known to be biologically heterogeneous, manifesting differences in clinical presentation and in the cytogenetic, immunologic and molecular features of their disease. The application of molecular biological methods to the study of drug resistance may ultimately provide valuable information regarding the mechanisms of treatment failure [9]. In addition to improving approaches with currently available antileukemic agents, there is a clear need for identification of new chemotherapeutic agents active against lymphoid leukemia. Several new approaches to intrathecal chemotherapy are already under preclinical and clinical study, including intrathecal 4-hydroperoxycyclophosphamide, intrathecal 6-mercaptopurine, and intrathecal Diaziquone. In addition, new lipophilic antifols (e.g., trimetrexate, piritrexim) may become useful agents for maintenance chemotherapy. The addition of other systemic agents which penetrate well into the CNS (intravenous 6-mercaptopurine, intravenous thiotepa) may add to our ability to approach both systemic and CNS disease simultaneously by the systemic route.

The role of bone marrow transplantation in the treatment of ALL is likely to increase. Recent success in the use of partially mismatched donors brings the possibility of totally crossing the human leukocyte antigen barrier closer to reality. In addition, the role of autologous marrow transplantation may expand as newer methods of in vitro purging (radiolabelled monoclonal antibodies, biologics, etc.) become available.

The recognition that some forms of adult leukemia (e.g., hairy cell, chronic myelogenous) respond to certain types of interferons has stimulated investigation of the role of biologics as a possible means of treating lymphoid leukemia. For example, recent studies with interleukin-2 have demonstrated that in vitro culture of T-cell lymphoblasts with interleukin-2 results in maturation and eventual death of leukemic blast cells [10]. In vivo studies of this approach have only recently been initiated. Another exciting potential use for biologics is in the area of molecularly cloned hematopoietic growth factors. Preclinical and early clinical studies with colony stimulating factors (GM and G) confirm the potential of these agents to shorten the duration and severity of chemotherapy-induced myelosuppression. The use of such agents may provide a means of intensifying chemotherapy (both dose and schedule) for patients with ALL at high risk of treatment failure.

Finally, as more children with ALL are cured, attention to avoiding late effects of ALL treatment will increase accordingly.

Ultimately, progress in the future will depend both upon continued basic research aimed at increasing our understanding of the biology of ALL as well as on the ability of clinicians to design innovative clinical studies.

References

1. Poplack DG (1985) Acute lymphoblastic leukemia in childhood. In: Altman AJ (ed) The pediatric clinics of North America. Saunders Philadelphia, pp 669–697
2. Hammond D, Sather H, Nesbit M, Miller D, Coccia P, Bleyer A, Lukens J, Siegel S (1986) Analysis of prognostic factors in acute lymphoblastic leukemia. Med Pediatr Oncol 14: 124–134
3. Hammond GD, Sather H, Bleyer WA, Coccia P (1987) Stratification by prognostic factors in the design and analysis of clinical trials for acute lymphoblastic leukemia. In: Büchner T, Schellong G, Hiddemann W, Urbanitz D, Ritter J (eds) Acute leukemias, Springer, Berlin Heidelberg, New York, pp 161–166 (Haematology and blood transfusion, vol 30)

4. Bleyer WA (1983) Acute lymphoid leukemia. Pediatr Ann 12: 277–292
5. Riehm H, Gadner H, Henze G et al. (1983) Acute lymphoblastic leukemia: treatment results in three BFM studies (1970–1981). In: Murphy SB, Gilbert JR (eds) Leukemia research: advances in cell biology and treatment. Elsevier, New York, pp 251–263
6. Zimm S, Collins JM, Riccardi R et al. (1983) Variable bioavailability of oral mercaptopurine: is maintenance chemotherapy in acute lymphoblastic leukemia being optimally delivered? N Engl J Med 308: 1005–1009
7. Linker CA, Levitt LL, O'Donnell M et al. (1987) Improved results of treatment of adult acute lymphoblastic leukemia. Blood 69: 1242–1248
8. Wright JJ, Poplack DG, Bakhshi A, Reaman G, Cole D, Jensen JP, Korsmeyer SJ (1987) Gene rearrangements as markers of clonal variation and minimal residual disease in acute lympho-blastic leukemia. J Clin Oncol 5(5): 735–741
9. Fojo AT, Ueda K, Slamon DJ, Poplack DG, Gottesman MM Pastan I (1987) Expression of a multidrug resistance gene in human tumors and tissues. Proc Natl Acad Sci USA 84: 265–269
10. Colamonici OR, Cole D, Trepel JB, Poplack DG, Neckers LH (1987) Induction of functional and phenotypic differentiation in immature T cell leukemias by treatment with IL-2. Abstract, 4th Intl. Symposium on Therapy of Acute Leukemias, Rome, February 1987.

44. Acute Nonlymphoblastic Leukemia

D.G. Poplack

Current Results and Therapeutic Issues

Acute nonlymphoblastic leukemia (ANLL) is the most common form of acute leukemia in adults and makes up approximately one-quarter of the cases of childhood acute leukemia. Although there has been significant improvement in the outlook of patients with this disease, the pace of therapeutic progress in ANLL has been slower than for acute lymphoblastic leukemia. Prior to the 1950s, ANLL was uniformly fatal, most patients surviving only 1–2 months from diagnosis. The initial introduction of effective single agents and the subsequent identification of active combination chemotherapy has, however, led to an improved outlook [1]. Presently, two therapeutic modalities are utilized to treat patients with ANLL. Combination chemotherapy, consisting of induction treatment, post-induction consolidation, and in some regimens maintenance chemotherapy, is the form of treatment for the majority of patients with ANLL. A smaller number of patients, following successful induction of remission, benefit from bone marrow transplantation. Because significant myelosuppression is induced in an attempt to obtain a complete remission in patients with ANLL, treatment of patients with this disease requires optimal supportive care techniques.

Complete remission can be obtained in most (approximately 70%–80%) patients with ANLL. In adults treated with chemotherapy, the median remission duration is approximately 1–2 years with a substantial fraction of patients (approximately 25%) achieving prolonged disease-free survival. Results are somewhat better in children; up to 45% may achieve long-term disease-free status.

Bone marrow transplantation has played an increasing role in the therapy of patients with ANLL [2]. It is most successful when applied to younger patients in their first complete remission. Bone marrow transplantation provides a means of restoring hematopoiesis following the delivery of very high doses of myelosuppressive chemotherapy (often administered in conjunction with total body radiation). In addition to being used as "post-remission" consolidative therapy in newly diagnosed patients, marrow transplantation has also been used in patients with various preleukemic states and in individuals with "high-risk" leukemia in whom conventional chemotherapy is unlikely to induce a remission. To date, the use of bone marrow transplantation has primarily been limited to those patients with histocompatible donors. Only approximately one-third of patients with ANLL, however, have histocompatible, allogeneic-matched, sibling donors.

Current Approaches Under Study

A number of current issues exist regarding the optimal mode of chemotherapy for ANLL. The standard, most effective form of remission induction treatment has been the combination of Cytarabine and the anthracycline daunorubicin. In most studies, addition of other agents to this combination has not been shown clearly to improve the remission induction rate. Recent evaluation of high-dose cytarabine suggests that this approach, combined with daunorubicin, may be associated with a higher remission induction rate. The toxicity associated with this approach, however, has led many investigators to reserve the use of high-dose cytarabine for post-remission consolidative therapy and for those patients refractory to the conventional combination of cytarabine and daunorubicin [3]. Recent attempts to improve remission induction have also included use of several anthracycline analogs, reportedly associated with less cardiotoxicity. Agents such as mitoxantrone and Idarubicin fall into this category.

Induction of remission is more difficult in patients who are elderly (over 60 years of age), who have certain cytogenetic abnormalities, and/or who developed their disease within the context of a preleukemic syndrome. The prognosis of patients with certain morphologic subtypes also may be different. Patients with the M2 or M3 subtype according to the French American British (FAB) morphologic classification may have a better prognosis than patients with monocytic, myelomonocytic, megakaryocytic, or erythroid subtypes. In addition, patients with higher initial white blood cell counts appear to fare poorly.

The value of post-remission consolidation chemotherapy has been confirmed by several studies. The longest remission durations have been reported in studies using at least two courses of consolidation chemotherapy. The use of high-dose Cytarabine, either alone or together with an anthracycline, has produced disease-free survival rates approximating 40% at 3 years. The value of maintenance chemotherapy has been a source of controversy and the focus of a number of different studies [4]. For adults with ANLL who have received intensive induction and consolidation therapy, the value of additional maintenance therapy has not been conclusively demonstrated, although the benefits of "late intensification" have been advocated by some. In childhood ANLL, some studies have demonstrated the value of continuation chemotherapy, but this issue continues to be reevaluated [5]. CNS preventive therapy is not routinely administered by many centers, primarily because the risk of CNS relapse is relatively low.

In addition to studies focusing on the value of intensified chemotherapy, attention has been directed toward defining the role of bone marrow transplantation in patients with ANLL and on improving bone marrow transplantation technology. Although patients in first remission generally fare better with bone marrow transplantation, some investigators still question the appropriateness of its use early in first remission. The apparently improved disease-free survival obtained with aggressive intensification regimens (e.g., high dose Cytarabine and daunorubicin) has led some investigators to suggests that marrow transplantation should be reserved for patients during second remission or at the time of relapse [6]. A prospective study comparing these approaches may be required to settle this issue. Results of a preliminary comparative study in children suggest that patients transplanted in first remission fare better than those treated with chemotherapy alone [7]. However, a larger, prospective study addressing this question is currently under way.

Future Approaches

Future advances in ANLL will require improvement in several areas. There is a need to identify more effective antileukemic agents than those currently available. In the absence of dramatic improvements in bone marrow transplantation technology or developments in other areas (e.g., biologic response modifiers), combination chemotherapy is likely to be the major form of treatment for ANLL in the forseeable future. Not only must new effective agents be developed, but investigators must achieve a better understanding of the causes of treatment failure, particularly the basis for the development of drug resistance. Promising leads, however, have been noted in the laboratory with regard to the use of differentiating agents and biological response modifiers. The concept of utilizing agents such as retinoic acid, which is capable of differentiating leukemia cells in vitro, as therapy for patients with this disease, is intriguing. Although clinical studies using differentiating agents have been unrewarding to date, this type of approach may have potential because of its unique mechanism of action.

The potential role for biological response modifiers, such as interferon and the interleukins, is not clear. Although recombinant α-interferon did not demonstrate activity in initial studies in patients with this disease, the possibility exists that newer biologics (e.g., interleukins, tumor necrosis factor) may be of value.

Considerable attention has focused on attempts to improve the applicability of bone marrow transplantation for patients with ANLL. Partial mismatched transplants are being actively evaluated in a number of centers and offer the possibility, if successful, of extending this modality to patients without histocompatible matched donors. Another approach of interest is autologous bone marrow transplantation. This strategy involves reinfusion of autologous bone marrow following high dose chemotherapy (with or without total body radiation). A variety of approaches are being investigated to eradicate residual leukemic cells from autologous bone marrow to circumvent the major problem associated with this approach—leukemic relapse. Both antileukemic monoclonal antibodies and pharmacologic agents have been used as marrow purging agents. In particular, promising results have been reported utilizing 4-hydroperoxycyclophosphamide, an analog of cyclophosphamide, as a means of purging marrow for autologous transplantation [8]. Whether this approach will ultimately prove of value or have wide applicability for patients with ANLL is presently unclear.

References

1. Frei E, Freireich EJ (1965) Progress and perspectives in the chemotherapy of acute leukemia. Adv Chemother 2:269
2. Champlin RE, Gale RP (1987) Bone marrow transplantation in acute leukemia: recent advances and comparison with alternative therapies. Semin Hematol 24:55
3. Herzig RH, Lazarus HM, Wolff SN et al. (1984) High dose cytosine arabinoside therapy with and without anthracycline antibiotics for remission reinduction of acute non-lymphocytic leukemia. J Clin Oncol 2:545
4. Champlin RE, Gale RP (1987) Acute myelogenous leukemia: recent advances in therapy. Blood 69:1551
5. Grier HE, Weinstein HJ (1985) Acute nonlymphocytic leukemia. Pediatr Clin North Am 32:653
6. Reece D, Phillips G, Herzig R, Buskard N, Benny B, Growe G, Vickars L, Herzig (1986) High dose cytosine arabinoside and daunorubicin as initial induction and consolidation therapy in acute adult nonlymphocytic leukemia. Blood 68:230
7. Sanders JE, Thomas ED, Buckner CD, Flournoy N, Steward P, Clift RA, Lum L, Bensinger WI, Storb R, Appelbaum FR, Sullivan KM (1985) Marrow transplantation for children in first remission of acute nonlymphoblastic leukemia: an update. Blood 66:460
8. Yeager AM, Kaizer H, Santos GW, Saral R, Colvin OM, Stuart RK, Braine HG, Burkee PJ, Ambinder RF, Burns WH, Fuller DJ, Davis JM, Karp JE, May WS, Rowley SK, Sensenbrenner LL, Bogelsang FG, Wingard JR (1986) Autologous bone marrow transplantation in patients with acute nonlymphocytic leukemia using ex vivo treatment with 4-hydroperoxycyclophosphamide. N Engl J Med 315:141

45. The Chronic Leukemias

G.P. Canellos

Current Results and Therapeutic Issues

Chronic Myelogenous Leukemia (CML)

This disease provides an interesting model for the study of human bone marrow stem cell physiology as well as for human neoplasia since, in most instances, it is a disease that will predictably pass from a status of hyperplasia to dedifferentiation blast cell leukemia [1]. A most interesting development in the treatment of this disease has been the discovery that the chronic phase of chronic granulocytic leukemia (CGL) can be effectively obliterated by high-dose chemoradiotherapy followed by an allogeneic or syngeneic marrow graft. The data clearly show that the results are superior if the patients are given a transplant in the chronic phase of the disease as opposed to the accelerated (or blastic) phase, since the disease becomes progressively refractory to the obliteration of the last neoplastic cell by chemoradiotherapy [2]. New developments in the treatment of donor grafts by techniques designed to remove T cells in general or specific T-cell subsets have resulted in a marked diminution in the incidence of graft-versus-host disease and the resulting mortality. However, an increased incidence of graft rejection has been noted, indicating that perhaps a small degree of graft-versus-leukemia is required for the successful obliteration of the last Philadelphia chromosome-bearing cell. If the patient lacks a suitable histocompatible donor, then occasional patients are given mismatched grafts, usually with poor results. The stable/chronic phase is managed very easily by conventional oral alkylating agents, such as busulfan and the more recently introduced hydroxyurea. The latter is probably the treatment of choice since it is not associated with any other visceral toxicity or long-term myelosuppression. Hydroxyurea is the drug with which all new therapies should be compared for the treatment of the chronic phase.

α-Interferon has recently been introduced for the treatment of the chronic phase. α-interferon, now an accepted agent for the treatment of hairy-cell leukemia, has been shown to have a cytotoxic effect against CGL in the chronic phase, both in vivo and in vitro, and is effective in reducing the blood counts. However, the toxicity, expense, and inconvenience of its use probably offset any practical application of interferon as compared with hydroxyurea [3]. Since interferon therapy, like all other chronic phase therapies, does not prevent the blastic phase, it does not appear to have replaced hydroxyurea.

Splenic irradiation and splenectomy in CML are reserved for selected complications of hypersplenism which are rare.

The blastic phase of the disease has been treated by intensive combination chemotherapy designed for the treatment of acute leukemia [4]. In most instances, it can be said to have been unsuccessful, except in the subtype of CGL in the blastic phase that has lymphoid characteristics, including lymphoblastic morphology, terminal transferase activity, and a positive common acute lymphocytic leukemia (ALL) antigen (CALLA). Patients having these lymphoid characteristics can be put into a satisfactory hematologic remission with treatment designed for acute lymphoblastic leukemia, including adriamycin, vincristine, and prednisone [5]. These remissions last considerably longer than those in patients with myeloblastic transformation but in most instances are terminated within 10 months by reversion to a more aggressive and refractory form of leukemia.

There have been a number of trials which include collection of marrow or peripheral stem cells during the chronic phase with cryopreservation for subsequent use during attempted ablation of the blastic phase with cytotoxic therapy. In almost all instances, engraftment can be achieved, but the regimens used to date, including high doses of alkylating agents, cytosine arabinoside (ara-C), and whole body irradiation, have not been effective in eliminating the last blast cell [6]. Engraftment is worthy of further investigation, especially with new therapeutic tools.

Myeloblastic transformation has usually been treated with ara-C in various dosages, including low-dose, continuous infusion and high-dose, intravenous pulses, with less than 20% remission. Recently, there has been some enthusiasm for the use of hydroxyurea plus mithramycin with some thought that it might induce differentiation of myeloid cells. In most instances, differentiating agents have not been successful in the conversion of the myeloblastic transformation to a more differentiated counterpart.

Chronic Lymphatic Leukemia (CLL)

CLL is a disease of older age groups, with a median age of between 60 and 65 years old. More recently, however, because of the widespread application of routine blood counts, younger patients in the early stages of this disease have been identified. Clearly, the early stage of CLL requires no therapy, and patients can be followed for a considerable amount of time without any treatment [7]. The approach to the early phase of CLL has been unchanged over the past 20 years and includes the judicious use of oral alkylating agents with or without prednisone. Patients with hypersplenism may have a splenectomy or splenic irradiation, the former being more effective in this event. The introduction of newer treatments, such as α-interferon, has not added to the cytotoxic armamentarium available for CLL.

Since patients with CLL are in the older age groups and may have a disease with a very long natural history, it has been difficult to justify intensive therapy

557

of stable CLL. However, patients with the disease in an accelerated form have been treated with a combination chemotherapy consisting of adriamycin, cytoxan, vincristine, and prednisone (CHOP), with some benefit in selected patients in whom the disease has assumed a more lymphomatous acceleration [8]. Low doses of weekly adriamycin may also prove useful in elderly patients with alkylating agent refractory disease. Leukopheresis for CLL, as for CML, has not proven to be a useful modality. Thus, the stable phase is probably best managed by a watch-and-wait policy, followed by the use of oral alkylating agents, with or without prednisone, for the treatment of progressive lymphadenopathy and leukocytosis. Almost any schedule of oral alkylating agents, usually chlorambucil, has proven effective. The pulse-dose technique does not seem to be superior to chronic daily oral medication. Other alkylating agents, such as L-phenylalanine mustard (L-PAM) and cyclophosphamide, are equally effective. The accelerated phase of the disease is complicated by the marked immunosuppression that is a consistent feature of the disease, with hypogammaglobulinemia and excessive accumulation of lymphoid cells with compromise of normal marrow function. The majority of patients die of infection in the advanced stages of the disease. A change in the character of the disease to a more lymphomatous type of transformation (Richter's syndrome) is worthy of treatment with combination chemotherapy designed for malignant lymphoma [9].

Current Approaches Under Study

Chronic Granulocytic Leukemia

Although the pilot trials with α-interferon have shown a marked cytotoxic effect in CGL, comparative trials are underway with hydroxyurea to evaluate the impact of α-inteferon on the natural history of the disease. Large numbers and careful stratification according to prognostic factors will be required since careful analysis of large numbers of patients has indicated that the height of the white count and the presence of thrombocytosis and hepatosplenomegaly are all negative prognostic factors [10]. Bone marrow transplantation continues, with newer techniques being introduced to ameliorate graft-versus-host disease. New technology will be required to explore intensive therapy of the chronic phase of the disease with a view toward resurrecting normal chromosome cell lines which might be harvested for subsequent transplantation. Because of the inevitable contamination by Philadelphia chromosome-positive cells, an investigation of techniques to eliminate these cells from autologous marrow is underway. This may include altering the temperature of the environment and introducing cytotoxic chemicals that may have a preferential effect against the more proliferative Philadelphia chromosome-bearing cell line. The blastic phase of the disease represents a frustrating and refractory form of leukemia, so most current investigations into this disease are directed to the stable or chronic phase.

Chronic Lymphatic Leukemia (CLL)

The use of biological response modifiers may have a significant future in CLL. There is certainly a need for a less toxic treatment, and an explosion of new knowledge in the biology of B-lymphoid cell growth should pave the way for the study of the use of new modalities, such as α-interferon and γ-interferon as well as the newer lymphokines. It is also a disease that is amenable to treatment with immunotoxins. Pilot trials with the antibody T101 (CD5) linked to the ricin A chain had only modest success [11]; this is an area for future investigation. As in CGL, treatment directed against the advanced refractory state of the disease is not likely to yield major benefits. The natural course of CLL might be altered through researching new treatments, prognostic factors, and aspects of the natural course of the disease, allowing for the application of these new treatments at a somewhat earlier stage. Bone marrow transplantation in CLL has not been attempted to any extent because of the advanced age of most patients.

Future Approaches

Chronic Granulocytic Leukemia (CGL)

Exciting new developments in understanding the pathogenesis of CGL may lead to therapeutic benefit to the patient. It is now clear that the translocation of the oncogene c-*abl* to chromosome 22, combining with the breakpoint cluster region (*bcr*) to form a hybrid ribonucleic acid (RNA) transcript and subsequently a hybrid protein, may play an important role in the pathogenesis of the disease. Identifying the nature of this protein and its function, which may have tyrosine kinase activity, would be a basis for the design of new treatments [12]. Whether this unique protein is on or close to the surface of the cell, which would permit the development of cytotoxic monoclonal antibodies against it, is unknown. Gene therapy may have a role to play in the treatment of CGL, especially if genetic material able to inhibit the action of the hybrid protein were discovered.

Chronic Lymphatic Leukemia (CLL)

The recent detection of younger sufferers in better health may prompt pilot trials designed to eradicate the disease completely. This may entail the use of autologous transplantation and monoclonal antibodies and complement in vitro to purge residual tumor cells from the normal marrow. CLL is very sensitive to cytotoxic agents and radiation, and if this regimen could safely be applied, then a pilot experiment to attempt obliteration of the disease would be justified. Since technology that allows identification of minimal numbers of monoclonal lymphoid cells exists, an assessment of the impact of treatment on the presence of residual disease would be possible. Similarly, in CGL, sensitive molecular biologic techniques, superior to routine cytogenetics, for the detection of abnormal genes would allow for the detection of minute quantities of residual malignant cells.

References

1. Champlin RE, Golde DW (1985) Chronic myelogenous leukemia: recent advances. Blood 65: 1039–1047
2. Thomas ED, Clift RA, Fefer A et al. (1986) Marrow transplantation for the treatment of chronic myelogenous leukemia. An Intern Med 104: 155–163
3. Talpaz M, Kantarjian HM, McCredie K et al. (1986) Hematologic remission and cytogenetic improvement induced by recombinant human interferon alpha$_a$ in chronic myelogenous leukemia. N Engl J Med 314: 1065–1069
4. Wiernik PH (1984) The current status of therapy for the prevention of blast crisis of chronic myelocytic leukemia. J Clin Oncol 2: 329–335
5. Bakhshi A, Minowada J, Arnold A et al. (1983) Lymphoid blast crises of chronic myelogenous leukemia represents stages in the development of B-cell precursors. N Engl J Med 309: 825–831
6. Karp DD, Parker LM, Binder N et al. (1985) Treatment of the blastic transformation of chronic granulocytic leukemia using high dose BCNU chemotherapy and cryopreserved autologous peripheral blood stem cells. Am J Hematol 18: 243–249
7. Rozman C, Montserrat E, Feliu E et al. (1982) Prognosis of chronic lymphocytic leukemia: a multivariate survival analysis of 150 cases. Blood 59: 1001–1005
8. Keller JW, Knospe WH, Raney M et al. (1986) Treatment of chronic lymphocytic leukemia using chlorambucil and prednisone with or without cycle-active consolidation chemotherapy. Cancer 58: 1185–1192
9. Harousseau JL, Flandrin G, Tricot G, Brouet JC et al. (1981) Malignant lymphoma supervening in chronic lymphocytic leukemia and related disorders. Cancer 48: 1302–1308
10. Sokal JE, Cox EB, Baccarani M et al. (1984) Prognostic discrimination in "good risk" chronic granulocytic leukemia. Blood 63: 789–799
11. Dillman RO, Shawler DL, Billman JB, Royston I (1984) Therapy of chronic lymphocytic leukemia and cutaneous T-cell lymphoma with T101 monoclonal antibody. J Clin Oncol 2: 881–891
12. Konopka JB, Watanabe SM, Witte ON (1984) An alteration of the human c-abl protein in K562 leukemia cells unmasks associated tyrosine kinase activity. Cell 37: 1035–1042

46. Hodgkin's Disease

D.L. Longo

Current Results and Therapeutic Issues

The high success rate in the treatment of patients with Hodgkin's disease is one of the greatest achievements in cancer therapeutics. The majority of patients with Hodgkin's disease can be cured with current state-of-the-art management, due to cooperation of surgeons, radiation therapists, and oncologists. It should be pointed out, however, that the proportion of patients cured is not as high as it could be, largely because of inadequate staging procedures, poorly designed radiation treatment portals, and ad hoc dose modifications that reduce the dose intensity of the standard chemotherapy treatment programs. Adherence to basic radiation therapy techniques and administration of the combination chemotherapy originally recommended would significantly increase the probability of cure.

As long as any subset of patients is best treated with a local treatment (i.e., with radiation therapy), and as long as intra-abdominal disease remains difficult to detect by nonivasive measures, staging laparotomy will be a crucial factor in the management of Hodgkin's disease. About one-third of patients with early stage disease have occult intra-abdominal Hodgkin's disease, which usually results in an increase to stage III. Although most stage III patients are now treated with chemotherapy, when radiation therapy is used, adjustments in treatment portals based on the laparotomy findings are often made.

Early Stage Disease (Stages IA, IB, IIA, IIB)

Since the pioneering studies of Henry Kaplan and Vera Peters were published [1, 2], radiation therapy has been the treatment of choice for early stage Hodgkin's disease; at Stanford University about 78% of patients with the disease in its early stages were cured by the initial treatment [3]. Since about half of the 22% of patients who relapse can be cured by salvage combination chemotherapy, nearly 89% of patients in whom the disease was detected in its early stages have been completely cured. Unfortunately, not all treatment centers achieve results comparable to those obtained at Stanford. In fact, documented relapse rates varying between 10% and 39% have been obtained for comparable patients treated at different centers. When reasons for this variability were sought, it was found that over one-third of randomly checked portal films failed to encompass the known extent of disease [4]. Thus, it is clear that technique is an important determinant of outcome in patients treated with radiation therapy for early stage Hodgkin's disease.

Because radiation therapy has for a long time been the standard treatment for early stage Hodgkin's disease, for subgroups of patients with an unacceptably high relapse rate, there has been a tendency simply to add combination chemotherapy to radiation therapy. However, the addition of combination chemotherapy is associated with synergistic toxicities, particularly the risk of developing acute nonlymphocytic leukemia as a second malignancy related to treatment. It would seem more reasonable to evaluate combination chemotherapy as the sole modality in patients with high relapse rates from radiation therapy. Only after radiation therapy alone has been tested and found inadequate and chemotherapy alone has failed to control primary disease is it appropriate to expose the particular patient group to both modalities. The only subgroup of patients for whom this has been done is patients with massive mediastinal Hodgkin's disease [chest mass greater than one-third of the largest posteroanterior (PA) chest diameter]. After treatment with either radiation therapy or chemotherapy, 50% or more of patients with massive mediastinal masses relapse, but fewer than 25% of patients relapse after combined modality therapy [5].

Advanced Stage Disease (Stages IIIA, IIIB, IVA, IVB)

The treatment of choice of advanced stage disease is combination chemotherapy with mechlorethamine, oncovin, procarbazine, and prednisone (MOPP) [6]. For the most part, clinical research into the treatment of advanced stage Hodgkin's disease in the last 15 years has been devoted to making small alterations in MOPP by deletion, substitution, or addition in an effort to reduce toxicity without compromising efficacy. However, to date no chemotherapy regimen has been shown to be clearly superior to MOPP. Recent reports of the superiority of MOPP with adriamycin, bleomycin, vinblastine, and dacarbazine (MOPP-ABVD) over MOPP alone require confirmation [7].

Salvage Therapy

The treatment of choice for patients relapsing from a radiation-induced complete remission is combination chemotherapy with MOPP, which will cure 50% of such patients. The treatment of choice for patients relapsing from a chemotherapy-induced complete remission depends upon the duration of initial response. In those patients whose first remission lasted longer than a year, there is a 95% chance of a second complete remission with a second course of MOPP chemotherapy. The median duration of the second remission is 3 years. If the first remission was shorter than a year, retreatment with MOPP is successful in less than 30% of patients; therefore, most researchers are attempting to develop more effective programs for such MOPP-resistant patients.

Although a number of combination chemotherapy programs have been established, they are minimally effective in well-defined MOPP-resistant patients (less than 20% long-term disease-free survival). The most successful treatment of MOPP—resistant patients is with high-dose combination chemotherapy with autologous bone marrow rescue. About 40%–50% of patients obtain durable complete remission with such an approach [8]. The success of high-dose chemotherapy with marrow rescue suggests that it may be very important to maximize dose intensity in front-line treatment programs.

Current Approaches Under Study

One major challenge in the management of Hodgkin's disease is the development of accurate noninvasive methods to detect intra-abdominal disease. The introduction of magnetic resonance imaging has improved intra-abdominal visualization to some degree, but it still is not as accurate at detecting lymph node disease as lymphography and is not more reliable than the quite unreliable computerized tomography (CT) scanning in detecting splenic disease. Perhaps with the development of better contrast-enhancing agents for magnetic resonance imaging this technique will be able to save some patients from undergoing laparotomy.

An excellent contrast-enhancing agent has been developed for use in conjunction with CT scanning. EOE-13 is a water soluble oil emulsion taken up by the Kupffer's cells of the liver and the sinusoidal lining cells of the spleen such that distortions in the normal architecture are much more readily detected. Hodgkin's disease cells do not take up EOE-13, and thus a tumor appears less dense on a CT scan than normal hepatic and splenic parenchyma. Tumors greater than 8 mm in diameter can be reliably detected. If systematically applied, it might save up to 25% of patients from undergoing an exploratory laparotomy.

The development of monoclonal antibodies like Ki-1 and Hefi-1 to Hodgkin's disease cell lines now makes it possible to perform radioimmunoimaging in patients with Hodgkin's disease. Injected into the web spaces of the feet, a radiolabled antibody can be used to perform radiolymphography, while intravenous administration may successfully visualize splenic and hepatic disease. Clinical imaging studies with labeled antibodies are just beginning, and may further refine the noninvasive staging procedure in patients with Hodgkin's disease. It is also possible that the antigen to which these antibodies are directed may be present in the serum of patients in proportion to the bulk (and, it is hoped, stage) of the tumor. Efforts to evaluate this antigen as a tumor marker are underway.

Combination chemotherapy alone has only recently been tested in patients with the disease in its early stages. Preliminary data from a prospective randomized study conducted at the National Cancer Institute, USA, suggest that patients treated with MOPP chemotherapy have a significantly lower relapse rate than those treated with subtotal lymphoid irradiation, but that the overall survival rate is similar with both treatments largely because of the success of

MOPP in treating radiation relapsers. Since radiation and chemotherapy treatments have distinct acute and chronic toxicities, long-term follow-up may be necessary before determining whether chemotherapy is actually superior to radiation therapy. However, there is no doubt that chemotherapy is at least as, and perhaps even more, effective than radiation therapy for treating early stage disease and that the use of combined modality therapy in early stage Hodgkin's disease (except for cases with large mediastinal masses) is unjustified. If combination chemotherapy proved to be as good as or better than radiation therapy, there would no longer be any reason to subject patients to exploratory laparotomy since all patients could be treated appropriately with systemic therapy.

Perhaps the most encouraging recent results in patients with advanced stage disease have been obtained in a pilot study by Klimo and Connors [9] with a regimen called MOPP-ABV in which patients are exposed to seven drugs in one week. It will be important to study this regimen in a randomized trial, comparing it with standard MOPP administered without ad hoc dose and schedule alterations.

The major problem in advanced stage disease is the treatment of patients with B symptoms, since a relapse from MOPP-induced remission in stages IIIA and IVA of the disease is quite rare. It may be appropriate to test the newer, more successful malignant lymphoma therapies, like ProMACE-CytaBOM (prednisone, doxorubicin, cyclophosphamide, etoposide, ara-C, bleomycin, vincristine) and MACOP-B (methotrexate, doxorubicin, cyclophosphamide, vincristine, prednisone, bleomycin), in stages IIIB and IVB of Hodgkin's disease.

Future Approaches

Hryniuk and Bush's [10] analysis of the outcome of breast cancer and ovarian cancer treatment as a function of the dose intensity of the chemotherapy program has provided a clinical paradigm for the development of more effective treatments for advanced stage and relapsed Hodgkin's disease. The remarkable success of using a single high-dose course of chemotherapy with marrow rescue suggests that there may well be a very steep dose-response curve in Hodgkin's disease. It seems quite reasonable to bring high-dose therapy plus autologous bone marrow rescue into the front-line treatment of advanced stage Hodgkin's disease. After obtaining a chemotherapy-induced complete response, patients may receive a course of high-dose combination chemotherapy to minimize relapse. Alternatively, the development of strategies to protect the bone marrow against the toxic effects of radiation and chemotherapy (for example, using the colony stimulating factors) raises the prospect that it may be possible to deliver combination chemotherapy at a full dose without any delays for six full cycles of chemotherapy. A study employing MOPP chemotherapy without dose modifications but with marrow protection by GM-CSF is soon to begin at the National Cancer Institute.

Rapid advances in biotechnology have also made it possible to consider a number of other treatment strategies. For example, Hodgkin's disease cells have a very high proportion of transferrin receptors. Attacking the receptor with monoclonal antibodies alone or conjugated to a toxin like the recombinant ricin A chain or *Pseudomonas* exotoxin should be high on the priority list for clinical testing. Furthermore, the study of Hodgkin's disease cell lines has revealed the production of autocrine growth factors which is may well be possible to block with an attendant therapeutic effect. The recombinant lymphokines, interferons, IL-2, and tumor necrosis factor are just beginning to be tested. It is likely that at least some of the constitutional symptoms accompanying Hodgkin's disease are related to some product of the Hodgkin's cell. The study of the cell biology of the Hodgkin's disease cell lines may reveal other characteristics that could be exploited by biological approaches to treatment.

One of the most exciting prospects for treating Hodgkin's disease involves attempting to recruit the many apparently normal T cells that infiltrate tumor deposits of Hodgkin's disease. Adoptive cellular therapy with lymphokine-activated killer cells plus IL-2 is currently underway at the National Cancer Institute. The possibility that the tumor will respond better to combined chemotherapy and immunotherapy is also under study. The data are too preliminary to evaluate this. However, it seems highly likely that chemotherapy and immunotherapy in some combination will be the standard treatment for patients with Hodgkin's disease within the next decade.

References

1. Peters MV (1950) A study of survival in Hodgkin's disease treated radiologically. Am J Roentgenol 62: 299–311
2. Kaplan HS (1962) The radical radiotherapy of regionally localized Hodgkin's disease. Radiology 78: 5533–561
3. Hoppe RT, Coleman CN, Cox RS et al. (1982) The management of stage I-II Hodgkin's disease with irradiation alone or combined modality therapy: the Stanford experience. Blood 59: 455
4. Kinzie JJ, Hanks GE, Maclean CJ, Kramer S (1983) Patterns of care study: Hodgkin's disease relapse rates and adequacy of portals. Cancer 52: 2223
5. Mauch P, Goodman R, Hellman S (1978) The significance of mediastinal involvement in early stage Hodgkin's disease. Cancer 42: 1039
6. Longo DL, Young RC, Wesley M, Hubbard SM, Duffey PL, Jaffe ES, DeVita VT (1986) Twenty years of MOPP therapy for Hodgkin's disease. J Clin Oncol 4: 1295
7. Bonadonna G, Valagussa P, Santoro A (1986) Alternating non-cross-resistant combination chemotherapy of MOPP in stage IV Hodgkin's disease. Ann Intern Med 104: 739
8. Jagannath S, Dicke KA, Armitage JO et al. (1986) High-dose cyclophosphamide, carmustine, and etoposide and autologous bone marrow transplantation for relapsed Hodgkin's disease. Ann Intern Med 104: 163
9. Klimo P, Connors JM (1985) MOPP/ABV hybrid program: combination chemotherapy based on early introduction of seven effective drugs for advanced Hodgkin's disease. J Clin Oncol 3: 1174
10. Hryniuk, W, Bush H (1984) The importance of dose intensity in chemotherapy of metastatic breast cancer. J Clin Oncol 2: 1281

47. Plasma Cell Myeloma

I.C. Quirt and D.E. Bergsagel

Current Results and Therapeutic Issues

Plasma cell myeloma is a chronic disease affecting mainly older patients. Although patients with a very low plasma cell mass survive for a long time, the median survival period for all patients presenting with plasma cell myeloma is still only 30 months. While the majority of patients respond to the administration of chemotherapy and radiation therapy, there is still no evidence that treatment is curative. The early recognition and prompt treatment of hypercalcemia, renal failure, neurological complications and infection is of paramount importance in improving the quality of life of patients with myeloma.

Some patients present with smoldering myeloma (serum M protein level greater than 3.0 g/dl, greater than 10% plasma cells in the bone marrow but no evidence of bone lesions, renal failure, or anemia). These patients do not require immediate treatment but must be kept under careful observation.

In patients with symptoms (bone lesions, renal insufficiency, anemia, thrombocytopenia, or a rising serum or urine M protein level) chemotherapy, with radiation to local painful bone lesions, is the standard treatment. The conventional treatment used throughout the 1960s and 1970s consisted of melphalan (0.25 mg/kg for 4 days or 0.15 mg/kg for 6 days) and prednisone (100 mg od for 4 days or 20 mg tid for 7 days) repeated every 4–6 weeks according to blood counts. With this approach 50%–60% of patients experienced an objective response. Varying response rates were seen depending on the definition of response and the patient population being studied.

Several groups have attempted to improve response and survival rates by using either combinations of alkylating agents and prednisone or combinations of doxorubicin, vincristine, alkylating agents, and prednisone.

The Southwest Oncology Group (SWOG) studied a combination of vincristine, melphalan, cyclophosphamide, and prednisone alternated with either a combination of vincristine, cyclophosphamide, doxorubicin, and prednisone or with a combination of vincristine, carmustine, doxorubicin, and prednisone in a prospective comparison with melphalan and prednisone alone. The combinations produced a 53% response rate and a median survival duration of 40 months, whereas melphalan and prednisone alone produced a 32% response rate and a median survival duration of 24 months.

The Cancer and Leukemia Group B (CALGB) compared a combination of melphalan, cyclophosphamide, carmustine, and prednisone with melphalan and prednisone alone. They obtained a 68% objective response rate with the combination and a 56% objective response rate with melphalan and prednisone alone. The statistical significance of this difference was borderline. The CALGB study demonstrated a slight improvement in survival the poor-risk patients treated with the combination, whereas in the good-risk patients a slight improvement in survival was seen when they were treated with melphalan and prednisone alone.

The Eastern Cooperative Oncology Group (ECOG) compared vincristine, carmustine, cyclophosphamide, melphalan, and prednisone with melphalan and prednisone alone. They observed an objective response rate of 72% with the combination and 51% with melphalan and prednisone. This difference was highly statistically singificant. However, the median survival was 31 months in patients treated with the combination and 30 months in patients treated with melphalan and prednisone. The ECOG's observations on overall survival contradicted those made by the CALGB. If high-risk elderly patients were excluded there was a trend to improved overall survival in patients treated with the combination [1]. Studies from Canada, Argentina, and the M.D. Anderson Hospital failed to demonstrate any improvement in response rate or in overall survival when combinations were compared with melphalan and prednisone alone [2].

While there is still a debate as to whether combinations can provide a marginal improvement in overall survival, no study has yet demonstrated a chemotherapy regimen that provides a major improvement in the survival period as compared with treatment with melphalan and prednisone alone. Comparison studies with several hundred patients per study arm will be required to determine the role of combination chemotherapy in subsets such as elderly patients, patients with renal failure, and patients with high- or low-plasma-cell mass. Major improvements in the overall survival outlook and perhaps even cure of the disease will require the advent of new chemotherapy drugs or the application of biological response modifiers.

Recent studies have demonstrated that maintenance chemotherapy can prolong remissions in patients who respond to it but that it will not alter the overall survival period. Patients may experience major and prolonged symptoms from relapse; therefore, the current recommendation is to discontinue chemotherapy when the patient has achieved a stable objective remission, to check the serum M protein level frequently, recommencing treatment when there is evidence that the serum or urine M protein level is rising, before symptoms develop.

Current Approaches Under Study

Although the majority of patients initially have an objective response to either combination chemotherapy or melphalan and prednisone, most patients will relapse and become resistant to their induction treatment. In addition, 30%–40%

of patients will be initially refractory to treatment. Much of the current clinical investigation is focused on these relapsed and refractory patients.

A 4-day continuous infusion of vincristine (0.4 mg/day) and doxorubicin (9 mg/m^2 per day) with dexamethasone (40 mg) each morning for 4 days beginning on day 1, 9, and 17 of each cycle (Vincristine, Adriamycin, Doxorubicin, VAD) produced a 63% objective response rate in patients relapsing after an initial response to other chemotherapy and a 25%–30% response rate in patients who were initially refractory to chemotherapy [3, 4]. The same dose of dexamethasone without the vincristine and doxorubicin gave a 21% response rate in patients relapsing after other chemotherapy and a 27% response rate in patients who were initially refractory to chemotherapy [4, 5]. The median relapse-free survival time had not been reached at the time of publication but the majority of responses will exceed 6 months. Two patients who relapsed 4 and 6 months after completion of VAD therapy experienced a second response when VAD treatment was recommenced. Infection is the most important complication of this regimen. Of 29 patients, 11 experienced episodes of fever, 9 required hospitalization, and 8 had documented infection. Because high-dose corticosteroid therapy is being given during the period of maximum myelosuppression, it is recommended that prophylactic cimetidine and trimethoprim-sulfamethoxazole be administered. If patients have received extensive previous chemotherapy and radiation, severe myelosuppression is observed; therefore, in this group of patients VAD must be used with extreme caution. This regimen deserves further evaluation as first-line treatment for myeloma.

The hypothesis that increasing the dose of an effective chemotherapy drug might increase the proportion of myeloma cells that were killed and hence improve the proportion and duration of responses has been tested by giving extremely high doses of melphalan, with and without autologous bone marrow transplantation, to patients with both untreated and refractory myeloma. In the original series, in all nine patients there was a rapid reduction in the serum or urine M protein level, but one patient died of a fungal infection in remission, and a second patient experienced rapid recurrence within 2 months of treatment [6]. In the second series, 16 patients were given 80–100 mg/m^2 of melphalan, and 7 were given 140 mg/m^2 followed by autologous bone marrow infusion. Six of the 16 patients treated without autologous bone marrow support responded to treatment, but 4 patients died because of marked and prolonged agranulocytosis and severe thrombocytopenia. Four of the seven patients receiving autologous bone marrow support responded, and only one patient died because of severe myelosuppression [7]. If methods can be found to purge the autologous bone marrow of the malignant clone of plasma cells, the technique of giving high-dose melphalan followed by autologous bone marrow transplantation may become more widely used in younger patients.

Both natural and recombinant α-2 interferon have been shown to have effect in patients with both relapsed and primarily refractory myeloma. The Myeloma Group of central Sweden observed objective remissions in five of eight previously untreated patients and two of six relapsed patients using human leukocyte interferon of the α type prepared from human leukocytes exposed to the Sendai

568

virus. They then compared this preparation of interferon to standard melphalan and prednisone as an induction treatment in untreated patients. Of the patients receiving melphalan and prednisone, 44% had objective responses, whereas 14% of the patients receiving interferon had objective responses. Since all the patients who failed to respond to one treatment received the opposite treatment as second-line therapy, no differences in overall survival duration were found [8].

A multicenter phase 2 study of recombinant α-2 interferon demonstrated objective responses in 2 of 19 patients with refractory myeloma and 5 of 19 patients with relapsed myeloma. In three of the seven patients who responded to treatment the disease is still in remission more than a year after the start of treatment [9].

Although the Swedish study indicated that interferon should not be used as induction therapy, it may be able to prolong remissions in patients who have initially responded to traditional chemotherapy. The Myeloma Subcommittee of the National Cancer Institute of Canada is currently testing this hypothesis in a randomized clinical trial.

Future Approaches

Other than natural and recombinant α-interferon, the biological response modifiers have not yet been adequately evaluated in patients with myeloma. Interleukin-1 can activate the resting B cell and therefore might temporarily increase the growth rate of myeloma cells. While theoretically this might have a deleterious effect on the clinical activity of the patient's disease, the alternative hypothesis is that the cells might be rendered more susceptible to being killed by chemotherapy. The temporary increase in clinical activity of the disease could be controlled with high-dose corticosteroid therapy. γ-Interferon may have similar effects. Interleukin-2 can stimulate the release of B-cell growth factor and B-cell differentiation factor from proliferating T cells and can also have a direct effect in causing the differentiation of B cells [10]. Tumor necrosis factor (TNF) will have to be used with extreme caution in patients with myeloma since TNF-beta appears to be the predominant osteoclast-activating factor in patients with multiple myeloma.

If any of the biological response modifiers can induce the differentiation of myeloma cells into more mature plasma cells, myeloma may then adopt the characteristics of monoclonal gammopathy of undetermined significance (MGUS), and the survival of patients may be prolonged. The evaluation of the biological response modifiers will be the next phase in the clinical investigation of myeloma.

References

1. Oken MM, Tsiati A, Abramson N, Glick J (1987) Evaluation of intensive (VBMCP) vs standard (MP) therapy for multiple myeloma. J Clin Oncol 6: 203 (abstr)
2. Bergsagel DE (1985) Controversies in the treatment of plasma cell myeloma. Postgrad Med J 61: 109
3. Barlogie B, Smith L, Alexanian R (1984) Effective treatment of advanced multiple myeloma refractory to alkylating agents. N Engl J Med 310: 1353
4. Alexanian R, Barlogie B, Dixon D (1986) Update of VAD for resistant multiple myeloma. Proc 5: 167
5. Alexanian R, Barlogie B, Dixon D (1986) High-dose glucocorticoid treatment of resistant myeloma. Ann Intern Med 105: 8
6. McElwain TJ, Powles RL (1983) High-dose intravenous melphalan for plasma-cell leukaemia and myeloma. Lancet 8353: 822
7. Barlogie B, Hall R, Zander A, Dicke K, Alexanian R (1986) High-dose melphalan with autologous bone marrow transplantation for multiple myeloma. Blood 67: 1298
8. Ahre A, Bjorkholm M, Mellstedt H, Brenning G, Engstedt L, Gahrton G, Gyllenhammar H, Holm G, Johansson B, Jarnmark M, Karnstrom L, Killander A, Lerner R, Lockner D, Lonnqvist B, Nilsson B: Simonsson B, Stalfelt AM, Strander H, Svedmyr E, Wadman B, Wedelin C (1984) Human leukocyte interferon versus intermittent high-dose melphalan-prednisone administration in the treatment of multiple myeloma: a randomized clinical trial from the Myeloma Group of Central Sweden. Cancer Treat Rep 68: 1331
9. Costanzi JJ, Cooper MR, Scarffe JH, Ozer H, Grubbs SS, Ferraresi RW, Pollard RB, Spiegel RJ (1985) Phase II study of recombinant alpha-2 inteferon in resistant multiple myeloma. J Clin Oncol 3: 654
10. Fauci AS (1987) Immunomodulators in clinical medicine. Ann Intern Med 106: 421

48. Follicular Non-Hodgkin's Lymphomas

S.J. Horning

Current Results and Therapeutic Issues

The follicular non-Hodgkin's lymphomas are B-cell neoplasms which typically present in an advanced stage, often with bone marrow involvement and diffuse adenopathy. Patients are usually middle aged and asymptomatic at presentation. Many give a history of adenopathy coming and going for several years preceding the pathologic diagnosis. There are three histologic subtypes of follicular lymphoma: follicular small cleaved cell (FSC), follicular mixed small cleaved and large cell (FM), and follicular large cell (FLC) (nodular poorly differentiated lymphocytic, nodular mixed poorly differentiated, and histiocytic or nodular histiocytic, respectively, in the Rappaport classification). Of these, FSC is the most common, comprising about 23% of all non-Hodgkin's lymphomas. Some studies suggest that there are important differences in the natural course of the disease and response to treatment between the three subtypes while others have failed to confirm these. It is important to recognize that there is great variability in the pathologic criteria and reproducibility in the subclassification of the follicular lymphomas, even among expert pathologists. Futhermore, multiple (discordant) histologic subtypes are found in as many as 20%–30% of patients when more than one biopsy is obtained at diagnosis.

A variety of systemic approaches including single alkylating agents, combination chemotherapy, whole body irradiation, and combined chemoradiotherapy have been used to treat advanced stage follicular lymphomas [1]. While complete response rates range from 40%–80%, recurrent lymphoma develops in the vast majority of patients with median remission durations of 2–4 years. There is data from small, uncontrolled trials which suggest that FM and FLC patients may enjoy prolonged initial remissions with four-drug combination chemotherapy; these have not been confirmed in randomized trials with a sufficient number of patients. In comparing treatment results, the documentation of remission duration by the ongoing assessment of occult disease sites such as bone marrow and abdominopelvic lymph nodes should be noted. The best measure of success, in the final analysis, is of course the impact therapy has on survival, and it is not clear whether any current treatment approach improves upon the median survival time of 6–10 years in patients with follicular lymphomas [2].

The failure of conventional therapy to effect cure, together with the frequently indolent course of recurrent lymphomas and the occasional spontaneous regression of the disease, has led some investigators to advocate no initial treatment of selected patients, as survival does not appear to be compromised by such an approach [3]. While first considered controversial, this approach has become standard practice for many patients with newly diagnosed follicular lymphoma. Patients in whom the disease is not bulky and is limited to fewer than five anatomic sites are an exception, as regional or total nodal irradiation may allow prolonged initial remission, especially among younger patients. Among all patients initially untreated or suffering a relapse after therapy, there is an increasing risk of the disease transforming to a more aggressive, diffuse histologic subtype. The challenge in new approaches to treatment is to prolong survival with curative therapy which may also eliminate the risk of developing an aggressive non-Hodgkin's lymphoma.

Current Approaches Under Study

Current clinical investigations of the follicular lymphomas can be divided into three groups: (a) studies which test the efficacy of intensive multidrug regimens with or without irradiation; (b) studies which test the efficacy of biological response modifiers alone or in combination, either with one another or with conventional therapy; and (c) studies which utilize new molecular tools to aid diagnosis and evaluation of response or to provide prognostic information.

Pilot studies of multidrug combination chemotherapy with additional agents such as doxorubicin, methotrexate, and bleomycin are underway in several institutions [4]. In an ongoing trial at the National Cancer Institute, USA, patients are randomized to an eight-drug combination with low-dose, total lymphoid irradiation at presentation, or to deferral of therapy until clinically indicated. While the preliminary results appear promising among the initial therapy group, longer follow-up is necessary to determine the curative potential and the impact on survival of this approach. High-dose chemotherapy and total body irradiation with autologous or allogeneic bone marrow rescue is also under investigation in follicular lymphoma. While there are only anecdotal preliminary data for this approach, it is an important study which will provide the ultimate test of intensive chemotherapy and radiotherapy for treating follicular lymphomas. If successful, greater enthusiasm for the study of additional chemotherapeutic agents in intensive multidrug regimens may be generated.

α-Interferon has been shown to act against follicular lymphomas in multiple studies, achieving partial remissions, usually of brief duration [5, 6], in about 40%–50% of patients. There are several, controlled, randomized trials underway which combine interferon with conventional chemotherapy with the goal of boosting response rates and increasing the duration of remission. Theoretically, interferon may cause regression of follicular lymphoma by its antiproliferative activity, by its enhancement of natural killer cells or of killer cell activity, or by a variety of effects on cell growth and regulation. Selection of the optimal dose and schedule for the desired effect may be critical for the successful use of interferon-chemotherapy combinations.

Another area of active clinical research among the biologicals is the use of therapeutic monoclonal antibodies. As virtually all follicular lymphomas are B-cell neoplasms, they have a unique surface immunoglobulin or idiotype. Monoclonal antibodies to these lymphoma-specific idiotypes prepared by murine hybridoma techniques are known as anti-idiotypes. Researchers at Stanford University have reported lymphoma responses in about half the patients treated with anti-idiotypic monoclonal antibodies [7]. As with interferon, the majority of responses have not been complete and have lasted only several months. Failure to respond completely to monoclonal antibody therapy is often related to the emergence of idiotype variants, a phenomenon in which there is mutation in the hypervariable region of the surface idiotypic immunoglobulin which in turn affects the binding of the monoclonal antibody [8]. Additional difficulties encountered with this approach have included the development of an immune response against mouse protein and the saturation of the therapeutic antibody by the circulating idiotype. Various strategies could be employed to overcome these problems. One under study in follicular lymphoma is based on a murine B-cell lymphoma model which demonstrates synergy between an anti-idiotypic monoclonal antibody and an α-interferon.

Another biological agent of interest in follicular lymphoma is interleukin 2 (IL-2). Several anecdotal responses have been reported by investigators at the National Cancer Institute using IL-2 together with lymphokine-activated killer cells. This is being pursued further at several centers. Trials of interest currently in development include those which use IL-2 alone, those which use combinations of IL-2 and interferon, or those which use multiple interferons.

Advances in molecular genetics, especially the understanding of immunoglobulin gene rearrangement, have greatly expanded our knowledge of the follicular lymphomas. Assessment of immunoglobulin gene rearrangements by Southern blot analysis can "fingerprint" individual malignant clones [9]. Given the ability of this technique to identify a 1% clonal population, a more sensitive diagnostic assay of the peripheral blood and bone marrow can be envisaged. The diagnostic sensitivity, specificity, and predictive accuracy of the Southern blot analysis is now under study in large populations of patients. Cytogenetic studies of the follicular lymphomas have yielded a characteristic karyotype, the 14;18 translocation. DNA probes encompassing a putative oncogene (bcl-2) have also been cloned. These are now being employed in research centers to characterize follicular lymphomas. Studies such as these may also improve understanding of critical events in the natural development of follicular lymphomas such as spontaneous regression, histologic transformation, and recurrence.

Future Approaches

Preliminary studies with radiolabeled antibodies, pan-B cell and anti-idiotypic, are in progress. In some instances, these have been combined with purged, autologous marrow. Additional studies with monoclonal antibodies will very probably utilize new techniques for the efficient development of antibodies directed against multiple idiotypic determinants and the conjugation of monoclonal antibodies to antineoplastic agents or toxins. It may prove desirable to introduce such treatments after initial cytoreduction with conventional therapy.

Recombinant DNA technology will undoubtedly provide additional biological agents for clinical study. Further advances in the understanding of the transcriptional and translational regulation of immunoglobulin genes will hopefully allow the identification of regulatory factors promising for clinical study. These are tremendously exciting avenues of basic and clinical research which should yield new approaches to the treatment of the follicular lymphomas [10].

References

1. Rosenberg SA (1985) Karnofsky Memorial Lecture: the low grade non-Hodgkin's lymphomas: challenges and opportunities J Clin Oncol 3: 299
2. Jones SE (1986) Follicular lymphoma—do no harm. Cancer Treat Rep 70: 1055
3. Horning SJ, Rosenberg SA (1984) The natural history of initially untreated low grade non-Hodgkin's lymphomas. N Engl J Med 311: 1471
4. Anderson KC, Skarin AT, Rosenthal DJ, MacIntyre JM, Pinkus GS, Case DC Jr, Leonard RC, Canellos GP (1984) Combination chemotherapy for advanced non-Hodgkin's lymphomas other than diffuse histiocytic or undifferentiated histologies. Cancer Treat Rep 68: 1343
5. Foon KA, Sherwin SA, Abrams PG, Longo DL, Fer MF, Stevenson HC, Ochs JJ, Bottino GC, Schoenberger CS, Zeffren J, Jaffe ES, Oldham RK (1984) Treatment of advanced non-Hodgkin's lymphoma with recombinant leukocyte A-interferon. N Engl J Med 311: 1148
6. Horning SJ (1984) Interferon and malignant lym ma. In: Zoon KC, Noguchi PD, Liu T-Y (eds) Interferon: Research, clinical application and regulatory consideration. Elsevier, New York, p 229
7. Miller RA, Maloney DG, Warnke R, Levy R (1982) Treatment of B-cell lymphoma with monoclonal anti-idiotype antibody. N Engl J Med 306: 517
8. Meeker T, Lowder J, Cleary ML, Stewart S, Warnke R, Sklar J, Levy R (1985) Emergence of idiotype variants during treatment of B-cell lymphoma with anti-idiotype antibodies. N Engl J Med 312: 1658
9. Cleary ML, Chao J, Warnke R, Sklar J (1984) Immunoglobulin gene rearrangement as a diagnostic criterion of B-cell lymphoma. Proc N' l Acad Sci USA 81: 593
10. Cheson BD, Wittes RE, Friedman MA (1986) Low-grade non-Hodgkin's lymphomas revisited. Cancer Treat Rep 70: 1051

49. Diffuse Aggressive Lymphomas in Adults*

W.J. Urba and D.L. Longo

Current Results and Therapeutic Issues

The aggressive lymphomas are nodular histiocytic (follicular, large cell), diffuse histiocytic (diffuse, large cell and diffuse, immunoblastic), diffuse undifferentiated (Burkitt's and non-Burkitt's) and lymphoblastic lymphoma [1]. In general, patients with aggressive lymphomas present with rapidly progressing tumor masses, often in nodal sites. There is also a high incidence of extranodal disease in the gastrointestinal tract, skin, bone, thyroid, testes, and other sites. If complete remission (CR) can be obtained in these patients, there is potential for cure. However, the failure to induce CR in approximately one-fourth of patients and the 30%–50% relapse rate mandate further research into the treatment of aggressive non-Hodgkin's lymphomas (NHLs).

Limited Stage Disease

In approximately 25%–30% of patients, extensive diagnostic efforts demonstrate that the disease is relatively localized, i.e., stage I or II. The current trend is toward the use of combination chemotherapy in these patients. Even with the benefit of staging laparotomy, radiation alone results in unacceptably high relapse rates in stage II patients. In one study, for example, 10 of 14 stage II patients relapsed less than 2 years after treatment with radiation alone. Chemotherapy alone in stage I patients gives results comparable to radiation, while results with chemotherapy alone in stage II disease are superior to those achieved with radiation alone.

The major question in patients with the disease in its early stages is whether any subset of clinically staged patients can be treated with radiation therapy alone with a nearly 100% probability of cure of whether all patients should receive chemotherapy. Other questions include: Can less aggressive (toxic?)

*Research sponsored, at least in part, by the National Cancer Institute, DHHS, under contract NO1-CO-23910 with Program Resources, Incorporated. The contents of this publication do not necessarily reflect the views or policies of the DHHS, nor does mention of trade names, commercial products, or organizations imply endorsement by the U.S. Government.

575

chemotherapy achieve the same high CR rates? Is there a need for combined modality therapy in these patients?

Advanced Stage Disease

The results for advanced stage aggressive lymphoma have improved steadily over the last 15 years (see Table 1). During the 1960s, 5-year survival with aggressive lymphoma was unusual. Complete remissions with single agents were rare, and it was not until combination chemotherapy was employed that long-term disease-free survival was obtained. Current regimens employ multiple drugs at frequent intervals and often alternate two effective and presumably non-cross-resistant chemotherapeutic regimens. Each successive treatment has led to an increase in CR and long-term survival rates such that there are now a number of regimens capable of inducing prolonged disease-free survival in 50%–60% of patients. These apparent improvements must be examined carefully, however, since these regimens have not been compared in prospective randomized trials and are therefore subject to the problems associated with the use of historical controls. The median follow-up period varies between studies, but all have included patients less than 2 years from remission induction who must be considered at risk of suffering a relapse. Some studies have included stage I and/or stage II patients who may have a more favorable prognosis while others have added radiation treatment to the combination chemotherapy. The studies also vary in their criteria for patient selection and stratification for known clinical prognostic variables. Clearly, long-term follow-up is needed for all the newer regimens. We eagerly await the results of a prospective randomized study being

Table 1. Evolution of combination chemotherapy for the treatment of aggressive non-Hodgkin's lymphomas

Treatment	CR (%)	Relapse (%)	3-year survival (%)
Single agent	5	NA	NA
CVP	10	NA	NA
C-MOPP/MOPP, BACOP	46	15	39
CHOP/HOP	67/60	60	25
BACOP	56	40	34
COMLA	55	15	47
COP-BLAM	73	17	61
M-BACOD	72	26	60
ProMACE-MOPP	74	18	61
CHOP/HOAP-Bleo/IMVP-16	82	20	71
MACOP-B	82	19	NA
ProMACE-CytaBOM	85	20	NA
F-MACHOP	81	19	NA

CR, complete remission
NA, not available

conducted by the Southwest Oncology Group investigating response rates, remission duration, and the toxicity of conventional and more aggressive regimens.

One question remaining is whether the prognosis of patients with large gastrointestinal masses can be improved by surgical debulking prior to treatment.

Current Approaches Under Study

Despite aggressive combination chemotherapy, almost 50% of patients still die of the disease. The regimens are complicated, not easily applied in a community hospital or general practice setting, and result in the death of 5%–10% of patients from treatment-related causes.

Recent work has focused on the identification of prognostic factors for predicting response and survival. One prognostic factor is histology. Lymphoblastic lymphomas, HTLV-I associated adult T-cell leukemia/lymphoma, and the undifferentiated lymphomas (Burkitt's and non-Burkitt's) respond less well than the other histologic subtypes to lymphoma regimens. Recently, the use of more aggressive leukemia-like treatment approaches with induction, consolidation, and late intensification components has resulted in a higher response rate and more durable remissions in patients with some of the high-grade histologic subtypes mentioned above, particularly in patients with lymphoblastic lymphomas.

The clinical features that predict response to therapy and the disease-free interval have been known for some time and basically relate to tumor burden. The major poor prognostic factors are elevated lactic dehydrogenase (LDH) and bulky disease, especially in the gastrointestinal tract. In addition, poor performance status and B symptoms (fever, night sweats or weight loss) are associated with a poorer response to treatment. Age has been called a poor prognostic factor but may relate more to the clinician's attitude than to the patient's tumor. In studies designed to address this point, it has been shown that given equal chemotherapy, CR and the survival rate for elderly patients need not be inferior to that attained in younger patients. While it is true that there may be more toxicity, low doses of therapy offer little prospect of cure.

A number of new treatment programs are being tested in patients with advanced stage aggressive lymphoma. The dominant ideas guiding the development of chemotherapy regimens have been the Goldie-Coldman hypothesis [2] and Hryniuk's dose-intensity hypothesis [3]. The Goldie-Coldman hypothesis predicts that the early use of the maximum number of agents at full dose will be associated with less emergence of drug resistance and superior disease control. Hryniuk's dose-intensity hypothesis proposes that the best treatment results will occur when a maximum rate of drug delivery is maintained. An oversimplified amalgamation of both ideas is that the use of more drugs at higher doses administered as soon as possible and as frequently as possible will achieve the best results.

Preliminary results with three regimens, MACOP-B [4], ProMACE-CytaBOM, and F-MACHOP [5], suggest that this may be true. MACOP-B emphasizes dose intensity, F-MACHOP early exposure to approximately twice as many drugs as the usual regimen, and ProMACE-CytaBOM both dose intensity and more drugs. All three programs have achieved complete responses in around 80% of patients with only 15%–20% relapsing within the first 2 years (the period of maximal risk of relapse). If these results hold true with longer follow-up, nearly two-thirds of patients may have been cured.

More support for the importance of dose intensity has been gained by studies employing autologus bone marrow transplantation (with or without purging of undetectable residual tumor with drugs or monoclonal antibodies) in patients with aggressive lymphoma who have suffered a relapse [6]. Such patients have a poor prognosis with conventional therapy. The use of high-dose chemotherapy with or without total body irradiation and with autologous marrow transplantation has resulted in second remissions lasting longer than a year in about 40% of patients; some of these patients may actually have been cured. The intensive therapy is clearly most beneficial to patients with no disease or minimal residual disease at the time of the high-dose therapy. Further increases in the doses of drugs in primary and salvage lymphoma treatment programs may be possible with the use of biological agents (e.g., hematopoietic growth factors) that may protect or enhance the recovery of marrow.

Future Approaches to Aggressive Lymphoma Management

The staging of patients with aggressive lymphoma and the definition of complete remission are already being refined experimentally by the application of molecular probes and monoclonal antibodies. The identification of persistent tumor at the level of one cell in 10^5 or 10^6 normal cells in marrow, spleen, or lymph nodes is possible with flow cytometric analysis of cell surface antigens. The detection of clonal rearrangements of immunoglobulin or T-cell antigen receptor genes and in situ hybridization with cDNA probes designed to detect chromosomal rearrangements specific for lymphomas [e.g., bcl-2 in nodular lymphomas with t(14;18)] have also been important for the understanding of the biology of these diseases.

Perhaps the most promising path for future investigation involves the application of strategies (usually employing biological agents) to protect or enhance the recovery of bone marrow while, at the same time, increasing the dose and frequency of administration of the chemotherapeutic agents that have been demonstrated to be active at the doses already being tolerated. Interleukin-1 pretreatment can convert an LD_{100} dose of radiation to an LD_5 dose, and can produce a dose-modifying factor of 1.25, an enormous protective effect in radiobiology. The cloning of the various colony stimulating factors has led to preclinical experiments demonstrating their capacity both to protect animals from lethal doses of chemotherapeutic agents and to accelerate recovery of the granulocyte count. Whether the antitumor effects of the drugs are affected by these marrow protection strategies remains to be determined.

The integration of biological antitumor therapies into combination chemotherapy programs also has enormous potential for improving the treatment of patients with aggressive lymphoma. Monoclonal antibody regimens (alone, in combinations or cocktails, and conjugated to toxins, isotopes, drugs, or other biological agents) are in various phases of clinical testing. A number of cytokines and lymphokines, especially interleukin-2 with or without lymphokine activated killer (LAK) cells, have potential as useful therapeutic tools [7]. Responses have now been seen in lymphoma patients.

Finally, it is likely that the ongoing intensive study of lymphoma biology will yield information leading to new ideas for lymphoma treatment. For example, it is clear that the antibody to T3 (CD3), a nonpolymorphic portion of the T-cell antigen receptor, can stimulate the proliferation of normal T cells, but paradoxically inhibits the proliferation of malignant T cells expressing T3. The antibody to T3 may be of therapeutic value for certain peripheral T-cell lymphomas. Other factors that regulate the proliferation of malignant lymphocytes, like oncogenes, growth factor receptors, and autocrine growth signals are under investigation and are likely to reveal vulnerabilities that are exploitable by the expanding therapeutic armamentarium of biological agents. The study of the responses of neoplastic cells to these agents or their antagonists is likely to be extremely rewarding.

References

1. Urba WJ, Longo DL (1985) Cytologic, immunologic, and clinical diversity in non-Hodgkin's lymphoma: therapeutic implications. Semin Oncol 12: 250
2. Goldie JH, Coldman AJ (1984) The genetic origin of drug resistance in neoplasms: implications for systemic therapy. Cancer Res 44: 3643
3. Hyrniuk W, Bush H (1984) The importance of dose intensity in chemotherapy of metastatic breast cancer. J Clin Oncol 11: 1281
4. Klimo P, Connors JM (1985) MACOP-B chemotherapy for the treatment of diffuse large-cell lymphoma. Ann Intern Med 102: 596
5. Amadori S, Guglielmi C, Anselmo AP, Cimino G, Ruco LP, Papa G, Biagini C, Mandelli F (1985) Treatment of diffuse aggressive non-Hodgkin's lymphomas with an intensive multi-drug regimen including high dose cytosine arabinoside (F-MACHOP). Semin Oncol [Suppl 3] 12: 218
6. Applebaum FR, Thomas ED (1983) Review of the use of marrow transplantation in the treatment of non-Hodgkin's lymphoma. J Clin Oncol 1: 1440
7. Rosenberg SA, Lotze MT, Muul LM, Leitman S, Chang AE, Ettinghausen SE, Matory YL, Skibber JM, Shiloni E, Vetto JT, Seipp CA, Simpson C, Reichert CM (1985) Observations on the systemic administration of autologous lymphokine-activated killer cells and recombinant interleukin-2 to patients with metastatic cancer. N Engl J Med 313: 1485

50. Childhood Non-Hodgkin's Lymphomas

I.T. Magrath

Current Results and Therapeutic Issues

Non-Hodgkin's lymphomas (NHL) account for approximately 10% of childhood cancers and have an incidence of 1–2 per 100 000 children under 15 years of age. The results of treatment have improved greatly in the last 10 years such that today some 60%–75% of all patients may be expected to enjoy long-term survival [1]. This result has primarily been achieved through the use of combination chemotherapy, including prophylactic therapy to the central nervous system (CNS). Radiation therapy has been gradually relegated to a secondary role, being used in only a small number of patients for emergency treatment of cord compression or cranial nerve palsies [1]. Even in these circumstances it is not clear that radiation adds to chemotherapy, since response to the latter is so rapid.

For treatment purposes, the childhood lymphomas are usually divided into lymphoblastic and nonlymphoblastic lymphomas, using the term lymphoblastic as in the National Cancer Institute (NCI) Working formulation scheme [1]. Standard therapy for lymphoblastic lymphomas, the majority of which are T-cell lymphomas, is based on intensive protocols designed for the treatment of high-risk acute lymphoblastic leukemia, the most widely used being modifications of the LSA2-L2 protocol originally designed at the Memorial Sloan Kettering Cancer Center [1–3]. Other protocols may be successfully used for subgroups of patients with lymphoblastic lymphomas, including patients with localized disease or mediastinal tumors without widespread peripheral disease such as generalized lymphadenopathy or bone marrow involvement [1, 4]. The nonlymphoblastic lymphomas, the vast majority of which are B-cell lymphomas histologically designated as small noncleaved lymphomas (undifferentiated lymphomas including Burkitt's lymphoma) and large cell lymphomas, are treated with repeated cycles of drug combinations containing cyclophosphamide, vincristine, prednisone, intermediate or high-dose methotrexate, and usually adriamycin. Some protocols include other drugs such as the epipodophyllotoxin (VM-26), cytosine arabinoside and 1,3-bis(2-chloroethyl)-1-nitrosourea (BCNU) (1,4–6). All protocols for childhood lymphoma employ prophylactic therapy against spread to the CNS. Cranial irradiation has not been shown to be necessary, and almost all protocols achieve good prophylaxis with intrathecal ara-C and methotrexate coupled with high-dose methotrexate.

580

In patients with localized NHL, almost all achieve complete remission and more than 90% can be expected to be cured with chemotherapy regimens. Some 25% of small non-cleaved lymphoma patients have all of their abdominal disease (usually in the right iliac fossa) resected prior to therapy, and these patients have an excellent prognosis. The main therapeutic issue in patients with localized disease is to find the lowest intensity and shortest duration of therapy consistent with excellent results.

In patients with extensive disease, more than 80% of the patients achieve complete remission. In patients with extensive intrathoracic disease (lymphoblastic lymphomas) or extensive abdominal disease (small noncleaved and large cell lymphomas), the cure rate is 60%–80%, but in most series, patients with marrow involvement (except lymphoblastic lymphomas), and especially those with CNS involvement at presentation, have a much worse prognosis (10%–50% are cured) [1,4–7]. Improved chemotherapy regimens need to be designed for these groups of patients. Improvements in the definition of risk groups in lymphoblastic lymphoma are also needed so that treatment can be refined.

Current Approaches Under Study

There is little innovation in the treatment of lymphoblastic lymphomas at present, since the general assumption is that the majority of patients do well with current regimens. However, in a Pediatric Oncology Group study, there was an indication that patients with extensive disease, including replacement of the bone marrow to greater than 25% as well as other mass lesions, have a poor prognosis, while patients with mediastinal masses had only a 40% chance of survival. The former group of patients would seem most appropriately treated with the most intensive acute lymphoblastic lymphoma protocols, which are continuously being refined (see Chap. 43). The possibility that those patients with mediastinal masses but no bone marrow involvement may do better with protocols more like those used for small noncleaved cell lymphomas [4] needs to be studied further.

In patients with nonlymphoblastic lymphomas there is increasing evidence that prolonged therapy is unnecessary, and in the most recently developed protocols only 3–8 months of treatment is stipulated, even in patients with extensive diease [1]. In stage IV nonlymphoblastic lymphomas (including bone marrow and/or CNS disease), two main approaches are currently under study: (a) refinement of conventional chemotherapy, usually by the introduction of additional drugs (including high-dose ara-C, epidophyllotoxins, and ifosfamide) [1] and (b) the use of transplantation procedures, either allogeneic or autologous, in patients in first remission (based on promising results in relapsed patients [8].) Initial results in this subset of patients treated with autologous marrow infusion after intensive therapy are promising [8], but few patients have been treated so far, and patients with bone marrow disease are excluded from autologous transplantation, even when purging procedures are undertaken. Patients who do not achieve complete remission after three cycles of therapy (surgically documented) are also considered high-risk patients by some, and these patients have done particularly well with autologous bone marrow transplantation [8]. However, what the outcome for these patients might have been with a more conventional approach is not entirely clear.

Some studies have been carried out using biological response modifiers, e.g., α-interferon, or targeted monoclonal antibodies, including the intrathecal administration of the latter [9–11]. These exploratory studies indicate that responses may be obtained, but the value of such approaches remains ill-defined.

Future Approaches

Future approaches to the treatment of childhood NHL will entail: (a) the further refinement of current approaches and (b) the utilisation of totally new therapies.

Improvements in Combination Chemotherapy

As discussed above, new combinations and doses of drugs, including very high-dose therapy, are currently under study. Since a high proportion of patients do well with the present treatment, the gradual replacement of currently used agents with newer drugs which are more efficacious and/or less toxic (or which at least have a toxic effect which is readily prevented) is likely to further improve the overall suvival rate. Agents of current interest in this regard include alkylating agents (e.g., ifosfamide) and anthracyclines with less cardiac toxicity (e.g., epirubicin). There is every reason to believe, as the ability to rationally modify the structure of drugs increases (see Chap. 11), that additional analogues with advantages over currently used agents will be synthesized. It seems likely that bone marrow transplantation will not provide an ultimate form of therapy, particularly not as evidence grows that in the B-cell tumors at least, total body irradiation is of limited value. This approach has demonstrated, however, that prolonged therapy is not necessary if the killing of tumor cells can be augmented sufficiently. Alternative high-dose combinations may be developed.

An additional area likely to be improved upon in the future is the management of CNS disease. New agents able to penetrate the blood-brain barrier effectively, or new agents for intrathecal use (e.g., hydroperoxycyclophosphamide or monoclonal antibodies [11, 12]) could dramatically alter the current poor prognosis of patients who present with CNS disease.

An exciting new possibility which could considerably increase the therapeutic index of chemotherapeutic agents is the use of molecularly cloned hemopoietic growth factors, such as the colony stimulating factor for granulocytes and macrophages (GM-CSF), as a means of significantly lessening the degree and duration of myelosuppression [13]. This is a particularly important facet in the treatment of tumors with short doubling times, like pediatric NHL, since tumor regrowth (possibly subclinical) after a cycle of effective but not curative therapy may occur before marrow recovery. Thus, the duration of myelosuppression may be one of the single most important factors in determining the outcome of treatment. Lessening the risk of serious infection resulting from prolonged neutropenia is another potential advantage of G-CSF or GM-CSF.

Totally New Approaches

With recent knowledge of the biochemical pathways relevant to cellular proliferation and differentiation, particularly with regard to lymphoid cells, it seems likely that new approaches to treatment in which these pathways provide the therapeutic target will be developed. A potential problem with such approaches is the effect on normal cells, and it will be necessary to determine the toxicity of biological response modifiers empirically. It is becoming clear, however, that there are unique aspects of the biochemistry of neoplastic cells, such as the structurally abnormal c-*myc* gene in most cases of Burkitt's lymphoma and the hybrid T cell receptor alpha chain/immunoglobulin hybrid protein described in some T cell neoplasms containing a chromosome 14 inversion [1]. In fact these unique genetic changes could provide the key to developing therapy which is truly specific for the malignant clone. Although much laboratory work needs to be done prior to any clinical studies, and there will be numerous problems to surmount, it is possible to envisage targeting systems based, for example, on antisense oligonucleotides, able to bind abnormal mRNAs specifically and inhibit their transcription. Alternatively, the use of the abnormal (e.g., hybrid) proteins as targets for immunotoxins, radionuclide-antibody conjugates, or drugs synthesized by using computer-generated models of the molecular structure of potential binding sites (see Chap. 11) could confer an element of specificity not attainable when molecules also expressed by normal cells are used as targets.

References

1. Magrath IT (1987) Malignant non-Hodgkin's lymphomas in children. In: Pizzo PA, Poplack DS (eds) Principles and practice of pediatric oncology. Lippincott, New York, (in press)
2. Anderson JR, Wilson JF, Jenkin RD et al. (1983) The results of a randomized therapeutic trial comparing a 4-drug regimen (COMP) with a 10-drug regimen (LSA2-L2). N Engl J Med 308: 559
3. Dahl GV, Rivera G, Pui CH et al. (1985) A novel treatment of childhood lymphoblastic non-Hodgkin's lymphoma: early and intermittent use of teniposide plus cytarabine. Blood 66: 1110
4. Magrath I, Janus C, Edwards B et al. (1984) An effective therapy for both undifferentiated (including Burkitt's) lymphomas and lymphoblastic lymphomas in children and young adults. Blood 63: 1102

5. Müller-Weihrich S, Ludwig R, Reither A et al. (1987) B-type non-Hodgkin's lymphomas and leukemia: the BFM study group experience. In: Cavalli F, Bonnadonna G, Rosencweig M (eds) Proceedings of the third international conference on malignant lymphoma.

6. Patte C, Philip T, Rodary C et al. (1986) Improved survival rate in children with stage III and IV B cell non-Hodgkin's lymphoma and leukemia using multi-agent chemotherapy: results of a study of 114 children from the French Pediatric Oncology Society. J Clin Oncol 4: 1219

7. Murphy S, Bowman, WP, Abromowitch M et al. (1986) Results of treatment of advanced stage Burkitt's lymphoma and B-cell (SIg+) acute lymphoblastic leukemia with high-dose fractionated cyclophosphamide and coordinated high-dose methotrexate and cytarabine. J Clin Oncol 4: 1732

8. Philip T, Biron P, Philip I et al. (1987) ABMT in Burkitt's lymphoma (50 cases in the Lyon protocol. In: Cavalli F, Bonnadonna G, Rosencweig M (eds) Proceedings of the third international conference on malignant lymphoma.

9. Ochs J, Abromowitch M, Rudnick S et al. (1986) Phase I–II study of recombinant alpha-2 interferon against advanced leukemia and lymphoma in children. J Clin Oncol 4: 883–887

10. Myers CD, Thorpe PE, Ross WC et al. (1984) An immunotoxin with therapeutic potential in T cell leukemia: WT1-ricin A. Blood 63: 1178–1185

11. Hertler A, Schlossman D, Lester C et al. (1987) Intrathecal administration of WT1-ricin a chain immunotoxin (Abstr). Proc ASCO 6: A989

12. Arndt C, Colvin M, Balis F et al. (1987) Intrathecal administration of 4-hydroperoxycyclophosphamide (hpc) (Abstr). Proc Annu Meet Am Assoc Cancer Res 28: 439

13. Giardyina SL, Fooy KA, Beatty SM, Morgan AC Jr (1986) Evaluation of clinical application of partially purified human urinary colony-stimulating factor. Immunobiology 172: 205–212

584

51. Osteosarcoma

M.P. Link

Current Results and Therapeutic Issues

The past 15 years have witnessed substantial advances in the treatment and outcome of patients with osteosarcoma which have in large part been attributed to
the application of effective adjuvant chemotherapy. However, the contribution
of adjuvant chemotherapy to this improvement in prognosis has been debated
for most of the past decade (reviewed in [1]). A retrospective review of the
results of studies from the Mayo Clinic and elsewhere suggested that the outcome for patients with osteosarcoma had improved over a period of time (after
1970) independent of the administration of adjuvant chemotherapy. In addition,
a randomized controlled trial of adjuvant high dose methotrexate (HDMTX)
conducted at the Mayo Clinic [2] between 1976 and 1980 failed to demonstrate
an advantage for patients treated with adjuvant chemotherapy. More than 40%
of patients in the control group from this trial survived without recurrence (compared with fewer than 20% in historical series), suggesting that the natural
history of osteosarcoma had changed over time, and challenging the apparent
benefits of adjuvant therapy demonstrated in the many uncontrolled trials of the
1970s and early 1980s.

Results from two recent trials addressing the role of adjuvant chemotherapy
of osteosarcoma may help to resolve this controversy. In both studies [1, 3, 4],
patients were randomly assigned to receive intensive adjuvant chemotherapy or
observation alone after definitive surgery of the primary tumor. Results for the
control groups in both studies duplicated the historical experience with fewer
than 20% of patients surviving without recurrence, whereas the adminstration of
adjuvant chemotherapy resulted in a significant improvement in relapse-free survival. Thus, it appears that the natural history of osteosarcoma has not changed
in the past 2 decades and that adjuvant chemotherapy has a favorable impact on
relapse-free survival for patients with this disease.

With the intensive adjuvant chemotherapy regimens currently in use, approximately 60%–70% of patients with nonmetastatic osteosarcoma of an extremity
will survive without recurrence [1], and a significant fraction of relapsing patients
may be salvaged by aggressive thoracotomy with or without the administration
of further chemotherapy. Although the dramatic improvement in outcome for
patients with osteosarcoma and the contribution of adjuvant chemotherapy to
this improvement now appear indisputable, refinements in therapy are needed.
Almost one-third of children presenting without metastases will relapse after

receiving the therapy currently available, and patients presenting with metastases continue to have a poor prognosis. Since osteosarcoma is resistant to conventional dose radiotherapy, the primary tumor in extremity lesions is controlled surgically; for the majority of patients, amputation has been the procedure of choice, resulting in numerous functional, cosmetic, and psychological problems. Patients with unresectable tumors of the axial skeleton have little hope of cure since local control of the primary cannot be achieved. Finally, the toxicity and expense of chemotherapy regimens currently in use are substantial, and the long-term effects of such therapy have not yet been assessed.

Current Approaches Under Study

With improvements in the survival rate of patients with osteosarcoma, surgeons have attempted subamputative surgery in the hope of reducing the functional and psychological problems of amputation by the use of limb-sparing resections. Limb-salvage surgery is being used with increasing frequency and enthusiasm and is one of the major new developments in the management of patients with osteosarcoma. However, the safety of limb-salvage surgery has been questioned by European investigators who found a significantly higher distant failure rate for patients treated by en bloc resection compared with patients undergoing amputation [5], although neither the local recurrence rate nor overall relapse rate appears to have been increased among American patients undergoing limb-salvage surgery. Furthermore, the long-term functional results achieved by limb-salvage surgery have not been adequently assessed. The durability of endo-prosthetic devices utilized for many patients undergoing limb salvage remains problematic, and late infection and graft failure may result in delayed amputation for patients treated by limb resection. While there is little doubt that limb salvage for upper extremity primary tumors results in a significant functional advantage for the patient, the functional advantage for patients undergoing limb salvage for lower extremity primary tumors continues to be debated. Current studies of patients undergoing limb salvage should clarify the safety and overall efficacy of limb-salvage surgery in the management of osteosarcoma.

Another of the important recent developments in the treatment of osteosarcoma has been the use of presurgical ("neoadjuvant") chemotherapy, i.e., the administration of chemotherapy for a period of 2–3 months prior to the definitive surgery of the primary tumor. This strategy is attractive because of several theoretical considerations [6]. Since chemotherapy is administered very soon after biopsy and diagnosis, treatment of micrometastases known to be present in the majority of patients can be instituted early. This represents a significant advantage over the traditional adjuvant approach where the administration of systemic chemotherapy is delayed by a month or more by surgery and the time necessary for wound-healing. Presurgical chemotherapy may also be important in facilitating limb-salvage surgery. One of the most compelling rationales for presurgical chemotherapy is the use of the period of presurgical chemotherapy as an in vivo drug trial to determine the drug sensitivity of an individual tumor to "customize" the postoperative adjuvant treatment. Data from several trials suggest that patients whose tumors are responsive to presurgical therapy will do well when the same therapy is continued postoperatively [5–7]. On the other hand, patients with tumors found to be unresponsive to the presurgical chemotherapy regimen (the majority of patients in most studies to date) have a much less favorable outlook and might benefit from a change in the agents used postoperatively. This customizing approach has been tested in trials from the Memorial Hospital with extremely favorable results (approximately 90% of patients remaining relapse-free) [6, 7], although these remain to be confirmed in follow-up studies. Such a confirmatory study is now being conducted by the Children's Cancer Study Group.

The strategy of presurgical chemotherapy has been accepted enthusiastically, although there are few data to suggest that this strategy is superior to the traditional adjuvant approach. Results from multi-institutional studies utilizing presurgical chemotherapy (with or without customizing of the treatment based on the response of the primary tumor) have resulted in 2-year relapse-free survival in 65%–70% of patients—results which may not be superior to those from adjuvant trials which utilize mutliagent regimens of similar intensity but without presurgical chemotherapy. The role of presurgical chemotherapy in facilitating limb salvage is also debated, although it appears that centers which utilize presurgical chemotherapy perform limb-salvage surgery on a higher percentage of patients than those centers which do not utilize presurgical chemotherapy. Thus the exact contribution of presurgical chemotherapy to the management of patients with osteosarcoma is still to be defined.

Future Approaches

Improvements in treatment for patients with osteosarcoma in the next 5–10 years will result primarily from the addition of new active therapeutic agents. The activity of ifosfamide against macroscopic osteosarcoma in phase II studies has been identified, and this agent is already being introduced into phase III studies. New platinum analogues (CHIP and carboplatin) are being tested in phase II trials and may prove to be active agents with reduced toxicity when compared with the parent compound.

Presurgical chemotherapy has increasingly been administered via the intra-arterial rout directly into the arterial supply of the tumor, to maximize both drug delivery to the tumor vasculature and drug extraction by the tumor. Adriamycin and cisplatin, in particular, have been delivered by prolonged intra-arterial infusion. High local drug concentrations have been achieved as documented by pharmacokinetic studies, and dramatic responses in primary tumors have been observed. Whether the responses achieved are superior to those resulting from systemic intravenous administration of the same agents, and whether systemic toxicity is ameliorated with intra-arterial administration of the drugs has not been demonstrated convincingly. To date, this technique has appropriately been limited to centers with excellent angiographic support facilities to administer repeated courses of therapy. The possibility of sterilizing the primary tumor site by the administration of intensive intra-arterial chemotherapy in the hope of avoiding surgery of the primary tumor altogether has been explored [8]; results indicate dramatic responses and durable local control in selected patients, but the local recurrence rate remains unacceptably high, and this approach cannot yet be recommended.

Surgical techniques for en bloc resection have greatly improved, increasing the proportion of patients eligible for limb salvage. In the past, limb salvage has not been suitable for lower extremity primaries in young patients who had not yet achieved full growth potential because of the leg-length discrepancy which would develop later in life. The development of an expandable prosthesis [9] based on the concept of a telescoping unit that can be expanded with a gear device permits the implantation of the endoprosthesis in skeletally immature individuals and gradual expansion of the overall length of the prosthesis to accomodate growth. Although an intriguing concept, experience with this device is limited.

The treatment of patients with unresectable axial skeleton primary tumors remains unsatisfactory because of the difficulty of obtaining clean surgical margins, which is a prerequisite for local control. More aggressive surgical approaches in conjunction with presurgical chemotherapy or irradiation to shrink the primary lesion have resulted in promising preliminary results. The use of hypofractionated radiotherapy with or without radiosensitizers to overcome the capacity of osteosarcoma cells to repair sublethal damage (a putative mechanism for radioresistance of osteosarcoma) may be particularly useful for the treatment of unresectable lesions, although the enhanced soft tissue injury which results may limit this approach [10].

Immunotherapy of osteosarcoma has been attempted in the past without success, but recent advances in technology have provided the immunotherapist with more active and more specific reagents. Monoclonal antibodies raised against osteosarcoma have been developed [11], and radiolabeled conjugates have been used successfully for imaging tumors in patients, and may prove useful in therapy for targeting drugs and toxins to tumor cells. Tumor-specific cytotoxic lymphocytes have been detected in the peripheral blood of patients with osteosarcoma, and recently T-cell clones which are cytotoxic to autologous tumors have been isolated from patients [12]. Such cytotoxic T cells can be expanded in vitro for reinfusion into patients. In a recent report, lymphocytic infiltration of the primary tumor was found to correlate with a longer relapse-free survival period in patients with osteosarcoma, suggesting the expression of potent, specific host immunity to the tumor in these patients. It is possible that lymphocytes with enhanced antitumor reactivity may be cloned directly from tumor specimens and provide a more potent source of immunoreactive cells for therapy.

References

1. Link MP (1986) Adjuvant therapy in the treatment of osteosarcoma. In: DeVita VT, Hellman S, Rosenberg S (eds) Important advances in oncology. Lippincott, Philadelphia, pp 193–207
2. Edmonson J, Green S, Ivins J et al. (1984) A controlled pilot study of high-dose methotrexate as post surgical adjuvant treatment for primary osteosarcoma. J Clin Oncol 2: 152–156
3. Link MP, Goorin AM, Miser AW et al. (1986) The effect of adjuvant chemotherapy on relapse-free survival in patients with osteosarcoma of the extremity. N Engl J Med 314: 1600–1606
4. Eilber F, Giuliano A, Eckardt J et al. (1987) Adjuvant chemotherapy for osteosacoma: a randomized prospective trial. J Clin Oncol 5: 21–26
5. Winkler K, Beron G, Kotz R et al. (1984) Neoadjuvant chemotherapy for osteogenic sarcoma: results of a Cooperative German/Austrian Study. J Clin Oncol 2: 617–624
6. Rosen G, Marcove RC, Caparros B, Nirenberg A, Kosloff C, Huvos AG (1979) Primary osteogenic sarcoma. The rationale for preoperative chemotherapy and delayed surgery. Cancer 43: 2163–2177
7. Rosen G, Marcove RC, Huvos AG, Caparros BI, Lane JM, Nirenberg A, Cacavio A, Groshen S (1983) Primary osteogenic sarcoma: eight-year experience with adjuvant chemotherapy. J Cancer Res Clin Oncol [Suppl] 106: 55–67
8. Jaffe N, Robertson R, Takaue Y (1984) Osteosarcoma: prolonged control of the primary tumor with chemotherapy. Proc ASCO 3: 77
9. Lewis MM (1986) The use of an expandable and adjustable prosthesis in the treatment of childhood malignant bone tumors of the extremity. Cancer 57: 499–502
10. Martinez A, Goffinet D, Donaldson S et al. (1985) Intra-arterial infusion of radiosensitizer (BUdR) combined with hypofractionated irradiation and chemotherapy for primary treatment of osteogenic sarcoma. Int J Radiat Oncol Biol Phys 11: 123–128
11. Baldwin R, Pimm M, Embleton M et al. (1984) Monocolonal antibody 791T/36 for tumor detection and therapy of metastases. In: Nicolson GL, Milas L (eds) Cancer invasion and metastases: biologic and therapeutic aspects. Raven, New York, pp 437–455
12. Slovin S, Lackman R, Ferrone S, Kiely P, Mastrangelo M (1986) Cellular immune response to human sarcomas: cytotoxic T cell clones reactive with autologous sarcomas. I. Development, phenotype, and specificity. J Immunol 137: 3042–3048

52. Ewing's Sarcoma

J.S. Miser

Current Results and Therapeutic Issues

Biology

In 1983 a study of tumor cells from both short-term tissue culture of Ewing's sarcoma cells and from tumor cell lines derived from Ewing's sarcoma revealed a t(11;22) chromosome translocation [1], as well as other chromosome abnormalities, often of chromosome 8. In spite of the relative constancy of these cytogenetic abnormalities, their significance is not yet known. A study of oncogene expression, translocation, and rearrangement has revealed: (a) c-*sis* is translocated from chromosome 22 to chromosome 11, but it is relatively distant from the breakpoint and is not expressed at high levels after translocation; (b) c-*ets* is located near the breakpoint on chromosome 11 and is variably expressed; (c) c-*myc*, present on chromosome 8, is expressed at high levels; and (d) c-*myb*, c-*mil/raf*, and c-*src* are all expressed and have a similar pattern to that of a related tumor, peripheral neuroepithelioma [2]. The significance of this relatively constant pattern of oncogene expression is not known at this time but it may be of diagnostic value.

In vitro studies have demonstrated that Ewing's cell lines produce type I, III, and IV collagen, data consistent with the interpretation that Ewing's sarcoma is derived from primitive mesenchymal cells [3]. Subsequent investigation, however, suggests that Ewing's sarcoma may, in fact, be of neural origin: Ewing's sarcoma has an oncogene expression that is indistinguishable from peripheral neuroepithelioma, a tumor of neural origin [2]; cell lines derived from Ewing's sarcoma exhibit a neural phenotype when treated with differentiating agents under controlled conditions [4]; and, choline acetyltransferase has been found within the Ewing's tumor cells. [2].

Therapy

At present, 50%–75% of patients with nonmetastatic Ewing's sarcoma can be expected to be disease-free 5 years after the development of the sarcoma, with the use of local therapy (radiation therapy or surgery) and adjuvant chemotherapy [5, 6]. The most effective chemotherapy regimens have emphasized the use of cyclophosphamide and doxorubicin; however, vincristine and dactinomycin have also been utilized [5–7]. Unfortunately, effective therapy for the majority of patients with metastatic disease, especially when it involves the bone or bone marrow, is not yet available. Although a 30% long-term survival rate of patients with metastatic disease has been reported, most of these long-term survivors have had only small amounts of metastatic disease limited to the lung [8].

Current Approaches Under Study

Biology

At this point in time there is no specific marker for Ewing's sarcoma that will distinguish it from other small round cell tumors of bone. Because the diagnosis of Ewing's sarcoma is arrived at only after the exclusion of other entities (e.g., peripheral neuroepithelioma and primitive sarcomas of bone), this diagnostic category includes a heterogeneous group of tumors. In ongoing studies of small round cell tumors of bone, immunocytochemical and ultrastructural features of these tumors are being analysed in an attempt to discern prognostic and biologic differences on the basis of pathologic differences. The development of specific tumor markers for Ewing's sarcoma, using monoclonal antibodies or molecular techniques, in order to provide more precise diagnostic criteria will be critically important for the analysis of future studies.

Therapy

Evaluation of New Agents

Recently, the combination of ifosfamide and etoposide has been demonstrated to have significant activity in the treatment of recurrent Ewing's sarcoma [9]. In the light of this information, the next important question in the treatment of Ewing's sarcoma will be whether the use of the combination of ifosfamide and etoposide can significantly improve the outlook for newly diagnosed patients. The addition of this "non-cross-resistant" regimen to the standard therapy is soon to be evaluated in a randomized study.

Evaluation of New Modalities

The use of very intensive therapy in the treatment of recurrent Ewing's sarcoma has demonstrated that both high-dose chemotherapy and total body irradiation (TBI) are effective against the disease [10, 11]. Unfortunately, in the treatment of recurrent disease, response to high-dose therapy is short-lived and toxicity is marked. Nevertheless, these studies have allowed the development of new therapies that may have application for newly diagnosed patients, especially those having a poor prognosis with standard therapy. Specifically, the use of high-dose melphalan followed by autologous bone marrow transplantation in patients with recurrent disease has resulted in a very high response rate (greater than 75%) but with responses being of very short duration [10]. The use of this modality in the consolidation of a first or second complete remission, however, may result in improvement in the outcome of treatment in this high-risk group of patients.

Total body irradiation (TBI) has been demonstrated to have some therapeutic effect in the adjuvant treatment of patients with pulmonary disease, and in the palliative treatment of patients with systemic disease [11]. Further, pulmonary irradiation has been proven effective in the prevention of pulmonary metastatic disease [6]. Pilot studies in patients with high-risk Ewing's sarcoma suggest that TBI may be of benefit [12]; however, randomized studies will be necessary to establish its efficacy in the treatment of patients in first or second remission.

Evaluation of Dose Intensity

One of the most controversial questions facing the therapist treating the patient with Ewing's sarcoma is determining the correct dose intensity of the therapy [5, 7]. Although many dose intensities of doxorubicin and cyclophosphamide-based regimens have been used in the adjuvant therapy of Ewing's sarcoma, the results with these regimens have been similar [5, 7]. In order to reduce toxicity while maintaining good tumor control, careful studies to define the optimal dose intensity, and thus refine the adjuvant therapy for patients without metastatic disease, will be important. Although markedly increasing the intensity of therapy for patients with metastatic disease has increased the complete remission rate, it has not resulted in a dramatically improved disease-free survival rate for patients with widespread metastatic disease [12]. It is important that the role of dose intensity in the treatment of Ewing's sarcoma be evaluated in randomized studies in the near future.

Evaluation of the Role of Local Management

Over the past 15 years radiation has been the standard therapy to control the primary disease, while surgery has been reserved for the control of extensive tumors with pathologic fractures or small tumors of the distal extremities. Recent retrospective reviews from large independent institutions have suggested that in patients selected for surgery the outcome has in fact been better than in those treated with radiation [13, 14]. However, the analyses are confounded by the fact that the patients selected for surgery generally have good prognostic features and do well regardless of the type of local management. The role of surgery in the treatment of Ewing's sarcoma must therefore be evaluated in carefully controlled prospective studies that evaluate not only the primary tumor control but also the functional outcome and the incidence of second tumors.

With the interaction of effective chemotherapy with both radiation treatment and surgery in the control of the primary tumor, it may be possible to achieve a favorable outcome with more limited surgery as well as with less extensive radiation therapy in the future. Randomized studies are needed to research these points. Further, new radiation therapy techniques such as hyperfractionation may result in equal or improved efficacy with reduced toxicity to normal tissues.

Staging

Although prognostic factors have been identified for patients with Ewing's sarcoma [i.e., the primary site of the disease, the presence of metastatic disease, the tumor size, lactic dehydrogenase (LDH) level], a formal staging system has not been widely applied. The current studies are addressing this issue because more and more data suggest that the size of the primary tumor has prognostic significance [15, 16].

Evaluation of Response to Primary Chemotherapy

The response to primary chemotherapy seems to have prognostic significance in the treatment of patients with nonmetastatic osteosarcoma. Recently, a small study suggested that this may also be true for patients with Ewing's sarcoma [17]. Pathologic response to primary chemotherapy and response as measured by nonivasive modalities [e.g., MRI, PET scanning] will be important areas of investigation in the next series of studies of this tumor.

Future Approaches

Biology

The major thrust of future investigations into Ewing's sarcoma will be to attempt to link observed molecular events with the pathogenesis and biology of this tumor. It is hoped as a result that molecular events (e.g., oncogene expression) can then: (a) be related to prognosis as an expression of the tumor biology (as has been seen with neuroblastoma), (b) provide a clue as to the cause and thus prevention of the tumor, and (c) provide a basis for innovative therapy. It is also hoped that molecular and biologic markers will be discovered that will definitively demonstrate the precise cell of origin of the "Ewing's cell."

Therapy

Finally, although there is no evidence that biologic therapies have had any impact on the treatment of sarcomas, the evaluation of these therapies has been limited thus far. Because most patients with Ewing's sarcoma, even those with extensive disease, will achieve a complete remission, the main area of investigation in the management of Ewing's sarcoma must be the development of new effective strategies aimed at maintaining the remission. This may require intensification of induction, the development of new effective agents to use in the initial therapy, improvement in the therapy of the primary tumor, and, finally, it may require the development of effective "maintenance" (immunologic or biologic) therapy.

References

1. Aurias A, Rimbaut C, Buffe D et al. (1983) Chromosomal translocation in Ewing's sarcoma. N Engl J Med 309: 496–497
2. McKeon C, Thiele CJ, Ross RA et al. (1987) Indistinguishable and predictable patterns of proto-oncogene expression in two histopathologically distinct tumors: Ewing's sarcoma and neuroepithelioma. (in press)
3. Dickman PS, Liotta L, Triche TJ (1982) Ewing's sarcoma: characterization in established cultures and evidence of its histogenesis. Lab Invest 47: 375–382
4. Cavazzana A, Triche TJ, Tsokos M et al. (1987) Experimental evidence for the neural origin of Ewing's sarcoma. (in press)
5. Rosen G, Caparros B, Nirenburg A, et al. (1981) Ewing's sarcoma: ten-year experience with adjuvant chemotherapy. Cancer 47: 2204–2213
6. Nesbit ME, Perez CA, Tefft M et al. (1981) Multimodal therapy for the management of primary non-metastatic Ewing's sarcoma of bone: an intergroup study. NCI Monogr 56: 255–262
7. Hayes FA, Thompson EI, Hustu HO et al. (1983) The response of Ewing's sarcoma to sequential cyclophosphamide and Adriamycin induction therapy. J Clin Oncol 1: 45–51
8. Vietti TJ, Gehan EA, Nesbit ME et al. (1981) Multimodal therapy in metastatic Ewing's sarcoma: an intergroup study. NCI Monogr 56: 279–284
9. Miser JS, Kinsella TJ, Triche TJ et al. (1987) Ifosfamide with mesna uroprotection and etoposide: an effective regimen in the treatment of recurrent sarcomas and other tumors of children and young adults. J Clin Oncol 5: 1191–1198
10. Graham-Pole J, Lazarus HM, Herzig RH et al. (1984) High-dose melphalan for the treatment of children with refractory neuroblastoma and Ewing's sarcoma. Am J Pediatr Hematol Oncol 6: 17–26
11. Jenkin RDT, Rider WD, Sonley MJ (1976) Ewing's sarcoma: adjuvant total body irradiation, cyclophosphamide, and vincristine. Int J Radiat Oncol Biol Phys 1: 407–413
12. Miser JS, Steis R, Longo DL et al. (1985) Treatment of newly diagnosed high risk sarcomas and primitive neuroectodermal tumors (PNET) in children and young adults. Proc ASCO 4: C-935
13. Wilkins RM, Pritchard J, Burgert EO et al. (1986) Ewing's sarcoma of bone: experience with 140 patients. Cancer 58: 2551–2555
14. Bacci G, Picci P, Gherlinzoni F et al. (1985) Localized Ewing's sarcoma of bone: ten years experience at the Istituto Ortopedico Rizzoli in 124 cases treated with multi-modal therapy. Eur J Cancer Clin Oncol 21: 163–173
15. Mendenhall CM, Marcus RB, Enneking WF et al. (1983) The prognostic significance of soft tissue extension in Ewing's sarcoma. Cancer 51: 913–917
16. Gobel V, Jurgens H, Etspuler G et al. (1987) Prognostic significance of tumor volume in localized Ewing's sarcoma of bone in children and adolescents. J Cancer Res Clin Oncol 113: 187–191
17. Oberlin O, Patte C, Demecoq F et al. (1985) The response to initial chemotherapy as a prognostic factor in localized Ewing's sarcoma. Eur J Cancer Clin Oncol 21: 463–467

53. Soft Tissue Sarcomas in Childhood

J.S. Miser

Rhabdomyosarcoma

Current Results and Therapeutic Issues

Biology

Rhabdomyosarcomas of childhood are divided into two major groups on the basis of histology: embryonal and alveolar. The distinction between these two groups is clouded by the observation that some cases have a mixed histologic pattern; however, embryonal rhabdomyosarcoma usually occurs in young children and the alveolar tumors, more often in older patients. Recently, chromosome abnormalities, primarily aneuploidies, have been observed in embryonal rhabdomyosarcoma; however, one single, consistent abnormality has not yet been associated with this tumor [1]. Abnormalities of chromosomes 2 and 13 including reciprocal translocation, t(2;13) (q37;q14), have been seen with rhabdomyosarcoma [2, 3].

The evaluation of the molecular events that are associated with rhabdomyosarcoma have only recently been investigated [4]. Because children with Beckwith-Wiedemann syndrome have an increased potential for the development of rhabdomyosarcoma, Wilms' tumor, and hepatoblastoma, a common pathogenetic mechanism has been hypothesized [4]. Indeed, the somatic development of homozygosity for a mutant allele at a locus on human chromosome 11 has been demonstrated without loss or deletion of the chromosome segment [4]. This finding suggests that the pathogenesis of embryonal rhabdomyosarcoma involves the loss of normal genetic material that had prevented the expression of a malignant phenotype.

Staging

Over the last 15 years the majority of children in the United States of America with rhabdomyosarcoma have been treated in the Intergroup Rhabdomyosarcoma Studies (IRS) [5]. Although major advances have been made by these studies, the patients have been grouped together for treatment purposes on the basis of postoperative characteristics. Thus, the group each patient is assigned to depends upon the surgical procedure or on the location of the tumor rather than on its size and extent. This system has led to patients with heterogeneous characteristics in Group I, II, and III.

595

Therapy

At present, between 60% and 70% of patients with rhabdomyosarcoma can be expected to be disease-free at 3–5 years after treatment [5]. Of patients with low stage embryonal tumors, which usually occur in younger children, more than 80% enjoy disease-free survival. Patients with larger tumors of the chest wall, trunk, and extremities, however, have a poorer chance of disease-free survival: 25%–50% in most studies. In patients with metastatic disease the outcome is poorer still: a 5%–30% disease-free survival rate [5–8]. The chemotherapy used for the treatment of rhabdomyosarcoma usually includes combinations of vincristine (VCR) and dactinomycin (AMD), with or without cyclophosphamide (CPM) and doxorubicin (DOXO) [5]. Patients with low stage disease (Group 1 and 2 tumors and selected group 3 tumors of the head) are usually treated with VCR and AMD without additional chemotherapy, and patients with completely resected disease do not require radiation therapy [5]. Recently, two newer agents, cisplatin and etoposide (VP-16) have been used; however, their role in the therapy of this disease is not yet clear [9]. European studies haverecently used a combination of ifosfamide (IFOS), VCR, and AMD with excellent results [10]. When radiation therapy is utilized, the majority of patients have required greater than 4000 cGy, and patients who have gross bulky disease have required greater than 5000 cGy in order to eradicate the tumor permanently [5].

Current Approaches Under Study

Biology

Cytogenetic and molecular studies of both embryonal and alveolar rhabdomyosarcoma are presently continuing, especially as they are associated with familial syndromes and are likely to uncover clues to the pathogenesis while elucidating similarities and differences between the two tumors.

Staging

Because of the success of therapy over the last 15 years, it is now especially important that true preoperative staging be evaluated and utilized in order that appropriate refinements in therapy can be made. The development and prospective evaluation of such a preoperative staging system will allow study of treatment strategies in more homogeneous subsets of patients with rhabdomyosarcoma, enhancing the chances of discovering ways of improving therapy.

Therapy

Evaluation of New Agents. Recently, the combination of ifosfamide and etoposide has been shown to have significant activity in the treatment of recurrent rhabdomyosarcoma [11]. The response rate has been approximately 75% (25% complete remission and 50% partial remission). Given this, one of the next important questions to answer in the treatment of patients with rhabdomyosarcoma who have not fared well on standard therapy is the evaluation of the role of ifosfamide alone and in combination with etoposide in newly diagnosed patients. A second combination under study, moderate doses of melphalan and vincristine, has been developed on the basis of the marked effect of melphalan in the human xenograft tumor model. A clinical assessment of this drug is currently being made in newly diagnosed patients with promising results.

Evaluation of Dose Intensity. In patients with metastatic disease treated in the IRS studies there were complete remission rates of approximately 50%–60% [5]. In a pilot study of high-risk sarcomas utilizing a significantly higher dose intensity of the chemotherapeutic agents, VCR, DOXO, and CPM, a complete remission rate of more than 90% was achieved [12]. In the light of this and other data, dose intensity will be prospectively evaluated in high-risk patients in the near future.

Evaluation of Duration of Therapy. The standard duration of therapy for most children with rhabdomyosarcoma is 2 years [5]. Because there is little evidence that "maintenance therapy" plays an important role in the treatment of rhabdomyosarcoma, once complete remission has been achieved and 6 months of adjuvant chemotherapy have been delivered, future studies, even of patients with metastatic disease, must establish the duration of therapy needed to reduce the morbidity among patients undergoing treatment.

Evaluation of New Modalities. Pilot studies of total body irradiation have not been promising in patients with rhabdomyosarcoma [10]; however, attempts to develop effective, high-dose regimens utilizing autologous bone marrow rescue are needed. Their use in the first remission of high-risk patients and in second remission of patients who have relapsed may result in an improvement in the relapse-free survival of these groups.

Evaluation of the Role of Local Management. The standard therapy for rhabdomyosarcoma has been initial surgery, if possible, followed by chemotherapy and then radiation therapy. This approach is being reconsidered. The role of more intensive chemotherapy regimens in the control of the primary disease is being evaluated and may allow for lower doses of radiation therapy and thus lower morbidity. It may also allow for delayed and less extensive surgery. It will be especially important to evaluate these strategies in the treatment of patients with genitourinary rhabdomyosarcomas.

New radiation therapy techniques, hyperfractionation schedules, interstitial radiation, and intraoperative radiation may improve local control and decrease morbidity, especially in patients with abdominal and genitourinary rhabdomyosarcomas. Pilot studies followed by randomized trials will be required to assess accurately the efficacy and toxicity of these new approaches.

Future Approaches

Biology. Further elucidation of the molecular events that are involved in the pathogenesis of both embryonal and alveolar rhabdomyosarcoma will be important in the future study of these tumors. It will facilitate the better understanding

of the similarities, the differences, and the relationship between the two histologic subtypes, give an insight into their pathogenesis, and allow the premorbid
detection of these diseases. The evaluation of molecular events associated with
progression of rhabdomyosarcoma will be especially important because it may
be possible to predict at diagnosis (as has been possible with neuroblastoma)
which patients with low stage disease will be at the highest risk of relapsing. This
would then allow intensification of therapy for these patients and hopefully an
improvement in prognosis.

Therapy. Biologic therapies for the treatment of sarcomas are only now being
developed and will most likely be evaluated in studies designed to prevent relapse. Human tumor model systems, such as the human xenograft tumor model,
promise to be important tools in the identification of new agents for the treatment of rhabdomyosarcoma.

Non-rhabdomyosarcoma Soft Tissue Sarcomas

Current Results and Therapeutic Issues

Biology. This group of tumors is heterogeneous in presentation, prognosis, and
biology. Molecular evaluation will provide important information about the
pathogenesis and biology of these tumors. Recently, for example, the loss of
genes on chromosome 22 associated with acoustic neuromas was discovered, and
this may provide a clue to the pathogenesis and biology of neurofibrosarcoma
and other tumors associated with von Recklinghausen's disease [13].

Therapy. Because the tumors are uncommon and the prognosis is good for most
patients when treated with surgery alone, trials of adjuvant chemotherapy have
not yet been undertaken in children.

Future Approaches

Biology. The evaluation of the molecular events that are associated with the
development and progression of nonrhabdomyosarcoma soft tissue sarcomas
will be an important part of the study of these tumors in the next 10 years.
Because the majority of the patients with these tumors have a relatively good
prognosis, careful evaluation of molecular events that are associated with a high
incidence of progression, will be needed to tailor therapy for each patient with a
nonrhabdomyosarcoma soft tissue sarcoma.

Therapy. The major questions to be answered in the treatment of this heterogeneous group of sarcomas are as follows. (a) What is the role of adjuvant

chemotherapy in patients without metastatic disease who have undergone gross removal of tumor? (b) What is the optimal chemotherapy regimen, especially for patients with advanced disease where the prognosis is, at present, very poor? (c) With effective chemotherapy, can the local management be more limited, thus reducing morbidity through radiation or increasing the number of limb-sparing procedures? (d) What is the role of aggressive surgical resection of metastases? Randomized trials will be needed to evaluate adjuvant therapy in patients without metastatic disease. Pilot studies will be required to develop new and better chemotherapy regimens to treat patients with advanced local or systemic disease.

References

1. Potluri R, Gilbert F (1985) A cytogenetic study of embryonal rhabdomyosarcoma. Cancer Genet Cytogenet 14: 169–173
2. Turc-Carel C, Lizard-Nacol S, Justrabo E et al. (1986) Consistent chromosome translocation in alveolar rhabdomyosarcoma. Cancer Genet Cytogenet 19: 361–362
3. Seidal T, Mark J, Hagmar B et al. (1982) Alveolar rhabdomyosarcoma: a cytogenetic and correlated cytological and histological study. Acta Pathol Microbiol Immunol Scand [A] 90: 345–354
4. Koufos A, Hansen MF, Copeland NG et al. (1985) Loss of heterozygosity in three embryonal tumors suggests a common pathogenetic mechanism. Nature 316: 330–334
5. Maurer HM (1982) The Intergroup Rhabdomyosarcoma Study. Cancer Bull 34: 108–110
6. Ransom JL, Pratt CB, Hustu HO et al. (1980) Retroperitoneal rhabdomyosarcoma in children. Cancer 45: 845–850
7. Raney RB, Ragab AH, Ruymann FB et al. (1982) Soft-tissue sarcoma of the trunk in childhood. Cancer 49: 2612–2616
8. Ruymann FB, Newton WA, Ragab AH et al. (1984) Bone marrow metastases at diagnosis in children and adolescents with rhabdomyosarcoma: a report from the Intergroup Rhabdomyosarcoma Study. Cancer 53: 368–373
9. Crist WM, Raney RB, Ragab AH et al. (1987) Intensive chemotherapy including cisplatin with or without etoposide for children with soft-tissue sarcomas. Med Pediatr Oncol 15: 51–57
10. Otten J, Flamant F, Rodary C et al. (1985) Effectiveness of combination of ifosfamide, vincristine, and actinomycin D in inducing remission in rhabdomyosarcoma in children. Proc ASCO 4: 236 (C-917)
11. Miser JS, Kinsella TJ, Triche TJ et al. (1987) Ifosfamide with mesna uroprotection and etoposide: an effective regimen in the treatment of recurrent sarcomas and other tumors of children and young adults. J Clin Oncol 5: 1191–1198
12. Miser JS, Steis R, Longo DL et al. (1985) Treatment of newly diagnosed high risk sarcomas and primitive neuroectodermal tumors in children and young adults. Proc ASCO 4: 240 (C-935)
13. Seizinger BR, Martuza RL, Gusella JF (1986) Loss of genes on chromosome 22 in tumorigenesis of human acoustic neuroma. Nature 322: 644–647

54. Wilms' Tumor

G.J. D'Angio*

Current Results and Therapeutic Issues

Much progress has been made in the management of children with Wilms' tumor [1]. Cure rates are excellent, and treatment can be modulated in intensity according to well-defined risks. This is because prognostic factors have been identified with accuracy. First among these is the cytohistopathology of the tumor [2]. The largest subset of children have tumors with pathologic features making up a "favorable histology" (FH) and have an excellent outlook [3]. Beckwith and Palmer [2] have also described children with an "unfavorable histology" (UH), comprising approximately 12% of the children registered in the National Wilm's Tumor Study (NWTS), who have a less encouraging prognosis. The UH category has been further subdivided into: (a) anaplastic tumors, (b) clear cell sarcoma of the kidney, and (c) rhabdoid tumor. Of these three UH subtypes, the anaplastic lesions are true Wilms' tumors; the other two are thought to be separate and distinct from the Wilms' tumor complex.

Criteria for staging have also been made more precise, so that treatments are now selected after taking stage and histology into account. The life expectancy for patients with FH lesions of any stage is very good; the overall 2-year survival rate is about 95% [3, 4]. These results are achieved with actinomycin D (AMD) plus vincristine (VCR) for stages I and II children who are not irradiated, and with the addition of Adriamycin (ADR) and postoperative radiation (RT) to appropriate areas for stages III and IV patients (Table 1). Children with stage I anaplastic tumors have the same outlook as their FH counterparts; the 2-year survival rate for these patients is 98% [4]. The outlook for children with more advanced anaplastic tumors, however, is poor, the 2-year survival rate being only about 45% despite management with AMD plus VCR plus ADR plus cyclophosphamide (CPM) [4]. In contrast, adding ADR to AMD plus VCR markedly improved the life expectancy of patients with clear cell sarcoma [5], all of whom also received postoperative RT. The prognosis stage by stage mirrors

* Reporting for all present and past members of the National Wilms' Tumor Study Committee, and is deeply grateful for their help.

Supported in part by USPHS Grant CA-11722. Principal investigators at participating institutions also receive independent support from the National Cancer Institute.

600

Table 1. Abbreviated staging system according to the National Wilms' Tumor Study

Stage	Characteristics of tumor
I	Tumor is confined to the kidney and is totally excised
II	Tumor extends into adjoining tissues and is completely excised
III	Lymph nodes involved and/or gross tumor spillage and/or tumor left behind grossly or microscopically
IV	Distant metastases present, e.g., lungs, liver, bones, or brain
V	Tumors present in both kidneys at diagnosis

Staging depends on findings at the time of surgery and as defined by the pathologist; it applies to both FH and UH tumors.

that seen with the FH patients, and the overall 2-year survival rate for stages I through IV clear cell sarcoma patient is about 88% [3, 5]. Children with the rhabdoid tumor, often infants, have an extremely poor life expectancy, in the 25% range after treatment with the four drugs mentioned above plus postoperative RT [2, 4].

The main aim over the years has been to identify categories of patients who require minimal therapy after surgical removal of the affected kidney, eliminating RT wherever possible. This has largely been achieved for most of those in the FH category, where RT dosage has been reduced from doses as high as 4000 cGy to zero. Clinical research has also shown that one of the effective drugs (ADR) with considerable potential for late cardiotoxicity in long-term survivors is not needed in stages I and II FH children [3, 4]. Much needs to be done, however, to improve matters for the children at high risk with stages II, III, and IV anaplastic tumors, and for all those with the rhabdoid neoplasm.

Current Approaches Under Study

Two major avenues are being explored. The first emphasizes early surgery, in the belief that treatment can best be individualized in this way [1]. The second focuses on preoperative therapy to minimize surgical difficulties and complications.

Early Surgery

The fourth NWTS is investigating whether the drug maintenance period after surgery can be reduced from 15 to 6 months for all patients. It is also investigating whether AMD, VCR, and ADR can be given in single doses during each course, rather than using the methods currently employed which entail five daily doses of AMD, three daily doses of ADR, and two doses a week of VCR. There will be important psychosocioeconomic gains if these simplified methods prove to be successful. For example, it has been estimated that a saving of approximately $8 million per year in dealing with children with cancer and their families would result, not to mention the significant saving in time and efficiency for the health care team. Wilms' tumor serves as a very good model for this kind of clinical research, because it is a single entity in a single organ, and predictably good results can be achieved using standard therapy in the control group.

Preoperative Therapy

The International Society of Pediatric Oncology (SIOP) has run serial clinical trials in patients without metastases at diagnosis [6, 7]. It has demonstrated that preoperative chemotherapy results in very good overall survival and lessens the frequency of intraoperative tumor spills. The overall survival rates are comparable to those cited by the NWTS. A recent problem is the apparently inappropriate downstaging of some patients occasioned by preoperative chemotherapy. A higher infradiaphragmatic relapse rate is being recorded for children found to have involvement consistent with stages I or II criteria at surgery, and who are therefore not irradiated [7].

High-Risk Patients

Standard drugs have not been successful in managing high-risk patients. Clinical research here is focused on identifying new drugs and new drug combinations. Because of the small numbers of patients in these categories, the attempt is being made to derive as much information as possible from each individual child. Thus, a "cascade" of retrieval regimens has been suggested for patients who relapse so that more than one drug can be tested for response rates in each such child. This entails moving to the next most promising set of drugs if the child fails to respond after an adequate trial of the first test regimen. The drugs under consideration are combinations of etoposide plus cisplatin or etoposide plus ifosfamide. Encouraging results in scattered patients are being recorded with both these regimens.

Future Approaches

Two surgical projects are being supervised by the surgical members of the NWTS Committee. The first of these deals with the use of subtotal nephrectomies to preserve as much kidney parenchyma as possible in children with bilateral tumors in whom it is clearly advantageous to do so [8]. Beyond that, if it can be shown that subtotal nephrectomies can be performed safely and with good results in these children, then it will be possible to extend these observations to children with unilateral tumors. That is, it may be feasible to perform local excisions in the future, with the objective of preserving as much kidney function as possible. This will have important implications if the evidence presented by Welch and McAdams [9] regarding late focal glomerulosclerosis after unilateral nephrectomy in children is substantiated.

The second surgical project deals with the role of surgery in the management of children with pulmonary metastases. Grundy et al. [10] reviewed NWTS-3 children with recurrent tumor and found that pulmonary irradiation seems to be an important adjunct to their care. It thus may not be possible to eliminate pulmonary irradiation despite its known long-term effects. Discernible changes in pulmonary function result, although these dysfunctions are not incapacitating. Rather, survival rates may be improved by employing surgical excision for chemo- and radioresistant foci.

There are no promising applications of biological response modifiers, with the possible exception of radioprotectors such as WR-2721. It, however, has not been tried in children. Bone marrow transplantation or autologous reconstitution methods (since the tumor does not metastasize to the bone marrow) have been attempted in a few Wilms' tumor patients with recurrent disease. There are relatively few children available for trial, because, happily, the overall survival rates are good. Also, most of these patients will have had pulmonary metastases that proved refractory to standard treatments, including lung irradiation. Therefore, additional radiation therapy to sites of metastases is precluded because of the high incidence of pneumonopathy in re-irradiated patients. There are a few children, however, who have not had radiation therapy of the lungs or have metastases to other sites. In these children, supralethal chemotherapy can be given, supplemented by irradiation to localized areas. The best drug combination for this has yet to be evolved.

References

1. D'Angio GJ (1985) Oncology seen through the prism of Wilms' tumor. Med Pediatr Oncol 13: 53
2. Beckwith JB, Palmer NF (1978) Histopathology and prognosis of Wilms' tumor. Results from the National Wilms' Tumor Study. Cancer 41: 1937
3. D'Angio GJ, Evans AE, Breslow N, Beckwith JB, Baum E, de Lorimier A, Farewell V, Fernbach D, Hrabovsky E, Jones B, Kelalis P, Othersen HB, Tefft M, Thomas PRM (1984) Results of the Third National Wilms' Tumor Study (NWTS-3): a preliminary report. Proc Am Assoc Cancer Res Abstract 25, 183
4. Statistical Report (1986) Third National Wilms' Tumor Study.
5. Beckwith JB, Norkool P, Breslow N, D'Angio GJ (1986) Clinical observations in children with clear-cell sarcoma of the kidney. Proc Am Assoc Cancer Res Abstract 200, 794
6. Lemerle J, Voute PA, Tournade MF, Rodary C, Delemarre JFM, Sarrazin D, Burgers JMV, Sandstedt B, Mildenberger H, Carli M, Jereb B, Moorman-Voestermans CGM (1983) Effective-

ness of preoperative chemotherapy in Wilms' tumor: results of an International Society of Paediatric Oncology (SIOP) clinical trial. J Clin Oncol 1: 604

7. Zucker JM, Tournade MF, Voute PA, Delemarre JFM, de Kraker J, Lemerle J, Perry HJM, Rey A, Ducourtieux M, Com Nougue C (1986) Report on SIOP 6 nephroblastoma trials. Proc SIOP 31
8. Blute ML, Kelalis PP, Breslow N, Beckwith JB, Offord KP, D'Angio GJ (1987) Bilateral Wilms' tumor. J Urol 138: 968–973
9. Welch TR, McAdams AJ (1986) Focal glomerulosclerosis as a late sequela of Wilms' tumor. J Pediatr 108: 105
10. Grundy P, Takashima J, Evans AE, Breslow N, D'Angio GJ (1985) Results of salvage therapy for relapsed third National Wilms' Tumor Study (NWTS-3) patients (Abstr). Proc ASCO Abstract C956, 245

55. Neuroblastoma

T. Philip and R. Pinkerton

Current Results and Therapeutic Issues

Neuroblastoma is the second most common solid childhood tumor and the outlook for patients with limited disease (25% of the cases) is good. However, with more advanced or metastatic disease, complex and demanding combinations of surgery, chemotherapy, and radiotherapy are required. Even with these treatment modalities the goal of cure remains frustratingly elusive in many patients.

The outcome with surgical treatment alone is good in the rare stage 1 patient (Table 1) and also in stage 2 cases where there is no associated lymph node involvement. Chemotherapy and/or radiation therapy is highly effective in the remaining stage 2 patients, raising chances of long-term survival to more than 75% [1]. With more advanced, initially unresectable disease (stage 3) the outcome appears to depend, to at least some extent, upon the completeness of surgical resection after primary chemotherapy [2]. The wide variation in the long-term survival rate for this stage (40%–70%) thus reflects both the activity of the chemotherapy and the surgical expertise. In stage 4 patients, age remains an important prognostic factor and for patients under 1 year old, even with metastatic disease, cure rates may exceed 60%. Between 1 and 2 years old the prognosis is intermediate, but for patients over 2 years old at diagnosis there is almost universal agreement that the likelihood of long-term survival with standard chemotherapy is only around 10%. The initial response to chemotherapy is often encouraging and with most modern regimens, up to 80%–90% will achieve at least a partial response with clearing or improvement of metastatic disease. Unfortunately, even with surgery and radiotherapy, this is rarely converted to a complete response, and disease progression usually occurs within the following year.

Apart from clinical staging, a number of other parameters have been introduced which may provide prognostic information. Elevated serum neurone-specific enolase (NSE), elevated serum ferritin, and a high copy number of N-*myc* oncogenes in tumor tissue all correlate with an adverse prognosis. The Shimada classification, based upon details of stromal elements, cell differentiation, mitotic index, and age has been shown to identify accurately poor prognosis subgroups within clinical stages. Such parameters are often helpful in making treatment decisions for the lower stages (such as 2 and 3) where more aggressive approaches may be warranted, but in stage 4 disease the outlook is so poor that

Table 1. Staging of neuroblastoma (after Evans) and the incidence and 5-year survival rate for the different stages

		Incidence	5-year survival rate
Stage 1	Localized tumor confined to the area of origin, completely resected, negative lymph nodes	5%	≥90%
Stage 2	Unilateral regional tumor, completely resected with or without either microscopic residue or ipsilateral node involvement	10%	70%–80%
Stage 3	Bilateral tumor invading in continuity across midline, with or without nodes	20%	40%–70% (depending on completeness of surgical resection)
Stage 4	Widespread tumor dissemination to distant nodes, bone, bone marrow, liver, or other organs	60%	>60% if age at diagnosis is <1 year 20% if age at diagnosis is >1 year and <2 years 10% if age at diagnosis is >2 years.
Stage 4s	Stage 1 or 2 primary, involvement of liver, marrow, skin, nodes. Under 1 year of age	5%	≥80%

there is little scope at the moment for a reduction in treatment intensity. Such subclassification does, however, permit better characterization of the small group of survivors. The improvement of therapy for stage 4 disease remains the major goal in the treatment of neuroblastoma.

Chemotherapy Regimens

Until recently, most chemotherapy regimens were variations of standard sarcoma combinations with Adriamycin, cyclophosphamide, and vincristine. The addition of cisplatin (CDDP) and the epidophyllotoxins (VP16, i.e., etoposide, and VM26, i.e., teniposide) has bad a significant impact on the initial response rate, but durable remissions remain difficult to achieve [3]. To date, the most effective drugs in the treatment of neuroblastoma are cyclophosphamide, CDDP, Adriamycin, VP16, VM26, vincristine, peptichemio, and melphalan. Investigators at St Jude, Memphis, United States of America, have clearly shown that combinations of drugs are more effective than single drugs and also that the sequence of drug administration plays a major role in the response rate (e.g., CDDP following by VM26 is superior to the reverse order). Despite clear evidence of efficacy in phase II studies as a single agent, the role of Adriamycin in drug combinations remains controversial. The dose-response relationship was clearly demonstrated by a trial conducted at Villejuif, Paris, in which a two- to threefold increase in the dose of cyclophosphamide and Adriamycin im-

606

proved response rates from 40% to 90%. Similarly, clear responses to a high dose of CDDP (200 mg/m²) are reported in patients whose tumors progress on a conventional dose of CDDP (100 mg/m²). The sequential administration of non-cross-resistant drugs, based on the Goldie-Coldman hypothesis (e.g., cyclophosphamide, Adriamycin, vincristine, alternating with CDDP and VP16), has not been shown to be superior to a standard combination. Drug combinations incorporating a number of agents, often studied in a randomized manner, [dacarbazine (DTIC), peptichemio, low dose melphalan at induction] have failed to show any survival advantage.

Current Approaches Under Study

Current directions of research are in three main areas: (a) phase II studies of new agents or new ways of using old agents, (b) megatherapy procedures with autologous or allogeneic bone marrow rescue and (c) targeted therapy using either radiolabeled methyl-iodo-benzyl-guanidine (MIBG) or semispecific monoclonal antibodies.

Phase II Studies

The results of introducing new agents into the therapy of neuroblastoma have been rather disappointing, with the exception of CDDP [4]. One approach which has been pursued vigorously in recent years, therefore, is to try and take advantage of the dose-effect relationship for this tumor, which has been clearly demonstrated in vitro and in vivo for several agents [5]. Using a divided dose and hypertonic saline regimen, much higher doses of CDDP can be given relatively safely, and studies of CDDP in combination with VP16 have been encouraging, both in relapsed and in untreated patients [6]. The cyclophosphamide analogue ifosfamide, when used with the uroprotective mesna, is well tolerated and allows dose escalation of this effective alkylating agent. Similarly, high-dose peptichemio, a drug resembling melphalan, has been reported to be effective in refractory cases, as have new combinations of alkylating agents such as busulphan and cyclophosphamide.

The development of non-nephro-ototoxic platinum analogues has inevitably aroused much interest. Phase II studies of carboplatin and iproplatin are currently underway, but it is too early to draw firm conclusions about either the relative activity of these agents or the optimum scheduling techniques. A major problem with carboplatin is its myelosupression, which limits its dose in combination. This may compromise its advantage over cisplatin in conventional therapy, but it is not a problem when used as part of a conditioning regimen prior to bone marrow transplantation.

607

Megatherapy

The ultimate use of dose effect is the administration of a single drug or combination chemotherapy at doses limited only by nonhemopoietic tissue tolerance by using bone marrow rescue procedures. Because of the limited availability of matched, related donors in this very young group of patients, experience with autologous marrow is greater than with allogeneic marrow. Moreover, unlike leukemia, neuroblastoma only secondarily involves the bone marrow which may be cleared of overt tumor by effective chemotherapy prior to marrow harvest. Various purging techniques have been developed which, in vitro, are capable of removing residual tumor cells from marrow [7]. The need for such purging procedures in practice remains a contentious issue, as the clonogenic potential of reinfused neuroblastoma cells is difficult to demonstrate (see Favrot and Philip, this volume). The main limiting effect in the use of megatherapy procedures remains the ability of such therapy to ablate completely the malignant cell population. The following are some of the high-dose chemoradiotherapy regimens in current use, but few of these ongoing clinical trials have yet been published: (a) melphalan 180 mg/m^2 (ENSG); (b) melphalan 180 mg/m^2, vincristine 4 mg/m^2, TB1 12 Gy (Philip et al.); (c) melphalan 140 mg/m^2, TB1/10 Gy (Graham Pole et al.); (d) Adriamycin VM26, CDDP, melphalan, TB1 (August et al.) (e) BCNU 300 mg/m^2, VM26 1 g/m^2, melphalan 180 mg/m^2 (Hartman et al.). (Details of references are in [7].)

The potential value of total body irradiation (TBI) is suggested by the finding of a 20% rate of 2-year progression-free survival in a group of highly selected patients with recurrent disease when TBI was used in the conditioning regimen. No progression-free survivors were reported when a non-TBI regimen was used (Houston, Autologous Bone Marrow Transplantation Meeting, December 1986). With or without TBI, with single or two sequential graft procedures, a 35%–40% rate of 2-year progression-free survival was reported in patients grafted in complete remission. No advantage was shown in this group for the TBI-containing regimen, but the mortality rate for this group was higher (20% versus 10%). In a Lyon-Marseille-Curie multicenter trial for patients in partial remission treated with a TBI-containing regimen, 20% of the patients on a single graft program are alive and progression free 36 months after the commencement of therapy. It is clear that in all studies, no plateau has yet been reached in the survival curves at or beyond 2 years.

Interest in the concept of a double graft procedure in neuroblastoma has been kindled by the timing of relapse post-BMT (i.e., between 3 and 12 months post graft in the majority of cases). Among selected patients in partial remission after induction therapy who received a double graft without TBI, there were no reported survivors at 2 years. This differs from the Lyon-Marseille-Curie current pilot study in which a double graft with TBI was used, instead of a single graft, with survivors reported up to 2 years.

The European Neuroblastoma Study Group (ENSG) has carried out a prospective randomized study of high-dose melphalan in patients with stages 3 and 4 disease who achieved at least partial remission after a standardized, platinum-containing induction regimen. There was a significant advantage at 2 years for the melphalan group, in terms of both median survival time and the period in which the disease does not progress. This provides a rational basis for the inclusion of this agent at high dose in future protocols [8]. TBI is still included in many pretransplant regimens because of in vitro radiosensitivity data and early clinical experience. However, because of concern about the contribution of this modality to both short- and long-term morbidity, its inclusion requires prospective evaluation. It is possible that the substitution of other drugs at high dose might provide a better therapeutic index. Late effects such as second malignancies are beginning to appear in the literature and avoidance of this problem, wherever possible, must be a consideration in the design of new regimens. However, for now, the first concern is to achieve prolonged good-quality remission in patients with neuroblastoma.

Targeted Therapy

The demonstration that effective imaging of pheochromocytoma could be achieved using radiolabeled MIBG was soon followed by therapeutic trials of this agent labeled with high doses of ^{131}I or ^{125}I. MIBG is also taken up by immature neuroblastoma cells, and this radioactive iodine-labeled MIBG has been recently evaluated in phases I and II studies. Some activity has been demonstrated, although patient numbers have been small and rather heterogeneous patients [9]. Myelosuppression, due to a "bystander" effect in infiltrated marrow, has been a significant problem. Moreover, the MIBG content of tumor cells is unpredictable and may not be uniform throughout the tumor cell population. It has been suggested that this approach may be most appropriate for the treatment of residual disease after surgery for stage 3 disease, allowing a less toxic but higher dose of radiotherapy to be delivered. A useful palliative effect of MIBG on bone pain has been reported by all groups studying the agent and is one of the major indications for its use in the future. Early studies with the radiolabeled monoclonal antibody, UJ13A, directed against tumor cells have been rather disappointing. Problems encountered include heterogeneity of antigen expression and reticuloendothelial tissue uptake [10]. The anti-ganglioside monoclonal antibody reported from Cleveland, USA, avoids the majority of these problems and is perhaps the most promising antibody for targeted therapy in the future. It is possible, however, that ultimately a combination of several treatment modalities may prove to be optimal.

Future Approaches

Future clinical advances will be closely linked to progress in laboratory investigation. In the absence of new, highly active agents, the immediate future in chemoradiotherapy lies in the more efficient use of currently available drugs. This approach has improved cure rates in other tumors and leukemia, and there is current evidence that, perhaps with bone marrow transplantation support, the same will apply to neuroblastoma. Surgical excision of the tumor, always emphasized by European groups but often refuted by American groups, could be one of the ways of improving results, especially in stage 3 disease. Targeted therapy is an appealing approach, but likely to always play an adjunctive role since effective induction chemotherapy will still, presumably, be required.

The current interest in biological response modifiers cannot be ignored in the context of neuroblastoma. Of all the childhood malignancies this is the one where such an approach might be effective. The unusual behavior of stage 4s disease with spontaneous regression, the better prognosis of advanced metastatic disease in infants, the regression of neuroblast "embryonal rests" in the newborn, and the spontaneous maturation of malignant tumor in some stage 2 patients all suggest that the disease may be treatable by exploiting the body's own defence systems. In the past, attempts to achieve tumor maturation, for example, with vitamin B_{12} or retinoic acid, have been singularly unsuccessful. Whether the tumor will be responsive to more aggressive measures such as IL-2-primed natural killer cell therapy remains to be evaluated but may be particularly difficult in the average, heavily pretreated, neuroblastoma patient. The hypothesis that neuroblastoma develops very early in life has led to a population screening for the early detection of the disease in Japan. Early detection and the prevention of disease progression will probably play a role in future approaches to this disease which has a biological behavior unique among pediatric tumors.

References

1. Rosen EM, Cassady JR, Frantz CN, Kretschmar C, Levey R, Sallan SE (1984) Neuroblastoma: the Joint Center for Radiation Therapy/Dana-Farber Cancer Institute/Children's Hospital experience. J Clin Oncol 2: 719
2. Le Tourneau JN, Bernard JL, Hendren WH, Carcassonne M (1985) Evaluation of the role of surgery in 130 patients with neuroblastoma. J Pediat Surg 3: 244
3. Shafford EA, Roger DW, Pritchard J (1984) Advanced neuroblastoma: improved response-rate using a multiagent regimen (OPEC) including sequential cis platinum and VM26. J Clin Oncol 2: 742
4. Carli M, Green AA, Hayes FA, Rivera G, Pratt CB (1982) Therapeutic efficacy of single drugs for childhood neuroblastoma: a review. In: Raybaud C (ed) Proceedings of the XIIIth SIOP Meeting, Marseille. Excerpta Medica, Amsterdam, pp 141–150
5. Hill BT (1986) Neuroblastoma—an overview of laboratory studies aimed at inducing tumor regression by initiation of differentiation or administration of antitumor drugs. Pediatr Hematol Oncol 3: 73
6. Philip T, Ghalie R, Pinkerton R, Zucker JM, Bernard JL, Leverger G, Hartmann O (1987) A phase II study of high dose-cis platinum and VP16 in neuroblastoma. J Clin Oncol 5: 941
7. Pinkerton R, Philip T, Bouffet E, Lashford L, Kemshead J (1986) Autologous bone marrow transplantation in paediatric solid tumors. Clin Haematol 15: 187
8. Pritchard J, Germond S, Jones D, De Kraker J, Love S (1986) Is high dose melphalan of value in treatment of advanced neuroblastoma? Preliminary results of a randomized trial by the European neuroblastoma study group. Proc ASCO 5: 205

9. Voute PA, Hoefnagel CA, De Kraker J, Marcuse HR (1986) ^{131}I-meta-iodobenzylguanidine (^{131}I-MIBG) as targeted radio-isotope in treatment of children with neuroblastoma. Proc ASCO 5: 213
10. Kemshead JT, Goldman A, Jones D, Pritchard J, Malpas JS, Gordon I, Malone JF, Hurley GD, Breatnach F (1985) Therapeutic application of radiolabelled monoclonal antibody UJ13A in children with disseminated neuroblastoma. A phase 1 study. Adv Neuroblastoma Res 4: 533–544

56. Retinoblastoma

B.L. Gallie

Current Results and Therapeutic Issues

Retinoblastoma (RB) is a rare, malignant tumor of the retina which arises in infants. If the tumor is diagnosed before it has spread from the eye, current management (removal of the eye, radiation, photocoagulation or cryotherapy) results in cure. If diagnosis and treatment are delayed, tumor cells spread intra-cranially and metastasize to bone marrow, with a severe effect on mortality. Thus, the overall mortality for RB is currently 6% in developed countries, but approaches 100% in areas with less readily available medical care.

Chemotherapy has been used almost exclusively for the treatment of metas-tatic RB, and only occasionally has control of intraocular tumors by chemother-apy been reported. Since penetration of chemotherapeutic drugs into the eye is generally poor, the systemic side effects are out of proportion to the effect on the intraocular tumor. Cyclophosphamide, vincristine, and Adriamycin have ben-eficial effects on hematogenous bone marrow metastasis of RB. Meningeal and brain metastases have been treated with combination intrathecal and systemic chemotherapy and radiation, with anecdotal suggestion of some cures. General-ly, metastatic RB treatment is palliative, and cure is not achieved.

Study of surviving RB patients demonstrates that in 40% of cases a germline mutation predisposing to RB is transmitted as an autosomal dominant trait with 95% penetrance. In 85% of these hereditary cases tumors arise in both eyes independently. The same individuals are at increased risk of developing sub-sequent second primary malignancies, particularly osteosarcoma. The reported incidence of second tumors ranges from 2%–90% [1], depending on follow-up treatment and the age of the patient. Radiation increases the frequency of sarcomas within the radiation field in patients with the genetic form of RB. There is no effective way to screen for these new malignancies in the predisposed individuals. Regular imaging using CT scans or bone scans is not effective enough to pick up early tumors.

The genetic locus leading to hereditary RB is located on chromosome 13q14. This was initially suspected because of the rare individuals in whom cytogenetic deletion involving 13q14 is associated with RB. Subsequently, the nondeletion heritable cases were shown to involve the same 13q14 locus by demonstration of close genetic linkage between RB and the polymorphic enzyme, esterase D^2. The recessive mechanism by which the RB mutation acts to produce tumors was predicted by Knudson [3], who suggested that the development of RB requires two mutations. In heritable RB, the first mutation occurs in the germline, while the second is a somatic mutation in a retinal progenitor cell. In nonheritable RB, both mutations are somatic and occur in the same retinal precursor cell. The recessive nature of the gene was demonstrated by the absence of one isoenzyme of esterase D in the tumors of constitutionally heterozygous individuals and by subsequent comparison of DNA from the normal, constitutional cells with DNA from RB tumor cells using restriction fragment length polymorphic markers around the RB locus [4]. The normal allele is lost from the tumor cells most commonly by major chromosomal rearrangements, including mitotic recombination, loss of the normal chromosome and reduplication of the mutant one, simple chromosome loss, or, presumably, by submicroscopic deletion or point mutation within the normal allele. The second primary tumors that develop in patients with hereditary RB also show homozygosity at the RB genetic locus, indicating that similar, if not identical, genetic mechanisms are involved in the second tumors [5].

Genetic counseling for individuals with RB is currently based on risk estimates for the germline presence of a mutant allele [6]. Any individual with bilateral RB must carry a germline mutation, which will be inherited by 50% of his offspring, most of whom will develop RB. Individuals with unilateral RB and relatives of RB patients who themselves do not develop RB tumors are unsure whether or not they also carry an RB mutation. The closely linked enzyme, esterase D, can be used to predict the inheritance of a mutant allele in families that have an informative polymorphism. However, this is not useful for individuals with no family history of RB, unless the mutant allele was identified by development of homozygosity of one chromosome in the RB tumor.

Current Approaches Under Study

The most effective way to control RB tumors is to diagnose and treat them early. Small retinal tumors noted at birth in familial cases are easily controlled with photocoagulation and cryotherapy prior to irreversible ocular damage. When intraocular tumors are too large to be controlled by local physical means, radiation must be given to save vision. Since radiation has the very significant side effect of increasing the frequency of second primary malignancies, in order to save eyes other ways of treating medium-sized tumors are needed. Photoradiation, with agents such as hematoporphyrin, theoretically has the potential to fill this role. Basic work on drug and light dosage, methods of delivery, and effectiveness against hypoxic, advanced, intraocular tumor cells is in progress. Some RB patients have been treated with this new modality, but a scientific basis for its use has not yet been established.

Medium-sized intraocular RB tumors are markedly hypoxic, particularly when growing in the vitreous without a direct blood supply, and tend to be resistant to radiation, resulting in loss of the eye. Hypoxic cell-sensitizing drugs have been studied for use in this situation. Misonidazole increases the radiation sensitivity of hypoxic RB tumor cells in vitro, at concentrations achievable systemically. However, the intraocular penetration of the systemically administered drug is poor. Derivatives of misonidazole may have significantly better ocular penetration when administered locally, and within the field of radiation, allowing increased effectiveness and decreased systemic toxicity [7]. The number of RB patients for whom this modality of therapy would be useful is limited. At present, no clinical trials have been proposed.

Studies of RB sensitivity to drugs suggests general sensitivity to dose levels obtainable systemically. A subset of RB tumors including tumors not previously exposed to chemotherapeutic agents, have shown multidrug resistance in vitro. This suggests that de novo multidrug resistance may be a characteristic of some RB tumors. Ongoing work will assess the means by which these RB tumors have acquired multidrug resistance and will be aimed at devising methods to detect multidrug resistance in tumor cells in histological preparations, for example, by antibody detection of P-glycoprotein, frequently amplified in the genome of multidrug resistant tumor cells.

The current exciting development in research into RB is the closeness of the approach to the RB gene. Recently, using a genomic probe mapped to chromosome 13q14, expression of a transcript was noted in an adenovirus-transformed human fetal retinal cell line; the genomic probe was used to isolate a cDNA clone, the putative RB gene recently reported by Friend et al. [8]. Although we find a low frequency of genomic rearrangements within this gene in RB tumors, and initial reports of its lack of expression in RB tumors are not correct, the presence of homozygous deletions within this gene in RB tumors suggests that either this is the RB gene or it is very close to it. Lee et al. [9] similarly derived overlapping genomic clones in this region covering at least 100 kb, using cDNA probes derived in a similar manner, and sequenced the cDNA. The sequence is reported to contain an open reading frame of 816 amino acids, with some characteristics of a DNA-binding protein.

Future Approaches

The remaining therapeutic problems in RB are delayed diagnosis, morbidity of therapy for intraocular RB that has not yet destroyed the anatomy of the eye, and inadequate treatment of metastatic RB. Early diagnosis will be assisted by family physicians and pediatricians being more aware of the early signs of RB and paying attention to what the parents describe. The results of careful studies of the role of photoradiation and hypoxic cell radiation sensitizers and greater understanding of multidrug resistance are needed for improved control of intraocular and metastatic RB.

It is not clear at present whether the cloned 13q14 gene is the RB gene or a near neighbor. The genomic rearrangements identified in RB and other tumors are not yet well characterized and may extend to involve adjacent genes within the region, only one of which is the true RB gene. Unequivocal identification of a candidate as the RB gene will require a functional assay or demonstration in affected families of germline mutation, somatic mutations within the gene, and association of the mutant germline allele with RB.

The recent demonstration by Weissman et al. [10] of a functional assay for the tumor-suppressing activity of chromosome 11p, the locus of the recessive Wilms' tumor gene, improves the chances that a functional assay for the RB gene can also be developed. Such an assay could conclusively identify the RB gene. When the RB gene is identified, its normal cellular and developmental function, and the way that the mutations lead to highly tissue-specific malignancies, will be of great relevance to the treatment of cancer in general. For many patients with RB, precise diagnosis of the presence of a germline mutation will be possible; however, for individuals with point mutations, genetic diagnosis may still be difficult. Application of the cloned RB gene to therapy for RB patients is a far more remote possibility but could be possible with knowledge of the cellular role of the gene. "Gene therapy" as treatment for RB presently appears unrealistic.

References

1. Draper GJ, Sanders BM, Kingston JE (1986) Second primary neoplasms in patients with retinoblastoma. Br J Cancer 53: 661
2. Sparkes RS, Murphree AL, Lingua RW, Sparkes MC, Field LL, Funderburk SJ, Benedict WF (1983) Gene for hereditary retinoblastoma assigned to human chromosome 13 by linkage to esterase D. Science 219: 971–972
3. Knudson AG (1971) Mutation and cancer: a statistical study of retinoblastoma. Proc Natl Acad USA 68: 820–823
4. Cavenee WK, Dryja TP, Phillips RA, Benedict WF, Godbout R, Gallie BL, Murphee AL, Strong LC, White RL (1983) Expression of recessive alleles by chromosomal mechanisms in retinoblastoma. Nature 305: 779
5. Hansen MF, Koufus A, Gallie BL, Phillips RA, Fodstad O, Brogger A, Gedde-Dahl T, Cavenee W (1985) Osteosarcoma and retinoblastoma: a shared chromosomal mechanism revealing recessive predisposition. Proc Natl Acad Sci USA 82: 6216
6. Musarella MA, Gallie BL (1987) A simplified scheme for genetic counselling in retinoblastoma. J Pediatr Ophthalmol Strabismus 24: 124
7. Rootman J, Gallie BL, Kumi C, Bussanich N, Rogers B, Palcic B (1986) Ocular penetration, toxicity and radiosensitization effects of two hypoxic cell radiosensitizers on retinoblastoma. Arch Ophthalmol 104: 1693
8. Friend SH, Bernards R, Rogelj S, Weinberg RA, Rapaport JM, Albert DM, Dryja RP (1986) A human DNA segment with properties of the gene that predisposes to retinoblastoma and osteosarcoma. Nature 323: 643
9. Lee WH, Bookstein R, Hong F, Young LJ, Shew JY, Lee EYHP (1987) Human retinoblastoma susceptibility gene: cloning, identification and sequence. Science 235: 1394
10. Weissmann BE, Saxon PJ, Pasquale SR, Jones GR, Geiser AG, Stanbridge EJ (1987) Introduction of a normal human chromosome 11 into a Wilms' tumor cell line controls its tumorigenic expression. Science 236: 175

Subject Index

620

621

624

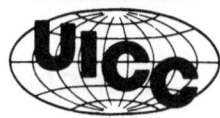

International Union Against Cancer

New edition accepted worldwide by all national committees

B. Spiessl, O. H. Beahrs, P. Hermanek, R. V. P. Hutter, O. Scheibe, L. H. Sobin, G. Wagner (Eds.)

TNM-Atlas

Illustrated Guide to the TNM/pTNM-Classification of Malignant Tumours

3rd edition. 1988. 452 figures.
Approx. 350 pages. ISBN 3-540-17721-3

The TNM Atlas follows the sound principles of the previous editions and includes a number of organs that were newly classified since the last edition. The present third edition takes into consideration all additions and changes made in the fourth edition of the TNM Classification of Malignant Tumours and, therefore, represents the current state of the TNM classification as **accepted worldwide by all national committees,** including the American Joint Committee on Cancer. Numerous illustrations help to visualize the anatomical extent of malignant tumours at the different stages of their development. The TNM Atlas is designed as an aid in the practical application of the TNM Classification for all doctors working in the field of oncology.

Springer-Verlag Berlin
Heidelberg New York London
Paris Tokyo Hong Kong

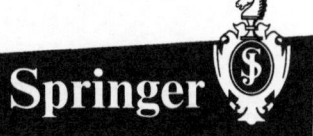

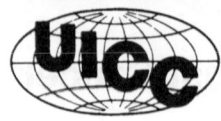

International Union Against Cancer

P. Hermanek, L. H. Sobin (Eds.)

TNM Classification of Malignant Tumors

4th fully revised edition. 1987. XVIII, 197 pages.
ISBN 3-540-17366-8

The TNM System is the most widely used classification of the extent of growth and spread of cancer. The anatomical extent of disease is the prime indicator of prognosis for most cancer patients and provides the main criterion for the selection of therapy. After four years of international collaborative activity, a revised, unified, fourth edition of the TNM Classification is published as the result of a joint venture by the American, British, Canadian, French, German, Italian and Japanese National TNM Committees. Of paramount importance is the adoption of identical criteria of classification in the fourth edition of the UICC TNM Classification and the third edition of the Manual of Staging of Cancer of the American Joint Committee on Cancer (AJCC).

Specific changes and additions to the fourth edition include the elimination of all differences between the AJCC and UICC TNM classifications of head and neck tumours and lung tumours; revision of the T classifications of esophageal and gastric carcinomas based on the Japanese studies of over 15,000 gastric and over 3,000 esophageal carcinomas; modification of the classification of colorectal tumours to provide direct congruence with the Dukes' classification, as well as allowing for a finer degree of subdivision; redrafting of the FIGO classification of gynecological tumours in the format of TNM, carried out in collaboration with FIGO; addition of TNM classification for sites not previously covered in earlier UICC editions, such as the pancreas, liver, gall bladder, biliary tract, salivary glands, maxillary sinus, bone and brain.

Springer-Verlag Berlin
Heidelberg New York London
Paris Tokyo Hong Kong

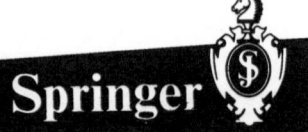